AF708318

GEORGE WASHINGTON UNIVERSITY
PAUL HIMMELFARB HEALTH SCIENCES LIBRARY
2300 EYE STREET N. W.
WASHINGTON, D.C. 20037
DISCARDED

OVARIAN CANCER

CONTROVERSIES IN MANAGEMENT

GEORGE WASHINGTON UNIVERSITY
PAUL HIMMELFARB HEALTH SCIENCES LIBRARY
2300 EYE STREET N. W.
WASHINGTON, D.C. 20037

OVARIAN CANCER

CONTROVERSIES IN MANAGEMENT

EDITED BY

DAVID M. GERSHENSON, M.D.
Professor and Deputy Chairman
Department of Gynecologic Oncology
The University of Texas M.D. Anderson Cancer Center
Houston, Texas

WILLIAM P. McGUIRE, M.D.
Clinical Professor
Department of Medicine
University of Mississippi School of Medicine
Jackson, Mississippi

CHURCHILL LIVINGSTONE

New York, Edinburgh, London, Madrid, Melbourne, San Francisco, Tokyo

Library of Congress Cataloging-in-Publication Data

Ovarian cancer : controversies in management / edited by David M.
Gershenson, William P. McGuire.
p. cm.
Includes bibliographical references and index.
ISBN 0-443-07804-1 (alk. paper) . — ISBN 0-443-07804-1 (alk.
paper)
1. Ovaries—Cancer. I. Gershenson, David M. (David Marc), date.
II. McGuire, William P., date.
[DNLM: 1. Ovarian Neoplasms—diagnosis. 2. Ovarian Neoplasms-
-therapy. WP 322 09645 1998]
RC280.080923 1998
616.99′465—dc21
DNLM/DLC
for Library of Congress 97-34798
CIP

© Churchill Livingstone Inc. 1998
Medical Division of Pearson Professional Limited

is a registered trademark of Pearson Professional Limited

All rights reserved. No part of this publication may be reproduced, stored in a retrieval system, or transmitted in any form or by any means, electronic, mechanical, photocopying, recording, or otherwise, without prior permission of the publisher (Churchill Livingstone, 650 Avenue of the Americas, New York, NY 10011).

Distributed in the United Kingdom by Churchill Livingstone, Robert Stevenson House, 1–3 Baxter's Place, Leith Walk, Edinburgh EH1 3AF, and by associated companies, branches, and representatives throughout the world.

Medical knowledge is constantly changing. As new information becomes available, changes in treatment, procedures, equipment and the use of drugs become necessary. The editors/authors/contributors and the publishers have, as far as it is possible, taken care to ensure that the information given in this text is accurate and up to date. However, readers are strongly advised to confirm that the information, especially with regard to drug usage, complies with the latest legislation and standards of practice.

The Publishers have made every effort to trace the copyright holders for borrowed material. If they have inadvertently overlooked any, they will be pleased to make the necessary arrangements at the first opportunity.

Acquisitions Editor: *Jennifer Mitchell*
Assistant Editor: *Jennifer Hardy*
Production Editor: *Elizabeth A. Plowman*
Production Supervisor: *Sharon Tuder*
Cover Design: *Jeannette Jacobs*

Printed in the United States of America

First published in 1998 7 6 5 4 3 2 1

RC
280
.O8
O92
1998

To our wives—Michelle Gershenson and Deborah McGuire—
and to our patients with ovarian cancer.
May women everywhere find solace in the
future elucidation of issues through
research presented herein

CONTRIBUTORS

Robert C. Bast, Jr., M.D.
Professor and Chief, Division of Medicine, The University of Texas M.D. Anderson Cancer Center, Houston, Texas

Ivor Benjamin, M.D.
Assistant Professor, Division of Gynecologic Oncology, Department of Obstetrics and Gynecology, University of Pennsylvania School of Medicine, Philadelphia, Pennsylvania

Jonathan S. Berek, M.D.
Professor and Vice Chairman, Chief of Gynecology and Gynecologic Oncology, Department of Obstetrics/Gynecology, University of California, Los Angeles, UCLA School of Medicine, Los Angeles, California

Joanna Mary Cain, M.D.
University Professor and Chair, Department of Obstetrics and Gynecology, The Milton S. Hershey Medical Center of Pennsylvania State University College of Medicine; Division Director, Division of Obstetrics and Gynecology, PennState Geisinger Health System, Hershey, Pennsylvania

David Cella, Ph.D.
Professor, Department of Psychology, Rush Medical College of Rush University; Director, Division of Psychosocial Oncology, Rush-Presbyterian-St. Luke's Medical Center, Chicago, Illinois

Nicoletta Colombo, M.D.
Deputy Director, Division of Gynecology, European Institute of Oncology, Milan, Italy

Larry J. Copeland, M.D.
Professor and Chair, Department of Obstetrics and Gynecology, James Cancer Hospital, The Ohio State University, Columbus, Ohio

Paul D. DePriest, M.D.
Associate Professor, Division of Gynecologic Oncology, Department of Obstetrics/Gynecology, University of Kentucky College of Medicine, Lexington, Kentucky

Holly H. Gallion, M.D.
Associate Professor, Division of Gynecologic Oncology, Department of Obstetrics/Gynecology, University of Kentucky College of Medicine, Lexington, Kentucky

David M. Gershenson, M.D.
Professor and Deputy Chairman, Department of Gynecologic Oncology, The University of Texas M.D. Anderson Cancer Center, Houston, Texas

Barbara A. Goff, M.D.
Associate Professor, Division of Gynecologic Oncology, Department of Obstetrics/Gynecology, University of Washington Medical Center, Seattle, Washington

Benjamin E. Greer, M.D.
Professor and Director, Division of Gynecologic Oncology, Department of Obstetrics/Gynecology, University of Washington Medical Center, Seattle, Washington

William J. Hoskins, M.D.
Professor, Department of Obstetrics/Gynecology, Cornell University Medical College; Deputy Physician in Chief, Disease Management Teams, Avon Chair in Gynecologic Oncology Research, Department of Gynecology, Memorial Sloan-Kettering Cancer Center, New York, New York

Ian Jacobs, M.D.
Director, Gynaecology Cancer Research Unit, Department of Gynaecological Oncology, St. Bartholomew's and The Royal London Medical College; Consultant, Department of Gynaecological Oncology, St. Bartholomew's and the Royal London Hospital, The Royal Hospitals Trust, London, England

Janne Kaern, M.D., Ph.D.
Senior Consultant, Gynecologic Section, University of Oslo, The Norwegian Radium Hospital, Oslo, Norway

Daniel S. Kapp, Ph.D., M.D.
Professor, Department of Radiation Oncology, Stanford University School of Medicine, Stanford, California

John Kavanagh, M.D.
Professor, Section of Gynecologic Medical Oncology, Division of Medicine, Department of Clinical Investigation, The University of Texas M.D. Anderson Cancer Center, Houston, Texas

Stan B. Kaye, M.D., B.S., F.R.C.P.
Professor, Department of Medical Oncology, University of Glasgow; Consultant in Medical Oncology, Beatson Oncology Center, Western Infirmary, Glasgow, Scotland

Sean Kehoe, M.R.C.O.G.
Senior Lecturer, Division of Gynaecological Oncology, Department of Gynaecological Oncology, University of Birmingham, Birmingham, United Kingdom

Elise C. Kohn, M.D.
Senior Investigator and Acting Chief of The Molecular Signaling Section, Laboratory of Pathology, National Cancer Institute, National Institutes of Health, Bethesda, Maryland

Andrzej P. Kudelka, M.D.
Assistant Professor, Section of Gynecologic Medical Oncology, Department of Gynecologic Medical Oncology, The University of Texas M.D. Anderson Cancer Center, Houston, Texas

Frank G. Lawton, M.D., F.R.C.O.G.
Consultant Gynecologic Cancer Surgeon, Department of Obstetrics/Gynecology, Gynecologic Cancer Unit, King's College Hospital, London, England

David M. Luesley, M.D., F.R.C.O.G.
Professor, Division of Gynecologic Oncology, Department of Obstetrics and Gynaecology, University of Birmingham, Birmingham, West Midlantic, United Kingdom; Professor, Department of Obstetrics and Gynecology, Dudley Road Hospital, Edgabaston, Birmingham, United Kingdom

Maurie Markman, M.D.
Director, The Cleveland Clinic Cancer Center; Chairman, Department of Hematology/Medical Oncology, The Cleveland Clinic Foundation, Cleveland, Ohio

William P. McGuire, M.D.
Clinical Professor, Department of Medicine, University of Mississippi School of Medicine, Jackson, Mississippi

Gordon B. Mills, M.D., Ph.D.
Professor and Chairman, Division of Medicine, Department of Molecular Oncology, The University of Texas M.D. Anderson Cancer Center, Houston, Texas

Bradley J. Monk, M.D.
Assistant Professor, Department of Obstetrics and Gynecology, Texas Tech Medical Center; Director, Division of Gynecologic Oncology and Associate Medical Director, Southwest Cancer Center, Lubbock, Texas

Hyman Bernard Muss, M.D.
Professor, Department of Medicine, University of Vermont College of Medicine; Physician, Division of Hematology/Oncology, Fletcher Allen Health Care, Burlington, Vermont

Jan P. Neijt, M.D., Ph.D.
Associate Professor, Department of Internal Medicine, University Hospital Utrecht, Utrecht, The Netherlands

Hextan Y. S. Ngan, M.D.
Professor, Division of Gynaecologic Oncology, Department of Obstetrics and Gynaecology, University of Hong Kong; Honorary Consultant, Division of Gynaecological Oncology, Department of Obstetrics and Gynaecology, Queen Mary Hospital, Hong Kong, China

James L. Nicklin, M.B.B.S., F.R.A.C.O.G., C.G.O.
Division of Gynaecologic Oncology, Department of Obstetrics and Gynaecology, University of Queensland; Gynaecologic Oncologist, Queensland Centre for Gynaecologic Cancer, Brisbane, Queensland, Australia

Jonathan M. Niloff, M.D., F.A.C.O.G., F.A.C.S., F.R.C.S.
Associate Professor, Department of Obstetrics, Gynecology, and Reproductive Biology, Harvard Medical School; Director, Division of Gynecologic Oncology, Department of Obstetrics and Gynecology, Beth Israel Deaconess Medical Center, Boston, Massachusetts

George A. Omura, M.D.
Professor Emeritus, Medicine and Gynecology, Departments of Medicine and Obstetrics and Gynecology, University of Alabama School of Medicine at Birmingham; Medical Director, Biocyst Pharmaceuticals, Inc., Birmingham, Alabama

Robert F. Ozols, M.D., Ph.D.
Senior Vice President, Medical Science, Fox Chase Cancer Center, Philadelphia, Pennsylvania

M. Steven Piver, M.D.
Clinical Professor, Division of Gynecologic Oncology, Department of Gynecology and Obstetrics, State University of New York at Buffalo School of Medicine and Biomedical Sciences; Chief, Department of Gynecologic Oncology, Roswell Cancer Institute, Buffalo, New York

Marcus E. Randall, M.D.
William A. Mitchell Professor and Chair, Department of Radiation Oncology, Indiana University School of Medicine, Indianapolis, Indiana

Emily G. Robinson, M.D.
Department of Hematology/Oncology, Mercy Health System, Janesville, Wisconsin

Barry Rosen, M.D.
Associate Professor, Division of Gynecologic Oncology, Department of Obstetrics and Gynecology, University of Toronto Faculty of Medicine; Director, Familial Ovarian Cancer Clinic, Department of Obstetrics and Gynecology, The Toronto Hospital, Toronto, Ontario, Canada

Stephen C. Rubin, M.D.
Professor and Director, Division of Gynecologic Oncology, Department of Obstetrics and Gynecology, University of Pennsylvania School of Medicine, Philadelphia, Pennsylvania

Peter E. Schwartz, M.D.
Professor, Division of Gynecologic Oncology, Department of Obstetrics/Gynecology, Yale University School of Medicine, New Haven, Connecticut

Robert E. Scully, M.D.
Professor, Department of Pathology, Harvard Medical School; Pathologist, Division of Anatomic Pathology, Department of Pathology, Massachusetts General Hospital, Boston, Massachusetts

Victoria L. Seewaldt, M.D.
Acting Assistant Professor, Division of Medical Oncology, Department of Obstetrics/Gynecology, University of Washington Medical Center, Seattle, Washington

Elvio Silva, M.D.
Professor of Pathology, Department of Pathology; Associate Director of Surgical Pathology, The University of Texas M.D. Anderson Cancer Center, Houston, Texas

John T. Soper, M.D.
Professor, Division of Gynecologic Oncology, Department of Obstetrics/Gynecology, Duke University Medical School, Durham, North Carolina

William J. Spanos, Jr., M.D.
Professor and Chairman, Department of Radiation Oncology, University of Louisville School of Medicine, Louisville, Kentucky

Kenneth D. Swenerton, M.D., F.R.C.P.C.
Clinical Professor, Department of Medicine, University of British Columbia Faculty of Medicine; Medical Oncologist, Gynecology Tumor Group, British Columbia Cancer Agency, Vancouver Clinic, Vancouver, British Columbia, Canada

J. Tate Thigpen, M.D.
Professor and Director, Division of Oncology, Department of Medicine, University of Mississippi School of Medicine, Jackson, Mississippi

Gillian M. Thomas, M.D.
Professor, Departments of Radiation Oncology and Obstetrics and Gynaecology, University of Toronto Faculty of Medicine; Head, Department of Radiation Oncology, Toronto Sunnybrook Regional Cancer Center, Toronto, Ontario, Canada

Edward L. Trimble, M.D.
Assistant Professor, Division of Gynecologic Oncology, Department of Gynecology and Obstetrics, Johns Hopkins University School of Medicine, Baltimore, Maryland; Head, Surgery Section, Cancer Therapy Evaluation Program, National Cancer Institute, National Institutes of Health, Rockville, Maryland

Claes Tropé, M.D., Ph.D.
Professor, Gynecologic Section, University of Oslo, The Norwegian Radium Hospital, Oslo, Norway

John R. van Nagell, Jr., M.D.
Professor and Director, Division of Gynecologic Oncology, Department of Obstetrics/Gynecology, University of Kentucky College of Medicine, Lexington, Kentucky

Paul A. Vasey, MB.ChB., M.Sc., M.D., M.R.C.P.
Senior Lecturer, Department of Medical Oncology, University of Glasgow; Honorary Consultant, Department of Medical Oncology, Beatson Oncology Center, Western Infirmary, Glasgow, Scotland

Ignace Vergote, M.D., Ph.D.
Professor, Gynecologic Section and Gynecologic Oncology, University and Hospital of Leuven, Leuven, Belgium

Claire F. Verschraegen, M.D.
Instructor and Assistant Internist, Section of Gynecologic Medical Oncology, Department of Gynecologic Medical Oncology, The University of Texas M.D. Anderson Cancer Center, Houston, Texas

Lari B. Wenzel, Ph.D.
Director, Psychosocial Research Programs, Center for Behavorial Sciences, A.M.C. Cancer Research Center, Denver, Colorado

Stephen Williams, M.D.
Professor, Department of Medicine, Indiana University School of Medicine; Director, Indiana University Cancer Center, Indianapolis, Indiana

Ling C. Wong, M.D.
Professor, Division of Gynaecological Oncology, Department of Obstetrics and Gynaecology, University of Hong Kong; Honorary Consultant, Division of Gynaecologic Oncology, Department of Obstetrics and Gynaecology, Queen Mary Hospital, Hong Kong, China

PREFACE

When the two of us met approximately two years ago to discuss the possibility of collaboration on a new book about ovarian cancer, we were seeking a different style. Rather than duplicate the standard format of other recently published books on the subject, we ultimately chose to develop a unique work that would highlight the major controversies in the field. William Hazlitt, the English essayist, stated, "When a thing ceases to be a subject of controversy, it ceases to be a subject of interest." Although controversy can be contentious and destructive, it can also be healthy and illuminating. By striving for the latter approach, we believe that dissection of important controversies in the field will allow physicians and scientists to identify opportunities and strategies for future research.

To this end, we have assembled the world's leading authorities, most of whom are from North America or Europe. These contributors are addressing some twenty different aspects of ovarian cancer management, including prevention, early detection, and therapy. In addition to the conventional topics of surgical, radiotherapeutic, and chemotherapeutic interventions, we have included chapters on the current status of screening, prophylactic oophorectomy, palliative care, quality of life, post-therapy surveillance, and the clinical relevance of laboratory investigations.

In most instances, each topic is discussed by two authors or sets of authors. No attempt was made to select authors with opposing points of view; we simply sought top experts in each area. We requested that each author address very specific questions that we provided. All authors were blinded to the answer provided by others. We selected the questions based on our joint perception of the most important controversies surrounding ovarian cancer management in the 1990s. Each chapter includes a brief introduction and editorial commentary by us.

As physicians who have devoted our careers to improving the status quo for women with ovarian cancer and their families, we are extremely pleased with the final product. We hope that the reader will find the information in *Ovarian Cancer: Controversies in Management* thought-provoking and helpful in future decision-making.

Finally, we would like to acknowledge the constant encouragement of our editors at Churchill Livingstone—Ms. Jennifer Mitchell, Vice President of Professional and Reference Publishing, Ms. Jennifer Hardy, Assistant Editor, and Ms. Betsy Plowman, Production Editor. We also acknowledge the tremendous assistance of our secretaries—Ms. Marta Abrams at The University of Texas M.D. Anderson Cancer Center and Ms. Debbie Quave at Emory University.

David M. Gershenson, M.D.
William P. McGuire, M.D.

CONTENTS

CHAPTER 1

SCREENING FOR EPITHELIAL OVARIAN CANCER

Ian Jacobs
John R. van Nagell, Jr.
Paul D. DePriest

EDITORS' INTRODUCTION

During the 1980s, it became obvious that, despite the introduction of the platinum compounds into the clinical management of ovarian cancer, little progress had been made in the fight against ovarian cancer over the previous two decades. This phenomenon was based on the fact that more than 70% of ovarian cancers are diagnosed after the disease has already spread beyond the ovaries. In such cases, although response to initial therapy was the rule, most patients developed progressive disease or relapsed after a disease-free interval of rather brief duration. It was only natural that investigators began to turn their attention to screening in an effort to detect the disease early enough to ensure a significantly greater probability of cure. In early-stage disease, the survival rate is significantly higher than that of women with advanced-stage disease.

With the discovery of serum CA 125 and advances in the technology of pelvic sonography, early screening trials in both Europe and the United States focused on these two modalities. In addition, many of these early studies involved the general population of women and did not concentrate on women at increased risk of ovarian cancer. Preliminary results of these trials indicated that, as stand-alone modalities, serum CA 125 screening was not sensitive enough, and sonography, either abdominal or transvaginal, was not specific enough.

In fact, at the 1994 National Institutes of Health Consensus Development Conference on Ovarian Cancer, there was considerable discussion about the futility of continuing to pursue research on the screening of ovarian cancer. Nevertheless, since the late 1980s, investigators have continued to study screening of ovarian cancer.

Furthermore, ovarian cancer screening clinics or programs have been developed in several major university and cancer centers. Currently, the atmosphere is somewhat more optimistic, and more investigators are targeting high-risk populations and using combinations of modalities in an effort to improve both the sensitivity and specificity of ovarian cancer screening. The experts selected for discussion of this subject are truly pioneers in this area of research and represent the best of both sides of the Atlantic Ocean.

QUESTIONS

1. What is the current status of screening for (1) the population as a whole, and (2) high-risk women?
2. What is the value of serum CA 125, other serum markers, or a panel of markers in screening, and what is the role of ultrasound and color flow Doppler in screening?
3. What effect will the availability of BRCA1 and BRCA2 have on recommendations for screening?
4. What future clinical trials should be designed based on the current knowledge and technology?

QUESTION 1

What is the current status of screening for (1) the population as a whole, and (2) high-risk women?

IAN JACOBS

Randomized controlled trials designed to determine the impact of ovarian cancer screening on mortality are currently in progress, but no results have been reported to date. Evidence for the efficacy of early detection of ovarian cancer by screening is limited to the following indirect observations:

1. Patients with ovarian cancers presenting clinically at an early stage have markedly better survival rates than those of patients diagnosed with advanced-stage disease. Whereas the small proportion of patients with accurately diagnosed stage I disease have 5-year survival rates in excess of 90%,[1] most patients have stage III disease, for which the outlook is extremely poor (5-year survival rate approximately 15%).
2. It is possible to detect a significant proportion of cases of ovarian cancer at a preclinical stage using the screening techniques discussed below.

It cannot be assumed, on the basis of this information, that a screening program for ovarian cancer will save lives. A number of important factors may limit the impact of screening. First, although the screening tests available detect ovarian cancer at a preclinical stage, this may still not be sufficiently early in the natural history of the disease to alter the outcome. Second, tumors detected at an early stage by screening may not behave in the same way as tumors presenting clinically at an early stage. For example, screen-detected tumors may be more aggressive and have worse survival rates than do clinically detected stage I cancers. Third, the duration of preclinical invasive disease in ovarian cancer is unknown. If it is short (e.g., 6 months), it will not be feasible to introduce a screening program with a sufficiently short screening interval, however sensitive and specific the screening tests are.

In addition to uncertainties about the benefits of screening, some rather definite disadvantages are associated with screening. As discussed below, all screening tests for ovarian cancer have a significant false positive rate, resulting in anxiety associated with recall for further tests and, in some cases, in unnecessary surgical intervention. In addition, the costs of screening are an increasingly important consideration that may prevent the introduction of ovarian cancer screening in many health care systems. Until the real benefit of screening is established by well-designed randomized controlled trials, a satisfactory assessment of the overall impact of screening will not be possible.

Against this background, the current status of screening for ovarian cancer can be summarized as follows:

1. *General population:* Screening of the general population for ovarian cancer should not be performed outside the research proto-

cols. If screening is introduced before it has been properly assessed, it might subsequently become impossible to perform a randomized controlled trial. Women in the general population should be informed that the risks of screening may outweigh any unproven benefit.

2. *Women at high risk:* A small proportion of women are at extremely high risk of ovarian cancer because they belong to ovarian cancer syndrome families. In view of the exceptional risk to this group of women, it is reasonable to provide screening despite the lack of evidence for a survival benefit. The screening strategy and the definition of this group of women are discussed further below. Women at increased risk due to a weak family history or other risk factors do not fall within this group.

JOHN R. van NAGELL, JR.
PAUL D. DePRIEST

The present evidence would suggest that ovarian cancer screening is not indicated for the population as a whole. Rather, screening should be applied to women at highest risk of ovarian cancer. The annual incidence of ovarian cancer in the United States increases from 20 per 100,000 in women aged 30 to 50 years to 50 per 100,000 in women over the age of 50.[2] Therefore, most screening studies are limited to women over the age of 50. Annual screening of a general population of women over the age of 50 should be performed only as part of a clinical research trial. Such a trial should be designed to evaluate the sensitivity, specificity, positive predictive value, and negative predictive value of each screening method in the trial.

Women with a documented family history of ovarian cancer are at high risk of developing the disease and should be considered for screening. Analysis of pooled data indicates that the relative risk of developing ovarian cancer for a woman with one affected relative (first or second degree) is 3.1 that of the general population.[3] This relative risk increases further to 4.6 with two or three affected relatives. Annual screening should be offered to all women aged 25 years or older with a family history of ovarian cancer. Again, such screening is optimal if it is part of a clinical trial. Sonographic screening of patients with a family history of ovarian cancer has been reported by Bourne and colleagues[4] in England. Screening was performed in 1,601 asymptomatic women, 88% of whom had at least one first-degree relative with ovarian cancer. Sixty-one ovarian tumors were detected, and six patients had ovarian cancer. Five of these patients had stage I disease, and all patients are alive and well following treatment.

QUESTION 2

What is the value of serum CA 125, other serum markers, or a panel of markers in screening, and what is the role of ultrasound and color flow Doppler in screening?

IAN JACOBS

CA 125

The biochemical marker that has been most thoroughly investigated in ovarian cancer is the CA 125 antigen. CA 125 is a high-molecular-weight glycoprotein recognized by the OC 125 monoclonal antibody (mAb), which is of established value in preoperative diagnosis and monitoring of ovarian cancer.[5,6] Serum levels of CA 125 are elevated (greater than 35 U/ml) in more than 85% of women with clinically apparent ovarian cancer. There is a correlation with stage, with serum levels elevated in more than 90% of people with FIGO stage II, III, and IV disease, but in only 50% with stage I disease.[6] In addition to ovarian cancer, a variety of physiologic conditions (e.g., pregnancy and menstruation), benign disorders (e.g., endometriosis, pelvic inflammatory disease, and hepatic failure) and other malignancies (e.g., breast, lung, pancreas, colorectal) are associated with elevated serum CA 125 levels. Fortunately, within the context of screening, most benign/physiologic causes of an elevated serum CA 125 are either clinically apparent or uncommon in the age group most likely to be selected for screening. Elevation of CA 125 levels in malignancies other than ovarian cancer is largely associated with advanced-stage clinically apparent disease.

Ultrasound techniques

Real-time ultrasonography is of established value in the clinical investigation and differential diagnosis of patients with a suspected pelvic mass. Ultrasonic features of pelvic masses associated with ovarian malignancy include a semisolid semicystic appearance, thick septae, surface papillations, and bilateral tumors. The potential of ultrasound in screening for preclinical ovarian cancer was first suggested by Campbell et al,[7] who demonstrated that accurate measurement of postmenopausal ovarian volume could be achieved by transabdominal ultrasonography. Subsequently, there has been important progress in ultrasound technology, and the transvaginal route is now considered superior for ovarian imaging. This approach improves the resolution and quality of ovarian imaging and avoids the need for a full bladder during scanning. The introduction of color doppler blood flow imaging has provided an additional method for ovarian imaging.[8] The process of neovascularization in ovarian carcinogenesis is associated with the development of a low-resistance blood flow pattern. The rationale for applying color flow doppler imaging in screening is evidence that it can distinguish the blood flow of benign and invasive tumors and consequently improve the specificity of screening.

Large studies of screening

Information concerning the efficacy of screening techniques has been derived from eight large studies. When comparing the sensitivity of tumor marker and ultrasound screening, several points should be noted. First, unlike ultrasonography, it is possible to perform tumor marker studies retrospectively because serum stored in serum banks can be analyzed. For this reason it has been possible to perform large retrospective studies, and more information and longer follow-up are available for tumor marker data than with ultrasound. Second, because ultrasound is relatively more expensive than tumor marker analysis, the prospective studies of tumor markers are larger than those of ultrasound. Overall, more information is available about the performance of tumor markers in screening than ultrasound.

Studies of Tumor Markers

The JANUS Study[9]: This retrospective study using the JANUS serum bank includes stored samples from 39,300 Norwegian women. Samples from 105 women who subsequently developed ovarian cancer up to 12 years after venepuncture and age-matched controls were assayed for serum CA 125 levels.

The Royal London Hospital (RLH) Study[10–12]: In the RLH ongoing prospective study of 22,000 apparently healthy postmenopausal women over 45 years of age, the screening protocol consists of serum CA 125 as a primary screen and ultrasound as a secondary test in women with elevated serum CA 125 levels.

The Stockholm Study[13]: In this study, 5,550 apparently healthy women underwent serum CA 125 estimation, those with elevated levels were followed clinically, with ultrasound and with serial CA 125 measurements.

The Maryland Study[14]: In this retrospective study involving a serum bank established in Maryland in 1975, samples from 37 women who subsequently developed ovarian cancer up to 14 years later and age-matched controls were assayed for CA 125.

Studies of Ultrasound and Color Flow Doppler

King's College Hospital Population Study[15]: In this prospective study of 5,479 apparently healthy women over the age of 45 years (pre- and postmenopausal), each volunteer was scanned transabdominally on one to three occasions, at approximately 18-month intervals.

King's College Hospital Family History Study[16]: This study involved 1,601 women with a family history of ovarian cancer and older than 25 years. Volunteers were screened with transvaginal ultrasonography and those with an abnormal result also underwent color flow doppler imaging.

University of Kentucky Study[17]: At the time this chapter was written, this study had reported on 3,220 postmenopausal women of whom 502 had a family history of ovarian cancer. Each volunteer was screened with transvaginal ultrasonography on an annual basis.

Zagreb Study[18]: This study has involved 5,013 asymptomatic pre- and postmenopausal women scanned by transvaginal color and pulsed doppler ultrasonography.

These are not the only studies of screening for ovarian cancer. Several smaller studies have been reported or are in progress.[19–21]

Sensitivity of screening tests

CA 125

In the JANUS study, 6 of 12 serum samples collected within 18 months of the diagnosis of ovarian cancer had serum CA 125 levels greater than 30 U/ml and 4 of 12 were greater than 65 U/ml. Of 59 samples collected more than 5 years before the diagnosis of ovarian cancer, 14 (25%) had a serum CA 125 level greater than 30 U/ml. The results of the RLH study are consistent with these findings. Eleven cases of ovarian cancer were detected at the prevalence screen, a further three presented as interval cases within 12 months of the screen, and five presented as interval cases 12 to 24 months after screening, giving a sensitivity at 1 year follow-up of 79% (11 of 14) and at 2-year follow-up of 58% (11 of 19). The estimated lead of CA 125 screening compared to clinical presentation was 1.4 years. In the Stockholm study, the median duration of follow-up was 32 months, and six of nine cases of ovarian cancer that occurred in the study population were associated with an elevated CA 125 (greater than 30 U/ml). In the Maryland study, the sensitivity of a CA 125 greater than 35 U/ml for detection of ovarian cancer at 3-year follow-up was 57% and at 6-year follow-up, sensitivity was still 40%. A reasonable conclusion from these studies is that CA 125 has a sensitivity at 1 year after screening of 70 to 80% and at 2 years after screening, 50–60%. It is clear from both the JANUS and Maryland studies that in at least a proportion of cases CA 125 provides several years lead time compared to clinical diagnosis of ovarian cancer. One obvious strategy for increasing the detection rate on screening with serum CA 125 measurement would be to reduce the cutoff for an abnormal result. Clearly such an approach will result in some sacrifice of specificity. Data from the RLH study indicate that the cutoff can be reduced to 25 U/ml, with significant increase in sensitivity and minimal loss of specificity. Below 25 U/ml, there is a considerable sacrifice in specificity for small increments of sensitivity. A recent analysis described by Skates et al[21] may be important in refining the sensitivity of CA 125 screening. Skates and colleagues described an algorithm that incorporates the change in CA 125 level with time, as well as absolute CA 125 levels. Whereas CA 125 levels in women who do not have ovarian cancer remain steady or fall with time, those in women with preclinical ovarian cancer rise with time. Retrospective analysis of the Stockholm data with this algorithm showed a sensitivity of 83% and a specificity of 99.7%. A recent analysis of the RLH data using the algorithm developed by Skates et al[22] confirms that this approach can achieve a sensitivity >80% (submitted for publication). Specificity is maintained at 99.8% by use of ultrasound as a secondary test. This important data suggest that a sensitive and specific screening strategy can be achieved using this approach. Intervention based upon a rising CA 125 (even if below 30 U/ml) considerably improves the specificity of CA 125. This is the basis for the randomized controlled trial described later in this chapter.

Other Tumor Markers

It may be possible to improve sensitivity by using additional markers that are complementary to CA 125. Even markers with a relatively low overall sensitivity may be of value if they are elevated in the serum of a significant proportion of ovarian cancer patients who do not have elevated serum CA 125 levels. In a recent study of 46 clinically detected stage I ovarian cancers, Woolas et al[23] found that the serum levels of either CA 125, OVXI, or M-CSF were elevated in 45 cases (98%). In order to assess the implications of these findings in screening for ovarian cancer Jacobs et al (unpublished data) analyzed stored preclinical serum samples from the RLH study for OVX1, MCSF, CA 15–3, and CA 19–9, in addition to CA 125. The most useful additional marker to CA 125 was OVX1. The combination of either a CA 125 (greater than 25 U/ml) or an OVX1 (greater than 12 U/ml) achieved a sensitivity of 80% and a specificity of 91%. Extending the panel to include additional markers resulted in a large decrease in specificity for a relatively small increase in sensitivity.

Ultrasound

The sensitivity of ultrasound screening for detection of preclinical ovarian cancer appears to be higher than that of CA 125. In studies of ultrasound screening, a total of 18 cases of primary epithelial ovarian cancer have been detected and only three false-negative cases reported.[15–20] However, there are a number of important caveats to this data. First, follow-up evaluation in these studies was not complete or was of short duration, or both. Second, it is surprising that 16 of the 18 cases detected were stage I ovarian cancers. As all these studies involved prevalence screens, the detection of some prevalent cases of advanced-stage ovarian cancer would have been expected. The fact that 16 of 18 cases detected were stage I cancers suggests either a degree of understaging or that ultrasound techniques may not detect cases of advanced-stage disease. Finally, only 11 of the 18 cases were invasive epithelial tumors. The remaining seven cases involving borderline or non epithelial tumors for which a good prognosis would be predicted, regardless of early detection by screening. It is unlikely that overall mortality from ovarian cancer will be significantly reduced by screen detection of borderline or other non epithelial ovarian tumors. On balance, the data are consistent with high sensitivity of ultrasound screening for ovarian cancer, but the available information is limited and should be interpreted with some degree of caution.

The specificity of screening tests

Even the most sensitive of tests will not be acceptable if it causes excessive morbidity due to false-positive results. The end point of a positive screening test for ovarian cancer is surgical investigation by laparoscopy or laparotomy. This requirement for an invasive procedure is inevitably associated with immediate physical and psychological morbidity, as well as considerable financial implications and the risk of long-term surgical/anesthetic complications in a small proportion of cases. The most useful measure of this morbidity is the positive predictive value (PPV), calculated as follows:

True-positive results/(true-positives + false-negatives) × 100%

The definition of an acceptable PPV is to some extent arbitrary, but it is unlikely that clinicians or patients would accept a minimum level of less than 10% (i.e., 9 false-positive procedures for each case of ovarian cancer detected).[10] As PPV varies with the incidence of disease, the target population selected for screening will have a major influence on the level of specificity required of the screening test. For a test with 100% sensitivity, the lower limit of specificity required to achieve a PPV of 10% on screening all women above 45 years age is 99.6%. For a test with 50% sensitivity in the same population, the lower limit of specificity to achieve a PPV of 10% would be 99.8%. The requirement for specificity on screening the general population is therefore extremely high. Lower levels of specificity would be required to screen women with a family history of ovarian cancer.

CA 125

In the Stockholm study, elevated CA 125 levels were detected in 2.4% of women above 50 years of age and in 5.7% of women under 50 years of age. Other studies have confirmed that CA 125 has lower specificity in premenopausal women than in postmenopausal women, presumably due to the rise in levels associated with menstruation and benign disorders. In the RLH study 340 of 22,000 postmenopausal volunteers had a serum CA 125 level greater than 30 U/ml, and the specificity of serum CA 125 estimation was 98.5%. This is similar to the specificity of ultrasound alone and, for the reasons outlined below, would not be sufficient to achieve an acceptable positive predictive value in general population screening. Data from both the Stockholm and RLH studies indicate that specificity can be improved substantially by serial measurement of CA 125 levels with time. CA 125 levels in patients with preclinical ovarian cancer rise during follow-up evaluation, whereas the levels in women with false-positive elevations either remain static or fall back into the normal range. As described above, this observation has provided a valuable approach to analysis of CA 125 results, which can be used to improve specificity without sacrificing sensitivity,[22] and a detailed analysis of the RLH data has confirmed the potential of this approach.

Ultrasound

The level of specificity of ultrasound screening as a one-stage test may be sufficient to achieve an acceptable PPV among women with a family history of ovarian cancer, but it is not satisfactory for screening the general population. False-positive results in the King's, Kentucky, and Zagreb studies were attributable largely to benign ovarian tumors or to other benign pelvic abnormalities, such as uterine fibroids or hydrosalpinx, but in a small proportion of cases no abnormality was detected. Overall, a total of 16,296 women participated in reported ultrasound studies, of whom 524 have undergone surgery and 18 have had primary epithelial ovarian cancer.[15–20] The overall specificity is 96.8% and the PPV 3.4%. It was noteworthy that Bourne et al[16] observed a much higher false positive rate amongst women with an artificial menopause, presumably because of the anatomic alterations resulting from previous surgery. Retrospective analysis of the women screened in the King's Population Study suggests that the specificity of TAS could be increased by the use of a morphologic index and analysis of the change in ovarian volume on serial scanning.[15] Bourne et al[16] found that the use of a defined ovarian volume change at repeat ultrasonography, a morphologic index, and color flow doppler imaging increased the specificity in the King's Family History Study to 99.1%. However, this was achieved at the expense of a reduction in sensitivity and may still result in a PPV of less than 10% if applied to general population screening.

Sequential Combination of CA 125 and Ultrasound

Both CA 125 and ultrasound have a significant false-positive rate that precludes their use alone as a one-stage screen of the general population. For this reason, the RLH study was designed to investigate the possibility that sufficient specificity could be achieved by incorporating both tests in a sequential screening strategy. Since obtaining samples for CA 125 analysis is logistically easier than organizing ultrasonography and the CA 125 test is substantially cheaper to perform, CA 125 was used as a first line test. Only women with an elevated serum CA 125 level (greater than 30 U/ml) were recalled for an ultrasound scan.[12] A total of 340 of the 22,000 postmenopausal volunteers screened had an elevated CA 125 level and underwent transabdominal ultrasonography. Only 41 of these volunteers had an abnormal ultrasound scan and underwent surgical investigation, of whom 11 had ovarian cancer and 31 either a benign abnormality or no abnormality. The overall specificity of this screening strategy was 99.9% and the PPV 26.8%.[12] This level of specificity would be acceptable in general population screening of a postmenopausal population.

Recommendations for current clinical use of screening

The efficacy of screening has not yet been demonstrated in a randomized controlled trial, and well-defined risks of screening are associated with false-positive results. Nevertheless, clinical decision making is being made against a background of increasing media interest in ovarian cancer, which has resulted in anxiety among some groups of women, and increasing pressure to provide access to screening techniques. Guidelines for the use of screening in clinical practice are required to achieve a balance between the long-term need to thoroughly assess potential screening tests in randomized controlled trials and the immediate need to assist women at high risk.

Women at High Risk

A small proportion of women can be defined as at high risk of ovarian cancer either on the basis of their family history (see above) or because they are known to have a BRCA1 or BRCA2 mutation. If, after thorough counseling, a woman in this group does not wish to undergo prophylactic oophorectomy, it is reasonable to provide annual screening with CA 125 and ultrasonography. Many women in this group will opt for screening until they have completed their families or as an interim measure pending the availability of BRCA1 and BRCA2 mutation testing during the next few years. It is difficult on practical and ethical grounds to propose a randomized controlled trial of screening in this group of women. Observational studies are in progress in the UK and elsewhere.

Women at Intermediate Risk

Women at intermediate risk include those with a single first-degree relative with ovarian cancer, several more distant relatives with ovarian cancer, or a personal history of breast cancer. The lifetime risk of ovarian cancer to this group of women is increased compared to the general population but remains low (less than 5% lifetime risk). Women in this group should be advised that their risk of ovarian cancer is low within the context of the risk of other cancers/illness and the limitations and risks of screening should be emphasized. The well-documented risks of screening may outweigh any possible benefit for this group of women, and screening should not be recomended. However, it is recognized that a significant proportion of women in this group will be particularly anxious because of their family history and will wish to undergo screening despite understanding the limitations and risks. If women in this group make an informed decision to proceed with screening, the use of a sequential strategy involving CA 125, followed by ultrasound only if CA 125 is elevated, will achieve a high specificity and PPV. Although the significance of a history of ovarian stimulation is currently controversial, women who have received this treatment and who have not subsequently conceived, may be included in the intermediate-risk group.

Women at Low Risk

Most women who request advice about screening for ovarian cancer do not have any major predisposing risk factors. The lifetime risk of ovarian cancer for this group of women is low (approximately 1%). The most important aspect of advising this group of women is a clear explanation of the current situation. First, their level of risk should be explained within the broad context of the risk of other cancers and other illness. Second, the limitations of the available screening techniques should be emphasized. Women in the low-risk group should not be screened as part of a clinical service, as the benefits of screening are unproved and the risk of false-positive results requiring surgical intervention is substantial. When possible, women in this group should be included in randomized controlled trials of screening.

JOHN R. van NAGELL, JR.
PAUL D. DePRIEST

Two studies have evaluated serum CA 125 as a screening method in large numbers of asymptomatic women. Einhorn and coworkers[24] evaluated CA 125 in 5,500 apparently healthy Swedish women over 40 years of age. Serum CA 125 was elevated (greater than 30 U/ml) in 175 of these women (3.2%) and six had an ovarian cancer confirmed clinically or sonographically. Unfortunately, four of the six ovarian cancer patients had advanced-stage disease at surgery. Three additional women with normal serum CA 125 levels also were found to have ovarian cancer. More recently, Jacobs and colleagues[25] examined serum CA 125 values in 22,000 asymptomatic postmenopausal women older than 45 years of age. Forty-one patients (0.2%) had an elevated (greater than 30 U/ml) serum CA 125 level and were investigated surgically. Eleven of these patients had ovarian cancer, but seven had advanced (stage III or IV) disease. An additional eight patients developed ovarian cancer despite having normal serum CA 125 values. The sensitivity of serum CA 125 in this trial was 78.6%, and the PPV was 26.8%.

When serum CA 125 has been used as the initial screening test, early-stage ovarian cancers have been missed, and stage at detection has not decreased appreciably. However, there is hope that the addition of other tumor markers, such as CA 15-3 or TAG 72.3, to CA 125 will increase its diagnostic accuracy.[26] To date, the lack of sensitivity of serum CA 125 in early stage disease has limited its usefulness as a primary screening method for ovarian cancer.

The most effective method for ovarian cancer screening is transvaginal sonography (TVS). TVS usually is performed using a standard ultrasound unit with a 5.0-MHz vaginal transducer. The test is painless and is best performed with the bladder empty. A complete screening examination can be performed in 5 to 10 minutes, and a permanent hard copy of each sonogram is generated for inclusion in the patient record. Each ovary is measured in three dimensions, and ovarian volume is calculated using the prolate ellipsoid formula:

$$L \times H \times W \times 0.523$$

An ovarian volume of 20 cm^3 or greater in premenopausal women and of 10 cm^3 or greater in postmenopausal women is considered abnormal. These values are two standard deviations (SD) above published values for normal ovarian volume in premenopausal and postmenopausal women.[27] In addition, any internal papillary projection from the tumor wall is considered abnormal.[28] The screening algorithm used at the University of Kentucky is illustrated in Figure 1-1. A woman with an abnormal screen is scheduled to have a repeat sonogram in 4 to 6 weeks. If the repeat examination is abnormal, she undergoes pelvic examination, color doppler assessment of tumor blood flow, a serum CA 125 determination, and morphologic indexing of the tumor. Operative removal of the tumor is then performed by laparoscopy or laparotomy. The tumor is photographed, measured in three dimensions, and sectioned for histologic examination. Patients with ovarian malignancies undergo total abdominal hysterectomy, bilateral salpingo-oophorectomy, tumor debulking, and complete surgical staging. If the screen is negative, the patient is asked to return in one year for the next screen.

Using this algorithm, screening results on 8,500 asymptomatic women were reported.[28] One hundred and twenty-one women (1.4%) had a persisting abnormality on TVS and underwent surgical tumor removal. Eight patients had ovarian cancer, and 57 had serous cystadenomas. Six of the patients with ovarian cancer had stage I disease, one patient had stage IIC disease, and one patient had stage IIIB cancer. Only one of these patients had palpable ovarian enlargement on clinical examination, and only one patient had an elevated serum CA 125. All patients whose cancers were detected on screening are alive and well 1 to 6 years after conventional therapy. There were 8,379 women with normal screens. One patient with a family history of ovarian cancer was noted to have ovarian cancer at prophylactic oophorectomy 11 months after a normal screen (false-negative result). This patient is alive and well 1 year after surgery and chemotherapy. There were approximately 20,000 patient screening years in this trial and no deaths from primary ovarian cancer in the screened population.

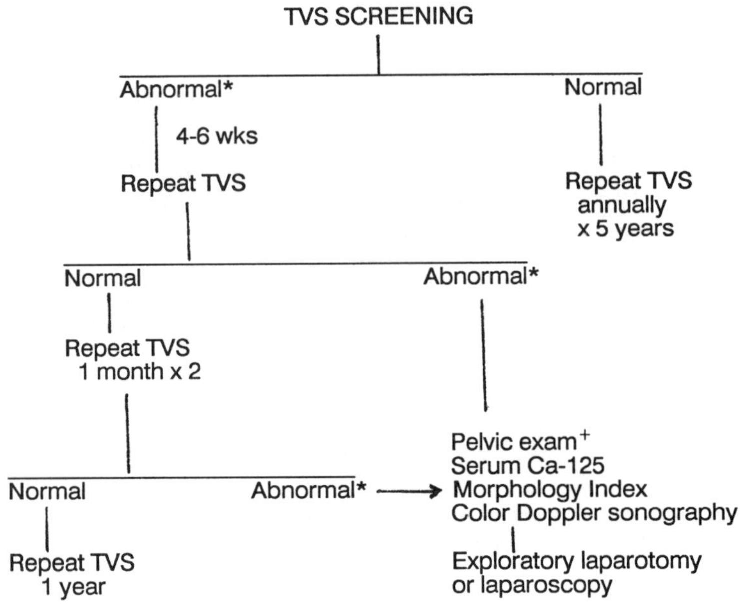

FIGURE 1-1. Algorithm for ovarian cancer screening. (*) Abnormal volume: ovarian volume > 10 cm^3–postmenopausal or (*) abnormal morphology: papillary projection into a cystic ovarian tumor. (+) Pelvic examination would be performed by physician without knowledge of transvaginal sonography (TVS) findings.

The use of Doppler flow sonography as a screening method in patients with a family history of ovarian cancer has been reported by Bourne et al[4] Screening was performed in 1,601 asymptomatic women, 88% of whom had at least one first degree relative with ovarian cancer. Sixty-one ovarian tumors were detected, and six patients had ovarian cancer. Five of these patients had stage I disease and all patients are alive and well following treatment. The prevalence of ovarian cancer in this group (390 of 100,000) was approximately 10-fold higher than that in patients from the general population (40/100,000).

Although screening with Doppler flow sonography is effective, the higher cost of this technology, as compared to conventional sonography, may preclude its use as a primary screening method. It is our policy to perform color flow studies only on women with a persisting ovarian tumor on TVS.

QUESTION 3

What effect will the availability of BRCA1 and BRCA2 have on recommendations for screening?

IAN JACOBS

Women at high risk of ovarian cancer, as judged by familial predisposition, require careful counseling and advice that should be provided with in the context of a well-organized familial cancer clinic. These clinics should have the resources to confirm the details of a family history, to provide advice about level of risk, methods of prevention, and early detection strategies, as well as facilities for psychosocial support. Since the familial cancer syndromes involving ovarian cancer usually involve other cancers (e.g., breast, colorectal, and endometrial cancer), screening for early detection of ovarian cancer is only one aspect of advising these women. For women in breast/ovarian cancer families, counseling will include an assessment of the level of risk and discussion about medical and surgical prevention, as well as screening for both breast and ovarian cancer. The availability of BRCA1 and BRCA2 mutation analysis will have a number of important implications for such clinics. First, a decision must be made about which group of women to offer direct gene testing. There are important ethical differences between providing testing to women in high-risk families who initiate the request, approaching women in these families to offer them the test, and offering the test to women with a weaker family history. Second, the psychosocial implications of testing positive or negative for mutations of BRCA1 or BRCA2 are largely unknown. Third, the BRCA1 and BRCA2 genes are large, and testing remains a laborious process. Organization and funding of direct gene testing will require careful consideration. Finally, the long-term financial and employment implications for women who test positive are unclear. These complex issues will need to be comprehensively addressed during the next few years. However, most of these issues do not impinge directly on recommendations for screening for ovarian cancer.

The availability of BRCA1 and BRCA2 mutation screening will not alter the recommendation that *screening should be confined to women at high risk*, until the efficacy of screening has been demonstrated in randomized controlled trials. The main impact of this technology will be to alter the group of women who are classified as at high risk. The definition of the high-risk group for screening is based on a family history that fulfills one of the following criteria:

Two or more women with ovarian cancer who are first-degree relatives

One woman with ovarian cancer and one woman with breast cancer diagnosed under 50 years who are first-degree relatives

One woman with ovarian cancer and two woman with breast cancer diagnosed before 60 years of age who are connected by first-degree relationships

Three women with colorectal cancer with at least one case diagnosed before 50 years as well as one case of ovarian cancer and all these women are connected by first-degree relationships

Women who are first-degree relatives of affected members of these families should be regarded as at high risk and may reasonably be offered screening. By limiting BRCA1 and BRCA2 mutation analysis to these high-risk families, the number of women requiring screening is likely to be reduced. First, individuals in families with a documented mutation who have not themselves inherited the mutation will be reallocated to the low-risk group. Second, many of the women who are found to have inherited the predisposing mutation will opt for prophylactic oophorectomy, rather than screening. If, however, BRCA1 and BRCA2 mutation screening is extended more widely (e.g., to women) with a weaker family history or no significant family history), some additional women with predisposing mutations will be identified as falling into the high-risk group. In summary, the direct implications of BRCA1 and BRCA2 testing for screening are limited and relate to the number of individuals who will be included in the high-risk group.

JOHN R. van NAGELL, JR.
PAUL D. DePRIEST

According to data from the Breast Cancer Linkage Consortium, germline BRCA1 mutations confer a 23% risk of ovarian cancer by age 30 and a 63% risk of the disease by age 70.[29] However, patterns of mutations in the BRCA1 gene may vary from one individual to another, and the risks associated with each specific mutation have yet to be determined.[30] Data concerning ovarian cancer risk in women with BRCA2 mutations are incomplete, but the risk is much lower than that associated with BRCA1 abnormalities. There is no evidence that annual ovarian cancer screening will reduce ovarian cancer mortality in women with BRCA1 mutations. Nevertheless, these patients theoretically could benefit from screening. Patients with BRCA1 mutations should be encouraged to participate in clinical research trials designed to determine the efficacy of screening in women with a genetic predisposition to ovarian cancer. Women with a documented family history of ovarian cancer should be provided information concerning the precision and specificity of genetic testing, their risk for ovarian cancer and ethical issues involved in such testing.[31] This information should be useful to women who may wish to participate in ovarian cancer screening trials before undergoing prophylactic oophorectomy. Perhaps the greatest benefit of genetic testing is in the identification of those members of an ovarian or breast cancer family who do not carry BRCA1 mutations. These members could then be spared unnecessary screening or prophylactic oophorectomy.

QUESTION 4

What future clinical trials should be designed based on current knowledge and technology?

IAN JACOBS

The information obtained from prospective studies during the past decade is sufficient to justify large randomized controlled trials to document the impact of screening for ovarian cancer on mortality. Three large trials are currently at an early stage and should provide mortality data in 8 to 10 years from now.

NIH PLCO study

Ovarian cancer screening is a component of the NIH PLCO study.[32] A total of 74,000 women older than 60 years of age will be randomized to a control group or to screening with each of clinical examination, CA 125, and ultrasound as first-line tests. Abnormal results for any of these tests will be referred to a gynecologic oncologist for further investigation at his or her discretion. The study duration to achieve 80% power for a 30% reduction in mortality is 16 years.

European multicenter study

The European Multicenter Study is a trial of 120,000 postmenopausal women randomized to a control group or two study groups to be screened with vaginal ultrasonography at intervals of either 1.5 or 3 years, for a total of 8 years. Women with abnormal ultrasound findings will have a color flow doppler examination and, if this is abnormal, will be referred for surgical investigation. The trial has a 78% ability to detect a significant difference between the combined ultrasound groups and the control group after 8 years assuming a 33% reduction in mortality for both screened groups.

Royal London/ St Bartholomew's study

The Royal London/St. Bartholomew's study trial involves 120,000 postmenopausal women over 50 years of age. Participants are randomized to a control group or to a study group to be screened with CA 125 as a primary test and ultrasound as a secondary test in women with an increased risk of ovarian cancer based on the pattern of CA 125 results. CA 125 results will be interpreted using a modification of the algorithm developed by Skates et al[22] The trial has an 80% ability to detect a 30% difference in mortality between the control and study groups.

In parallel with these randomized controlled trials, it will be important to perform studies of the health economic and psychosocial implications of screening, so that a balanced view of the costs and benefits of early detection will ultimately emerge. In addition, ongoing efforts should be made to refine current screening modalities using the data obtained from earlier prospective trials of tumor markers and ultrasound. It may be possible to use the serum banks from previous studies to identify new markers that are complementary to CA 125. Finally, the progress in understanding the molecular basis of ovarian carcinogenesis is only just beginning to have an impact in clinical practice. It is difficult to predict where major progress will occur, but the identification of a precursor lesion for ovarian cancer that will be a target for screening is an exciting possibility for the future.

JOHN R. van NAGELL, JR. PAUL D. DePRIEST

Ideally, there should be a randomized double-armed trial comparing stage at detection, case-specific ovarian cancer mortality, and site-specific ovarian cancer mortality in a population of women participating in annual screening versus a control population not exposed to screening. Nevertheless, ethical or medico-legal issues, and patient failure to participate in the control arm may limit the success of such a trial. In the absence of such a trial, it may be necessary to have a trial in which all participants receive some type of screening. We believe that screening should be evaluated in three populations of asymptomatic women: (1) all women over the age of 50, (2) women over the age of 25 with a documented family history of ovarian cancer, and (3) women who are members of an ovarian cancer family or those who are BRCA1 mutation carriers. Ovarian cancer mortality rises significantly above the age of 50, the population of women found to include the vast majority of ovarian cancer cases.[3] Ovarian cancer risk rises further in women with one or more relatives who have this disease;[3] data concerning the protective effect of screening in this population are needed. Finally, women who are members of ovarian cancer families or who have documented BRCA1 mutations are at highest risk for the development of ovarian cancer.[33,34] Although prophylactic oophorectomy will be recommended in most of these cases, screening should be evaluated as a means to monitor BRCA1 mutation carriers who choose to retain their childbearing function.

Primary screening tests that should be evaluated include CA 125 or other markers and TVS. My preference would be a TVS-driven trial, as TVS has been shown to demonstrate high sensitivity in the detection of small, curable ovarian cancers. The major issue to be evaluated in a TVS trial is the lack of specificity and the low PPV of this method. The use of doppler flow sonography,[35,36] biochemical markers,[37] and a morphology index[38] are being evaluated as means to increase the PPV of TVS screening (see the algorithm illustrated in Fig. 1-1). Another trial design would be to use CA 125 or a panel or markers in the initial screen and to employ TVS in patients with a persisting or rising serum marker level. The optimal interval for screening in various at-risk populations has not been established and must be evaluated.

In any trial, it will be imperative to assess the sensitivity, specificity, positive predictive value, and negative predictive value of each screening method. It will also be necessary to generate reliable data concerning the direct and indirect costs of each screening test.

EDITORS' COMMENTARY

We agree with the recommendation of the authors that ovarian cancer screening of the normal population be conducted in a clinical research setting. Drs. van Nagell and DePriest also recommend that screening of high-risk populations be performed in a research setting. Such a strategy is important if we are to enhance our understanding of this effort.

As outlined by both groups, studies to date do not give us much encouragement that either serum CA 125 or pelvic sonography will emerge as a useful single-modality screening tool for ovarian cancer. CA 125 lacks both sensitivity and specificity. Only about 50% of those women with stage I disease will have abnormal CA 125 values. On the other hand, the algorithm method of CA 125 assessment may ultimately prove to be of benefit. By contrast, ultrasound lacks sufficient specificity. Estimates range from 40 to 100 operations for every ovarian cancer detected on the basis of sonographic findings. The authors nicely outline strategies being employed in second-generation screening studies to overcome these deficits: (1) multimodality approaches using both serum CA 125 and ultrasound in a sequential fashion, (2) the use of a panel of serum tumor markers designed to enhance sensitivity, and (3) the use of the longitudinal study of serum CA 125 based on samples from serum banks. Dr. Jacobs proceeds to make recommendations about ovarian cancer screening based on current technology and the reality of media interest and pressure from women to provide access to screening techniques, however flawed. He classifies women into low-, intermediate-, and high-risk groups, on the basis of available information.

Both groups discuss the societal and ethical implications of genetic susceptibility testing. They emphasize the fact that, even if a women does have a BRCA1 or BRCA2 mutation, she may elect to forego prophylactic oophorectomy in favor of screening. It will be key to study these women to learn more about the efficacy of screening of women with genetic susceptibility. In addition, testing will allow us to identify women who would otherwise be classified as high-risk based on family history but who do not have a mutation; they will be reclassifed as low risk.

Finally, both groups agree that future clinical trials in this area should include prospective randomized studies comparing screening with no screening. In fact, Dr. Jacobs briefly outlines three trials that are already under way. Concomitantly, attention will be paid to the cost-benefit ratio associated with ovarian cancer screening strategies. Based on the excellent summaries presented here, it appears that within the next decade we may have sufficient information about screening to determine its ultimate fate.

References

1. Young RC, Decker DG, Wharton JT et al: Staging laparotomy in early ovarian cancer. JAMA 250:3072, 1983
2. Carlson KJ, Skates SJ, Singer D: Screening for ovarian cancer. Ann Intern Med 121:124, 1994
3. Kerlikowske K, Brown JS, Grady DG: Should women with familial ovarian cancer undergo prophylactic oophorectomy? Obstet Gynecol 80:700, 1991
4. Bourne TH, Campbell S, Reynolds KM et al: Screening for early familial ovarian cancer with transvaginal ultrasonography and colour blood flow imaging. BMJ 306:1025, 1993
5. Bast RC, Klug TL, St John E et al: A radioimmunoassay using a monoclonal antibody to monitor the course of epithelial ovarian cancer. N Engl J Med 309:169, 1983.
6. Jacobs IJ, Bast RC: The CA 125 tumour associated antigen; a review of the literature. Hum Reprod 4:1, 1989
7. Campbell S, Goswamy R, Goessens L et al: Real time ultrasonography for determination of ovarian morphology and volume. Lancet 1:425, 1982
8. Bourne T, Campbell S, Steer C et al: Transvaginal colour flow imaging: a possible new screening technique for ovarian cancer. BMJ 299:1367, 1989
9. Zurawski VR, Orjaseter H, Andersen A, Jellum E: Elevated serum CA 125 levels prior to diagnosis of ovarian neoplasia; relevance for early detection of ovarian cancer. Int J Cancer 42:677, 1988
10. Jacobs IJ, Stabile I, Bridges J et al: Multimodal approach to screening for ovarian cancer. Lancet 1:268, 1988
11. Jacobs IJ, Oram DH, Bast R Jr: Strategies for improving the specificity of screening for ovarian cancer with tumor-associated antigens CA 125, CA 15-3, and TAG 72.3. Obstet Gynecol 80: 396, 1992
12. Jacobs I, Davies AP, Bridges J et al: Prevalence screening for ovarian cancer in postmenopausal women by CA 125 measurement and ultrasonography. BMJ 306:1030, 1993

13. Einhorn N, Sjovall K, Knapp RC et al: Prospective evaluation of serum CA 125 levels for early detection of ovarian cancer. Obstet Gynecol 80:14, 1992

14. Helzlsouer KJ, Bush TL, Alberg AJ et al: Prospective study of serum CA 125 levels as markers of ovarian cancer. JAMA 269:1123, 1993

15. Campbell S, Bhan V, Royston P et al: Transabdominal ultrasound screening for early ovarian cancer. BMJ 299: 1363, 1989

16. Bourne TH, Campbell S, Reynolds KM et al: Screening for early familial ovarian cancer with transvaginal ultrasonography and colour blood flow imaging. BMJ 306:1025, 1993

17. DePriest PD, van Nagell JR, Gallion HH et al: Ovarian cancer screening in asymptomatic postmenopausal women. Gynecol Oncol 51:205, 1993

18. Kurjak A, Shalan H, Kupesic S et al: An attempt to screen asymptomatic women for ovarian and endometrial cancer with transvaginal color and pulsed doppler sonography. J Ultrasound Med 13:295, 1994

19. Karlan BY, Raffel LJ, Crvenkovic G et al: A multidisciplinary approach to the early detection of ovarian carcinoma: rationale, protocol design, and early results. Am J Obstet Gynecol 169:494 1993

20. Muto MG, Cramer DW, Brown DL et al: Screening for ovarian cancer: the preliminary experience of a familial ovarian cancer center. Gynecol Oncol 51:12, 1993

21. Schwartz PE, Chambers JT, Taylor KJ et al: Early detection of ovarian cancer: preliminary results of the Yale Early Detection Program. Yale J Biol Med 64:573, 1993

22. Skates SJ, Feng-Ji X, Yin-Hua Y et al: Towards an optimal algorithm for ovarian cancer screening with longitudinal tumour markers. Cancer 76:2004, 1995

23. Woolas RP, Xu FJ, Jacobs IJ et al: Elevation of multiple serum markers in patients with stage I ovarian cancer. J Natl Cancer Inst 85:1748, 1994

24. Einhorn N, Sjovall K, Knapp RC et al: Prospective evaluation of serum Ca- 125 levels for early detection of ovarian cancer. Obstet Gynecol 80:14, 1992

25. Jacobs I, Davies AP, Bridges J: Prevalence screening for ovarian cancer in postmenopausal women by Ca-125 measurement and ultrasonography. BMJ 306:1030, 1993

26. Jacobs I, Oram D, Bast R: Strategies for improving the specificity of screening for ovarian cancer with tumor associated antigens Ca-125, Ca 15-3, and TAG 72.3. Obstet Gynecol 80:396, 1992

27. Goswamy RK, Campbell S, Whitehead MI: Screening for ovarian cancer. Clin Obstet Gynecol 10:621, 1983

28. van Nagell JR, Gallion H, Pavlik E, De-Priest PD: Ovarian cancer screening. Cancer 76:2086, 1995

29. Easton DF, Ford D, Bishop PT, and the Breast Cancer Linkage Consortium: Breast and ovarian cancer incidence in BRCA-1 mutation carriers. Am J Hum Genet 56:265, 1995

30. Shattuck-Edens D, McClure M, Simard J et al: A collaborative survey of 80 mutations in the BRCA1 breast and ovarian cancer susceptibility gene. JAMA 273: 435, 1995

31. Statement of the American Society of Human Genetics on Genetic Testing for Breast and Ovarian Cancer Predisposition. Am J Hum Genet 55:i, 1994

32. Kramer BS, Gohagan J, Prorok PC, Smart C: A National Cancer Institute sponsored screening trial for prostatic, lung, colorectal, and ovarian cancers. Cancer 71:589, 1993

33. Amos CI, Shaw GL, Tucker MA, Hartge P: Age at onset for familial epithelial ovarian cancer. JAMA 268:1896, 1992

34. Lynch HT, Watson P, Bewtra TA et al: Hereditary ovarian cancer. Heterogene-

ity in age at diagnosis. Cancer 67: 1460, 1991

35. Fleischer AC, Rodgers WH, Kepple DM et al: Color Doppler sonography of ovarian masses: a multiparameter analysis. J Ultrasound Med 12:41, 1993

36. Weiner Z, Thaler I, Beck D et al: Differentiating malignant from benign ovarian tumors with transvaginal color flow imaging. Obstet Gynecol 79:159, 1992

37. Gadducci A, Ferdeghini M, Prontera C et al: The concomitant determination of different tumor markers in patients with epithelial ovarian cancer and benign ovarian masses: relevance for differential diagnosis. Gynecol Oncol 44:147, 1992

38. DePriest PD, Shenson D, Fried A et al: A morphology index based on sonographic findings in ovarian cancer. Gynecol Oncol 51:7, 1993

CHAPTER 2

THE ROLE OF PROPHYLACTIC OOPHORECTOMY

M. Steven Piver
Barry Rosen

EDITORS' INTRODUCTION

Over the past two decades, an increasing amount of attention has been paid to familial ovarian cancer. Until recently, information regarding this entity was restricted to a discussion of family pedigrees. With the advent of genetic susceptibility testing in the form of BRCA1 and BRCA2, awareness of genetic predisposition to the development of ovarian cancer has been raised further.

Consequently, questions about prophylactic oophorectomy have assumed even greater importance in daily practice. Our patients are turning to us for answers regarding this very complex subject. As physicians, we know that there are no easy answers to these questions. Included in our responses must be a thorough discussion of risk assessment based on detailed family pedigree, hormone replacement therapy, alternatives, risks of surgical procedures, and the ramifications of genetic susceptibility testing. The individual patient's menopausal status and reproductive status continue to be the key factors in the ultimate decision about prophylactic oophorectomy.

QUESTIONS

1. Should prophylactic oophorectomy be recommended to women undergoing a laparotomy or laparoscopy for (1) hysterectomy or (2) a nongynecologic surgical procedure?
2. Should prophylactic oophorectomy be recommended to women with two or more first-degree relatives with epithelial ovarian cancer?
3. Should prophylactic oophorectomy be recommended to women with one first-degree relative with epithelial ovarian cancer?
4. What are the surgical options for prophylactic oophorectomy, and what is your recommended method? Should hysterectomy also be performed routinely?
5. What should women be counseled about regarding the protective effects of prophylactic oophorectomy? What are the alternatives to prophylactic oophorectomy?

QUESTION 1

Should prophylactic oophorectomy be recommended to women undergoing a laparotomy or laparoscopy for (1) hysterectomy or (2) a nongynecologic surgical procedure?

M. STEVEN PIVER

Approximately 600,000 women undergo hysterectomy each year in the United States; many more have other surgical procedures that allow access to the pelvis. All these patients have an opportunity to eliminate their future risk of ovarian cancer almost completely by undergoing prophylactic oopherectomy at the primary procedure. Schwartz[1] recently published a review of the literature from the past six decades summarizing the incidence of prior hysterectomy in women with ovarian cancer (Table 2-1). Over the years, the reported incidence has ranged from 1% to 18%, with a mean of 8%. Sightler et al[2] were able to pool their data with three other studies in the literature to determine the number of ovarian cancer patients who underwent hysterectomy at age 40 or older. Of 2,362 cases of ovarian cancer, these investigators predicted that 138 (5.2%) could have been prevented if all women in the series who underwent hysterectomy beyond age 40 had also had a prophylactic bilateral oophorectomy. Finazzo et al[3] reviewed a series of 291 women with ovarian cancer for history of prior laparotomy. Seventy-one patients had undergone previous laparotomy, at least 43 of whom had undergone surgery after age 35. Finazzo and colleagues predicted that prophylactic oophorectomy in all women in this group who had a laparotomy at age 36 or older would have prevented 15% of the ovarian cancer cases and 10% of the mortality. In a more recent report, Boike et al[4] reviewed 12,316 cases of ovarian cancer from an American College of Surgeons patterns of care study. Of the

TABLE 2-1
Incidence of Prior Hysterectomies in Women With Ovarian Cancer

AUTHOR	YEAR	NO. OF OVARIAN CANCERS	NO. OF PRIOR HYSTERECTOMIES	%
1. Pemberton	1940	149	3	2.0
2. Rollins	1951	106	1	0.9
3. Golub	1953	210	16	7.6
4. Counseller	1955	1,500	67	4.5
5. Fagan	1956	172	7	4.1
6. Bloom	1962	141	15	10.6
7. Terz	1967	624	32	5.1
8. Gibbs	1971	236	28	11.9
9. McGowan	1979	197	2	1.0
10. Stapleton	1985	392	43	11.0
11. Scottolini	1986	95	17	17.9
12. McGowan	1987	291	41	14.1
13. Finazso	1988	291	46	15.8
14. Sightler	1991	755	95	12.6
Total		5,159	413	8.0

(From Schwartz,[1] with permission.)

2,241 women in the series who had previously undergone hysterectomy, 1,286, or just over 10% of the total group, had the procedure performed at age 40 or above and could have potentially been spared their disease had they undergone routine prophylactic oophorectomy. Assuming an annual incidence of 26,000 cases and a rate of prior hysterectomy at age 40 or beyond of 5 to 10%, an estimated 1,300 to 2,600 cases of ovarian cancer could potentially be prevented each year if prophylactic oophorectomy at the time of hysterectomy were widely recommended.

Despite the potential for reduction of disease and mortality, routine salpingo-oophorectomy at hysterectomy is not widespread. During the 3-year period 1988 to 1990, only 61% of women in the United States who underwent hysterectomy after age 40 had a bilateral salpingo-oophorectomy.[4] Schwartz[1] surveyed members of the Society of Gynecologic Oncology and obstetrician-gynecologists in the state of Connecticut, asking "What percentage of women could be saved from ovarian carcinoma by removal at hysterectomy of both ovaries?" Approximately one-half of all obstetrician-gynecologists responding with a quantifiable answer believed that the answer was only 2% or less. Similar attitudes seem to prevail in Great Britain, where 52% of 1,142 gynecologists surveyed felt that prophylactic oophorectomy would prevent less than 5% of cases of ovarian cancer.[5] Furthermore, only 65% of respondents said they routinely discuss prophylactic oophorectomy with their patients before a planned procedure, and only 44% said they would perform prophylactic oophorectomy as a primary procedure in women with a strong family history of ovarian cancer.

Historically, approximately 10 to 30% of hysterectomies have been performed vaginally.[2] However, avoidance of laparotomy does not preclude prophylactic oophorectomy, nor does desire for prophylactic oophorectomy mandate abdominal or even laparoscopically assisted vaginal hysterectomy. Sheth and Malpani[6] reported the feasibility of routine prophylactic oophorectomy in women undergoing vaginal procedures. Of 150 women who underwent vaginal hysterectomy, successful bilateral oophorectomy or salpingo-oophorectomy was accomplished in 145. When compared to 200 controls, the mean additional operative time was 15 minutes. There was no major morbidity in either group, and no increased minor morbidity in patients undergoing vaginal oophorectomy. It is expected that with the present level of utilization of laparoscopy in the United States, any oophorectomy that could not be completed vaginally could be completed laparoscopically under the same anesthetic, if the patient so desired.

There are other potential benefits to prophylactic oophorectomy besides prevention of ovarian cancer. When the ovaries are left in situ after hysterectomy, up to 20% of patients may have residual ovarian syndrome, subsequent neoplasm, or other pathology, and approximately 5% will require reoperation for subsequent oopherectomy.[7,8] Oophorectomy may confer a protection against breast cancer.[9] However, this benefit is most pronounced in younger women and is partially negated by use of estrogen replacement therapy, such that breast cancer risk returns to baseline or above in women undergoing oopherectomy after age 40 who take lifelong estrogen. Siddle et al[10] reported that women who undergo a hysterectomy with ovarian conservation experience menopause approximately 4 years earlier than expected, possibly due to circulatory or other factors. Thus, patients who decide to retain their ovaries because of a desire to maintain endogenous estrogen production may obtain less benefit than anticipated. There is no known benefit to routine unilateral removal of an ovary.[11,12]

BARRY ROSEN

Ovarian cancer is the most lethal gynecologic malignancy. During the past 15 to 20 years, there has been no significant improvement in the overall survival rate.[13] This is disappointing because extensive efforts have been made to improve diagnostic techniques and treatment strategies. With little or no change in the incidence rate during this period, we can expect to see a larger number of women presenting with ovarian cancer as the population ages and more women enter the high-risk years.[14] Thirty percent of ovarian cancers occur in women aged 70 years and older.[13] As the median life expectancy for women has increased to more than 80 years, we can expect to see even more cases of ovarian cancer in this group.[14]

As a result of these predictions, issues such as prevention and screening have become very important. Possible preventive strategies for ovarian cancer include use of oral contraceptive pills (OCP), lowering of dietary fat intake,[15] and prophylactic surgery.[16]

This chapter considers the controversial issues related to concurrent prophylactic oophorectomy at hysterectomy and other non-gynecologic surgery. A primary focus is the use of prophylactic surgery in women with familial ovarian cancer history. Over the past 2 to 3 years, considerable new information has been published regarding familial ovarian and breast cancer, especially since the identification of the BRCA1 and BRCA2 genes.[17] Earlier, most papers on familial ovarian cancer classified families on the basis of pedigree. These classifications included ovarian site-specific, breast-ovarian, and Lynch type II families. Another definition of these families included such terms as *familial* for those with a family history and *hereditary* for those with an autosomal dominant pattern of inheritance. Availability of genetic testing provides another way to classify women at risk—as BRCA1 mutation positive or negative. This categorization most accurately reflects risk compared to the other classifications, which include both BRCA1-positive and -negative women. Those with a BRCA1 mutation have a lifetime risk (to age 70) of ovarian cancer as high as 44%[18] to 56%,[19] whereas gene mutation negative women have a risk slightly less than that of the general population, of 1.4%. Genetic testing is still limited, however, and for those families in which no mutation is found and in those who cannot be tested, family history will continue to be used to determine risk of ovarian cancer. This chapter evaluates how genetic testing has changed the approach to prophylactic oophorectomy.

Before addressing these questions, it is useful to provide you with a definition of prophylactic oophorectomy:

> It is a surgical procedure whose primary intent is to prevent future development of ovarian cancer. It includes removal of the ovary (ovaries) in situations where the woman is asymptomatic and has no clinical or surgical abnormality of either ovary. In other words, the ovaries are clinically and grossly normal.

Prophylactic oophorectomy does not include situations in which an oophorectomy is undertaken in patients with conditions such as endometriosis, pelvic pain, and endometrial or breast cancer. In these latter situations, oophorectomy is a therapeutic procedure whose primary intent is to solve a clinical problem, not prevent ovarian cancer. If one were to propose a clinical trial designed to evaluate the effectiveness of prophylactic oophorectomy to prevent ovarian cancer, its main end points of analysis would be a comparison of incidence and mortality rates between the study (prophylactic oophorectomy) and control groups.

Issues to consider when deciding whether to recommend concurrent removal of normal ovaries in women undergoing hysterectomy or other surgery include menopausal status, hormone replacement therapy, family history, added surgical morbidity, and patient preference. In 1989, Jacobs and Oram[5] surveyed 2,817 Fellows of the Royal College of Obstetricians and Gynecologists in the United Kingdom. When asked their recommendations about oophorectomy at hysterectomy, less than 1% advocated it in women under age 40, whereas 85% recommended this approach for those who were postmenopausal. Since most gynecologists recommend oophorectomy to postmenopausal women undergoing hysterectomy, it is controversial whether to recommend a concurrent oophorectomy during surgery for women aged 40 to menopause. The issue is whether the risks and consequences of ovarian cancer are greater than the benefits of ovarian preservation. Schwartz,[1] surveyed gynecologic oncologists and found within this group that only 8.4% of them considered prophylactic oophorectomy was 95 to 100% protective. To answer this question, evidence that prophylactic oophorectomy prevents ovarian cancer in both the general population and in those with a family history of ovarian cancer is reviewed.

Evidence that prophylactic oophorectomy protects against ovarian cancer in the general population

Three papers and one abstract have been published since 1985 that evaluate this question by determining the number of women with ovarian cancer who previously had a hysterectomy. Sightler et al[2] found that 12.6% of women presenting with ovarian cancer previously had a hysterectomy, 7.9% of whom had undergone surgery after age 40. In reviewing 291 cases of ovarian cancer, McGowan[20] found that 14.1% had had a previous hysterectomy, whereas Jacobs and Oram[21] found the rate in the United Kingdom to be 6.9% for women undergoing hysterectomy but 9.1% for any pelvic surgery. Fung Kee Fung[22] noted that 11.4% of women presenting with ovarian cancer had had previous pelvic surgery over age 40 and that an additional 15.6% had had upper abdominal surgery for a combined rate of 27%. On the basis their studies, these investigators[2,20–22] propose that concurrent oophorectomy during hysterectomy in women over age 40 could lead to a reduction in the incidence of ovarian cancer.

Howe[23] took a different approach in evaluating whether prophylactic oophorectomy lowered incidence rates for ovarian cancer. Using a mailed questionnaire, she established oophorectomy rates for each 5-year age group from 25 to 74. Age-specific incidence rates for ovarian cancer were taken from the New York State Cancer Registry and she calculated the incidence rates for ovarian cancer after excluding those who had previously undergone bilateral oophorectomy. Howe[23] found that the overall incidence rate for ovarian cancer increased by 12% when only women with at least one intact ovary were considered. The combined data from the case series[2,20–22] and Howe,[23] suggest that there are opportunities to offer prophylactic oophorectomy to women over age 40 and, if performed, the incidence of ovarian cancer may decrease. Although suggestive of a benefit from prophylactic oophorectomy, these studies do not consider all the important issues, such as added surgical risk, effects of castration, long-term hormone replacement therapy, or risk of postoophorectomized carcinomatosis.

Evidence that prophylactic oophorectomy protects against ovarian cancer in those with a familial cancer risk

Struewing et al[24] reviewed 12 families ascertained at the National Cancer Institute (NCI) between 1969 and 1980. Each family had a minimum of three cancers (at least two ovarian) diagnosed before age 50. These families are considered at high risk of carrying a BRCA1 gene mutation. Cancer rates were calculated for unaffected first- and second-degree relatives at inception and compared to incidence rate data from the Connecticut Cancer Registry. Struewing et al[24] found a 24-fold excess rate of ovarian and a 7-fold excess rate of breast cancer in nonoophorectomized women compared to the general population. When Struewing (personal communication) combined his families with those from Creighton University, he compared the rate of ovarian carcinoma in nonoophorectomized women to the rate of peritoneal carcinomatosis for women whose ovaries had been removed. For first-degree nonoophorectomized relatives, the rate of ovarian cancer in this high-risk group was 20.3 times greater than that in the general population. Women who had undergone oophorectomy had an 8.4-fold increased risk of peritoneal carcinomatosis, compared to the general population. Oophorectomized women had a relative risk (RR) of 0.44 (95% confidence interval [CI] 0.1, 1.3) of developing peritoneal carcinomatosis compared to nonoophorectomized women who developed ovarian cancer. This is an important piece of direct evidence suggesting a benefit for oophorectomy in prevention of ovarian cancer. This benefit is not absolute, and in some women, postoophorectomy carcinomatosis will develop.

What is the risk of postoophorectomy carcinomatosis?

Despite evidence that prophylactic oophorectomy is protective against ovarian cancer, it is not 100% effective. Tobacman et al.[25] found that 3 of 28 (10.7%) women from 16 different high-risk families ascertained by NCI developed postoophorectomy carcinomatosis that was indistinguishable histologically from ovarian cancer. Struewing and colleagues'[26] update of 12 of the 16 NCI families in 1994 detected a peritoneal carcinomatosis rate of 4.6% in women who had undergone prophylactic oophorectomy. Piver et al[27] reported that 6 of 324 (1.8%) women developed peritoneal carcinomatosis 1 to 27 years after prophylactic oophorectomy. These case report calculations are low, however, because they evaluated all at-risk family members as being at equal risk, when only one-half of them will be BRCA1 mutation carriers. Consequently, the rate of posthysterectomy carcinomatosis is probably higher than stated in these papers. Even with a postoophorectomy rate as high as 10%, there still is a potential preventive benefit from prophylactic oophorectomy.

Role of prophylactic oophorectomy at hysterectomy

With data supporting a cancer prevention benefit, the role of prophylactic oophorectomy will be reviewed for women undergoing a hysterectomy for a noncancer indication. Most gynecologists do not recommend a concurrent oophorectomy at hysterectomy before age 40 because they believe the benefits of normal ovarian function outweigh the benefits of oophorectomy. These benefits include protection against both cardiovascular disease and osteoporosis, in addition to maintenance of secondary sexual characteristics. The risk-benefit analysis must also be balanced by the risks attributable to exogenous hormones related to the development of breast cancer. Whether real or not, there is a strong public perception in our patient community that hormone replacement therapy increases risk of breast cancer, and this risk weighs heavily in the decisions made by our patients. As a result of these factors, the recommended age for prophylactic oophorectomy during hysterectomy has changed in our community from age 40 years, 15 years ago, to age 50 years, and some gynecologists recommend waiting until menopause.

In women with a strong family history of ovarian or breast cancer, or both, when undergoing hysterectomy or other pelvic surgery, prophylactic oophorectomy should be considered. The potential benefit in this population is high, and there is no justification for missing an opportunity that will reduce risk. The issue regarding at what age to offer prophylactic oophorectomy is difficult, but it would be reasonable for any women over age 35 who has completed her family and has a proven familial autosomal dominant pattern of inheritance for breast/ovarian cancer to consider prophylactic oophorectomy. The ideal situation would be for that woman to undergo BRCA1 or BRCA2 testing before making that decision. Testing an individual with no known mutation in her family may be unreliable if negative. However, if there is a known mutation in the family, either a positive or negative test would be reliable and the result would help the women make a decision regarding the impending surgery.

Prophylactic oophorectomy in women undergoing nongynecologic surgery

Surgery in this category includes cholecystectomy, hernia repair, appendectomy, genitourinary surgery, and vascular surgery. A significant proportion of this surgery is now undertaken laparoscopically, and it is unlikely that we would be able to convince our surgical colleagues, nor would it be appropriate to perform an oophorectomy in women with no significant risk factors for ovarian cancer.

In the situation in which nongynecologic abdominal surgery is being undertaken in known BRCA1 or BRCA2 mutation positive women whose lifetime risk of ovarian cancer is 44 to 56%,[18,19] prophylactic oophorectomy should be offered and recommended. For women in whom genetic testing is not possible who have either an autosomal dominant pattern of inheritance in their family or two first-degree relatives with ovarian cancer, prophylactic oophorectomy should be considered as well.

In summary, prophylactic oophorectomy in women over age 40 is unlikely to gain widespread acceptance among either gynecologists or general surgeons because the overall benefit in the general population is small. In those with a strong family history, or who are BRCA1 or BRCA2 mutation positive, the likelihood of benefit is greater, and therefore probably more acceptable, to both surgeons and patients. It becomes our responsibility to educate both patients and physicians of this potential benefit, so that an opportunity to prevent ovarian cancer is not missed.

QUESTION 2

Should prophylactic oophorectomy be recommended to women with 2 or more first-degree relatives with epithelial ovarian cancer?

M. STEVEN PIVER

In 1979, and again in 1982, the Department of Gynecologic Oncology at Roswell Park Cancer Institute, Buffalo, New York, separately reported two extended families seen within a 2-year span, each with five members with epithelial ovarian cancer.[28,29] A review of the literature revealed only five reports of familial ovarian cancer between 1929 and 1969, but an additional 26 cases between 1970 and 1979. Because of this apparent increase in frequency, a Registry was formed in 1981 for further evaluation of familial ovarian cancer syndrome. This Registry, renamed the Gilda Radner Familial Ovarian Cancer Registry in 1989, in memory of the late comedienne, has accessioned through 1994 more than 1,000 families comprising more than 2,425 cases of ovarian cancer (Fig. 2-1). All families in the Registry have two or more first- or second-degree relatives with ovarian cancer, and 40% have three or more first-degree relatives. There are 400 cases of breast cancer in the Registry, including 78 patients with both breast and ovarian cancer. The demographics of the women in the Registry have most recently been reported in 1996,[30] it is hoped that this information will be useful in the prospective evaluation of interventions such as early detection and prophylactic oophorectomy.

The definition of familial ovarian cancer syndrome has never been clearly established. The estimated lifetime risk of any woman developing ovarian cancer is 1.8%, or 1 in 55.[31] Therefore, the chance of any two women developing ovarian cancer is 0.018^2 or 1 in 3,086. The Gilda Radner Familial Ovarian Cancer Registry always required two or more first- or second-degree relatives with ovarian cancer for inclusion into the Registry. The National Institutes of Health (NIH) consensus conference on ovarian cancer stated that "less than 0.05% of women are at a significantly increased risk because of three heredi-

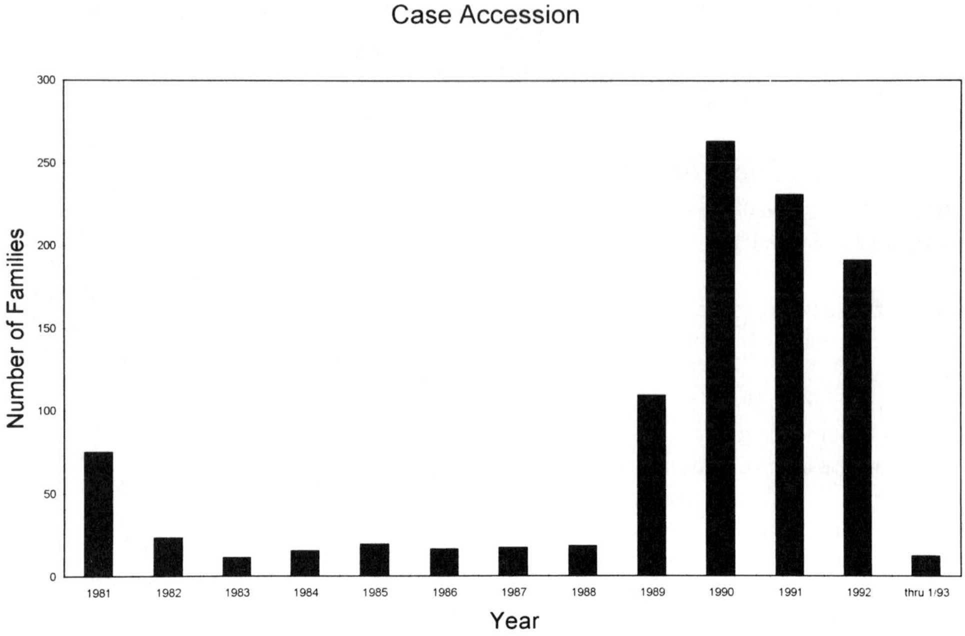

FIGURE 2-1. Number of cases accessioned into the Gilda Radner Familial Ovarian Cancer Registry by year. (From Piver,[30] with permission.)

tary ovarian cancer syndromes: breast/ovarian cancer syndrome, site-specific ovarian cancer syndrome, and hereditary non-polyposis colorectal cancer (Lynch Syndrome II), which includes early onset non-polyposis colorectal cancer, endometrial cancer, cancer of the gastrointestinal system (including biliary ducts, pancreas and possible small bowel), urothelial carcinomas of the renal pelvis and ureter and ovarian cancer."[32] The NIH consensus does not define breast/ovarian cancer syndrome or site-specific ovarian cancer, and to date there is no uniform agreement on the definition of either of these syndromes in the scientific community. Because of the lack of agreement on definitions of these syndromes, the practicing physician lacks guidelines as to who is a candidate for prophylactic oophorectomy. According to the Breast Cancer Linkage Consortium "families with three or more cases of ovarian cancer is generally considered to be examples of hereditary ovarian cancer.

Families with a total of five or more breast or ovarian cancers in first- or second-degree relatives qualifies having hereditary breast/ovarian cancer syndrome."[33] The confusion is highlighted in a recent report by Narod et al,[34] who stated that "our distinction between hereditary and familial ovarian cancer is arbitrary. We have included families with three ovarian cancers or five or more cases of ovarian or breast cancer in the hereditary group; the number was chosen because it is unlikely that this many cancers could arise by chance and because it has been estimated that 100% of all families would satisfy these criteria have been linked to BRCA1. Clearly, a proportion of smaller families may be hereditary, but there may be too few carrier females in the family for a cluster to be identified, or the proband may be unaware of the diagnosis in relatives." The reality of the latter is exemplified in the 1993 letter to the Registry.

Thank you for your letter of kindness and information and for registering me with the Gilda Radner Familial Ovarian Cancer Registry (because of my own history of ovarian cancer). I'm so very pleased that there is such an organization for this type of cancer. I want to express some thoughts that I feel important to other women who may be in the same situation that I am in with my family history. My mother's family came from Czechoslovakia in the 1800s, they were a farming family, and records of births and deaths are rare from that time up until maybe 50 years ago. I just want to stress that I do not know if my family has a history of cancer. Most died on their farms and no autopsies were done at that time. Many believe that family members just died of whatever was going around at that time or of natural causes. I believe that there were some members who did die of certain cancers, but no one remaining in my mother's family knows. I hope you consider these facts and not think of excluding women who have a family history such as mine.

As our understanding of the molecular genetics involved in hereditary ovarian cancer has evolved, it has become more apparent that site-specific and breast-ovarian cancer syndromes may actually be phenotypic variations of the same genetic abnormality. Expanding on earlier epidemiologic data, Hall et al[35] reported the first convincing evidence for localization of a breast cancer gene on chromosome 17q by linkage analysis. Narod et al[36] subsequently presented confirmation of linkage to chromosome 17q in five families with breast and ovarian cancer. This was designated the BRCA1 gene by Solomon and Ledbetter.[37] In a more recent study that included members of the Gilda Radner Familial Ovarian Cancer Registry, an analysis of 132 breast/ovarian cancer families with no breast cancer in males demonstrated that an estimated 88% of the families were linked (95% confidence interval [CI] = 74–95%) to the BRCA1 gene.[38] Of the 81 families in which there were two or more cases of breast cancer below the age of 60 and two or more cases of ovarian cancer, 92% of the 81 families were linked to the BRCA1 gene (95% CI = 76–100%). These latter 81 families would clearly fit a definition of a hereditary breast/ovarian cancer syndrome. In a subsequent study in which members of the Gilda Radner Familial Ovarian Cancer Registry participated, which included only families with three or more cases of ovarian cancer and no breast cancer below the age of 50 years, 78% (7 of 9) were linked to the BRCA1 gene.[39] These families with three or more cases of ovarian cancer and no breast cancer below the age of 50 would fall under the category of site-specific ovarian cancer. Regrettably, the BRCA1 linkage analysis on families with only two or more first degree relatives is not available. Therefore, at this point, to exclude these women as not being in the site-specific ovarian cancer category by "an arbitrary definition" would prejudice them from the availability of prophylactic oophorectomy and the prevention of epithelial ovarian cancer.

Concerning the recommendations for prophylactic oophorectomy in women with Lynch Syndrome II, the data are even less clear. Although Watson and Lynch in studying 23 hereditary nonpolyposis colon carcinoma families estimate the risk of ovarian cancer to be increased four fold greater than the general population, we were only able to find a total of 33 women in the world literature with ovarian cancer who also were part of hereditary nonpolyposis colon cancer kindreds.[40–45] Moreover, the data show that the ovarian cancer risk differed among families. Finally, an estimate that hereditary nonpolyposis colon carcinoma syndrome accounts for only 1% or less of colorectal cancer makes the number of women eligible for prophylactic oophorectomy in this syndrome exceedingly rare.[46]

Based on the above discussion, the Gilda Radner Familial Ovarian Cancer Registry recommends that women with a family history of epithelial ovarian cancer in two or more first- or first- and second-degree relatives undergo prophylactic oophorectomy as soon as childbearing is completed and preferably before age 35. These same criteria would be applicable to women with breast/ovarian cancer syndrome when there are at least two cases of epithelial ovarian cancer as well as breast cancer.

BARRY ROSEN

The decision of when to offer a woman prophylactic surgery is not black and white. Prior to the discovery of the BRCA1 and BRCA2 genes, clinical management decisions were based on family history and when available, linkage analyses performed by a research laboratory. Evidence supporting the use of family history to make surgical treatment decisions includes Schildkraut's and Thompson's[47] analysis of the cancer and steroid hormone study, and Parazzini and colleagues'[48] case-control study. These investigators assessed the degree of aggregation of ovarian cancer in families, and Schildkraut and Thompson[47] found a 3.6-fold increased susceptibility to develop ovarian cancer if a women had a first-degree relative affected with ovarian cancer whereas Parazzini et al[48] found only a 1.9-fold increase in risk. In the OPSC study, Ponder et al[49] evaluated the cause of death in first-degree relatives of women who had previously died from ovarian cancer. Ponder's group found an increased rate of death from ovarian cancer in first-degree degree relatives, as compared to the general population. The risk in the general population was approximately 1 in 100, whereas the risk in a first-degree relative increased to 1 in 40. Even though the numbers were small, the risk when two first-degree relatives were affected increased dramatically to 1 in 3. This risk of ovarian cancer is exceedingly high and, as a result, it was a logical next step for clinicians to recommend prophylactic oophorectomy in women with two first-degree relatives affected with ovarian cancer. An unaffected woman with two to three relatives with ovarian cancer had a 4.6 times (95% CI = 1.1, 18.4) increased risk compared to the general population risk.[50] This translates into a 7.2% lifetime probability of developing ovarian cancer for a 35-year-old woman.[50] For those with hereditary ovarian cancer who are BRCA1 positive, the lifetime risk climbs to a range of 44%[18] to 56%.[19] For women with more than two relatives affected with ovarian cancer, Kerlikowske et al[50] consider prophylactic oophorectomy reasonable because a small percentage of will be BRCA1 positive, and their risk of cancer is very high. Kerlikowske and colleagues thought the benefit of surgery for women with this hereditary pattern outweighed the surgical risks and future morbidity associated with surgical menopause and hormone therapy. Based on ovarian cancer incidence data, these investigators believed that surgery could be delayed until the woman was in her 40s. Piver[51] recommended that women with a family history of ovarian cancer who have completed childbearing undergo a prophylactic oophorectomy by age 35. Piver's age recommendation is lower than that recommended by Kerlikowske and colleagues[50] because he believes that these cancers occur at younger ages than in the general population.

Using family history as the only criterion on which to make management decisions was acceptable until specific genetic testing became available. Not all families with a history of ovarian cancer will be BRCA1 or BRCA2 carriers and, in those mutation-positive families, on average, only one-half of at-risk women will be carriers. Therefore, within these families some women will have an ovarian cancer risk as high as 44%[18] to 56%,[19] whereas the non-BRCA1 or BRCA2 carriers lifetime risk will be less than the 1.4% risk figure used for the general population. In the past, when family history was the only information available, it was acceptable to offer all women from high-risk families the option of surgery, realizing that one-half of these women would undergo the surgery unnecessarily because they would be BRCA mutation negative. Since the discovery of the BRCA1 gene in 1994, testing has become possible, especially for the well-known gene mutations. Once a mutation is identified in a family, the other at-risk members can now be tested reliably and decisions regarding prophylactic surgery can be made after test results. Testing therefore provides us with the opportunity to offer prophylactic surgery only to those women who are BRCA1 positive and to avoid surgery in women who test negative. Outcome analyses in this group will allow us to establish whether prophylactic oophorectomy is beneficial.

Genetic testing has not yet become widely accepted, one reason being that the accuracy of testing negative with no known mutation in the family is not yet fully established. There are a number of reasons why a test may be negative: (1) there may not be a mutation present, (2) the individual being assessed could be a sporadic case not familial, (3) the technique used to do the test for the mutation may not be sensitive enough,[52,53] and (4) the mutation may be outside the coding regions. Consequently, a negative test when there is no known family mutation is not in any way an absolute guarantee that no mutation exists. In addition, others claim that social, ethical, legal, and psychological issues are not yet fully understood and consequently it is suggested that genetic testing for cancer may be premature at this time.[55]

There will also be a percentage of the population in which it is not possible to identify a mutation but in which there is a significant family history that places family members at high risk of both ovarian and breast cancer. Reasons for being unable to test individuals include those having a small family, those with no living affected relatives, and those who have no access to testing in their community. In these situations, family history continues to play a major role in determining management.

Shattuck-Eidens et al[53] evaluated the risk of BRCA1 carrier status based on family history and age of affected relatives. She found that when two sisters were affected with ovarian cancer under age 50, the probability of the family having a BRCA1 mutation was 61%. In families in which there were two or more breast cancers, as well as two or more ovarian cancers, the probability rose to 91%. Similar data related to breast cancer were published by Claus et al.[56] She found a woman's lifetime risk of breast cancer with one or two first-degree relatives affected by ovarian cancer to be 13% and 31%, respectively. In women who have one first-degree relative with ovarian cancer at any age and one first-degree relative with breast cancer diagnosed under age 40, the estimated lifetime risk of breast cancer is 40%. Publications by Claus et al[56] and Shattuck-Eidens et al[53] support the consensus that women with two first-degree relatives with ovarian or breast cancer, or both, have a high likelihood of belonging to a family that carries a BRCA1 mutation. Consequently, when testing is not possible, we should offer the same medical advice and care to at-risk women in these families as we do to those who are gene positive. We need to realize, however, that when recommending prophylactic oophorectomy to all at-risk women based only on their family history, only one-half will be BRCA mutation positive and only 44 to 56% of these will develop ovarian cancer.[18,19]

In the familial Ovarian Cancer Clinic at The Toronto Hospital, 850-plus women from more then 450 families have been evaluated over the past 5 years. It has been unusual for a proband to present who has two first-degree relatives affected by ovarian cancer. More commonly, women present from families in which several affected women with breast or ovarian cancer are spread throughout the pedigree. Risk evaluation is not always straightforward and to evaluate the family adequately, the overall familial inheritance pattern should be assessed before management is recommended.

At our clinic, family assessment is based on the overall pattern of breast, ovarian, and other cancers. To make an accurate assessment, we obtain as much of the pedigree information as possible by extending it out to include uncles, aunts, cousins, and grandparents, and when possible even more distant family branches. The next step is to confirm the pathology of affected relatives. There have been situations in which a presumed diagnosis of ovarian cancer was, in fact, a bowel or pancreatic cancer. In addition, it is possible that there is confusion about previous gynecologic surgery and a misinterpretation of a benign cyst for a malignancy.[50] Although very important, pathology confirmation is labor intensive and not always successful, especially when affected relatives are from different parts of the world or when they were affected 20 plus years ago. The local cancer registry in our province has been an excellent source of confirmatory data in some of these families.

Once all the information is collected and confirmed, we assess the family's risk of BRCA1 or BRCA2 carrier status. In high-risk families that demonstrate an autosomal dominant pattern of inheritance, not all at-risk women will have two first-degree relatives affected. Consequently, even though two first-degree relatives affected with ovarian cancer is highly predictive of a positive BRCA1 mutation carrier status, this specific situation is uncommon and does not predict for the vast majority of at-risk women. Completion of a detailed pedigree is the most reliable method to assess risk of BRCA1 or BRCA2 status and confirmation of pathology is necessary because it can have a dramatic effect on risk assessment.

The question of what age to recommend prophylactic oophorectomy has not yet been answered. There are data[19] now suggesting that BRCA1-positive women develop ovarian cancer at an earlier age than do those in the general population. It is therefore necessary to recommend prophylactic surgery early enough so as not to miss a cancer, but at the same time not so early that it will affect childbearing or needlessly extend the exposure to hormone replacement therapy. Narod et al[19] recently published a study of 333 North American women found by haplotype analysis to carry BRCA1 mutations. These investigators found the incidence of ovarian cancer to be highest at ages 51 to 55, and it was uncommon for ovarian cancer to be diagnosed before age 40. The cumulative incidence for ovarian cancer before age 50 was only 19.5%, whereas for breast cancer before age 50 it was 52.2%.[19] This new information is helpful because it will guide recommendations regarding the age at which women should be offered prophylactic oophorectomy. In the past, based solely on family history, prophylactic oophorectomy was recommended at age 35.[51] At our clinic, prophylactic surgery is recommended 5 to 10 years earlier in age than their closest affected relative was diagnosed, but we realize this is based on circumstantial data. On average this will be when the woman is in her early 40s. The decision to proceed with surgery will ultimately depend on the woman's wishes and their perception of long-term hormone replacement.

It is also critically important that we address the need for breast cancer screening and discuss the option of prophylactic mastectomy in gene-positive women, since their lifetime risk of breast cancer is greater than that of ovarian.[19] In terms of family history, Narod et al[34] conducted a population-based study in which they found a positive family history in 71 of 450 unselected ovarian cancer cases, with 80% reporting a family history of breast cancer. Fitzgerald et al[57] found a 27-fold increased risk of early-onset breast cancer among Askenazi Jewish women with a 185delAG mutation. All these factors support the need for us to promote breast cancer screening in this population who may initially enter the medical system because of their risk of ovarian cancer. The risk of breast cancer begins at a younger age than the risk of ovarian cancer.[57]

Our current approach is to recommend prophylactic oophorectomy in gene-positive women only. We acknowledge that other at-risk women may wish to have surgery, and we will honor that request when the patient's anxiety is affecting her quality of life. For others, in whom gene testing is not yet available, we recommend screening in the short term until such time as testing may be possible. We believe that these high-risk women are at increased risk, but that increased risk over the next 1 to 2 years is probably very small, taking into account their age and the age of their affected relatives.

In summary, we have found few women at our clinic who present with two first-degree relatives affected by ovarian cancer. Instead, it is more common to have one first-degree degree relative with ovarian cancer and other relatives with either ovarian or breast cancer. We have developed a policy of recommending prophylactic oophorectomy only to gene-positive women. We expect testing to become more readily available and reliable in the near future, subsequently, we recommend that women who cannot be tested now undergo screening every 6 months with transvaginal ultrasound and CA 125. We feel that the risk of the development of ovarian cancer in the short term while waiting for genetic testing is probably less than the risk involved in undergoing an unnecessary surgery. In our 5 years, experience with the Familial Ovarian Cancer Clinic at The Toronto Hospital, only one woman has developed an ovarian cancer, detected at stage 1 on an interval screen, and four women have developed breast cancer. These cases demonstrate that it is imperative that our approach involve breast cancer screening as well as consideration of prophylactic mastectomy in appropriate situations.

QUESTION 3

Should prophylactic oophorectomy be recommended to women with one first-degree relative with epithelial ovarian cancer?

M. STEVEN PIVER

Women with one first- or second-degree relative with ovarian cancer appear to be at a modest increased risk of ovarian cancer. Schildkraut and Thompson[47] studied 493 cases of ovarian cancer and compared them to 2,465 matched controls. The relative risk (RR) of ovarian cancer was 3.6 for any first-degree relative, resulting in a lifetime risk of 6.5% (3.6 × 1.8%). This increased to a relative risk of 4.3 if that first-degree relative was a mother, resulting in a lifetime risk of 7.5%. This 7.5% lifetime risk for this subset of women with only one first-degree relative with ovarian cancer begins to approach the 10% lifetime risk of breast cancer, a significant risk of a disease that, unlike breast cancer, has no highly effective and practical screening method.

I do not consider routine prophylactic oophorectomy justified in this entire group. However, because this group likely harbors some BRCA1 gene defect carriers, I do recommend that they be followed every 6 months with a pelvic examination, transvaginal ultrasound, and CA 125 level. Bourne et al[58] have reported good results using transvaginal ultrasound in a similar population. A group of 1,601 women with at least one first- or second-degree relative with ovarian cancer were screened using transvaginal ultrasound. Sixty-one (3.8%) of these women were found to have abnormal ovarian morphology and were evaluated surgically. Six were found to have malignancies (although three were low malignant potential tumors), and five of the six were FIGO stage IA tumors. Four of the six women had pedigrees strongly suggestive of hereditary ovarian cancer syndrome, whereas two of the six did not appear to have a clear pattern of inheritance. Five of the six women were premenopausal, with ages ranging from 30 to 54 years. If only patients with complex ovarian masses were surgically evaluated, the number of false-positives would have dropped from 55 to 33, while sensitivity would have remained at 100%. Therefore, I believe that routine screening with transvaginal ultrasound in a population at slightly increased risk of ovarian cancer has the potential to diagnose early-stage disease, with higher expected cure rates, while holding the false-positive rate and screening-related morbidity to an acceptable minimum.

One possible exception in the management of women with one family member with ovarian cancer is the patient with a first-degree relative in whom ovarian cancer developed at a young age. Houlston et al[59] studied 391 ovarian cancer family pedigrees by complex segregation analysis evaluating the observed number of ovarian cancer cases, as compared with an expected number of ovarian cancer cases in England and Wales during that same time period. If her mother developed ovarian cancer before age 45, a patient's RR was 14.2, resulting in a lifetime risk of 26% (14.2 × 1.8%). This decreased to a lifetime risk of 9% (RR = 5.2) if the first-degree relative developed ovarian cancer at age 45 to 54 and to approximately 7% (RR = 3.7) if ovarian cancer developed after age 55. For all 391 pedigrees, the relative risk was 4.5, yielding a lifetime risk of 8%, not dissimilar to that reported by Schildkraut and Thompson in their case-control study.[47] Confirmation of Houlston and colleagues' data on one first-degree relative with ovarian cancer developed prior to age 45 could dramatically change those eligible for prophylactic oophorectomy with only one first-degree relative. These results suggest that women who carry a BRCA1 abnormality may develop malignancy at a younger age than is seen in the general population, a finding reported in the Gilda Radner Familial Ovarian Cancer Registry.[30] However, such findings must be interpreted with caution, particularly when used to justify prophylactic oophorectomy in women with only one first-degree relative with ovarian cancer. These data are based on self-reported cases, rather than on a broad, population-based study. In fact, using data from the CASH study, Amos et al[60] reported no significant difference in age at onset of ovarian cancer in women with or without one first-degree relative with ovarian cancer. Therefore, prophylactic oophorectomy should only be undertaken in a woman with a single first-degree relative diagnosed with ovarian cancer before age 45, when there are other considerations, such as cancer phobia, concomitant surgery for other indications, or additional risk factors.

BARRY ROSEN

It is important to approach these women in a similar way to those with two first-degree relatives by first constructing an extended pedigree followed by pathology confirmation. When only one woman from a family is affected with ovarian cancer and there are no breast cancers, it is unlikely that she will carry a BRCA1 gene mutation.[49–52] In our clinical setting this family would be classified as low risk. Kerlikowske et al[50] pooled odds ratios for five case-control studies with a family history of one first-degree relative with ovarian cancer. The pooled OR of 3.1 (95% CI-2.1–4.5) predicts a 5% lifetime risk of ovarian cancer. For this group, Kerlikowske et al[50] did not recommend prophylactic oophorectomy.

Fitzgerald et al[57] reported on eight Askenazi Jewish women with a 185delAG mutation and found germline mutations in some who did not belong to families with multiple affected relatives. Langston et al[61] recently reported six BRCA1 mutations from 80 women with early-onset breast cancer. Two of the six women reported no family history of either breast or ovarian cancer, confusing the situation, because it demonstrates that we may not be able to identify all at-risk women based on their family history. Even though the risk of being a BRCA1 carrier with one affected first-degree relative is lower than among women with multiple affected relatives, there will be BRCA1 mutation positive women from low-risk families.[57] In addition, when families with one first-degree relative are evaluated, the initial assessment may not be final. For example, if one other close relative were to subsequently develop breast or ovarian cancer, our risk assessment would change, especially if that relative was less than 45 years old. Consequently, patients are advised to notify our clinic of any changes within the family.

In the future, as specific BRCA1 and BRCA2 mutations become linked to certain cultural and ethnic groups, it may be possible to test women in in low-risk situations (i.e., those with one first-degree affected relative). For example, an Askenazi Jewish woman with one first-degree relative affected with ovarian cancer could reliably be tested for three BRCA1 and one BRCA2 mutations. In this situation, it is unknown exactly how informative a negative test will be, but it will most likely convey a significant degree of risk reduction. Prophylactic surgery could then be recommended to those with a gene mutation.

In summary, it does not appear that the risk associated with one first-degree relative is more than 5% and subsequently it is not recommended to offer prophylactic oophorectomy in this situation. In the future, however, it may be possible to provide some of these women with a simple, inexpensive, and reliable genetic test if they are from an ethnic or cultural group in which specific mutations have been previously identified.

QUESTION 4

What are the surgical options for prophylactic oophorectomy, and what is your recommended method? Should hysterectomy also be performed routinely?

M. STEVEN PIVER

The preferred method of prophylactic oophorectomy is laparoscopic salpingo-oophorectomy. In experienced hands, this technique can be accomplished rapidly, with very little morbidity, and on an outpatient basis.[62] Because early-stage ovarian cancer and primary peritoneal malignancy have been reported in patients undergoing prophylactic oophorectomy for a family history of ovarian cancer[27] pelvic washings should be obtained at laparoscopy to rule out occult metastatic disease, after which a thorough visual survey of the peritoneal cavity should be conducted. The ovaries should be serially sectioned to look for the presence of early malignancy. While such disease may not require adjuvant therapy or any change in recommended surveillance, it is important that patients at risk of hereditary ovarian cancer be properly classified, so that all family members may be given the best possible counseling.

When laparoscopic salpingo-oophorectomy is contraindicated due to severe pelvic adhesive disease or other reasons, the risk of ovarian cancer must be weighed against the cost, inconvenience, and possible increase in morbidity of laparotomy. In patients who have first- or second-degree relatives with hereditary ovarian cancer syndrome, laparotomy, if required, is clearly justified. For patients at less risk, the decision must be individualized.

Some women may request concomitant hysterectomy at oophorectomy, either to remove any risk of endometrial cancer, to obviate the need for progestational agents accompanying estrogen replacement therapy, to end menstrual discomfort or irregularities, or other reasons. Routine hysterectomy has been advocated in the past.[63] However, the addition of even a vaginal hysterectomy to prophylactic oophorectomy adds operating time, convalescence, slight additional morbidity and considerable expense to the procedure. Abdominal hysterectomy and bilateral salpingo-oophorectomy add these disadvantages to an even greater extent. The potential benefits to be gained from routine hysterectomy are questionable. Endometrial cancer nearly always presents with bleeding while still confined to the uterus and highly curable. Combination estrogen and progesterone therapy is usually well tolerated and, if not, can be substituted with unopposed estrogen and annual endometrial sampling. Dysmenorrhea and menometrorrhaghia can often be managed pharmacologically until menopause. In my view, hysterectomy, either vaginally or abdominally, should only be undertaken if specific indications would justify the procedure in the absence of the need for prophylactic oophorectomy.

BARRY ROSEN

Once the decision to provide prophylactic surgery has been made, the decisions regarding the type of surgery and method are dependent on both your patient's past surgical and medical history in addition to your own skills. Since the primary objective of surgery is to remove the ovaries, the technique you choose must be able to satisfy that requirement. To accomplish this, you need to be certain to remove the entire ovary. To do this, you need to place your clamp across the infundibulopelvic ligament above the ovary, which requires identification of the ureter. If the ovary is adherent to the pelvic side wall, you will need to dissect it free and be certain not to leave any remnant of ovarian tissue behind. This will require identification, and possibly dissection of the ureter.

In recent years, laparoscopic surgery has become acceptable and very safe. It is often the preferred choice of patients and can be recommended for prophylactic oophorectomy, provided the surgeon is capable of removing the entire ovary. A limited surgical staging is recommended because, even though it is rare, microscopic foci of ovarian cancer can be found. Surgical staging at oophorectomy could avoid a second staging surgery.

The written recommendations regarding prophylactic oophorectomy are unclear with respect to whether a concurrent hysterectomy should also be performed. In a review of five papers,[21,27,64–66] only Piver et al[27] make a specific recommendation that only an oophorectomy is necessary. They also recommend cytologic washings and complete evaluation of the abdominal and pelvic peritoneum by visualization, through the laparoscope. These workers then recommend combination hormone replacement therapy consisting of estrogen and progesterone. Since their publication and most others on this subject, the BRCA1 and BRCA2 genes have been cloned. Simard et al[67] subsequently reported in their family number 279, that there was a woman with a fallopian tube cancer who had a 5,382 insC BRCA1 mutation. Others have similarly reported BRCA1 mutations found in women with fallopian tube cancer (Narod SA: personal communication.) This is relevant because when doing an oophorectomy without a concurrent hysterectomy, it is impossible to remove all the tubal epithelium. If the association between fallopian tube cancer and BRCA1 status is real,[68] concurrent hysterectomy with oophorectomy may provide further benefit. Since the epithelium of the fallopian tube has the same embrylogic origin as the surface epithelium of the ovary, it is also plausible that it could be the source of malignant change as the result of a BRCA1 or BRCA2 mutation.

Most gynecologists would recommend combination hormone replacement therapy following bilateral oophorectomy, especially in a 35 to 45- year-old woman. The benefits with respect to osteoporosis and cardiovascular disease are well known. The addition of progesterone to estrogen protects against development of endometrial carcinoma.[69] However, recent publications suggest adding progesterone to estrogen also increases the risk of breast cancer over use of estrogen alone.[70,71] Another recent publication suggests no increased risk associated with combined therapy.[72] This controversy has reached the lay press, making many women aware of a potential risk of breast cancer in association with hormone replacement therapy. Unfortunately, the lay press does not always present a balanced view of this subject, and patients who have personally witnessed the effects of breast cancer in a close relative may not be willing to accept any increased breast cancer risk despite hormone replacement benefits. These women may therefore have established biases against hormone replacement therapy before you have had a chance to provide your perspective. This is important because you will need to be prepared to have a full discussion about hormone replacement therapy before proceding with a prophylactic oophorectomy.

Progesterone has also been reported to have a negative effect on the cardiovascular benefit of estrogen replacement therapy by neutralizing the effect on high-density lipoproteins.[73] The new micronized progesterone may negate this detrimental effect somewhat, but the most advantageous therapy for increasing high-density lipoproteins in The Pepi Trial was use of estrogen alone.[73] Furthermore, the long-term studies on improved life expectancy from hormone replacement therapy are based on estrogen therapy alone, and not on estrogen-progesterone combined therapy.[74–76] In general, hormone replacement therapy is an extremely important issue when considering prophylactic oophorectomy. Women need to become very well informed on this subject, as their beliefs will affect their willingness to make use of the therapy. As a result, when doing a prophylactic oophorectomy, a concurrent hysterectomy will probably be beneficial because the women will only need to use estrogen replacement, and the benefits to her cardiovascular system and life expectancy will be maximized.

Another factor to consider when deciding to leave the uterus in situ is the lifetime risk of uterine cancer. When placed on both estrogen and progestin therapy the risk is less than the general population.[69] However, Jishi et al[77] reviewed 143 families from the Gilda Radner Familial Ovarian Cancer Registry in whom there were three or more reported cases of ovarian cancer. These investigators compared the rate of uterine cancer in this population to an expected rate in the Connecticut Cancer Registry and found a five fold increase over the general population. If the lifetime risk of uterine cancer in the general population is just over 2%, women in high-risk families are at increased risk of greater than 10% for the development of uterine cancer.

In summary, the method of surgical procedure is dependent on both the surgeon and the patient, and in my view laparoscopy-assisted surgery is acceptable. In terms of the procedure, a concurrent hysterectomy is indicated for three reasons: (1) removal of entire fallopian tube reduces the risk that cancer will develop in it,[67] (2) these women have an increased risk of uterine cancer,[77] and (3) hormone replacement therapy is simpler because only estrogen is needed, and its beneficial effects are well documented. Furthermore, by eliminating progesterone, it is possible to avoid the potential adverse effects on cardiovascular disease and breast cancer.

QUESTION 5

What should women be counseled about regarding the protective effects of prophylactic oophorectomy? What are the alternatives to prophylactic oophorectomy?

M. STEVEN PIVER

The only widely accepted measure for definitive prevention of ovarian cancer is prophylactic oophorectomy. Admittedly, a reduction in mortality has yet to be demonstrated in a clinical trial, and in fact primary peritoneal carcinoma has still been reported to occur following prophylactic oophorectomy in women with a family history of hereditary ovarian cancer syndrome. However, prophylactic oophorectomy remains the single best theoretical method for dramatically reducing the risk of premature death from hereditary ovarian cancer. In view of the lack of an acceptable test to detect early disease, and the poor results associated with standard treatment of metastatic disease, there are really no acceptable therapeutic alternatives to prophylactic oophorectomy.

However, in women at increased risk of ovarian cancer who are unwilling or unable to undergo prophylactic oophorectomy, modification of certain risk factors may be possible. Whether any such modification will be effective in reducing the risk of ovarian cancer in women who harbor a BRCA1 abnormality is unknown.

The benefits of oral contraceptive use in reducing the risk of ovarian cancer are well established, with prolonged use resulting in up to a 40 to 50% reduction in risk.[78–81] However, a protective effect in women with hereditary ovarian cancer has not been established. In Kerber's report from the Utah population database, increasing parity was highly protective in women without a strong family history of ovarian cancer, with an OR of 0.56 and 0.29 for the development of ovarian cancer in women with four to five children and women with six or more children, respectively.[82] However, increasing parity was not protective in women who had a strong family history of ovarian cancer. Although the mechanism of protection against ovarian cancer by oral contraceptives and increased parity is unknown, speculation centers on interruption of ovulation as being a possible common mechanism. If increasing parity does not confer a protective effect in women with a strong family history, oral contraceptive use may also not have any effect.

For reasons that are not well understood, tubal ligation appears to have a protective effect against ovarian cancer.[83,84] The use of fertility drugs has been reported to increase the risk of ovarian neoplasm among women who subsequently failed to conceive.[85,86] However, the number of reported cases of ovarian cancer after the use of fertility drugs is small, and the precise level of increased risk, if any, has not been firmly established. Pending further studies, women with infertility should be cautioned regarding possible increased risk of ovarian cancer, and women with a family history of ovarian cancer may wish to consider avoiding use of fertility drugs if possible. The use of talc, high dietary fat intake, and high consumption of galactose has been reported to be associated with an increased risk of ovarian cancer.[87–91] Women at increased risk of ovarian cancer may wish to pay particularly close attention to modifying these risk factors.

BARRY ROSEN

The main alternatives to surgery are screening, and prevention. The purpose of screening is to detect the cancer at a stage at which it is more likely curable. Chapter 1 presents the issues regarding screening. We caution the reader on two points regarding screening, which you may want to share with your at-risk patients: (1) screening has not yet proved effective in high-risk populations, and (2) screening, itself, is not without risk. The false-positive screen rate is significant[76,93] and consequently a certain percentage of women will undergo surgery, when in fact they do not have cancer. The morbidity and potential mortality in this false-positive group needs to be balanced against the benefit of screening. At our clinic, we include a short paragraph about the risks of screening in our consent form.

Prevention alternatives to prophylactic oophorectomy include use of oral contraceptives and dietary changes. Risch et al[15] studied the relationship between diet and ovarian cancer in a population-based case-control study. These workers found that saturated fat intake was associated with an increased risk of ovarian cancer. For every 10 of saturated fat consumed, the risk of ovarian cancer increased with an OR of 1.2 (95%Cl-1.03, 1.4)[15] By contrast, consumption of vegetable fiber was associated with a decreased risk (OR = 0.6 95%Cl 0.49, 0.8) for every 10 per day. Risch and colleagues[94] concluded that diet modifications may allow women to lower their ovarian cancer risk but cautioned the reader that their studies need to be confirmed by others. The same study showed a risk reduction with the use of the birth control pill, with an OR of 0.92 per year of use. This latter finding is consistent with other published studies.

Data on the protective effects of prophylactic oophorectomy were included in response to the first question. In summary, prophylactic oophorectomy is not 100% effective at eliminating a post oophorectomy carcinomatosis. Piver et al[27] described a 1.8% risk, and Struewing et al[26] a 4.6% risk of the development of a post oophorectomy peritoneal carcinomatosis. The estimates given by these investigators may be low. They included all at-risk women from families with a history of ovarian cancer in their denominator. Since not all at-risk women are BRCA1 carriers, Piver and Struewing and their colleagues have potentially underestimated the risk by 50%. Furthermore, even though they have chosen high-risk families to make their calculations, it is likely that not all these families are BRCA1 positive. Consequently, the real number of women who are BRCA1 positive in whom postoophorectomy carcinomatosis will develop is unknown, but it could be estimated to be 5 to 10%.

In summary, alternatives to prophylactic oophorectomy include lowering percentage of intake of dietary saturated fats, the use of oral contraceptives, and screening with ultrasound and CA 125. The postoophorectomy peritoneal carcinomatosis rate, which is not yet known for BRCA1 carriers, may be as high as 5 to 10%.

This chapter identified some of the controversial issues regarding prophylactic oophorectomy. There is evidence that prophylactic oophorectomy will protect against the development of ovarian cancer, and this evidence is strongest in the familial cancer group. Since the discovery of the BRCA1 and BRCA2 genes, the approach to prophylactic surgery should change from being offered to all at-risk women to only those who have a BRCA1 or BRCA2 gene mutation. In cases in which gene testing is not possible, family history will still be used to determine the need for surgery. The procedure recommended in this chapter includes a concurrent hysterectomy because of the risk of both fallopian tube and endometrial cancer and the possible negative effects of progesterone on the cardiovascular system and the risk of breast cancer risk. There is also evidence that dietary changes and the use of the birth control pill will provide some protection against the development of ovarian cancer.

EDITORS' COMMENTARY

In response to the question about prophylactic oophorectomy at hysterectomy or nongynecologic surgical procedure, both authors underscore the fact that there are no universal guidelines governing indications for this operation. Drs. Piver and Goldberg approach the question from the viewpoint of the general population and make several compelling arguments for its serious consideration. Dr. Rosen approaches the issue based on the patient's individual risk factors. Clearly, preoperative counseling of a woman undergoing hysterectomy for benign disease or a woman undergoing a nongynecologic procedure, particularly an abdominal operation, should include discussion of the patient's own risk factors based on her family history, alternatives for ovarian cancer prevention, risks and benefits of estrogen replacement therapy (including possible increased risk of breast cancer), possible ovarian pathology postsurgery, and the potential risk of peritoneal carcinomatosis.

In answer to the question about prophylactic oophorectomy in women with two affected first-degree relatives, the authors emphasize the fact that the introduction of BRCA1 and BRCA2 genetic susceptibility testing has had a major influence in the decision-making process in these women. Dr. Rosen also points out the possibility of a false-negative test and its implications. Women with two first-degree relatives certainly fit into a high-risk category until proved otherwise. We would recommend that these women participate in a comprehensive ovarian cancer screening program in a major university or cancer center, so that they can receive state-of-the-art counseling and for analysis of the outcomes, in an effort to advance our knowledge in this area.

In response to the question about the role of prophylactic oophorectomy in women with one first-degree relative with epithelial ovarian cancer, the authors agree that, in general, the increased risk in these women is only modest. As noted, however, this group will include some women with a BRCA1 mutation. Therefore, these women are also excellent candidates for risk assessment and counseling in a comprehensive ovarian cancer screening program.

The authors also agree that, unless there are extenuating circumstances, operative laparoscopy is the preferred approach for prophylactic oophorectomy. As Dr. Rosen indicates, however, the issue of concomitant hysterectomy is intimately linked to the effects of hormone replacement therapy after prophylactic oophorectomy. Of major concern in women who do not undergo concomitant hysterectomy are the effects of the addition of a progestational agent on the risk of breast cancer and on the cardiovascular system. In the former instance, current information is conflicting.

The authors indicate that the potential alternatives to prophylactic oophorectomy include screening and other forms of prevention, including oral contraception and tubal ligation. The role of dietary changes remains unclear. Interestingly, as Drs. Piver and Goldberg point out, the efficacy of oral contraceptives in ovarian cancer risk reduction among women who harbor a BRCA1 mutation is unknown. Likewise, as Dr. Rosen observes, screening is not without risk and has not yet proved effective in a high-risk population.

In summary, the role of prophylactic oophorectomy will continue to be modified and refined as we continue to learn more about the genetic predisposition to ovarian cancer. Already, the cloning of the BRCA1 and BRCA2 genes have had a major impact on the manner in which we approach this entire issue.

References

1. Schwartz PE: The role of prophylactic oophorectomy in the avoidance of ovarian cancer. Int J Gynaecol Obstet 39: 175, 1992

2. Sightler SE, Boike GM, Estape RE, Averette HE: Ovarian cancer in women with prior hysterectomy: a 14 year experience at the University of Miami. Obstet Gynecol 78:681, 1991
3. Finazzo MS, Hoffman MS, Roberts WS, Cavanagh DM: Previous pelvic surgery in patients with ovarian cancer. South Med J 81:1518, 1988
4. Boike G, Averette H, Hoskins W et al: National Survey of ovarian carcinoma. IV. Women with prior hysterectomy: a failure of prevention? Gynecol Oncol 49:112, 1993
5. Jacobs I, Oram D: Prevention of ovarian cancer: a survey of the practice of prophylactic oopherectomy by fellows and members of the Royal College of Obstetricians and Gynaecologists. Br J Obstet Gynaecol 96:510, 1989
6. Sheth S, Malpani A: Routine prophylactic oopherectomy at the time of vaginal hysterectomy in postmenopausal women. Arch Gynecol Obstet 251:87, 1992
7. Christ JE, Lotze EC: The residual ovary syndrome. Obstet Gynecol 46:551, 1975
8. Ranney B, Abu-Ghazaleh S: The future function and fortune of ovarian tissue which is retained in vivo during hysterectomy. Am J Obstet Gynecol 128:626, 1977
9. Meijer WJ, Lindert ACM: Prophylactic oopherectomy. Eur J Obstet Gynecol Reprod Biol 47:59, 1992
10. Siddle N, Sarrel P, Whitehead M: The effect of hysterectomy on the age at ovarian failure: identification of a subgroup of women with premature loss of ovarian function and literature review. Fertil Steril 47:94, 1987
11. Randall CL, Hall DW Armenia CS: Pathology in the preserved ovary after unilateral oopherectomy. Am J Obstet Gynecol 84:1233, 1962
12. Randall CL: Background of statistical data on ovarian cancer. p. 211. In HRK Barber, EA Graber (eds): Gynecologic Oncology, A Comprehensive Review and Evaluation. Williams & Wilkins, Baltimore, 1970
13. Canadian Cancer Statistics 1994: Produced by National Cancer Institute of Canada, Statistics Canada, Provincial Cancer Registries and Health Canada
14. Wingo PA, Tong TMS, Bolden BA: Cancer statistics. CA Cancer J Clin 45:1, 1995
15. Risch HA, Jain M, Marrett LD, Howe GR: Dietary fat intake and the risk of epithelial ovarian cancer. J Natl Cancer Inst 86:1409, 1994
16. NIH Consensus Development Panel on Ovarian Cancer: Ovarian cancer: screening, treatment, and follow up. JAMA 273:491, 1995.
17. Miki Y, Swensen J, Shattuck-Eidens D et al: A strong candidate for breast and ovarian cancer susceptibility gene BRCA 1. Science 266:66, 1994
18. Ford D, Easton DF, Bishop DT et al, and the Breast Cancer Consortium: Risks of Cancer in BRCA1-Mutation carriers. Lancet 343:692, 1994
19. Narod SA, Goldgar D, Canon-Albright L et al: Risk modifiers in carriers of BRCA1 mutations. In J Cancer 64:394, 1995
20. McGowan L: Ovarian cancer after hysterectomy. Obstet Gynecol 69:386, 1987
21. Jacobs I, Oram D: Prophylactic ophorectomy. Br J Hosp Med 38:440, 1987
22. Fung Kee Fung M, Rosario D et al: Is incidental prophylactic oophorectomy an acceptable means to reduce the incidence of ovarian cancer?, abstracted. Society of Obstetricians and Gynecologists of Canada, Annual Meeting, Calgary, Alberta, 1995
23. Howe H: Age-specific hysterectomy and oophorectomy prevelance rates and the risks for cancer of the reproductive system. Am J Public Health 74:560, 1984
24. Struewing JP, Watson P, Easton DF et al: Prophylactic oophorectomy in in-

herited breast/ovarian cancer families. J Natl Cancer Inst 17:33, 1995

25. Tobacman J, Tucker MA, Kase R et al: Intra-abdominal carcinomatosis after prophylactic oophorectomy in ovarian cancer prone families. Lancet 2:795, 1982
26. Struewing JP, Watson P, Easton DF: Effectiveness of prophylactic oophorectomy in inherited breast/ovarian cancer families. Am J Hum Genet, suppl. 55:A384, 1994
27. Piver MS, Jishi MF, Tsukada Y, Nava G: Primary peritoneal carcinoma after prophylactic oophorectomy in women with a family history of ovarian cancer: a report of the Gilda Radner Familial Ovarian Cancer Registry. Cancer 71: 2751, 1993
28. Lurain JR, Piver MS: Familial ovarian cancer. Gynecol Oncol 8:185, 1979
29. Piver MS, Barlow JJ, Sawyer DM: Familial ovarian cancer: increasing in frequency? Obstet Gynecol 60:397, 1982
30. Piver MS, Goldberg JM, Jishi MF et al: Characteristics of familial ovarian cancer: a report of the first 1000 families in the Gilda Radner Familial Ovarian Cancer Registry. Eur J Gynaecol Oncol 17:169, 1995
31. Ries LAG, Hankey BF, Miller BA et al: Cancer Statistics Review: 1973–1988. NIH Publ No. 91–2789. National Cancer Institute, Bethesda, 1991
32. National Institute of Health Consensus Development Conference Statement. Ovarian cancer: treatment and follow-up. Gynecol Oncol 55:S4, 1994
33. Easton DF, Bishop DT, Ford D, Crockford GP and the Breast Cancer Linkage Consortium: Genetic linkage analysis in familial breast and ovarian cancer: results from 214 families. Am J Hum Genet 52:678, 1993
34. Narod SA, Madlensky L, Bradley L et al: Hereditary and familial ovarian cancer in southern Ontario. Cancer 74:2341, 1994
35. Hall JM, Lee MK, Morrow J et al: Linkage analysis of early onset familial breast cancer to chromosome 17q21. Science 250:1684, 1990
36. Narod SA, Feunteun J, Lynch HT et al: Familial breast-ovarian cancer locus on chromosome 17q12–23. Lancet 338: 82, 1991
37. Solomon E, Ledbetter DH: Report of the committee on the genetic constitution of chromosome 17. Cytogenet Cell Genet 58:686, 1991
38. Narod SA, Ford D, Devilee P et al: An evaluation of genetic heterogeneity in 145 breast-ovarian cancer families. Am J Hum Genet 56:254, 1995
39. Steichen-Gersdorf E, Gallion HH, Ford D et al: Familial site-specific ovarian cancer is linked to BRCA1 on 17q12–21. Am J Hum Genet 55:870, 1994
40. Watson P, Lynch HT: Extra-colonic cancer and hereditary non-polyposis colorectal cancer. Cancer 71:677, 1993
41. Itoh H, Houlston RH, Harcopos C, Slack J: Risk of death in first degree relatives of patients with hereditary non-polyposis colon cancer (Lynch type II): a study of 130 kindred in the United Kingdom. Br J Surg 77:1367, 1990
42. Lynch HT, Cavalieri RG, Lynch JF, Casey MJ: Gynecologic cancer clues to Lynch Syndrome II diagnosis: a family report. Gynecol Oncol 44:198, 1992
43. Love RR: Small bowel cancers, B-cell lymphatic leukemia and six primary cancers with metastases and prolonged survival in the cancer family syndrome of Lynch. Cancer 55:499, 1985
44. Mecklin JP, Jarvinen HJ: Clinical features of colorectal carcinoma in cancer family syndrome. Dis Colon Rectum 29:160, 1986
45. Vasen HFA, Taal BG, Griffioen G et al: Clinical heterogeneity of familial colorectal cancer and its influence on screening protocols. Gut 35:1262, 1994
46. Ford D, Easton DF: The genetics of breast and ovarian cancer. Br J Cancer 72:805, 1995

47. Schildkraut JM, Thompson WD: Familial ovarian cancer. A population-based case-controlled study. Am J Epidemiol 128:456, 1988

48. Parazzini F, Negri E, La Vecchia C: Family history of reproductive cancers and ovarian cancer risk. An Italian case controlled study. Am J Epidemiol 135:35, 1992

49. Ponder BAJ, Peto J, Easton DF: Familial ovarian cancer. In Sharp F, Mason WP, Creasman W (eds): Ovarian Cancer. Chapman & Hall, London, 1992

50. Kerlikowske K, Brown JS, Grady DG: Should women with familial ovarian cancer undergo prophylactic oophorectomy? Obstet Gynecol 80:700, 1992

51. Piver MS: Prophylactic oophorectomy and ovarian cancer mortality. In Cancer Prevention. JB Lippincott, Philadelphia, 1992

52. Offit K: BRCA1: a new marker in the management of patients with breast cancer. Cancer 77:599, 1996

53. Shattuck-Eidens D, McClure M, Simard J et al: A collaborative survey of 80 mutations in the BRCA1 and ovarian susceptibility gene. Implications for presymptomatic testing and screening. JAMA 273:535, 1995

54. Serova O, Montagna M, Torchard D et al: A high incidence of BRCA1 mutations in 20 breast-ovarian cancer families. AJ Hum Geneti 58:42, 1996

55. MacDonald KG, Doan B, Kelner M, Taylor KM: A sociobehavioral perspective on genetic testing and counselling for hereditable breast, ovarian, and colon cancer. Can Med Assoc J 154:457, 1996

56. Claus EB, Risch N, Thompson WD: The calculation of breast cancer risk for women with a first-degree family history of ovarian cancer. Breast Cancer Res Treat 28:115, 1993

57. Fitzgerald M, MacDonald DJ, Krainer M, Hoover I: Germ-line BRCA1 mutations in Jewish and non-Jewish women with early onset breast cancer. N Engl J Me 334:143, 1996

58. Bourne TH, Campbell S, Reynolds KM et al: Screening for early familial ovarian cancer with transvaginal ultrasonography and colour blood flow imaging. BMJ 306:1025, 1993

59. Houlston RS, Bourne TH, Collins WP et al: Risk of ovarian cancer and genetic relationship to other cancers in families. Hum Hered 43:111, 1993

60. Amos Cl, Shaw GL, Tucker MA, Hartge P: Age at onset for familial epithelial ovarian cancer. JAMA 268:1896, 1992

61. Langston AA, Malone E, Thompson JD et al: BRCA1 mutations in a population based sample of young women with breast cancer. N Engl J Me 334:137, 1996

62. Nehzat F, Nezhat C, Silfen SL: Video laparoscopy for oophorectomy. Am J Obstet Gynecol 165:1323, 1991

63. Wright RC: Hysterectomy: past, present and future. Obstet Gynecol 33:560, 1969

64. Meijer WJ, van Lindert ACM: Prophylactic oophorectomy. Eur J Obstet Gynecol Reprod Biol 47:59, 1992

65. Schwartz PE: The role of prophylactic oophorectomy in the avoidance of ovarian cancer. Int J Gynecol Obstet 39: 175, 1992

66. Averette HE, Nguyen HN: The role of prophylactic oophorectomy in cancer prevention. Gynecol Oncol 55:s38, 1994

67. Simard J, Tonin P, Durocher F: Common origins of BRCA 1 mutations in Canadian breast and ovarian cancer families. Nature Genet 8:392, 1994

68. Massad LS, Mutch DG: Fallopian tube neoplasms. In Copeland L (ed): Textbook of Gynecology. WB Saunders, Philadelphia, 1993

69. Gambrell RD: Use of progesten therapy. Am J Obstet Gynecol 156:1304, 1987

70. Colditz GA, Hankinson SE, Hunter DJ et al: The use of estrogens and progestins and the risk of breast cancer in postmenopausal women. N Engl J Me 332:1509, 1995
71. Schairer C, Byrne C, Keyl PM et al: Menopausal estrogen and estrogen-progestin replacement therapy and risk of breast cancer. (United States). Cancer Causes Control 5:491, 1994
72. Stanford JL, Weiss NS, Voight LF et al: Combined estrogen and progestin hormone replacement therapy in relation to risk of breast cancer in middle-aged women. JAMA 274:137, 1995
73. The Pepi Trial: Effects of estrogen or estrogen/progestin regimens on heart disease risk factors in postmenopausal women JAMA 273:199, 1995
74. Bush TL, Cowan LD, Barrett-Connors E et al: Estrogen use and all cause mortality. JAMA 249, 1983
75. Petitt DB, Perlman JA, Sidney S: Noncontraceptive estrogens and mortality: long term follow up of women in the Walnut Creek Study. Obstet Gynecol 70:289, 1987
76. Ettinger B, Friedman GD, Bush T, Quesenberry CP: Reduced mortality associated with long term postmenopausal estrogen use. Obstet Gynecol 87:6, 1996
77. Jishi MF, Itnyre JH, Oakley G et al: Risks of cancer among members of families in the Gilda Radner Familial Ovarian Cancer Registry. Cancer 76:1416, 1995
78. Cancer and Steroid Hormone Study of the Centers for Disease control and the National Institute of Child Health and Human Development: The reduction in risk of ovarian cancer associated with oral contraceptive use. N Engl J Med 316:650, 1987
79. Schlesselman JJ: Cancer of the breast and reproductive tract in relation to use of oral contraceptives. Contraception 40:1, 1989
80. Prentice RL, Thomas DB: On the epidemiology of oral contraceptives and disease. Adv Cancer Res 49:385, 1987
81. Rosenberg L, Palmer JR, Zauber AG et al: A case-control study of oral contraceptive use and invasive epithelial ovarian cancer. Am J Epidemiol 139:654, 1994
82. Kerber RA, Slattery ML: The impact of family history on ovarian cancer risk. Arch Intern Med 155:905, 1995
83. Hankinson SE, Hunter DJ, Colditz GA et al: Tubal ligation, hysterectomy, and risk of ovarian cancer: a prospective study. JAMA 270:2813, 1993
84. Cornelison TL, Natarajan N, Piver MS, Mettlin CJ: Tubal ligation and the risk of ovarian carcinoma. Cancer Detection Prev 21:1, 1997
85. Whittemore AS, Harris R, Itnyre J: Characteristics relating to ovarian cancer risk: collaborative analysis of 12 U.S. case-control studies. II. Invasive epithelial ovarian cancers in white women. Am J Epidemiol 136:1184, 1992
86. Rossing MA, Daling JR, Weiss NS et al: Ovarian tumors in a cohort of infertile women. N Engl J Med 331:771, 1994
87. Cramer DW, Welch WR, Scully RE, Wojciechowski CA: Ovarian cancer and talc: a case-control study. Cancer 50: 372, 1982
88. Harlow BL, Cramer DW, Bell DA, Welch WR: Perineal exposure to talc and ovarian cancer risk. Obstet Gynecol 80:19, 1992
89. Cramer DW, Welch WR, Hutchinson GB et al: Dietary animal fat in relation to ovarian cancer risk. Obstet Gynecol 63:833, 1984
90. Mettlin C, Piver MS: A case-control study of milk drinking and ovarian cancer risk. Am J Epidemiol 132:871, 1990
91. Cramer DW, Harlow BC, Willett WC et al: Galactose consumption and metabolism in relation to the risk of ovarian cancer. Lancet 2:66, 1989

92. Bourne TH, Whitehead MI, Campbell MI et al: Ultrasound screening for familial ovarian cancer. Gynecol Oncol 43: 92, 1991

93. Grover S, Quinn MA, Weideman P et al: Screening for ovarian cancer using serum CA125 and vaginal exam:report on 2550 females. Int J Gynecol Cancer 5:29, 1995

94. Risch H, Marrett LD, Howe GR: Parity, contraception, infertility, and the risk of epithelial ovarian cancer. Am J Epidemiol 140:585, 1994

CHAPTER 3

ADJUVANT THERAPY FOR EARLY-STAGE EPITHELIAL OVARIAN CANCER

Claes Tropé
Janne Kaern
Ignace Vergote

EDITORS' INTRODUCTION

An understanding of the issues surrounding treatment of early-stage ovarian cancer requires an understanding of the problems associated with performing clinical trials in this area. First, only 20% of all presentations are stage I or II, and as a result, accrual to well-powered studies takes years or completion of the study in a timely fashion often finds the results underpowered. Second, and related to the first issue, the outcome for these patients is generally good, and even large trials may not develop enough events (recurrence and death) to allow firm conclusions. Third, studies from the 1960s and 1970s include many patients who were understaged (cryptic stage III), making outcomes worse than they actually were. Fourth, all studies of early-stage disease include some patients (as high as 20%) with borderline tumors, making outcomes better than they actually were. Finally, only in the past decade has a clear appreciation emerged of the risk factors within FIGO stages. Thus, in 1997 early-stage disease is subdivided into high-risk (all stage II, all stage IC, and stages IA and IB with high-grade tumors) and low-risk groups (all other types), and separate trials have been developed for each. Studies prior to 1985 frequently evaluated all these patients in one protocol. Thus, about 25 years after the first trials in early ovarian cancer were initiated, less is known about how best to treat these patients than there should be. We have asked Drs. Tropé, Kaern, and Vergote, to comment on which patients should be candidates for protocol therapy in stage I disease and what prognostic factors are important in separating patients into high and low-risk groups. Further, we have asked him and his colleagues to summarize the results of trials over the past 20 years and to give his opinion regarding what we have learned from these studies.

To complicate this matter further, many trials have not included a control arm because of both physician and patient bias. This may be acceptable if there is a clear "winner" in one of the intervention arms, however, most studies have shown equivalency in efficacy, leaving open the question of whether any therapy is better than no therapy. It is also important in such studies to explore therapeutic index. For example, single-agent alkylating therapy is just as good as intraperitoneal therapy with ^{32}P, but patients treated with alkylating therapy have a chance of developing a fatal myeloid leukemia as a result. Additionally, as many trials now appropriately explore quality-of-life issues, it will be very important in future studies to include this parameter also.

We asked our expert to comment on the advisability and ethics of including a control arm in future trials. This very controversial topic will likely remain just that for many years to come unless biases can be set aside and a control trial performed in the high-risk population. It is important to note that the current recommendation for the low-risk population is no additional therapy if an adequate surgical staging procedure was performed. Is it not possible that the same applies to the high-risk population?

We have asked our expert to outline his recommendations for treatment of a high-risk patient outside a clinical trial (although we hasten to discourage this practice). We have also asked Dr. Tropé to recommend an approach to the difficult and all too frequent situation involving management of a patient who is operated on by a person inexperienced in ovarian cancer who refers the patient as early-stage disease but who has not adequately staged her by modern criteria. This is not uncommon, particularly with the increasing use of laparoscopic pelvic surgery where complete staging is often not feasible even if the physician suspects a malignancy. Finally, we have asked our expert to make any recommendations for future trials that may further help us elucidate the proper therapy for this all too uncommon ovarian cancer patient.

QUESTIONS

1. Please define high-risk disease within the stage I category based on prognostic factors.
2. What have we learned from clinical trials of early-stage epithelial ovarian cancer over the past 20 years?
3. Do you believe that ongoing or future clinical trials in this area should include an observation arm? Do you believe that this approach is ethical? Do any of the existing adjuvant therapies benefit patients?
4. What is your current recommendation for treatment of a high-risk stage I patient outside a protocol setting?
5. What are the management options for a patient referred to you after surgery for epithelial ovarian cancer apparently confined to the ovary but without adequate surgical staging? What is your recommendation?
6. Please discuss ongoing clinical trials and any recommendations you may have for future trials.

CLAES TROPÉ

Ovarian carcinoma is the second most common gynecologic cancer and is the leading cause of death from gynecologic malignancy and overall fourth behind lung, breast, and colorectal cancer. Although important advances in surgery, chemotherapy, and radiotherapy have been made, the overall survival for patients with ovarian cancer has not changed significantly—even for those with early-stage disease—over the past 20 years.[1] Worldwide, 42,000 new cases of early ovarian cancers are diagnosed each year.[2] Approximately one-third of the 500 new epithelial ovarian cancers reported annually in Norway present with FIGO I and II. The prognosis for these 150 women is much better than that for patients with stages III and IV.[3,4] The 5-year survival rates reported for patients with early-stage disease have varied considerably: for stage I patients it ranges from 50% to 95%, and for stage II patients from 30% to 80%.[1-3] The reason for these variable results probably depends on the heterogeneity of prognostic factors for patients in the published studies. Survival might be improved if high-risk patients with early-stage disease could be identified and treated with more intensive regimens and those with low risk could be spared treatment. In some cases operations to preserve fertility might even be possible.

QUESTION 1

Please define high-risk disease within the stage I category based on prognostic factors.

CLAES TROPÉ
JANNE KAERN
IGNACE VERGOTE

Traditional clinical and pathologic prognostic factors in early-stage disease are FIGO substage, degree of differentiation, histologic type, dense adhesions, large-volume ascites, and age of patient, which have been identified as independent prognostic characters with multivariate analysis.[5] Residual tumor (relevant only for stages IIB and IIC) has moderate prognostic value.[6] Several studies elucidating multivariate analysis for ovarian cancer have been published. Since many of these publications analyze too many factors on nonhomogeneous materials of too few patients, the results should be interpreted with caution. In the literature[5–8] there are only five multivariate studies with more than 200 patients.

The reliability of analyses for prognostic factors depends on the number of cases analyzed, the number of prognostic variables analyzed, and the internal consistency of the factors analyzed. The number of patients analyzed can be increased by including patients over a very long time or by analyzing series from several centers or from several studies together (meta-analysis). Both methods have a negative effect upon the reliability of the results by increasing the heterogeneity of the material. Staging, histopathology, and treatment vary over time and from one trial to another.[9]

Stage varies with the applied stage classification and with the guidelines for the staging procedure. Only patients staged according to uniform guidelines should be grouped in a multivariate analysis. Many patients staged 10 years ago as stage I or II would today be classified as stage III. Even uniform guidelines for stage classification can be altered by different interpretations and applications of the guidelines.[10] There are no exact, well-defined criteria for histologic grading. A classification based on architectural pattern is recommended by WHO,[11] but even well-defined grade criteria are difficult to apply in the same way from one observer to another, and even from one time to another by the same observer. Bertelsen et al.[9] analyzed the reproducibility of grade, the most important prognostic factor in 410 patients with early-stage disease. The agreement rate between primary and review grading according to the architectural classification was reasonable (69%, κ value 0.52), but the agreement rate between primary and review grading according to a combined classification was poor (52%, κ value 0.28). The agreement rate between review grading according to the two classifications was poor (62%, kappa value 0.44).

A detailed knowledge of prognostic factors is essential for the clinician to assess the prognosis and individualize the treatment of ovarian cancer patients. However, as mentioned above, these prognostic factors have important shortcomings. Therefore, factors that can be measured objectively with better reproducibility should be used. Most of those in current use have too low predictive power. The cellular DNA content in the tumor cells has been used for 25 years,[12] but the time-consuming measurements employing absorption cytometry have kept it from being clinically useful. The introduction of flow cytometry with high-speed measurements and better reproducubility has facilitated the analysis and has verified to some extent, the prognostic value of such determination.[13] The classic prognostic parameters such as FIGO stage, histologic type and grade, amount of residual tumor after primary surgery, age, and performance status are far from sufficient for predicting the prognosis of an individual ovarian cancer patient with early-stage disease. These parameters contain a touch of the subjective, and the reproducibility is too low.[14] In an attempt to improve the predicability of the patient's prognosis, there has been a search for more objective and more reproducible prognostic variables including DNA ploidy and proliferation acitivity (S-phase fraction), (SPF). In a Norwegian Radium Hospital study traditional clinical and morphologic prognostic factors and flow cytometry DNA ploidy were analyzed in 290 stage I patients.[15] The median follow-up for living patients was 60 months, with a range of 36 to 112 months. The overall actuarial 5-year survival and disease-free survival were 80% and 78%, respectively. Twenty-one percent of the patients had relapsed. Fifty-one percent of the tumors were diploid and 49% aneuploid. Of the aneuploid tumors 65% were single aneuploid, 34% were tetraploid, and 11% multiploid. Diploid tumors were often stage IA, well-differentiated, and of the mucinous or endometroid type with patient age under 50 years. Aneuploid tumors were more frequently stage IC, poorly differentiated, and of the serous or clear-cell type with patient age above 50 years. Clear-cell tumors made up 50% of the tetraploid tumors, and two-thirds of the aneuploid clear-cell tumors were tetraploid. No difference in disease-free survival was observed among the subgroups of aneuploid tumors. The 5-year disease-free survival for patients with diploid tumors was 90% compared to 64% for patients with aneuploid tumors ($P < 0.0001$). Degree of differentiation, DNA ploidy, FIGO stage (1986), FIGO stage (1973), histological type, presence of dense adhesion, age, and extracapsular growth proved to be prognostic in the univariate analyses. In patients with graded tumors multivariate analysis identified degree of differentiation as the most powerful prognostic indicator of disease-free survival, followed by DNA diploid tumors and finally FIGO (1996) substage. When the effects of the three most important factors were considered, none of the following factors was prognostic: histologic type, dense adhesion, extracapsular growth, ascites, rupture during surgery, FIGO (1973) stage, tumor size, age, and type of adjuvant treatment. None of 77 patients with DNA diploid and well-differentiated tumors and only 2 out of 55 patients (3%) with stage IA diploid tumor relapsed (Tables 3-1 and 3-2). Tumors with clear-cell carcinoma elements were not graded. In this subgroup FIGO stage was the most important prognostic characteristic.

Based on this Norwegian study early ovarian cancer could be divided into two risk groups: low risk consisting of well-differentiated and DNA diploid tumors; none of these patients relapsed. The high-risk group consisted of all moderate and poorly differentiated tumors and well-differentiated and nondiploid tumors; in this group 25% of patient relapsed. The clear-cell tumors in stages IB and IC belong to a very high-risk group as 54% of patients relapsed (Table 3-3, Fig. 3-1).

These results strongly indicate that DNA ploidy and morphometric criteria, compared to the classic parameters, add important prognostic information in patients with early ovarian carcinoma. By combining the independent prognostic variables identified by multivariate

TABLE 3-1
Stage I Epithelial Ovarian Cancer Relapse Rate Versus DNA Ploidy and Degree of Differentiation[a]

DIFFERENTIATION	DIPLOID	NONDIPLOID	TOTAL
Total	15/143 (61)	46/136 (34)	61/279 (22)
Degree of differentiation I	0/77 (0)	6/36 (14)	6/113 (5)
Degree of differentiation II	2/23 (9)	6/23 (26)	8/46 (16)
Degree of differentiation III	7/23 (30)	15/37 (41)	22/60 (36)
Differentiation unknown	7/20 (35)	19/40 (48)	26/60 (43)

[a] *Numbers in parentheses denote percentages.*

TABLE 3-2

Stage I Epithelial Ovarian Cancer Relapse Rate Versus DNA Ploidy and FIGO Stage (1986 Definition)[a]

STAGE	DIPLOID	NONDIPLOID	TOTAL
Total	15/143 (11)	46/136 (33)	61/279 (22)
FIGO stage IA	2/55 (3)	5/34 (15)	7/89 (8)
FIGO stage IB	1/6	5/8	6/14
FIGO stage IC	12/82 (15)	36/94 (38)	48/176 (27)

[a] *Numbers in parentheses denote percentages.*

analysis it is possible to calculate the relative risk for individual patients, allowing the separation of patients into risk groups for treatment decisions. Proliferative activity, SPF is currently not a reliable prognostic factor. It can be estimated in only a selected part of the tumor, the SPF of diploid and aneuploid tumors cannot be compared, and the SPF of a tumor cannot be judged from the analysis of only one sample. SPF is not reliable when paraffin-embedded tissue is used; in such material, DNA ploidy assessments are not possible in about 10% of tumors mainly because of poor fixation and preparation techniques. When fresh tumor is used, the main source of error is not poor sampling but poor preparation and technique. About 10% of diploid samples do not contain sufficient tumor cells for adequate analysis compared to the amount of normal cells. There is a need for international standards for the calculation and use of SPF. By complementary flow cytometry measurements with morphology/imagecytometry (ICM) (cross-checked with cytologic and histologic information) an improved sensitivity and specificity in the detection of aneuploid cells is possible. Together with a more biologically, correct subclassification of tumors, improved prediction of prognosis and response to treatment can hopefully be achieved.[16]

Histopathologic analysis of DNA ploidy by flow cytometry, image cytometry, and morphometric analysis should be performed on selected patients with ovarian cancer, especially those who have borderline, low-grade and/or early-stage tumors. An effort should be made to increase the availability of this test and the training of pathologists in the technique. When these biologic assays suggest a good prognosis, as in borderline tumors, well-differentiated early-stage invasive tumors (Stages IA, IB, IC), postoperative treatment can be omitted.[16]

Other biologic prognostic factors are less well characterized. The expression of

TABLE 3-3

Relapse in Stage I Epithelial Ovarian Carcinoma According to Prognostic Groups

	DEGREE OF DIFFERENTIATION[a]			
	WELL	MODERATE	POOR	NOT GRADED (CLEAR CELL)[b]
Diploid	0/77 (0)	High		
Nondiploid		Risk	35/142 (25)	
Stage IA				1/15 (7)
Stages IB to IC				25/46 (54)

Note: Shaded areas show high risk group.

[a] *Numbers in parentheses denote percentages.*

[b] *Including mixed epithelial tumors with clear cell elements.*

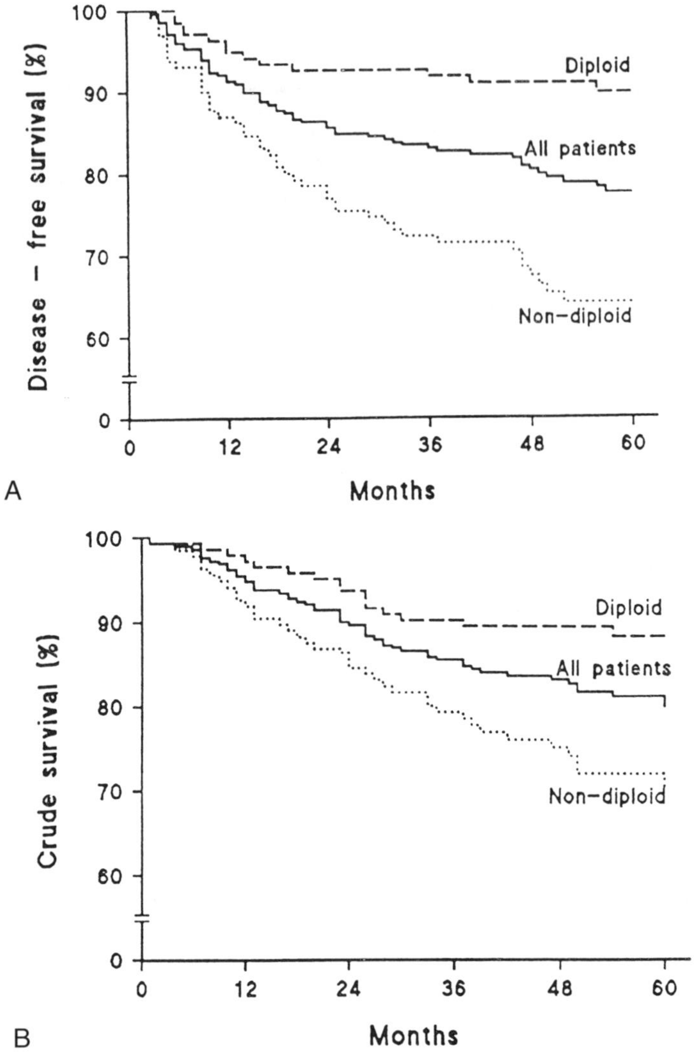

FIGURE 3-1. (A) Actuarial disease-free survival in patients with DNA diploid tumors (n = 136) versus DNA nondiploid tumors (n = 130). (Log-rank test; diploid versus nondiploid, $P < 0.0001$; patients dying of intercurrent disease are excluded). All patients (n = 277) (patients with undeterminable DNA ploidy are included). (B) Actuarial crude survival in patients with DNA diploid tumors (n = 143) versus DNA nondiploid tumors (n = 136). (Log-rank test; diploid versus nondiploid, $P = 0.0004$). All patients (n = 290) (patients with undeterminable DNA ploidy are included).[15]

platelet-derived growth factor (PDGF), platelet-derived growth factor alpha receptor (PGDFR-α) and PDGF-beta receptors, (PDGF-β) was studied by Henriksen et al[17] in normal ovaries and ovarian neoplasms by immunohistochemical analysis. PDGF was detected in tumor cells in 33 of 45 malignant tumor samples but in none of 20 benign tumors or 11 normal ovaries. PDGFR-α was detected in tumor cells in 16 of 45 malignant tumors, while no epithelial staining was found in 16 benign tumors or in 10 normal ovaries. Patients with ovarian cancer stages I through IV and PDGFR-α-positive tumor cells demonstrated an overall shorter survival compared to those who had negative staining of tumor cells. Thus, concomitant expression of PDGF and PDGFR-α in tumor cells is related to the progression of malignant ovarian tumors, indicating the functional role of PDGF via autocrine growth stimulation.[17] Cell kinetic data are other important indicators of the aggressiveness of the tumor and the treatment response. Tumor growth is determined by a balance between tumor cell proliferation and cell loss, and proliferation is dependent on the fraction of proliferating cells and cell cycling time. Therefore, determination of an ovarian tumor's proliferating activity may be of prognostic value. Several methods exist for this purpose; for example, Ki- 67 expression and flow cytometry SPF. Henriksen et al[18] examined malignant epithelial ovarian tumors for the expression of Ki-67, DNA ploidy, and SPF. In addition, normal ovaries and benign and borderline tumors were immunostained with Ki-67 to examine its role in ovarian carcinogenesis and to estimate its prognostic significance. Ki-67, DNA ploidy, and SPF showed a significant correlation with survival in malignant tumors, and furthermore, SPF greater than 10% showed a significant correlation with decreased survival in stages I and II.

The p53 protein is a nuclear phosphoprotein recently discovered in virus-transformed cells.[19–21] It was classified as an oncogene product, but there is substantial evidence that it has a tumor suppressor function. Studies on p53 gene expression in several tissues have indicated a role in carcinogenesis. A few studies have shown that p53 mutation is quite common in ovarian cancer,[22–24] but the significance of abnormal p53 protein production for tumor development and survival has not been examined in depth. Henriksen et al[25] showed that p53 may be involved in tumorigenesis, as its expression was detected in both borderline and malignant tumors while normal ovaries and benign ovarian tumors had no expression. The presence of p53 was also related to dissemination of disease, residual tumor bulk, and poor differentiation, as well as the presence of a proliferation variable, Ki-67. Its presence in malignant ovarian tumors was related to a significant decrease in patient survival, with only 36% alive compared to 70% in the p53-negative group. At the Norwegian Radium Hospital 374 early-stage ovarian tumors, including 27 borderline and 347 stage l carcinomas, were investigated immunohistochemically for overexpression of p53. Alterations in p53 were detected in 15% of borderline tumors and in 15% of stage l carcinomas, respectively. The mutations in the p53 gene (exons 5 through 8) were demonstrated in 29 of the 50 stage l carcinomas studied using denaturing gel electrophoresis followed by direct sequencing. Our results indicate that p53 abnormalities play a crucial role in the development of early-stage ovarian carcinoma. There was, however, no significant association between p53 and survival in multivariate analyses[26] (Fig. 3-2).

Bcl-2 is an oncoprotein which apparently inhibits apoptosis.[27,28] In a recent study in ovarian tumors Bcl-2 expression was positively correlated with survival.[29] Furthermore, in patients with early ovarian cancer with residual tumor bulk, Bcl-2 expression showed a significant positive correlation with survival.

Nevertheless, until further studies are performed, as well as the above-mentioned biological assays, as well as HER-2/neu, C-erbB-2, ras, c-myc, and p53 oncogenes and EGFR should be confined to the research setting and not applied routinely in the clinical management of early ovarian cancer patients.

QUESTION 2

What have we learned from clinical trials of early-stage epithelial ovarian cancer over the past 20 years?

CLAES TROPÉ
JANNE KAERN
IGNACE VERGOTE

Adjuvant chemotherapy involves the administration of chemotherapeutic agents, most often systemically after removal of the primary tumor, at which point no evidence of residual tumor remains. This approach is based on data from the 1950s and 1960s which noted an inverse relationship between response to chemotherapy and number of tumor cells. The possibility of improved survival in patients with minimal disease after surgery, coupled with poor response in advanced disease, provided a good rationale using adjuvant therapy.

The role of adjuvant treatment in patients with early epithelial ovarian cancer is still controversial. There is, however, little argument about the role of platinum-based chemotherapy after primary surgery in all patients with FIGO stage II disease.[30] In addition, since many of these cases are understaged FIGO

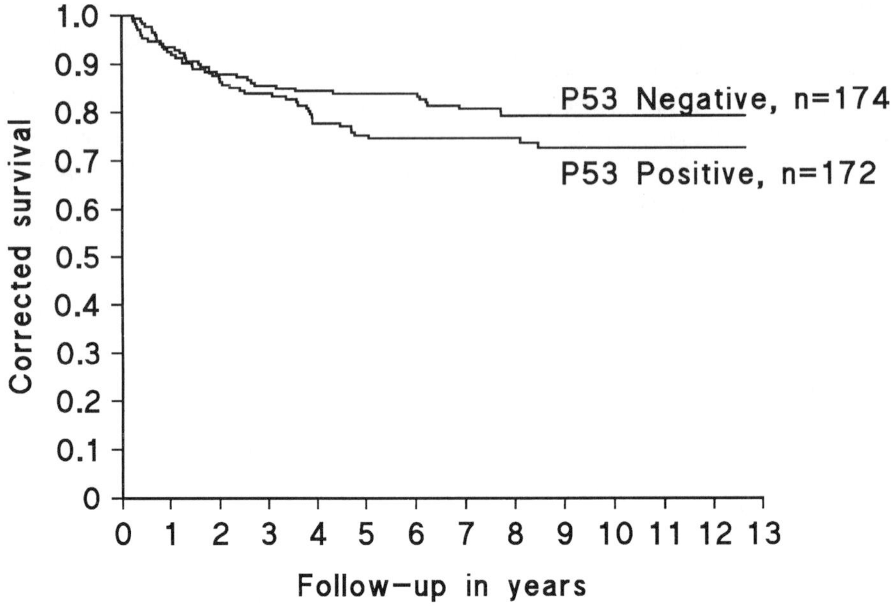

FIGURE 3-2. Correlated survival related to p53 expression in 346 ovarian cancer patients. FIGO stage I (1986) treated at the Norwegian Radium Hospital.[26]

stage III disease, it seems appropriate to recommend chemotherapy rather than pelvic irradiation, particularly because there are data showing that systemic chemotherapy may be less hazardous than radiotherapy following lymphadenectomy.[31–32] Postoperative adjuvant treatment with alkylating agents or irradiation either as intraperitoneal isotope [radioactive gold (^{198}Au) or phosphorus (^{32}P) colloid] installation or whole-abdomen teletherapy has been evaluated in various prospective randomized trials, but the value of postoperative adjuvant treatment is still controversial.[33–41] The unsettled questions regarding adjuvant therapy of ovarian cancer are (1) What therapeutic options for adjuvant treatment are reasonable and justifiable (2) Which patients have a prognosis poor enough to justify adjuvant therapy? (3) Do any of the existing adjuvant therapies benefit patients? (4) Is it possible to develop a new therapy that might be more effective.[33]

What therapeutic options are reasonable and justifiable for adjuvant treatment?

In a randomized study including 418 patients with stage I and II disease, Kolstad et al[34] compared the results of postoperative external beam irradiation with intraperitoneal installation of radioactive ^{198}Au. There was no significant difference in 5-year survival for patients with stage I disease, although that for patients with stage II disease was 54.1% for those treated with ^{198}Au compared with 40% for those treated with radiotherapy. The morbidity in the former group was, however, considerably worse. In another trial from the Norwegian Radium Hospital the addition of thiotepa to adjuvant ^{32}P therapy did not improve survival.[35]

The first randomized trial on adjuvant treatment of ovarian carcinoma comparing alkylating agent therapy with whole-abdomen or pelvic irradition was a randomized study from the M.D. Anderson Cancer Center which showed no benefit for whole-abdominal irradiation when compared with oral melphalan. However, this study was criticized for not irradiating the diaphragm adequately, for giving quite low doses to the liver and kidney areas, and for an imbalance in stage distribution between the two treatment arms.[36] In 1979, Dembo and Bush[37] published a randomized study showing a 25% improvement in survival for patients treated with whole-abdomen irradiation postoperatively. These findings initiated two other studies testing the effect of whole-abdomen irradiation. These two trials failed to show an advantage for whole-abdomen irradiation over the use of alkylating agents and concluded that whole-abdomen irradiation should not be recommended as adjuvant therapy in early ovarian cancer.[38,39] A randomized study of a Gynecological Oncology Group (GOG) suggested that all FIGO stage I patients, except for those with FIGO stage IA well-differentiated tumors, appeared to benefit from adjuvant treatment with melphalan compared with no treatment or radiotherapy to the pelvis. However, in this study only 86 patients were available after randomization to three arms and 49% of the patients entered were removed from the analysis.[40] Young et al[41] reported on two trials of the Ovarian Cancer Study Group/GOG for FIGO stage I and II ovarian cancer. In the first trial 81 patients with well-differentiated or moderately differentiated tumors (FIGO 1973) with stage IA or IB were assigned to either no treatment or melphalan, while in the second trial 141 patients with FIGO stage IC or II or poorly differentiated tumors in FIGO stage IA or IB were randomized between ^{32}P and melphalan. In both trials no difference in survival between the two randomized arms was observed.[41] However, deaths due to alkylating agent– induced leukemia were seen in both arms involving melphalan. Cisplatin is the most active chemotherapeutic agent for treatment of advanced ovarian cancer. However, so far only two trials testing it as an adjuvant treatment in early disease have been published, one from the Norwegian Radium Hospital, Oslo, Norway, and one from Italy.[31,42]

In the Norwegian Radium Hospital study we compared adjuvant intraperitoneal ^{32}P therapy with six cycles of cisplatin, in a group of 347 patients without residual tumor following primary laparatomy.[31] No difference in actuarial survival or disease-free survival was observed in the two treatment groups. However, late bowel obstruction occurred more often in the group treated with ^{32}P compared with the cisplatin group. In a second trial[43] we studied treatment complications in 313 patients treated with intraperitoneal ^{32}P therapy. It was concluded that morbidity was substantial since 2 patients died of complications that could be at least partly attributed to ^{32}P therapy and 22 (7%) of the patients suffered from small bowel complications treated surgically or medically. In earlier series no deaths due to treatment complications were observed, but in these studies a maximum of 100 patients were treated with ^{32}P. Small bowel complications requiring laparotomy have been reported in the literature in 23 (4%) of 576 patients[44,45] treated with ^{32}P without the addition of external irradiation therapy and were observed in 13 (4%) of 313 patients in the Norwegian Radium Hospital study. Furthermore, no significant relation existed between the incidence of small bowel complications and ^{32}P dose, the ^{32}P distribution scintigram, treatment with ^{32}P after primary surgery or at second-look laparotomy, type of surgery at installation, number of prior laparotomies, or whether ^{32}P was given on the same day as surgery or the next day.

Because of the well-established risk of leukemia after adjuvant treatment with alkylating agents,[46–48] Young et al[49] recommended ^{32}P as standard treatment in subsequent studies. Recently it has been suggested that cisplatin might also induce leukemia or other secondary cancer.[50–53] But this risk seems to be much lower than that with alkylating agents. In the absence of therapeutic differences in the Norwegian Radium Hospital report between the ^{32}P and cisplatin groups, in addition to a low frequency of serious toxicity following cisplatin therapy and a higher occurrence of bowel complications after ^{32}P therapy, we suggest that cisplatin (or eventually other platinum analogs) be the standard treatment in stage I and II ovarian carcinoma.

The Italian study by Gruppo Italiano Collaborativo Oncologica Ginecologica (GICOG) performed between October 1983 and October 1990, two multicenter randomized clinical trials.[42,54] After surgical staging and stratification by center, eligible patients in study 1 (n = 92, eligible 83, stages IA and IB, grades 2 and 3) were randomized to either cisplatin 50 mg/m^2 every 28 days for six cycles or no further treatment (control). Patients in study 2 (n = 186, eligible 176, stage IC, any grade) were randomized to cisplatin 50 mg/m^2 every 28 days or intraperitoneal ^{32}P (15 mCi of chromic phosphate). The median follow-up was 69 months in both studies. The disease-free survival showed similar patterns in the two studies, favoring cisplatin. In study 1, 5-year disease-free survival (DFS) was 83% for cisplatin and 64% for the control group. However, no difference in overall survival could be detected (5-year survival in the cisplatin group 87% and in the control group 81%) (Fig. 3-3). In study 2, 5-year disease-free survival was 81% for the cisplatin group and 66% for the ^{32}P group. This was the first randomized study to show the impact of any therapy on disease-free survival (that for cisplatin being better than that for ^{32}P in early ovarian cancer). Again, however, there was no difference in the 5-year survival: 83% in the cisplatin group and 79% in the ^{32}P group (Fig. 3-4).

These two studies interestingly showed that cisplatin-treated patients had a poorer outcome at relapse than non-cisplatin-treated patients. This could be explained by a different response rate to second-line therapy since non-cisplatin-treated patients were crossed over to cisplatin while no effective second-line therapy existed for cisplatin-treated patients. Alternately, the adjunctive cisplantin may have selected a resistant population of cells at recurrence. The above-mentioned studies for high-risk groups lack a control group comparing surgery alone with surgery plus postoperative treatment. Therefore, we still cannot consider these results sufficient to answer the question regarding the need for adjuvant therapy.[54]

Controversial issues and unsettled questions in the management of early epithelial cancer

Conservative Surgery

There is a steep rise in the incidence of ovarian epithelial cancer after 40 years of age. Most clinicians are seldom faced with the problem of preserving ovarian function in the presence of malignant ovarian tumors. As stated above, optimal surgical procedures have been standardized to ensure correct staging, which is of great importance in defining prognosis and planning subsequent therapies. However, one controversial issue concerns the possibility of a conservative surgical approach in young patients who want to retain fertility.[54] Stage I ovarian cancer and borderline tumors can frequently be observed in women of childbearing age for whom preservation of reproductive function is important. Because of the increase in the number of such women referred to the Norwegian Radium Hospital during the last two decades, it has been necessary to revise some of our earlier radical treatment principles for selected cases of ovarian malignancies found in women under 40.[55] We feel that the question of conservative surgery should not be considered in cases of clear-cell, mixed, or undifferentiated carcinomas, and we agree with most gynecologic oncologists that conservative surgery should be performed in young patients with borderline tumors, endometroid, mucinous, and serous stage I, grade I ovarian cancer. However, the literature lacks prospective studies with adequate numbers of patients to assess the cost/benefit ratio of conservative surgery in ovarian cancer. When is it advisable to perform unilateral oophorectomy in fertile women with one of these types of epithelial malignancy? Both serous and endometroid highly differentiated tumors are

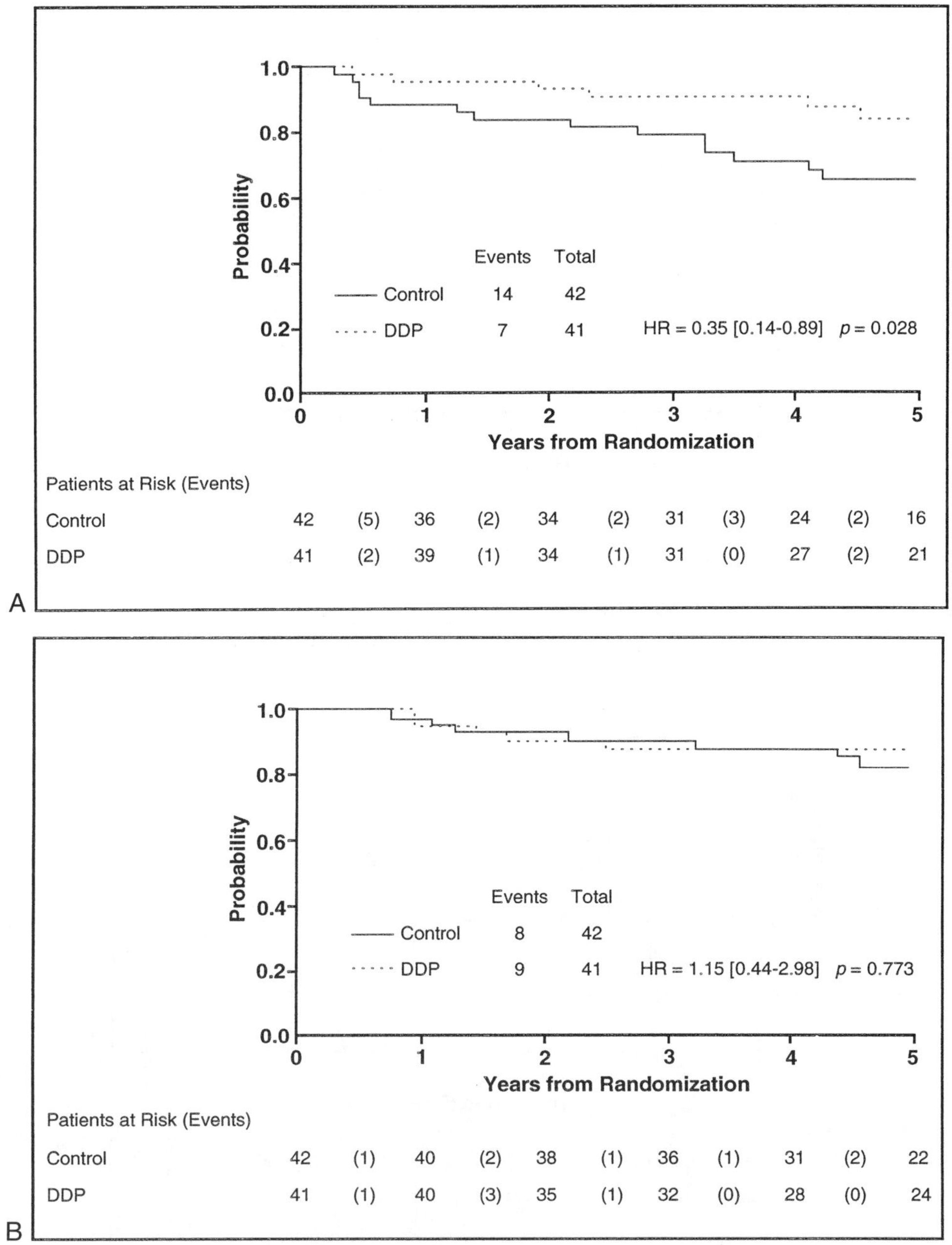

FIGURE 3-3. GICOG Study I: DDP vs Control. (A) Disease free survival. (B) Overall survival.[42]

frequently bilateral. In a large series of 2,800 early-stage ovarian cancers treated at the Norwegian Radium Hospital, 15% of mucinous and endometrioid cancers were bilateral, and 30% of serous.[55] Thus, it should be emphasized that even when the contralateral ovary is macroscopically normal, a microscopic lesion may be found in the stroma. Therefore, biopsy of the remaining ovary should be performed. However, this issue is still controversial because it has been reported that wedge biopsies may cause mechanical infertility.[56] Currently,

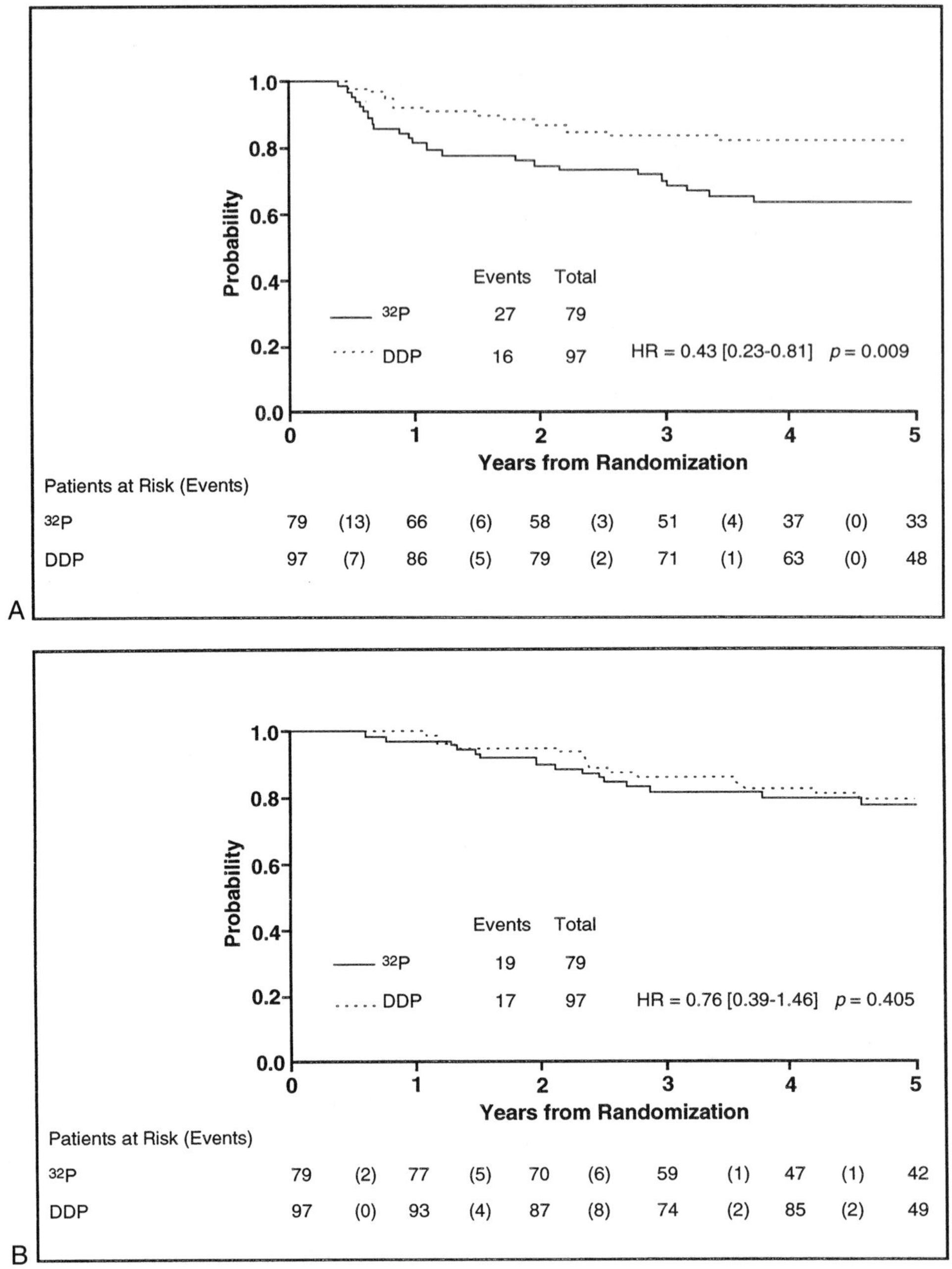

FIGURE 3-4. GICOG Study II: ^{32}P vs DDP. (A) Disease free survival. (B) Overall survival.[42]

we perform careful inspections of ovarian surfaces and biopsies of any suspicious lesion or cystectomy if it can be done radically, but we have stopped performing random wedge biopsies in normal-appearing ovaries. If the tumor ruptures during surgery, or if ascites is present, our policy has been to avoid performing conservative surgery. Peritoneal washings may not contain cancer cells. Using this strategy we have observed 10 normal pregnancies. Data from Colombo et al[54] have suggested the possibility of some extension of the traditional conservative approach to patients with unfavorable factors. In the 10-year period between 1982 and 1992, Colombo et al[54] treated 99 patients younger than 40 years of age with stage I epithelial ovarian cancer, using a conservative approach in 56 cases. More specifically this approach was carried out in 36 of 56 stage IA patients (24 grade 1, 8 grade 2, and 4 grade 3), in 1 of 5 stage IB patients, and in 19 of 35 stage IC patients. Cisplatin as a single agent was given as adjuvant therapy. During a follow-up of 75 months they observed three relapses and two deaths. There were three relapses in 36 patients with conservative treatment, compared to two relapses in a group of 23 patients of the same age and with the same stage who underwent radical pelvic surgery. None of 20 patients with stage IB or IC tumors conservatively operated on relapse versus three relapses in 20 patients of the same age who underwent radical operations. Seventeen patients desired children, and there were 15 uncomplicated pregnancies with 16 healthy babies. It is probably advisable in both borderline lesions and highly differentiated invasive carcinomas to perform an annual laparoscopic examination with peritoneal washing until the woman has completed her family. Unfortunately, a common observation is that such women often have fertility problems.

QUESTION 3

Do you believe that ongoing or future clinical trials in this area should include an observation arm? Do you believe that this approach is ethical? Do any of the existing adjuvant therapies benefit patients?

CLAES TROPÉ
JANNE KAERN
IGNACE VERGOTE

The comparison of survival results in nonrandomized studies using different types of adjuvant treatment and no adjuvant treatment at all is difficult. Most prior randomized trials compared two or three different treatment modalities. However, without an untreated observation group, the efficacy of any adjuvant treatment cannot be firmly established. Only two randomized studies including a control arm have been published thus far.[41,54] In the first study of the gynecologic oncology group (GOG), only 81 patients with well or moderately differentiated tumor (FIGO 1973, stage IA or IB) were randomized between adjuvant melphalan therapy and no treatment.[41] Unfortunately, 30% of patient, were later declared on central pathology review to have tumors of borderline malignancy. The estimated 5-year survival rates for untreated patients and patients treated with melphalan were 94% and 98%, respectively (not statistically significant). This might have been expected since approximately 1,000 patients are required to detect a difference in survival of 5% at a significance level of 5% and a power of 90% when expected survival is 90%.[57]

The second study by GICOG[42,54] showed a significant disease-free survival advantage in the cisplatin group: 83% versus 64% in the untreated group. But when the control group patients were treated with cisplatin at relapse, they had the same 5-year survival as the immediate cisplatin group. This suggests that 8 of 10 women in the cisplatin group had been overtreated.[54] Since for early stages, long-term survival is the only appropriate end point, it is important to perform large, multicenter studies with long-term follow-up and quality-of-life measurements.

Only a large, prospective trial of poor-prognosis early ovarian cancer patients with an untreated control arm will be able to resolve the question of whether any adjuvant therapy contributes to survival. However, it has been very difficult to conduct such studies since patients hesitate to be randomized to a control arm with no active treatment when they are informed about the increased disease-free survival (the banana effect) with cisplatin. We find that many patients refuse to participate in such trials which include the important control arm. In spite of these difficulties, there are now three ongoing very important trials in Europe trying to determine if adjuvant treatment in high-risk patients significantly improves long-term survival.

QUESTION 4

What is your current recommendation for treatment of a high-risk stage I patient outside a protocol setting?

CLAES TROPÉ
JANNE KAERN
IGNACE VERGOTE

Prospective studies examining the effect of adjuvant treatment in early stages of ovarian cancer are few and generally include a limited number of patients. At present there is no consensus about which subgroups benefit from adjuvant therapy. When such therapy is recommended, chemotherapy is preferred. All agree that we must identify the subsets of women at highest risk of relapse who may most benefit from adjuvant therapy. Precise definition of these subsets on the basis of surgical findings, histologic grade, and tumor biology is not yet agreed upon. Treatment recommendations outside a protocol setting in stage I low- and high-risk patients from the Norwegian Radium Hospital are as follows.

1. Complete surgical staging should be performed to establish a population of patients with FIGO stage IA to IIC disease.
2. Prognostic findings should be evaluated to assess the risk of relapse. Patients with stage IA, grade 1, stage IB, grade 1, and diploid tumors do not require adjuvant therapy. On relapse we treat patients who are inoperable with paclitaxel combined with cisplatin.
3. For all grade 2 and grade tumors 3 and grade 1 aneuploid tumors the relapse rate is 25%. When clear-cell tumors are added, FIGO (1986) stage IB and IC, 32% of the patients relapsed. This rate is sufficiently high for most gynecologic oncologists to advise adjuvant chemotherapy. At the Norwegian Radium Hospital we treat these high-risk patients outside the protocol setting with paclitaxel combined with cisplatin.
4. Many but not all women with stage IC, disease require adjuvant therapy (paclitaxel combined with cisplatin).
5. Stages, IIB and IIC should be treated like stages III and IV with paclitaxel combined with cisplatin.

However, at the Norwegian Radium Hospital we try to include all high-risk patients in prospective, randomized clinical trials with active treatment versus no adjuvant treatment, since the majority of published studies have failed to demonstrate an overall survival advantage for any adjuvant approach. The Italian group (GICOG) has conducted a new large-scale prospective randomized study in stage I ovarian cancer comparing cisplatin therapy directly after surgery versus waiting until relapse.[54] In 1991, international collaborative ovarian neoplasm study group started ICON I, a trial to determine whether adjuvant platinum-based chemotherapy improves the survival of patients with early-stage epithelial ovarian cancer. ICON I will be analyzed in conjunction with the similar ACTION study being conducted by the European Organization for Research and Treatment of Cancer (EORTC). ICON I and ACTION have participating centers in Brazil Denmark, Eire, France, Italy, the Netherlands, Poland, Portugal, Spain, Switzerland, and the United Kingdom A total of 604 patients have been entered through May 1997.

In an effort to answer the question concerning the benefits of adjuvant treatment in high-risk stage I patients, we started a Scandinavian randomized trial in May 1992 in which high-risk FIGO stage I ovarian cancer patients are included. We are comparing carboplatin with a no treatment arm (Fig. 3-5). Carboplatin is used instead of cisplatin because it has been shown to be equally effective in advanced ovarian cancer and has lower ototoxic, nephrotoxic, and neurotoxic properties than cisplatin.[57–64] The carboplatin dose is set to an AUC of 7 based on the Calvert[65] formula. By December 1996 160 patients had been randomized. It has

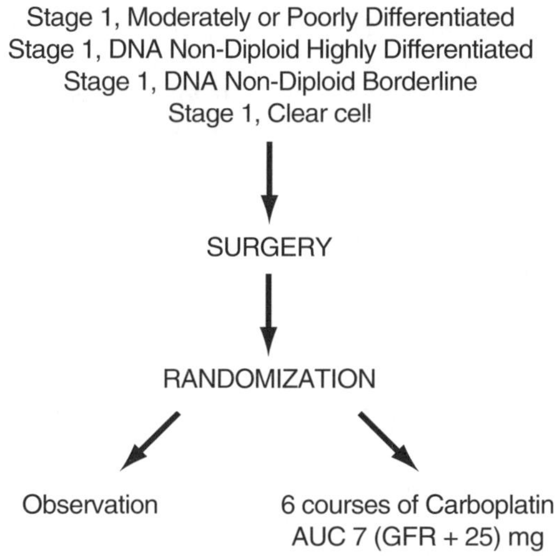

FIGURE 3-5. Study design of the Scandinavian randomized adjuvant trial on stage I ovarian carcinoma.

been very difficult to recruit patients for this study because 15 to 20% of them refuse participation because they do not want to be randomized to a control arm. It may be necessary in the future to pool all the European studies to achieve an adequate number of patients to show any significant difference in survival. This should be possible since the active treatment arm is similar in the Scandinavian, ICON I, and ACTION trials.

QUESTION 5

What are the management options for a patient referred to you after surgery for epithelial ovarian cancer apparently confined to the ovary but without adequate surgical staging? What is your recommendation?

CLAES TROPÉ
JANNE KAERN
IGNACE VERGOTE

There is little doubt that surgical resection of early-stage ovarian cancer can be curative, but there is little evidence that cytoreductive surgery improves the prognosis in advanced disease in spite of numerous studies showing that the most important independent prognostic factor is residual tumor.[66] All these data are insufficient because of selection bias. Extension of the surgical procedures required for staging of early ovarian cancer as stated above give better prognostic information.[67] In a study from Yale University[67] with FIGO stage I and II invasive ovarian carcinoma, it was shown that the strongest negative prognostic indicator was the specialty of the surgeon, with the best survival occurring in the group of patients surgically treated by a gynecologic oncologist. Considering the increased complications caused especially by pelvic and paraaortic lymph node dissection, it is questionable whether extension of a surgical procedure is always justified in stage I patients without adequate lymph node surgical staging. At the Norwegian Radium Hospital such patients have their pathological slides reviewed with DNA ploidy examined both with flow cytometry and image cytometry, postoperative 2-week CA 125 values, liver ultrasound, MR/CT pelvis and abdomen. We have shown that none of 77 patients with stage I well differentiated diploid tumors with normal liver ultrasound and pelvis/abdomen MR/CT, and normal CA 125 relapsed. This low-risk group had significantly better survival than patients with well-differentiated DNA nondiploid tumors or moderately differentiated DNA diploid tumors. At the Norwegian Radium Hospital we have performed complete staging procedures in low-risk stage I patients and found only 1% with positive nodes. Therefore, we claim that performing another laparotomy in that particular group of patients is overtreatment which also harms the patient. After the tumor has been reviewed by our pathologist, if it appears to be moderately or poorly differentiated and highly differentiated aneuploid tumors or clear-cell tumor or with a postoperative 3-week positive CA 125 value, we perform a second laparotomy within 3 weeks with a complete restaging procedure. In our experience, 40% of these patients have positive nodes and 32% of these high-risk patients relapse. This rate should be high enough for most investigators to feel that a trial of adjuvant therapy is warranted. Morphometric analysis, DNA ploidy measurements, and new prognostic factors determined by molecular biological techniques may provide prognostic information, making extensive surgical staging unnecessary.

QUESTION 6

Please discuss ongoing clinical trials and any recommendations you may have for future trials.

CLAES TROPÉ
JANNE KAERN
IGNACE VERGOTE

Intraperitoneal chemotherapy in early ovarian cancer

After the reports of Dedrick et al[68] in 1978 and Hovell et al[69] in the early 1980s, there was a trend to ward a change from palliative to curative treatment, and an increasing number of experimental and clinical reports analyzed the technique, pharmacokinetics of the different drugs used, response rate, survival and feasibility after intraperitoneal administration. Dedrick et al[69] and others[70,71] have shown that there is a great pharmacologic advantage in using intraperitoneal compared to intravenous administration of drugs defined as the ratio of peak peritoneal concentration to peak plasma concentration. Depending on several factors this advantage varies from 1 to 3 logs for different drugs.[69–72] Malmstrøm et al[72] treated 19 patients with stage I or II not previously treated with chemotherapy in a phase 1 study with the purpose of determining the maximal tolerable dose for intraperitoneal carboplatin. Seventeen patients were evaluable for toxicity. The maximum tolerable dose of carboplatin was determined to be 500 mg/m^2 which is comparable to that for previous phase-I studies. Myelosuppression, specifically thrombocytopenia, was the dose-limiting toxicity. The same group performed phase II study of intraperitoneal carboplatin as adjuvant treatment in early-stage ovarian cancer.[73] They recruited 47 patients with the purpose of determining the relapse-free interval and the toxicity. Recurrent disease was documented in 10 patients (23%); the relapse site was intra-abdominal in 7 and extra-abdominal in 1, and patients had combined intra- and extra-abdominal relapse. In this phase II study, myelosuppression, especially thrombocytopenia, was dose-limiting. The authors concluded that intraperitoneal carboplatin as a single agent in adjuvant chemotherapy for early-stage ovarian cancer showed moderate activity since the 23% relapse rate was lower than the average relapse for early-stage ovarian tumors treated with conventional techniques at their clinic. Paclitaxel has been demonstrated to produce objective antitumor response in approximately 50% of previously untreated patients with stage III disease.[74] It is an important drug to be examined for its potential role in intraperitoneal delivery. Experimental models have suggested that the activity of paclitaxel against solid human cancer depends on the concentration and duration of exposure. These features can potentially be optimized following intraperitoneal drug delivery.[75] GOG Protocol 151[76] is a phase II study of intraperitoneal paclitaxel as salvage therapy in patients with small-volume residual ovarian carcinoma after initial platinum-based chemotherapy. The results of this study can be important and can serve as a basis for future regimens using paclitaxel intraperitoneally. If this study shows positive results, paclitaxel should be investigated in patients with completely staged high-risk stage I or II ovarian carcinoma.

Is it possible to develop a new therapy that might be more effective?

A number of new treatment modalities might be used as adjuvant therapy for ovarian carcinoma, for example, monoclonal antibody–

guided therapy, intraperitoneal chemo- or immunotherapy, and treatment with new, more effective chemotherapeutic agents or radioisotopes. At our hospital we have studied α emitters such as ^{211}At, ^{212}Bi, and ^{212}Pb (which decays to the α-emitter ^{212}Bi), and they might be a useful additions in the future treatment of small clusters of cancer cells. The high linear energy transfer and five to seven cell-diameter pathlength of the α particles ejected by ^{211}At or ^{212}Bi make these radionuclides interesting for the treatment of tumors in which most clonogenic cells are accessible after intracavitaru injection of the isotopes. The choice of a suitable α-emitter is limited largely because many have unsuitable physical half-lives or highly toxic daughter products. ^{211}At decays with a half-life of 7.2 hours and has two acceptable daughters,^{211}Po and ^{207}Bi, both of which decay to stable lead.[77] In order to investigate whether the physical advantage of α emitters might lead to better treatment, Vergote et al[78,79] developed an intraperitoneal tumor model using hybridoma cells in mice, established a method for labelling polymer microspheres with ^{211}At, investigated the distribution of intraperitoneally injected ^{211}At microspheres in comparison with ^{32}P and ^{90}Y colloids in mice, and compared the therapeutic efficacy of ^{211}At microspheres with that of ^{32}P and ^{90}Y colloids in the hybridoma tumor model. The study showed that the labelling of polymer microspheres with ^{211}At was successful, that the intraperitoneal distribution of ^{211}At microspheres in mice was favorable, and that the therapeutic efficacy in an intraperitoneal hybridoma tumor model was encouraging compared with that of ^{32}P and ^{90}Y colloids. However, caution is warranted because the results obtained in a hybridoma tumor model in mice may not be transposable to humans. Future studies on ^{211}At microspheres will have to evaluate their efficacy on human-derived tumor cells in vitro and in vivo, compare the results with those for ^{211}At-labelled monoclonal antibody treatment and determine their toxicity in other animal species.[79–80]

The relapse rate for high-risk stage I or II patients is noted above, to be as high as 60%. Despite different postoperative adjuvant chemotherapy regimens, a significant improvement in long-term survival in these patients has not been achieved during the past 20 years. Therefore, we should look into other systemic treatment modalities. Ovarian carcinoma is an extremely chemosensitive tumor, and several studies have demonstrated a clinically important dose-response relationship for cisplatin.[80] Dose intensity of chemotherapeutic agents with autologous bone marrow transplantation (ABMT) is important to achieve long-term survival in chemosensitive malignancies such as Hodgkins and non-Hodgkins lymphoma. However, the morbidity and mortality of ABMT has steered investigators away from using high-dose chemotherapy as part of the initial treatment for ovarian cancer. High-dose chemotherapy with peripheral hematopoietic cell support (PBPC) should be tested upfront in patients with stage I poor prognosis. Results from trials using PBPC[81–82] in patients with recurrent disease has encouraged the use of such aggressive treatment upfront. High-dose chemotherapy with PBPC stem cell support should be tested in patients with high-risk stage IA and II ovarian cancer. At the Norwegian Radium Hospital we are planning to test high-dose chemotherapy carboplatin approaches requiring cytokines, autologous bone marrow support, or peripheral blood stem cell transfusion in patients with stage I and II cancer.

EDITORS' COMMENTARY

Dr. Tropé and his collegues have masterfully outlined the various prognostic factors currently used to separate patients into low and high-risk groups. They demonstrate the problem with the current system which uses factors that are poorly reproducible (stage and grade) and Dr. Tropé cites his own data in which DNA ploidy is second only to grade in terms of prognosis. We agree that the current system for defining risk groups in early disease is suboptimal, at best, and encourage an international forum on this area, perhaps under the auspices of FIGO, to clarify these issues and move toward a more standard classification of risk using, as much as possible, reproducible and easily measurable parameters. While we agree that the use of molecular biologic probes (p53, PGDF, and BCL-2/BAX ratios) is of interest, there are insufficient data relating to prognosis and a lack of widespread availability of these tests, making it inappropriate to recommend them at this time.

A quick synopsis of the trials leads Dr. Tropé et al to conclude that patients with early stage (IA or IB) and low- or moderate-grade tumors not be further treated after a *complete* staging procedure. With this we agree. They also state that all patients with stage II disease deserve adjunctive therapy. Although there is an obvious tendency to do this since 40 to 60% of these patients eventually relapse and die, there still is *no* firm randomized data suggesting that one therapy is better than another therapy, bringing into question the value of each. Only the recently published Italian study, which needs several more years of maturity, begins to suggest an outcome benefit for patients treated with systemic therapy. We feel a safe approach with such patients is to put them on a study protocol to learn more about proper treatment of this disease. When this is not possible, the use of platinum-based chemotherapy seems to have a better therapeutic index than treatment with single alkylating agents (nonrandomized data) and may delay or prevent recurrence in a small subset of patients. To date there are *no* data supporting the routine use of combination therapy in early stage, high-risk patients, however, as paclitaxel becomes more firmly established as part of primary therapy, the use of platinum and paclitaxel together will likely be tried. This seems reasonable because each is active as a single agent and there is evidence of synergism between the two in combination.

For the treatment of patients outside a protocol setting, the authors recommend a combination of paclitaxel and cisplatin. It is important to note that this is an extrapolation from data on much more advanced disease and should (if our understanding of cytotoxic therapy is correct in concluding the low tumor burdens are more successfully treated than larger ones) be very active in the high-risk early-stage patient. Randomized studies incorporating paclitaxel, however, are only 3 to 4 years old and none has matured to a degree to allow a comment about efficacy. Although there is good scientific rationale for this approach, there are not as yet supportive data from the literature. We agree, however, with Dr. Tropé et al that it is ethically difficult to recommend no therapy to a patient with a 50% chance of recurrence and death even without data indicating that the proffered therapy alters the prognosis.

In terms of re-exploring the early-stage patient who had inadequate staging before referral, Dr. Tropé's approach is a unique one. If the patient has a well-differentiated tumor, the tumor is diploid, the CA 125 is normal, and ultrasound of the abdomen and liver are normal, then no further surgery and no further treatment are offered. None of 77 patients in this group has relapsed in his series. Aneuploid tumor, persistent elevation of CA 125, and moderate to poor differentiation lead to re-exploration and complete staging. Approximately 32% of this latter group develops recurrent disease. What is not discussed in regard to this group of patients is whether data generated by the second surgical procedure ever dictates subsequent therapy. If the answer is no, then the value of the procedure must be called into question. The only situation in which re-exploration may be of help is in determining response to therapy. If a third laparotomy discloses disease that was not there after the second procedure, then the patient has drug-resistant persistence and needs alternate therapy. If the residual disease at third look is at the same site as before and smaller, then drug-sensitive disease is present and high-dose approaches (ABMT or IP therapy) may be indicated. This is a very rare situation in clinical practice. Thus, we feel the role for re-exploring improperly staged patients is seldom.

We agree with the authors that the use of intraperitoneal therapy is rational in patients with high-risk early disease. The recent report from Alberts showing survival advantage for small-volume stage III patients when intraperitoneal cisplatin was substituted for intravenous cisplatin is interesting and may require further study. It makes sense to try such therapy in even earlier disease, particularly now that emerging data show that systemic platinum results in modestly improved disease-free survival when compared to more conventional therapy. Likewise, paclitaxel has good activity and safety by the intraperitoneal route and also should be explored for use in early disease. It appears that the therapeutic index of paclitaxel will be better than that of cisplatin. Dr. Tropé and collegues also mention ABMT in the setting of small-volume disease. We agree that autologous transplant is feasible, however, there are as yet no randomized trials showing that it is superior to more standard forms of salvage therapy. A recently activated intergroup study, GOG protocol 164, selects patients with both drug-sensitive and small-volume disease disease following primary therapy and randomizes them to six additional courses of standard salvage therapy or ABMT following very high doses of carboplatin (AUC 28), cyclophosphamide (120 mg/kg), and mitoxantrone (75 mg/m^2). We encourage investigators worldwide to participate in this or similar trials to answer the important question of whether this approach is worth the toxicity and expense in terms of improving long-term survival.

It would be preferable to know best how to treat early-stage ovarian cancer. Unfortunately, because of the reasons enumerated above, we still have much to learn. Extrapolating from the breast cancer story, however, the use of active drugs in an advanced disease setting in a high-risk adjuvant setting has now clearly shown a reduction in recurrence in some subsets of patients. Such studies are much easier in breast cancer where there are seven to eight times the number of patients available for study, making trials quick to accrue and generate outcomes. Of interest, in the last early-stage ovarian trial the GOG has noted an accrual three-fold higher than in previous studies. Whether this a real shift in investigator commitment to such trials, a shift of the disease to more early presentations, or an internet effect (patients armed with data demand trial participation from physicians) is an unclear but happy state of affairs. We encourage all physicians to consider early ovarian cancer in a woman 40+ years old with an adnexal mass and make certain the appropriate surgery is performed to allow the patient to enter one of the important on-going trials so that a decade from now we will have a more in-depth understanding of how best to treat this disease.

References

1. Boring CC, Squires TS, Tong T: Cancer statistics 1993. Ca Cancer J Clin 43:7–26, 1993
2. Petterson F: Annual report on the results of treatment in gynecological cancer. Vol. 21: Statements of the results obtained in patients, 1982 to 1986, inclusive 3- and 5-year survival upto 1990. Int J Gynecol Obstet suppl:238–255, 1991.
3. Cancer Registry of Norway, Institute for epidemiological cancer research, 1990
4. Makar A: Prognostic studies in cancer of the ovary and fallopian tube with emphasis on the CA125 antigen and c-erB 2 oncogene. Thesis. The University of Oslo, Norway, 1993
5. Dembo AJ, Davy M, Stenwig AE, Berle EJ et al: Prognostic factors in patients with stage I epithelial ovarian cancer. Obstet Gynecol 75:263, 1990
6. Bertelsen K, Hølund B, Andersen JE, Nielsen K et al: Prognostic factors and adjuvant treatment in early epithelial ovarian cancer. Int J Gynecol Cancer 3:211, 1993
7. Finn CB, Luesly DM, Buxton EJ, Blackledge GR et al: Is stage I epithelial ovarian cancer treated both surgically and systematically? Results of a 5-year cancer registry review. Br J Obstet Gynecol 99:54, 1992
8. Young RC, Walton LA, Ellenberg SS et al: Adjuvant therapy in stage I and stage II epithelial ovarian cancer: Results of two prospective randomized trials. N Eng J Med 322:1021, 1990

9. Bertelsen K, Hølund B, Andersen JE: Reproducibility and prognostic value of histologic type and grade in early epithelial ovarian cancer. Int J Gynecol Cancer 3:72, 1993

10. Trimbos JB, Bolis G, Pecorelli S: The surgical staging of ovarian cancer—current practice in 15 European countries. Int J Gynecol Cancer 1:89, 1991

11. Russell P, Bannatyne P: Surgical pathology of the ovaries. Churchill Livingstone Edinburgh, 1989

12. Atkin NB, Kay R: Prognostic significance of modal DNA value and other factors in malignant tumors, based on 1465 cases. Br J Cancer 10:210, 1979

13. Iversen OE, Skaarland E: Ploidy assessment of benign and malignant ovarian tumors by flow cytometry: a clinicopathologic study. Cancer 60:82, 1987

14. Baak LJ, Lindeman J, Overdiep SH, Langley FA: Disagreement of histopathological diagnosis of different pathologists in a ovarian tumors—with some theoretical considerations. Eur J Obstet Gynecol Reprod Biol 13:51, 1982

15. Vergote IB, Kaern J, Abeler VM, Pettersen OE et al: Analysis of prognostic factors in stage I epithelial ovarian cancer. Importance of degree of differentiation and deoxyribonucleiod acid ploidy in predicting relapse. Am J Obstet Gynecol 169:40, 1993

16. Allen DG, Baak J, Belpomme D, Derek J et al: Advanced epithelial ovarian cancer: 1993 consensus statement. Ann Oncol 4 (suppl 4):S83, 1993

17. Henriksen R, Runa K, Wilander E, Bäckstöm T et al: Expression and prognostic significance of platelet-derived growth factor and its receptors in epithelial ovarian neoplasms. Cancer Res 53:4550, 1993

18. Henriksen R, Strang P, Bäckstöm T et al: Ki-67 immunostaining DNA flow cytometry in epithelial ovarian cancers as determinants of tumor proliferation and prognosis. Anticancer Res 14:603, 1994

19. Lane DP, Crawford LV: T antigen is bound to a host protein in SV40-transsformed cells. Nature 278:261, 1991

20. Linzer DIH, Levine AJ: Characterization of a 54K dalton cellular SV40 tumor antigen present in SV40-transformed cells and uninfected embryonal carcinoma cells. Cell 17:43, 1979

21. Deleo AB, Jay G, Apella E, Dubois GC, et al: Detection of a transformation-related antigen in chemically induced sarcomas and other transformed cells of the mouse. Proc Natl Acad Sci USA 76:2420, 1979

22. Jacobs IJ, Kohler MF, Wiseman RW, Marks JR et al: Clonal origin of epithelial ovarian carcinoma: analysis by loss of heterozygosity, p53 mutation and X-chromosome inactivation. J Natl Cancer Inst 84:1793, 1992

23. Mok CH, Tsao SW, Knapp RC, Fishbaugh PM et al: Unifocal origin of advanced epithelial ovarian cancers. Cancer Res 53:2128, 1993

24. Milner BJ, Allan LA, Eccles DM, Kitchener HC et al: p53 mutation is a common genetic event in ovarian carcinoma. Cancer Res 53:2128, 1993

25. Henriksen R, Strang P, Wilander E, Bäckström T et al: p53 expression in epithelial ovarian neoplasms: relationship to clinical and pathological parameters, Ki-67 expression and flow cytometry. Gyn Oncol 53:301, 1994

26. Skomedal H, Kristensen G, Abeler V, Børresen AL et al: TP53 protein accumulation and gene mutation in relation to overexpression of MDM 2 protein in ovarian borderline tumors and stage I carcinoma. J of Pathology 181:158, 1997

27. Hockenbery D, Nunez G, Milliman C, Schreiber RD et al: Bcl-2 is an inner mitochondrial membrane protein that blocks programmed cell death. Nature 358:334, 1990

28. McDonnel TJ, Deane N, Platt FM et al: bcl-2 immunoglobulin transgenic mice demonstrate extended B cell survival and follicular lymphoproliferation. Cell 57: 79, 1989

29. Henriksen R, Wilander E, Öberg K: Expression and prognostic significance of Bcl-2 in ovarian tumors. Cancer Res 53:4550, 1993

30. Piver MS, Malfetano J, Hempling RE, Baker TR et al: Cisplatin-based chemotherapy for stage II ovarian adenocarcinoma: a preliminary report. Gynecol Oncol 39:249, 1990

31. Vergote IB, Vergote-De Vos LN, Abeler VM et al: Randomized trial comparing cisplatin with radioactive phosphorus or whole abdominal irradiation as adjuvant treatment of ovarian cancer. Cancer 69:741, 1992

32. Sigurdsson K, Johansson JE, Tropé C: Carcinoma of the ovary stage I and II: a prospective randomized study of the effects of post-operative chemotherapy and radiotherapy. Ann Chir Gynaecol 71:321, 1982

33. Young RC: Editorial. Gynecol Oncol 43:193, 1991

34. Kolstad P, Davy M, Hoeg K: Individualised treatment of ovarian cancer. Am J Obstet Gynecol 128:617, 1982

35. Davy M, Stenwig AE, Kjoerstad KE et al: Early stage ovarian cancer. Acta Obstet Gynecol Scand 64:531, 1985

36. Smith JP, Rutledge FN, Declos L: Postoperative treatment of early cancer of the ovary: a random trial between posoperative irradiation and chemotherapy. J Natl Cancer Inst 42:149, 1975

37. Dembo AJ, Bush RS, Beale FA, Bean HA et al: Ovarian carcinoma: Improved survival following abdominopelvic irradiation in patients with a completed pelvic operation. Am J Obstet Gynecol 134:793, 1979

38. Klaassen D, Shelley W, Starrevel A, Kirk M et al: Early stage ovarian cancer: a randomized clinical trial comparing whole abdominal radiotherapy, melphalan, and intraperitoneal chromic phosphate: a National Cancer Institute of Cancada Clinical Trials Group Report. J Clin Oncol 6: 1254, 1988

39. Sell A, Bertelsen K, Andersen JE, Stryer I et al: Randomized study of whole-abdomen irradiation versus pelvic irradiation plus cyclophosphamide in treatment of early ovarian cancer. Gynecol Oncol 37:367, 1990

40. Hreshenchyshyn MM, Park, RC, Blessing JA, Norris HJ et al: The role of adjuvant therapy in stage I ovarian cancer. Am J Obstet Gynecol 138:139, 1980

41. Young RC, Walton LA, Ellenberg SS, Homesley GD et al: Adjuvant therapy in stage I and II epithelial ovarian cancer: results of two prospective randomized trials. N Engl J Med 322:1021, 1990

42. Bolis G, Colombo N, Pecorelli S, Torri V et al: Randomized multicenter clinical trial in stage I epithelial cancer. Ann Oncol 9:887, 1995

43. Vergote IB, Winderen M, De Vos L, Tropé C: Intraperitoneal radioactive phosphorus therapy in ovarian cancer: analysis of 313 patients treated primarily or by second-look laparotomy. Cancer 71:2250, 1993

44. Hester LL, White L: Radioactive colloidal chromic phosphate in the treatment of ovarian malignancies. Am J Obstet Gynecol 103:911, 1968

45. Soper JT, Berchuk A, Clarke Pearson DL: Adjuvant intraperitoneal chromic phosphate therapy for women with apparent early ovarian carcinoma who have not undergone comprehensive surgical staging. Cancer 68:725, 1991

46. Reimer RR, Hoover R, Fraumeni JF Jr, Young RC: Acute leukemia after alkylating-agent therapy of ovarian cancer. N Engl J Med 297:177, 1977

47. Greene MH, Boice JD, Greer BE, Blessing JA et al: Acute nonlymphocytic leu-

kemia after therapy with alkylating agents for ovarian cancer. N Engl J Med 307:1416, 1982

48. Kaldo RHM, Day NE, Petterson F, Clarke EA et al: Leukemia following chemotherapy for ovarian cancer. N Engl J Med 322:1, 1990
49. Young RC, Walton LA, Ellenbergh SS, Homesley H et al: Prognostic factors for survival in stage I epithelial carcinoma. Cancer 65:2349, 1990
50. Leopold WR, Miller EC, Miller EA: Carcinogenicity of antitumor cis-platinum (II) coordination complexes in the mouse and rat. Cancer Res 39:913, 1979
51. Pedersen-Bjergaard J, Røorth M, Avnstrøom S, Philip P et al: Acute nonlymphocytic leukemia following treatment of testicular and gastric cancer with combination chemotherapy not including alkylating agents: report of two cases. Am J Hematol 18:425, 1985
52. Kempf SR, Ivankovic S: Chemotherapy-induced malignancies in rats after treatment with cisplatin as single agent and in combination: preliminary results. Oncology, 43:187, 1986
53. Chambers SK, Chopyk RL, Chambers JT, Schwartz PE et al: Development of leukemia after doxorubicin and cisplatin treatment for ovarian cancer. Cancer 64:2459, 1989
54. Colombo N, Chari S, Maggioni A, Bocciolone L et al: Controversial issues in the management of early epithelial ovarian cancer: conservative surgery and role of adjuvant therapy. Gynecol. Oncol. 55:47, 1994
55. Kolstad P, Tropé C: Preservation of ovarian function in the treatment of epithelial and specialized malignant tumors of the ovary: atti del convegno internazionale i tumori della gonadi. Workshop “Inuovi Farmaci” Ancona-Jesi 23–26 Sept, 1987. Ed Monduzzi 321, 1987
56. Weinstein D, Polishuk WZ: The role of wedge resection of the ovary as a cause for mechanical sterility. Surg Obstet Gynecol 141:417, 1975
57. Freedman LS: Tables of the number of patients required in clinical trials using the long rank test. State Med 1:121, 1982
58. Perren TJ, Gore ME, Fryatt I, Wiltshaw E: High dose (hd) carboplatin (jm8) for stage 4 ovarian carcinoma: a preliminary analysis of response, toxicity and survival (meeting abstract). Proc Annu Meet Am Soc Clin Oncol 7:A568, 1988
59. McVie JG, Ten Bokkel Huinink WW, Hilton A et al: Carboplatin and cylcophosphamide in relapsing ovarian cancer patients (meeting abstract) Proc Annu Meet Am Soc Clin Oncol 8:A629, 1989
60. Ten Bokkel Huinink WW, van der Burg ME, Van Oosterom TT, Neijt JP et al: Carboplatin in combination therapy for ovarian cancer. Cancer Treat Rep 15: suppl B9, 1988
61. Advanced Ovarian Cancer Trials Group. Chemotherapy in advanced cancer: an overview of randomized trials. Br Med J 303:884, 1991
62. Alberts D, Green S, Hannigan E, O’Toole R et al: Improved efficacy of carboplatin (carbop)/cyclophosphamide (cpa) vs cisplatin (cisp)/cpa: preliminary report of a phase III, randomized trial in stages III–IV, suboptimal ovarian cancer (ov ca) (meeting abstract). Proc Annu Meet Am Soc Clin Oncol 8:A588, 1989
63. Pater J: cyclophosphamide (c)/cisplatin (cddp) versus c/carboplatin (cbdca) in macroscopic residual ovarian cancer: initial results of a national cancer institute of Canada clinical trials group trial (meeting abstract). Proc Annu Meet Am Soc Clin Oncol 9:A602, 1990
64. Meerphol HG, Sauerbrei W, Kuhnle H, Pfleiderer A: Cyclophosphamide/carboplatin (CTX/Carbo PT) versus cisplatin (CTX/PT) in patients with small volume stage III/IV ovarian cancer: an interim analysis report by the German Ovarian Cancer Study Group (GOCA). In Hacker N (ed) 3rd Biennial Meet Int Gynecol Cancer Soc. Cairns: Gynecol Cancer Soc, Abstr 199, 1991.

65. Calvert AH, Newell DR, Gumbrell LA, Burnell M et al: Prospective evaluation of a simple formula based on renal function. J Clin Oncol 7:1748, 1989
66. Girling JC, Souter WP: Cytoreductive surgery in the primary management of advanced epithelial ovarian carcinoma: a topic for debate. Int J Gynecol Cancer 6:81, 1996
67. Mayer AR, Chamber SK, Graves E, Holm C et al: Ovarian cancer staging: Does it require a gynecological oncologist? Gynecol Oncol 47:223, 1992
68. Dedrick RL, Myers CE, Bungay PM et al: Pharmacokinetic rationale for peritoneal drug administration in the treatment of ovarian cancer. Cancer Treat Rep, 62:1, 1978
69. Howell SB, Zimm S, Markman M et al: Long-term survival of advanced refractory ovarian carcinoma patients with small volume disease treated with intraperitoneal chemotherapy. J Clin Oncol 5:1607, 1987
70. Howell SB, Zimm S, Cleary S, Andrews PA et al: Phase I/pharmacokinetic study of intraperitoneal (IP) cisplatin (DDP) and etoposide (VP-16). Abstr 5th NCI-EORTC Symp, Amsterdam, 1988
71. Collins JM: Pharmacokinetic rationale for regional drug delivery. J Clin Oncol 2:498, 1984
72. Malmström H, Larsson D, Simonsen E: Phase I study of intraperitoneal carboplatin as adjuvant therapy in early ovarian cancer. Gynecol Oncol 39:289, 1990
73. Malmstöm H, Simonsen E, Westberg R: A phase II study of intraperitoneal carboplatin as adjuvant treatment in early stage ovarian cancer patients. Gynecol Oncol, 52:20, 1992
74. Tropé C, Sorbe B, Simonsen E, Bertelsen K et al: A phase II, nonrandomized study of single-agent paclitaxel (Taxol) in patients with previously untreated FIGO stage III, suboptimally resected ovarian cancer: a preliminary report. Int J Gynecol Cancer suppl 1 4:7, 1994
75. Rowinsky EK, Donehower RC, Jones RJ et al: Microtubule changes and cytotoxicity in leukemic cell lines treated with taxol. Cancer Res 48: 4093, 1990
76. Thigpen T, Vance R, McGuire W, Hoskins W et al: The role of paclitaxel in the management of coelomic epithelial carcinoma of the ovary: a review with emphasis on the gynecology group of experience. Semin Oncol 22:6, suppl 14:23, 1995
77. Munzel F: Nuclear properties of astatine isotopes. In Pietsch EHE, Kotowski A, Becke-Goering M (eds) Gmelin handbook of inorganic chemistry: astatine, atomic number 85. Springer Verlag, Berlin, 15:1985
78. Vergote I, Larsen R, DeVos L, Nesland J et al: Distribution of intraperitoneally injected microspheres labelled with the α-emitter astatine (^{211}A) compared with phosphorus (^{32}P) and yttrium ^{90}Y] colloids in mice. Gynecol Oncol 47:358, 1992
79. Vergote I, Larsen R, De Vos L, Nesland J et al: Therapeutic efficacy of the α-emitter ^{211}At bound on microspheres compared with ^{90}Y and (^{32}P) colloids in a murine intraperitoneal tumor model. Gynecol Oncol 14:366, 1992
80. Levin L, Hryniuk WM: Dose-intensity analyses of chemotherapy regimens in ovarian cancer. J Clin Oncol 5:757, 1987
81. Benedetti-Panici P, Greggi S, Scambia G et al: Very high dose chemotherapy (VHDC) with autologous peripheral stem cells (SPSC) as hematologic support (HS) in previously untreated ovarian cancer (AOC). Proc Soc Gynecol Oncol 30, 1995
82. Fenelly D, Schneiden J, Bengala C et al: Escalating-dose Taxol Plus high-dose (HD) cyclophosphamide (C) carboplatin (CBDCA) plus C rescued with peripheral blood progenitor cells (PBP) in patients with stage IIC-IV ovarian cancer (OC). Gynecol Oncol 56:121, 1995

CHAPTER 4

PRIMARY CYTOREDUCTIVE SURGERY FOR ADVANCED-STAGE DISEASE

William J. Hoskins
Frank G. Lawton

EDITORS' INTRODUCTION

For a patient suspected of having ovarian cancer, primary surgery accomplishes the following goals: (1) confirmation of the diagnosis of ovarian cancer, (2) precise determination of extent of disease (i.e., comprehensive surgical staging), and (3) maximum cytoreductive surgery in patients with advanced disease. Primary cytoreductive or debulking surgery refers to a surgical procedure for which the goal is to reduce the amount of tumor as much as possible in a patient with metastatic ovarian cancer. Early studies suggested a relationship between the completeness of the surgery or the extent of residual tumor and survival. Subsequently, Griffiths and others confirmed an inverse relationship between residual tumor diameter and survival; patients having residual disease no greater than 1 to 2 cm in diameter had a significantly improved survival compared with patients with bulky residual disease. As the philosophy about cytoreductive surgery has evolved over the last two decades, *optimal debulking* has come to denote minimal residual disease no greater than 1 to 2 cm in diameter; *suboptimal debulking* denotes bulky residual disease greater than 1 to 2 cm in diameter.

Several reports have described the accomplishment of optimal cytoreductive surgery in a high percentage of patients, as high as 98% of those operated on by gynecologic oncologists, although the overall estimate is probably closer to 50%. The primary question concerning the efficacy of primary cytoreductive surgery is whether improved survival is related more to the biology of the tumor or to the skill and aggressiveness of the surgeon. In other words, are those tumors that can be debulked optimally also tumors that are less invasive, less infiltrative, and more indolent? Although most experts currently assume that both tumor biology and surgical intervention have an effect on survival, very little is understood about the relative influence of these factors.

Unfortunately, prospective information is insufficient to permit resolution of important issues in this area. Moreover, prospects for randomized clinical trials are limited because of several factors, including deeply established biases, the multiplicity of associated prognostic factors, and the highly individualized nature of each procedure. On the other hand, major academic centers and cooperative research groups are beginning to re-examine the role of primary cytoreductive surgery.

The questions posed to our experts attempt to address several important issues, including selection of patients for primary treatment other than surgery (i.e., neoadjuvant chemotherapy), the relative influences of tumor biology and surgery, the role of primary debulking in patients with presumed stage IV disease, optimal guidelines for referral of patients with possible ovarian cancer to gynecologic oncologists, and degree of aggressiveness of primary debulking.

QUESTIONS

1. Are there any factors that may be identified in the preoperative evaluation of a woman with probable epithelial ovarian cancer that would cause you to recommend against primary surgery (i.e., neoadjuvant chemotherapy instead)?
2. In patients with advanced-stage disease, which factor is more important—tumor biology or surgical intervention? Are there clinical trials that could be designed to determine the relative effects of these two factors?
3. Which women with a pelvic mass should be referred to a gynecologic oncologist for primary surgery? What is the role, if any, of diagnostic laparoscopy prior to referral?
4. Is there any role for cytoreductive surgery in patients with stage IV disease? If so, which stage IV patients?
5. What factors should influence the degree of aggressiveness during primary cytoreductive surgery? How does one balance the desire to achieve optimal cytoreduction and the risk of morbidity? If, at the time of surgical exploration, one determines that optimal cytoreduction is not possible, should any surgical cytoreduction be performed?

QUESTION 1

Are there any factors that may be identified in the preoperative evaluation of a woman with probable epithelial ovarian cancer that would cause you to recommend against primary surgery? (i.e., neoadjuvant chemotherapy instead)

WILLIAM J. HOSKINS

The currently accepted management of epithelial ovarian cancer is primary cytoreductive surgery followed by combination chemotherapy with paclitaxel and a platinum compound.[1] Although there are no hard data to support this particular regimen, it is usually administered in five to six courses. The theoretical value of primary cytoreductive surgery has been outlined by several investigators.[2–9] The central feature of the theoretical benefit is the removal of large tumor masses, which have a poor blood supply and are in the portion of the Gompertzian growth cycle where growth has slowed, leaving small tumors that are more sensitive to chemotherapy. This has been proved by multiple studies documenting improved response rates (Table 4-1), longer progression-free survival (Table 4-2), improved survival (Table 4-3), and more frequent negative second-look surgical evaluations (Table 4-4) in patients with minimal residual disease. Figure 4-1 is a composite of Gynecologic Oncology Group (GOG) protocols 52 (optimal disease) and 97

TABLE 4-1
Effect of Residual Disease After Primary Cytoreductive Surgery on Response Rate in Advanced Ovarian Cancer

STUDY/YEAR	AGENT	NO.	RESIDUAL (CM)	RESPONSE (%) COMPLETE	TOTAL
Young et al (1978)	HexaCAF vs L-PAM	19	<2		84
		58	≥2		53
Ehrich et al (1979)	PAC	14	<3	46	78
		25	≥3	32	54
Wharton and Herson (1981)	L-PAM	45	<2	12	29
		59	≥2	8	24
Conte et al (1986)	CAP vs CP	37	<2	70	76
		38	≥2	32	82
Total/mean		115	Optimal	42.7	66.8
		180	Suboptimal	24.0	53.3

Abbreviations: HexaCAF, hexamethylmelamine, cyclophosphamide, amethopterin, 5-fluorouracil; PAC, Platinol cisplatin, Adriamycin, cyclophosphamide; L-PAM: melphalan; CAP vs CP, cisplatin, Adriamycin, cyclophosphamide versus cisplatin, cyclophosphamide. (From Hoskins,[8] with permission.)

(suboptimal disease) that demonstrate the clear relationship of residual disease to survival.[7,10,11] These survival curves do not address the issue of biology versus surgery. By contrast, in reviewing GOG protocol 97, Hoskins and colleagues[11] showed that only initial surgical cytoreduction of ovarian cancer to a residual disease volume of less than 2 cm had a significant effect on survival; there was no benefit for patients who underwent cytoreduction but who were left with residual disease of greater than 2 cm. This implies that if initial cytoreductive surgery to "optimal" disease is not possible, patients will not benefit from initial surgical cytoreduction. The importance of residual tumor volume has been further underscored by

TABLE 4-2
Effect of Primary Cytoreductive Surgery on Progression-Free Interval in Advanced Ovarian Cancer

STUDY/YEAR	AGENT	NO.	RESIDUAL (CM)	MEDIAN PROGRESSION-FREE INTERVAL
Vogl et al (1983)	CHAP	32	<2	38
		68	≥2	12
Redman et al (1986)	CAP	34	<3	23
		51	≥3	14
Piver et al (1988)	PAC	35	<2	25
		5	≥2	13
Omura et al (1989)	CAP vs CP	99	<1	48
		250	≥1	21
Total/mean		200	Optimal	33.5
		374	Suboptimal	15.0

Abbreviations: CHAP, cyclophosphamide, hexamethylmelamine, Adriamycin, cisplatin; CAP, cisplatin, Adriamycin, cyclophosphamide; PAC: cisplatin, Adriamycin, cyclophosphamide; CP, cisplatin, cyclophosphamide. (From Hoskins,[8] with permission.)

TABLE 4-3
The Effect of Residual Disease at the Conclusion of Primary Cytoreductive Surgery on Survival

STUDY/YEAR	AGENT	NO.	RESIDUAL (CM)	SURVIVAL (MO)
Griffiths (1975)	L-PAM	29	0	39
		28	0–0.5	29
		16	0.6–1.5	18
		29	>1.5	11
Hacker et al (1983)	Varied	7	≤0.5	40
		24	0.6–1.5	18
		16	>1.5	6
Vogl et al (1983)	CHAP	32	<2	>40
		68	≥2	16
Pohl et al (1984)	Varied	37	<2	45
		57	≥2	16
Delgado et al (1984)	Varied	21	<2	45
		54	≥2	16
Redman et al (1986)	CAP	34	<3	38
		51	≥3	26
Conte et al (1986)	CAP vs CP	37	<2	>40
		38	≥2	16
Neijt et al (1987)	CHAP vs CP	88	<1	40
		219	≥1	21
Piver et al (1988)	PAC	35	<2	48
		5	≥2	21
Total/mean		388	Optimal	36.7
		537	Suboptimal	16.6

Abbreviations: L-PAM, melphalan; CHAP, cyclophosphamide, hexamethylmelamine, Adriamycin, cisplatin; CAP, cisplatin, Adriamycin, cyclophosphamide; CP, cisplatin, cyclophosphamide; PAC, cisplatin, Adriamycin, cyclophosphamide. (From Hoskins,[8] with permission.)

phase II trials from Memorial Sloan-Kettering Cancer and phase III trials by the European Organization for Research on Treatment of Cancer (EORTC), which seem to indicate that "interval" cytoreduction can result in improved progression-free intervals and improved overall survival. In the Memorial Sloan-Kettering series, Brown et al[12] showed that initial cytoreduction, or the combination of initial cytoreduction and induction chemotherapy, or interval cytoreduction resulted in equal survival providing the patient's disease was rendered optimal by one of these modalities. In a randomized trial, the EORTC showed that interval cytoreduction improved both progression-free survival and overall survival.[13]

The logical conclusion from these studies is that if it is not possible to perform initial surgical cytoreduction to an optimal level, initial surgery should be foregone, with induction chemotherapy administered instead followed by interval cytoreduction. This leads to the critical question: can we identify a population of patients who may not benefit from primary cytoreductive surgery? On the basis of the report by Hoskins et al[7] if one accepts the lack of benefit of less than optimal cytoreduction, any presurgical evaluation that indicates an inability to cytoreduce the patient to optimal disease would permit identification of a group of patients for whom initial cytoreduction is inadvisable. There will certainly be the occasional patient for whom preoperative evaluation will

TABLE 4-4
The Effect of Primary Cytoreductive Surgery on the Result of Second-look Surgical Reassessment in Ovarian Cancer

STUDY/YEAR	NO.	PERCENT NEGATIVE		
		NONE	OPTIMAL	SUBOPTIMAL
Curry (1981)	27	76	33	33
Webb (1982)	59	95	36	20
Cohen (1983)	73	73	35	34
Barnhill (1984)	96	67	61	14
Podratz (1985)	135	82	44	39
Smirtz (1985)	88	75	37	19
Cain (1986)	177	76	50	28
Dauplat (1986)	51	85	73	19
Gallup (1987)	65	71	63	13
Carmichael (1987)	146	62	30	25
Lund (1990)	131	77	55	25
Ayhan (1991)	49	92	61	15
Total/mean	1,097	77.6	48.2	23.7

(From Hoskins,[8] with permission.)

FIGURE 4-1. Survival by residual disease, GOG protocols 52 (optimal disease) and 97 (suboptimal disease). (From Hoskins,[7] with permission.)

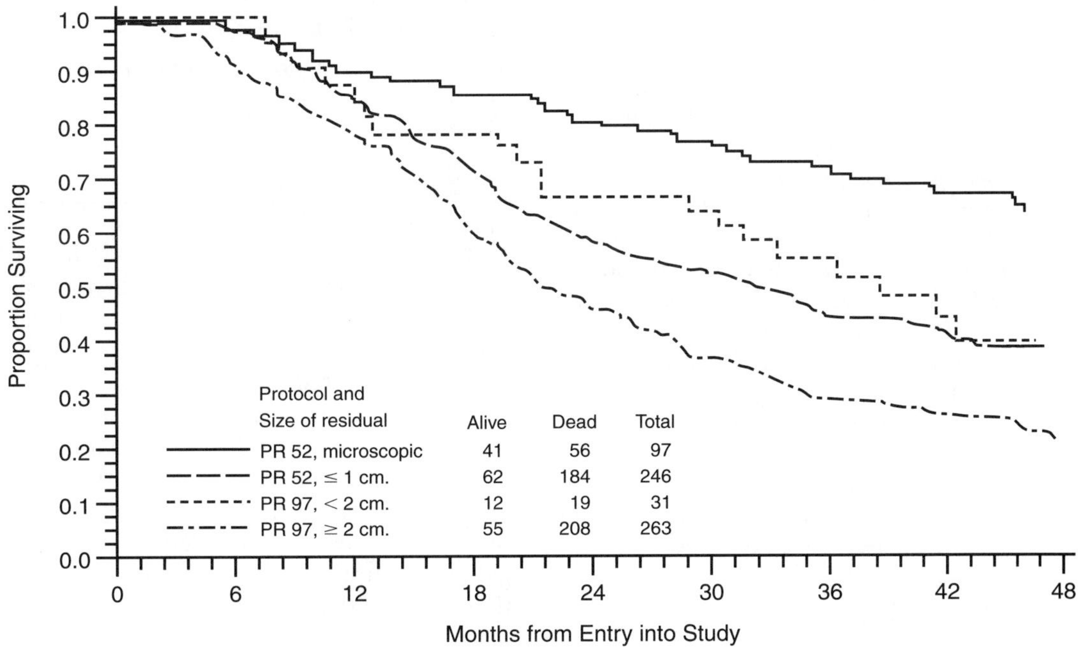

document unrespectable disease, such as liver metastases or parenchmal lung involvement. Fortunately, such cases are rare. In the vast majority of patients, disease is limited to the abdominal cavity, and in these cases, preoperative determination of respectability is more difficult. Despite several attempts to use preoperative evaluation, no study to date has demonstrated a reliable ability to predict which patient can undergo successful cytoreduction and which patient cannot. Certainly, the presence of pleural effusions or the findings on a preoperative computed tomography (CT) scan have been less than satisfactory.

It appears that most patients will benefit from an attempted initial surgical cytoreductive operation. The exception to this position is the occasional patient with multiple liver metastases or the patient that has significant comorbid problems. In the latter category, in which the medical status precludes a proper initial operation, there may be a role for neoadjuvant chemotherapy. This group of patients is quite small, however.

FRANK G. LAWTON

The mean age of patients with ovarian cancer and the incidence of concomitant illness in this group means that not all such patients could be subjected to aggressive debulking surgery. An important consideration, however, should be the expectation of being able to carry out optimal debulking. It would be inappropriate to subject a 65-year-old patient with a history of previous cardiovascular disease to a prolonged aggressive surgical procedure if there were little chance of achieving optimal tumor resection. The case to do so, however, would be easier to support if the chances of an optimal surgical outcome were in the order of 70% or greater. Abdominal palpation cannot determine the resectability of an upper abdominal mass, and the place of imaging in assessing resectability is minimal. A realistic appraisal of the degree of surgery possible can really be made only after exploration of the abdomen. Clearly, by virtue of old age or concomitant ill health, some patients are poor operative risks, but old age per se should not be a contraindication to radical pelvic surgery.

That chronologic, rather than biologic, age is used by clinicians to exclude some patients from aggressive treatment schedules is seen in a recent report regarding the management of 12,316 patients with ovarian cancer, of whom 1,115 were 80 years of age or older.[14] The 5-year survival for older patients and for all stages was significantly less than that for their younger counterparts. In addition, older patients were more likely to be treated by general surgeons and nonspecialist gynecologists than by gynecologic oncologists and, as such, had less extensive and less optimal surgery. They also were less likely to receive chemotherapy.

However, old age is not a contraindication to radical pelvic surgery per se and, with appropriate patient selection, optimal surgical cytoreduction can be carried out in older women as successfully as, and with no more morbidity or mortality than, in younger patients.[15]

QUESTION 2

In patients with advanced-stage disease, which factor is more important—tumor biology or surgical intervention? Are there clinical trials that could be designed to determine the relative effects of these two factors?

WILLIAM J. HOSKINS

The relative importance of tumor biology versus surgical cytoreduction on the response rate, progression-free interval, and survival of patients with epithelial ovarian cancer has long been debated. Those who point to the benefits of surgical cytoreduction use the multiple clinical trials that demonstrate improved outcome based on the diameter of the largest residual disease. There is little doubt that these studies have clearly demonstrated that patients with small residual disease have a better prognosis than patients with large residual disease. In fact, in a GOG review, Hoskins et al[7] demonstrated a clear difference in survival among patients with advanced ovarian cancer based on the categories of microscopic disease, optimal disease (residual diameter < 2 cm), and residual disease (diameter > 2 cm) (Fig. 4-1). These investigators found that surgical cytoreduction that did not result in a residual tumor diameter of less than 2 cm failed to have a significant effect on survival. Other authorities point out that these effects may be due to the inherent biology of the disease and unrelated to the results of surgical cytoreduction. They contend that those patients who are cytoreduced to small-diameter residual disease simply have tumors with "better biology," making them more amenable to surgical cytoreduction.

The ideal trial to settle this issue would be to make the diagnosis of ovarian cancer by fine-needle biopsy or laparoscopy and then randomize the patients to surgical cytoreduction followed by chemotherapy or chemotherapy without surgical resection, and to follow the patients for response, progression-free interval, and survival. Ideally, subsequent therapy in the event of failure would be constant in each arm of the trial. To date, such a trial has not been conducted. There appears to be too much investigator bias regarding the importance of initial cytoreductive surgery. The GOG attempted such a trial in patients subjected to laparotomy and biopsy at outside institutions and subsequently referred to GOG institutions. Unfortunately, most investigators refused to participate and re-explored these patients for attempted cytoreduction. The protocol was eventually closed for lack of accrual.

In an attempt to answer the question indirectly, Hoskins et al[6] designed a retrospective analysis of an optimal disease protocol. These investigators from the GOG chose GOG protocol 52, designed to answer the question of whether the addition of Adriamycin added to cisplatin and cyclophosphamide provided any survival benefit. Since this was a negative trial, the entire population could be considered a single population. Their theory was as follows: since the protocol required all patients to have 1 cm or less of disease to be eligible for entry, there would be two categories of patients entered in the study: those who at exploration were found to have 1 cm or less of disease in the abdomen and those found to have large-volume abdominal disease but who could be cytoreduced to 1 cm or less of tumor. Pelvic disease was not considered, except that all disease had to be resected to 1 cm or less before entry into the study. The authors theorized that if cytoreductive surgery was the only important factor, survival in the two populations of patients would be equal. Final analysis demonstrated an improved survival in the group of patients found to have 1 cm or less of disease at exploration, compared to those cytoreduced to 1 cm or less. Thus, failing to prove their hypothesis, the investigators appeared to implicate tumor biology as an important factor. As can be seen in Table 4-5, factors that were important included the age of the patient at diagnosis, number of tumor nodules, and tumor grade. Hoskins and colleagues point out that their study does not indicate that surgical cytoreduction is not important but that tumor biology plays a key role. Until an investigative group is able to conduct a prospective trial as outlined above, it is unlikely that this question will be answered in any reliable fashion. Given the pressure to test new agents in ovarian cancer, it is not likely that a trial will be conducted.

FRANK G. LAWTON

The lack of any prospective randomized study remains the major criticism of cytoreductive surgery in ovarian cancer. Without this, it is impossible to determine whether the survival advantage seen for patients with small-volume residual disease is a function of surgical resection or of the favorable biology demonstrated by tumor that can be resected. Such a study would have to be designed to compare survival of patients who underwent debulking surgery followed by chemotherapy with survival of a group who had a biopsy-only procedure followed by chemotherapy. Attempts to conduct such research, in the

TABLE 4-5
Results of the Cox Modeling of Survival

FACTOR	RELATIVE RISK	NO. OF PATIENTS
Age (yr.)[a]		
30	1.0	22
40	1.2	64
50	1.5	89
60	1.9	104
70	2.4	56
80	3.0	7
Grade		
1	1.0	83
2–3	2.0	265
Number of residual lesions		
0–15	1.0	156
20	1.3	53
>20	1.5	138
Omental disease status		
None/microscopic		
Abdomen		
None/microscopic	1.0	58
Gross	1.3	59
Gross		
Abdomen		
None/microscopic	1.5	47
Gross (except below)	2.3	139
Omentum and abdomen >1 cm	3.2	45

[a] *Includes ages from 4 years less to 5 years greater than the indicated decade. (From Hoskins,[6] with permission.)*

United States and Europe, have proved futile. A number of studies have shown that even when experienced gynecologic oncologists undertake surgical debulking, a proportion of patients still leave the operating room with bulky residual disease. It is apparent not only that patient status after primary surgery is affected by surgical skill and diligence but also that tumor biology or the host-tumor relationship is also a major determinant of surgical outcome.

The importance of the host-tumor relationship has been suggested by two studies. Both Hacker[16] and Hoskins and colleagues[6] have shown that patients presenting with large-volume disease (perhaps primary masses >10 cm) do not fare as well as those with smaller-volume disease even if optimal surgical cytoreduction is completed in both groups. An intriguing paper suggested that biologic differences in tumor characteristics between patient groups do exist.[17] A comparison between Dutch and Danish patients with stage III ovarian cancer found that even in those receiving suboptimal surgery (i.e., >2-cm residual disease), the median survival for Dutch patients was 24 months, compared with 17 months for Danish patients ($P = 0.008$). This difference was not associated with the use of different chemotherapy regimens in both countries, nor was it associated with differences in patient age or tumor grade.

Logistic regression analysis showed that these survival differences were associated with differences in tumor mean-nuclear area (MNA). Survival was similar in the two groups for patients with similar MNAs, but the median MNA was significantly higher in Danish patients compared with their Dutch counterparts (78 v63, $P < 0.00001$).

Other studies have indicated that a number of tumor-associated factors, oncogenes, tumor antigens, steroid hormone receptor levels, growth factors, and DNA ploidy—all essentially, markers of tumor biology—may be of prognostic significance.[18]

QUESTION 3

Which women with a pelvic mass should be referred to a gynecologic oncologist for primary surgery? What is the role, if any, of diagnostic laparoscopy prior to referral?

WILLIAM J. HOSKINS

It is unlikely that all patients with an adnexal mass will be referred to a gynecologic oncologist, although one could argue that, with the continuing sacrifice of surgical and oncology training in obstetrics and gynecology residency programs, this might be the best option for them. Nevertheless, this is not likely to happen over the next few years, and so it is best to establish referral, guidelines for patients. Obviously, the principal reason to refer such patients is the risk of cancer of the ovary, which requires the expertise of a trained oncologic surgeon. In those situations in which an oncologist is available on standby to come to the operating room, requirements for referral can be more flexible.

Table 4-6 presents clearly outlined guidelines for referral. These guidelines are based on the likelihood of malignancy in an adnexal mass. In some cases, referral of patients to a gynecologic oncologist is dependent on the location of the practice, as a gynecologic oncologist may not be readily available in some areas of the United States. In these cases the gynecologist should counsel the patient with great deliberation. Some patients may prefer to remain in their own community and take a calculated risk that the mass will be malignant. In such cases, the gynecologist should outline the planned extent of the procedure and explain that if a cancer is found, the procedure may be limited and the patient will in all likelihood require a second operation. This action is better than employing the assistance of a general surgeon or urologist who may provide the necessary technical skills without the necessary knowledge of the spread patterns of the disease or the necessary operative procedure. There is never an indication to perform a less-than-adequate surgical procedure for the patient.

The question of the role of laparoscopy is developing even as this chapter is being written. In the hands of a trained gynecologic oncologist, many adnexal masses can be managed by laparoscopy, and most gynecologic oncologists agree on the patient-selection criteria. For general gynecologists, the indications for referral remain the same as those listed in Table 4-6; although they may define the type of masses they feel comfortable managing by laparoscopy, this should never exceed the guidelines in Table 4-6. The one advantage of laparoscopy for general gynecologists is the possibility of defining a mass at diagnostic laparoscopy with which they do not feel comfortable because it appears malignant, affecting referral without the morbidity and discomfort of a complete laparoscopy. Certainly the discovery of any mass that appears to be malignant at diagnostic laparoscopy mandates termination of the procedure, followed by proper referral.

While the above criteria may seem to restrict the scope of the general gynecologist, the current level of gynecologic oncology training in obstetrics and gynecology and general surgery training programs mandates this approach. With the current availability of trained gynecologic oncologists in most communities, a less restricted approach cannot be justified.

FRANK G. LAWTON

Failure to refer patients with ovarian carcinoma to a gynecologic cancer center remains one of the most controversial issues about the

TABLE 4-6
Characteristics for Referral of Patients with an Adnexal Mass to a Gynecologic Oncologist

CHARACTERISTIC	GYNECOLOGIC ONCOLOGIST	GENERAL GYNECOLOGIST
Size		
Postmenopausal	>10 cm	<10 cm
Premenopausal	>6 cm	<6 cm
Complex	All	>6 cm
Elevated CA 125	All	No fibroids, endometriosis
Ascites	All	All
Family history of ovarian cancer	All	All
Personal history of breast cancer	All	All

disease in many countries. The fact that fewer than one-half of patients entered into studies have undergone optimal surgical cytoreduction attests not only to surgical ineptitude but also to doubt by nonspecialist gynecologists about the value of debulking.[14]

A recent study examined which factors influenced gynecologists' referral of a patient with suspected ovarian cancer to a gynecologic oncologist.[19] Two hundred and forty-nine Canadian obstetricians and gynecologists were given five theoretical case histories and asked if they would operate on such a patient themselves or re-refer to a gynecologic cancer center. Interestingly 15% said they would operate on a 67-year-old patient with bilateral solid ovarian tumors, bilateral hydronephroses, and bowel obstruction, which again may be a reflection of doubt as to the value of debulking. Yet 43% would be prepared to operate on a 56-year-old woman with ascites, a 10-kg weight loss, and a 12-cm solid right ovarian mass. The investigators' concern that 43% of gynecologists would operate on a patient with obvious ovarian cancer was highlighted by their conclusion that "this practice pattern can only be explained by ignorance of the medical literature, disbelief of the medical literature, or a belief that the conclusions of the medical literature do not apply to the individual physician answering the questionnaire." Also of interest was the finding that while gynecologic oncologists estimated that 18% of their patients had no macroscopic residual disease after surgery, the figure for nonspecialists was 43%.

The question arises as to the criteria to be used by clinicians in deciding which patients should be referred to a gynecologic oncologist for primary surgery. In essence, these criteria relate not only to the potential operability of these patients but also to the degree to which the referring clinician believes that optimal debulking is desirable and achievable. The report discussed above and data from other countries suggest that most patients are not given the benefit of a concerted debulking attempt. It is difficult to believe that clinicians are ignorant of the mass of data relating to debulking surgery.

The excuse that absence of data from a prospective trial means that clinicians remain unconvinced of the benefits of debulking surgery is difficult to uphold. No multivariate analysis of prognostic factors has ever shown that optimal debulking has an adverse effect on patient survival. Likewise, multivariate analysis of factors affecting survival has not shown that the use of chemotherapy can overcome the adverse effect of bulky residual tumor.

Are poor referral patterns a reflection of indifference on the part of gynecologists or medical oncologists who do not believe the mass of data regarding debulking? It is worth noting that patient referral to fetal medicine or infertility centers for specialist treatment seems much less influenced by such medicopolitical factors.

Recently the goal of primary cytoreductive surgery was further refined. A study by Lawton et al[20] reported a greater than 80% 3-year survival rate for women with stage III ovarian cancer in whom the initial surgical procedure had left no macroscopic cancer. This result, however, could be achieved in only 16 of 124 patients (13%). A report from Sydney showed that the only women with a better than 50% chance of survival of longer than 4 years are those with no macroscopic tumor after primary surgery.[16] This was achieved in 7 out of a total of 59 patients (11.9%), a proportion strikingly similar to that reported by Lawton et al. Despite continuing controversy as to the role of laparoscopy in reassessing patients with apparent early-stage disease or as a second-look procedure, it may have use in determining the operability of a patient with ovarian cancer, and preliminary experience with laparoscopic cytoreductive surgery has been reported.[21] The resectability of upper abominal disease may be assessed using modern laparoscopic instruments and techniques. Such an approach in cases in which the surgical outcome is unclear may sometimes avoid more extensive exploratory surgery. It is my fervent belief, however, that the laparoscopist should also be a trained gynecologic oncologist for proper assessment of the operability of the patient.

QUESTION 4

Is there any role for cytoreductive surgery in patients with stage IV disease? If so, which stage IV patients?

WILLIAM J. HOSKINS

Stage IV cancer is a wide spectrum of disease and must be dealt with on an individual basis when considering the question of resectability. There is no simple answer as to which patient is a candidate for initial surgical cytoreduction. A patient with early ovarian cancer with an abdominal wall metastasis may have totally resectable disease with a relatively simple ovarian cancer operation that includes resection of the abdominal wall metastasis. By contrast, a patient with multiple large liver metastases clearly may not be a candidate for surgical resection and may benefit from initial chemotherapy with interval cytoreduction, provided the liver metastases respond to chemotherapy. Even patients with unifocal resectable liver metastases may be candidates for surgical resection.

Curtin and associates[22] evaluated 97 patients with stage IV ovarian cancer who underwent attempted surgical cytoreduction at Memorial Sloan–Kettering Cancer Center. They found equivalent survival for stage IV ovarian cancer patients who underwent optimal surgical resection compared to stage III patients undergoing optimal surgical cytoreduction. This study appears to indicate that stage IV patients should undergo the same or a similar operative procedure as patients with stage III disease.

Of particular note are patients with stage IV ovarian cancer based only on positive pleural effusions. In the study conducted by Curtin et al,[22] these patients had survival similar to that of stage III patients. In fact, most gynecologists tap pleural effusions in patients with advanced ovarian cancer only if such a procedure is necessary for preoperative pulmonary management. Thus, it is quite likely that many patients carried as stage III actually have stage IV disease on the basis of pulmonary effusions that would have been positive if tapped for cytology.

FRANK G. LAWTON

The role of debulking surgery in patients with stage IV disease is controversial. How aggressive should abdominal surgery be in a patient with intrahepatic or extra-abdominal disease? Since late 1993 the protocol for all patients with stage IV ovarian cancer at King's College Hospital has included an expectation that they would undergo debulking surgery. Of 16 such patients, 4 were excluded from surgery because of medical complications, but an exploratory laparotomy was carried out in the rest. Patient details are given in Table 4-7. Neoadjuvant chemotherapy comprising of one to three cycles of weekly carboplatin was given to 7 patients. The response to such therapy was not used as a marker of the possible success of debulking surgery, but it is interesting to note that lack of response to neoadjuvant chemotherapy seems to predict a poor outcome. This might indicate that an aggressive surgical intent is not indicated in such patients who show little or no response to preoperative chemotherapy.

QUESTION 5

What factors should influence the degree of aggressiveness during primary cytoreductive surgery? How does one balance the desire to achieve optimal cytoreduction and the risk of morbidity? If, at the time of surgical exploration, one determines that optimal cytoreduction is not possible, should any surgical cytoreduction be performed?

WILLIAM J. HOSKINS

How extensive an attempt at surgical cytoreduction is feasible is one of the most difficult decisions that any gynecologic oncologist must make. Judging the degree to which a patient can tolerate an extended operation is often difficult, and failure to make the correct decision may result in a reduced chance of cure or excessive morbidity for the patient. In general, every effort should be made to remove as much tumor as possible since, as

TABLE 4-7
Patients with Stage IV Ovarian Cancer—King's College Hospital, 1993–1995

AGE (YR)	DISEASE SITE[a]	NEOADJUVANT CHEMOTHERAPY, NO. OF CYCLES, AND RESPONSE[b]	SIZE OF MAXIMUM INITIAL ABDOMINAL TUMOR (CM)	SIZE OF MAXIMUM RESIDUAL TUMOR (CM)	STATUS[c]
63	PE	Yes, 3, pr	6	1.5	dod 16 mo
52	H	No	10	4	dod 8 mo
44	H	Yes, 2, pr	8	<1	dod 11 mo
52	H	Yes, 2, none	15	10	dod day 4
59	PE	Yes, 3, cr	30	<1.5	ned 16 mo
72	H/PE	No	15	12	dod 1 mo
56	PE	Yes, 2, r	6	2	prog 12 mo
81	PE	No	20	1.5	ned 11 mo
52	PE	No	6	1	ned 9 mo
30	H	Yes, 2, none	20	8	dod 8 mo
56	H	Yes, 1, prog	8	6	dod 6 mo
79	H/PE	No	10	10	dod 2 mo

[a] *Abbreviations: PE, Pleural effusion; H, Intrahepatic or porta hepatis disease.*
[b] *Abbreviations: pr, 50% reduction in intra-abdominal tumor volume; cr, complete clinical resolution of intra-abdominal disease; prog, progressive disease.*
[c] *Abbreviations: dod, Died with evidence of progressive or recurrent disease; prog, evidence of disease progression, patient remains alive; ned, alive with no clinical disease.*

pointed out previously, progression-free interval and survival are related to the largest diameter of residual disease.

It is our practice at Memorial Sloan-Kettering to perform extended primary surgical cytoreduction with resection of bowel, spleen, or portions of other structures only if that surgical resection will result in resection of all tumor larger than 1 to 2 cm. We also perform a total pelvic and para-aortic lymphadenectomy to achieve optimal cytoreduction if there is extensive nodal disease. However, if it is determined that optimal cytoreduction is not possible, we generally avoid such radical procedures as described above. In those cases, we remove only large masses that can be removed without major organ resection.

In a study of the GOG, Hoskins and colleagues[7] reported that cytoreduction of tumor masses to less than 2 cm resulted in improved survival, but resection that did not achieve that goal had little influence on survival (Fig. 4-2). In that same paper, they showed that survival can be related to three categories of residual disease: microscopic disease, gross disease less than 2 cm, and disease greater than 2 cm (Fig. 4-1).

Although some surgeons find ultrasonic dissectors (CUSA) and argon beam lasers helpful, there is no good data in the literature indicating that this is more than surgeons' preference. No randomized or well-controlled studies have shown a survival benefit. At Memorial Sloan-Kettering, we generally utilize electrocautery dissection but have found little additional benefit with the CUSA. Again, our choices probably relate primarily to surgeon preference.

FRANK G. LAWTON

Achieving a balance between the desire to leave a patient with minimal or no macroscopic residual disease and the morbidity that such an attempt might produce is problematic. In order to complete such surgery, bowel resection might be needed in 13 to 36% of patients, and urinary tract resection in about 5%.[23–25] Heintz reported that the mean op-

FIGURE 4-2. Survival rates by maximum diameter of residual disease. (From Hoskins,[7] with permission.)

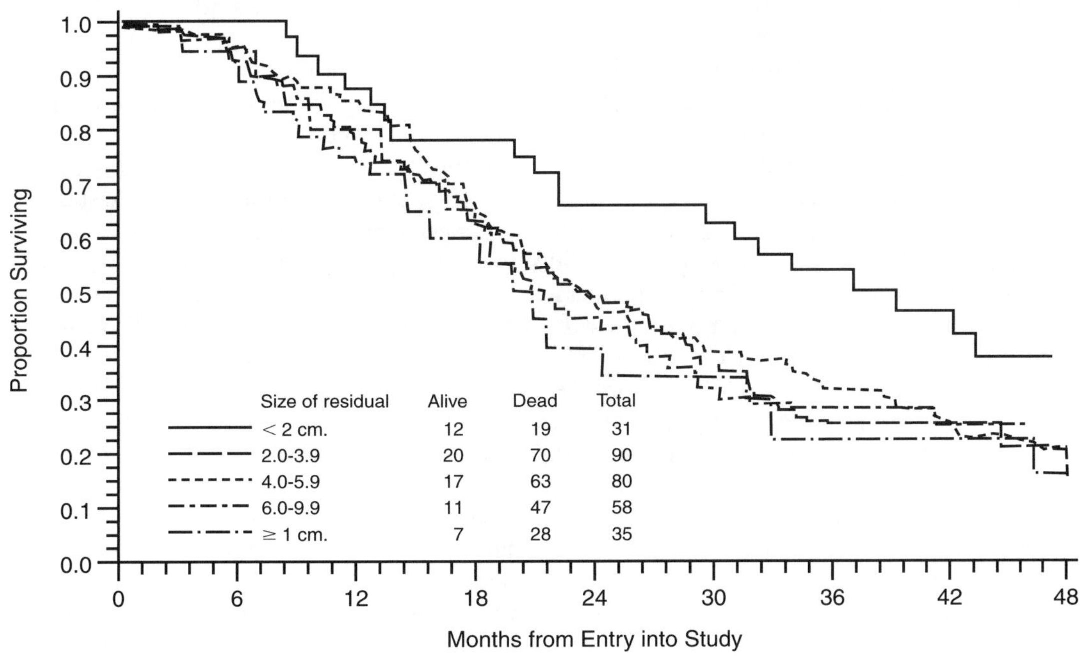

erating time required to achieve optimal cytoreduction was 3.5 hours (range 2 to 9 hours), the mean blood loss 1.1 liters (range 2.15 to 4 liters), and the mean postoperative stay 12 days (range 5 to 24 days). Serious morbidity, defined as pneumonia, cardiac failure, wound dehiscence, or hemorrhage requiring reoperation, occurred in 23% of patients. There were two postoperative deaths—one of a cerebrovascular accident (CVA) 2 weeks after surgery and one due to septicemia secondary to necrosis of the terminal bowel. Piver[24] reported a 12% serious morbidity rate with no mortality; Chen and Bochner had one postoperative death in 84 patients.[23]

There can be little argument that a patient should not be subjected to a prolonged procedure, possibly including bowel resection and reanastomosis or surgery to the lower urinary tract, if there is little or no prospect of optimal surgery being completed. In any case, it seems that if bowel surgery is needed to achieve optimal tumor clearance, such patients have a poorer prognosis than those who require no bowel surgery but have residual disease.[26]

It is important to emphasize the effect that debulking surgery may have on a 1-kg stage III ovarian cancer. Such a mass may contain 10^{12} cells, a size achieved after perhaps 40 tumor doublings of the initial malignant cell. Therefore, even a 50% extirpation of the tumor mass would in effect achieve only one log cell kill. Only one extra doubling would be required for the tumor to regain its former mass. This surgery is unlikely to have any effect on the natural history of the disease at all. On the other hand, surgery leaving a residual nodule of about 1 cm, which would require 10 doublings to regain its former mass, would have a 25% effect on tumor growth. Therefore, when the patient is not at risk of bowel obstruction, surgeons should consider what impact, if any, extensive upper abdominal surgery or multiple bowel resections with reanastomoses may have on the prognosis. It makes no sense to contemplate such surgery if, despite it all, the patient leaves the operating theater with bulky residual disease.

The pattern of tumor spread in the abdominal cavity may also be an important factor in patient survival. Patients presenting with widespread intraperitoneal seedlings seem to have a poorer survival than those who present with predominantly bulky disease.[27] Could this be a function of different tumor biology? Or is it that, even after debulking surgery, the total mass of the multiple peritoneal seedlings in these patients is far greater than the volume of residual disease in patients presenting with bulky disease? Such a finding needs further study, as it may be that in cases where a preliminary laparoscopic examination reveals a "miliary"-type spread pattern, consideration should be given to primary chemotherapy rather than an initial attempt at debulking surgery.

The report from Heintz[25] showed that in about 50% of cases, residual disease in patients who had undergone suboptimal surgery consisted of unresectable upper abdominal disease. Sites included the hilum of the spleen, the stomach and transverse colon, the porta hepatis, the lesser sac, the retroperitoneal space above the renal vessels, and the mesentery of the small bowel. Piver[24] reported that a similar proportion of patients with suboptimal surgery had upper abdominal disease or lymph node metastases. Clearly an aggressive surgical intent at the outset is necessary if these sites are to be explored adequately and tumor excised.

Whether lymphadenectomy in ovarian cancer is a diagnostic or a therapeutic procedure remains controversial. About 10 years ago the first reports began to appear regarding the incidence of lymph node metastases in advanced ovarian cancer.[28,29] These early studies essentially related to node biopsy, but at the time Burghardt suggested that lymphadenectomy might be therapeutic. His group reported that the 5-year survival for patients with stage III disease after radical lymphadenectomy was 53%, compared with a historic control group with the same stage of disease who had debulking surgery without lymphadenectomy and had a survival of only 13%. However, the results were complicated by the fact that the two groups were not comparable: the former had undergone more aggressive surgical procedures and, probably more importantly, had been treated with cisplatin-containing cytotoxic regimens.

That nodal disease may be a site relatively immune to chemotherapy, and therefore a reason to consider lymphadenectomy a therapeutic procedure, comes from a large study from Italy.[30] Eighty-eight patients underwent radical lymphadenectomy after treatment with cisplatin-containing chemotherapy. Positive nodes were found in 33 patients, and in 4 the nodes were the only site of residual cancer. An international randomized study of the effects of lymphadenectomy is currently underway. In it, patients with optimal surgical cytoreduction, defined as residual disease less than 1 cm in diameter, will be randomized intraoperatively to undergo systemic para-aortic and pelvic lymphadenectomy or resection of only bulky nodes. The results of the study are awaited not only so that the role of lymphadenectomy may be defined more accurately but also as an indication that large prospective studies of ovarian cancer surgery can be completed. I doubt, however, that such cooperation would then lead to a prospective study of primary debulking surgery.

With appropriate surgical training it is rare that all macroscopic pelvic disease cannot be removed or at least a state achieved where only small-volume peritoneal disease remains. Even if the pelvic anatomy is grossly distorted, a retroperitoneal approach more often than not facilitates total tumor resection. In many cases, where large bowel resection is necessary, a low anterior resection of the colon, en bloc with the pelvic tumor, can be accomplished.[31] The use of stapling devices, particularly the EEA stapler, has resulted in primary bowel reanastomosis being achieved in the vast majority of cases.

An interesting report has recently documented the proportion of patients with gastrointestinal metastases from ovarian cancer who have disease within mesenteric nodes.[32] In a series of 100 separate bowel resections, 55% of patients had lymphvascular space invasion in the bowel mesentery. In addition, median survival for patients with positive mesenteric nodes was 20 months, compared with 32 months for node-negative patients. The investigators suggest that since spread of ovarian cancer within the gastrointestinal tract appears similar to that of colon cancer, wedge resection of the adjacent mesentery in a manner similar to that used for primary bowel cancer may be appropriate. Extensive upper abdominal disease is a much greater surgical challenge. Usually, despite the appearance of invasion of the transverse colon from an omental cake, access to the lesser sac and transverse mesocolon, allowing dissection of the omentum from the transverse colon and greater curvature of the stomach, can be achieved.

Problems may be encountered with tumor spread to the hilum of the spleen. Careful dissection may be possible to mobilize tumor at this site; in rare cases splenectomy may be needed. In a recent study it was reported that splenectomy was necessary to achieve optimal cytoreduction in 18 of 210 cases (8.6%).[33]

A number of innovations in surgical technology have recently been applied in an attempt to intensify the degree of cytoreduction possible where disease is present at "problem" sites. The Cavitron ultrasonic surgical aspirator (CUSA) is a hand-held device with a 2-mm hollow titanium tip which vibrates at a frequency of 23,000 Hz. Stroking or dragging the tip over tumor nodules fragments them, allowing dissection away from, and without damage to, underlying tissue such as blood vessels and ureters. Deppe et al[34] showed that diaphragmatic metastases can be safely fragmented using this technique.

Brand and Pearlman[35] reported use of the argon beam coagulator (ABC) to destroy tumor nodules in patients with stage III and IV disease at sites essentially inaccessible to standard surgical techniques—the diaphragm, bowel, presacral space, ureters, vagina, and iliac vessels. Despite extensive disease, optimal debulking was achieved in all seven patients in the study with complete tumor excision in four.

An initial report of treatment employing the loop electrosurgical excision procedure (LEEP) has also demonstrated its use in intensifying the degree of surgical cytoreduction.[36] In this study 20 consecutive patients with stage IIIB to IV ovarian cancer underwent standard surgical cytoreduction followed by LEEP to excise nodules involving intestines (18 patients), peritoneal surfaces (18), liver (6), and diaphragm and spleen (3 each). All macroscopic peritoneal disease was excised in all patients, as it was in all cases of liver and splenic metastases and in 17 patients with intestinal disease. The median time of LEEP treatment was 9 minutes (range 3 to 27 minutes). Blood loss secondary to LEEP was no greater than 20 ml. Since the ultimate goal of cytoreductive surgery, in terms of improving long-term survival, must be to remove all macroscopic disease, techniques such as CUSA, ABC, and LEEP need further evaluation. The inexpensive and robust nature of LEEP equipment may give it an important advantage.

A recent study concluded that cytoreductive surgery had probably only a small effect on survival, producing only a 4.1% increase in survival time, whereas the type of chemotherapy had more impact.[35] A meta-analysis of 58 studies, comprising 97 treatment cohorts of 6,962 patients, was reported. Studies were included if they contained "predominantly" patients with stage III and IV disease and if they included the overall median survival and the proportion of patients undergoing maximum cytoreduction. The study can be criticized on a number of counts. First, maximum cytoreductive surgery was variously defined in terms of residual disease as less than 3 cm (5.2% of cohorts), less than 2 cm (78.4%), less than 1.5 cm (4.1%), less than 1 cm (2%), or as a verbal description of "no palpable tumor" (10.3%). Consequently, at least 15% of patients had suboptimal residual disease or a suboptimal description of it, or alternatively, only 6.1% of cohorts had less than a 1.5 cm tumor residuum.

These definitions notwithstanding, the proportion of patients in the cohorts who had undergone optimal cytoreduction varied from 2.9% (a study of 20 patients with stage IV disease, none of whom had had optimal surgery, was included) to 87%, with a median of only 31.5%. This is a much lower proportion than would be expected if truly aggressive cytoreductive surgery had been undertaken.[23–25] In addition, in 23 cohorts optimal cytoreduction was achieved in 20% or less of patients, and greater than 50% was achieved in only 11 cohorts. Since, as already stated, a 50% reduction in tumor volume by surgery has so little impact on tumor doubling, the conclusions of this report are not surprising. It can be stated that this meta-analysis did not address the question of the impact of *optimal* debulking surgery, merely that of surgery in general, and inadequate surgery in particular.

Apart from the morbidity of the actual surgical procedure, the criticism that debulking surgery may actually be harmful to the patient has never really arisen. However, an intriguing study from Birmingham, United Kingdom, has shown that after debulking surgery there is an increase in proliferative activity of aneuploid malignant cells in the peritoneal cavity as detected by flow cytometry of peritoneal lavage samples.[38]

The case for or against the benefit afforded patients with advanced ovarian cancer who undergo optimal primary surgical cytoreduction has not been proved with a prospective randomized trial, but retrospective data support overwhelmingly the belief that patients do benefit from such surgery. In a disease where in most cases cure is not possible, but a reasonable disease-free palliation and quality of life are likely after adequate primary surgery, it is difficult to uphold the position advocating "open and close, take a biopsy, and refer for chemotherapy."

In a recent editorial Hacker wrote, "To suggest that the role of cytoreduction is a subject for debate is to suggest that patients with advanced ovarian cancer may be managed in a community hospital by laparoscopic biopsy followed by chemotherapy. Such an approach would set progress in this disease back 20 years and would be a gross disservice to all patients who suffer from this disease."[39]

If a gynecologist, either ignorant or dismissive of the data, is not prepared or able to attempt optimal cytoreduction, the patient should be referred to a gynecologic oncology center. Likewise, if a gynecologist, aware of the data, is unsure as to the degree of debulking that he or she can achieve, the patient ought to be referred. The economic demands on health care in many countries, with those purchasing that care requiring evidence of value for money for their patient population, will have a major impact on referral patterns. In light of the data available to those organizations paying for health care, either in a state-funded or a private system, a center with little or no expertise in debulking surgery is unlikely to receive funding for such cases. In the end, the socioeconomic argument regarding debulking may be more important than the medical one.

EDITORS' COMMENTARY

Current standard practice regarding primary cytoreductive surgery for patients with advanced ovarian cancer has largely evolved from information collected from retrospective studies and the development of consensus among experienced experts rather than from data accumulated from prospective randomized clinical trials.

As pointed out by both experts, primary cytoreductive surgery remains the standard for the vast majority of patients with suspected advanced ovarian cancer. Selection of primary therapy other than surgery is based on experience and common sense rather than on scientific data. Most experts agree that primary surgery should not be performed on patients with debilitating effusions or severe comorbid conditions. In the former, however, interval debulking may be both feasible and prudent after a few cycles of neoadjuvant chemotherapy.

As indicated, the relative influences of primary debulking and tumor biology remain elusive. But hints from retrospective studies suggest that tumor biology is important in determining patient survival. Over the next few years, future studies will hopefully elucidate the complex interactions between these two factors. As outlined by Dr. Hoskins, one clinical trial design that would help resolve some of our questions would be one in which the diagnosis of ovarian cancer is made by fine-needle biopsy or laparoscopic biopsy followed by randomization between the standard practice of surgery plus chemotherapy and chemotherapy alone. However, investigator bias has led to premature closure of similar studies in the past because of lack of patient accrual. Such a study is therefore unlikely in the foreseeable future.

The issue of referral of women with suspected ovarian cancer has several economic, political, and social overtones. Criteria for appropriate referral of a woman with a pelvic mass to a gynecologic oncologist are being developed by several groups. In this era of health care reform, however, it is difficult to predict whether referral patterns will improve or not. Obviously, the optimal surgeon for a woman with ovarian cancer is an individual who understands the biology of ovarian cancer and who has the experience and skill to perform the indicated procedure. Our approach in changing the environment surrounding this issue includes a multipronged approach aimed at establishing practice guidelines; establishing criteria for appropriate referral; and educating elected officials, insurance and managed care executives, and the public about the best care for women with ovarian cancer.

Primary cytoreductive surgery remains the standard for patients with suspected stage IV ovarian cancer. Moreover, a growing number of studies are demonstrating that optimal debulking in patients with stage IV disease results in better survival when compared to suboptimal debulking in stage IV patients. Nevertheless, overall survival for patients with stage IV disease regardless of residual disease status remains quite poor. The ideal study to resolve the role of surgery in this population would be a randomization of standard surgery plus chemotherapy versus neoadjuvant chemotherapy, interval debulking, and further chemotherapy, versus chemotherapy alone. Of course, initial diagnosis suggesting stage IV ovarian cancer would require fine-needle aspiration biopsy or laparoscopic biopsy.

And finally, there remains a wide range of opinions among gynecologic oncologists regarding the optimal degree of aggressiveness of primary cytoreductive surgery. When is it appropriate and clearly beneficial to the individual patient to resect the rectosigmoid colon, to debulk para-aortic lymph nodes, to perform a splenectomy, or to cytoreduce diaphragmatic tumor implants? Such issues are not easily resolved, and the individual nature of each patient's tumor distribution and each surgeon's skill and opinions concerning benefit to the patient obviously complicate the situation.

References

1. McGuire WP, Hoskins WJ, Brady MF et al: Cyclophosphamide and cisplatin compared with paclitaxel and cisplatin in patients with Stage III and Stage IV ovarian cancer. N Engl J Med 334:1, 1996
2. Griffiths CT: Surgery at the time of diagnosis in ovarian cancer. p. 60. In Blackledge G, Chan KK (eds): Management of Ovarian Cancer. Butterworths, London, 1986
3. Griffiths CT: Surgical resection of tumor bulk in the primary treatment of ovarian cancer. Natl Cancer Inst Monogr 42:101, 1975
4. Redman JR, Petroni GR, Saigo PE et al: Prognostic factors in advanced ovarian cancer. J Clin Oncol 4:515, 1986
5. Neijt JP, van der Burg MEL, Vriesendorp R et al: Randomized trial comparing two combination chemotherapy regimens (Hexa-CAF vs. CHAP-5) in advanced ovarian carcinoma. Lancet 2:549, 1984
6. Hoskins WJ, Bundy BN, Thigpen JT, Omura GA: The influence of cytoreductive surgery on recurrence-free interval and survival in small-volume Stage III epithelial ovarian cancer: a Gynecologic Oncology Group study. Gynecol Oncol 47:159, 1992
7. Hoskins WJ, McGuire WP, Brady MF et al: The effect of diameter of largest residual disease on survival after primary cytoreductive surgery in patients with suboptimal residual epithelial ovarian carcinoma. Am J Obstet Gynecol 170: 974, 1994
8. Hoskins WJ: Primary cytoreduction. p. 163. In Markman M, Hoskins WJ (eds).: Cancer of the Ovary. Raven Press, Philadelphia, 1993
9. Hoskins WJ: Primary surgical management of advanced epithelial ovarian cancer. p. 241. In Rubin SC, Sutton GP (eds): Ovarian Cancer. McGraw-Hill, New York, 1993
10. Omura GA, Bundy BN, Berek JS et al: Randomized trial of cyclophosphamide plus cisplatin with or without doxorubicin in ovarian carcinoma: a Gynecologic Oncology Group study. J Clin Oncol 7:457, 1989
11. McGuire WP, Hoskins WJ, Brady MF et al: Assessment of dose-intensive therapy in suboptimally debulked ovarian cancer: a Gynecologic Oncology Group study. J Clin Oncol 13:1589, 1995
12. Brown C, Hakes T, Wong G et al: Chemosurgical cytoreduction followed by intraperitoneal cisplatin/etoposide in advanced ovarian cancer. (in preparation)
13. van der Burg ME, van Lent M, Kobierska et al: Intervention debulking surgery (IDS) does improve survival in advanced epithelial ovarian cancer (EOC): an EORTC Gynecological Cancer Cooperative Group (GCCG) study, abstract 818. Proc Am Soc Clin Oncol 1993
14. Hightower RD, Nguyen HN, Averette HE et al: National survey of ovarian carcinoma IV: patterns of care and related survival for older patients. Cancer 73:377, 1994
15. Lawton FG, Hacker NF: Surgery for invasive gynecologic cancer in the elderly female population. Obstet Gynecol 76:287, 1990
16. Hacker NF, Wain GV, Trimbos JP: Mangagement and outcome of stage III epithelial ovarian cancer. p 351. In Sharp F, Mason WP, Creasman W (eds): Ovarian Cancer. 2. Biology, Diagnosis and Management. Chapman & Hall, London, 1992

17. Brinkhuis M, Baak JPA, van Diest PJ et al: In Dutch and Danish patients with FIGO III ovarian carcinoma, geographic differences are associated with differences in quantitative pathologic features. Int J Gynecol Cancer 6:108, 1996

18. Beale PJ, Friedlander ML: Prognostic variables in ovarian cancer. p. 96. In Epithelial Cancer of the Ovary. Lawton FG, Neijt JP, Swenerton KD (eds): Epithelial Cancer of the Ovary. BMJ Publishing Group, London, 1995

19. Prefontaine M, Gruslin A. Referral patterns for suspected ovarian cancer: a survery of practicing gynecologists. Int J Gynecol Cancer 5:381, 1995

20. Lawton FG, Luesley DM, Redman CWE et al: Feasibility and outcome of complete secondary tumor resection for patients with advanced ovarian cancer. J Surg Oncol 45:14, 1990

21. Surwit EA, Childers JM: Minimal access surgery in ovarian cancer. p. 248. In Epithelial Cancer of the Ovary. Lawton FG, Neijt JP, Swenerton KD (eds): BMJ Publishing group, London, 1995

22. Curtin J, Malik R, Venkatraman E et al: Surgical debulking of patients with Stage IV ovarian cancer: impact on survival, abstract 76. Gynecol Oncol 56:129, 1995

23. Chen SS, Bochner R: Assessment of morbidity and mortality in primary cytoreductive surgery for advanced ovarian carcinoma. Gynecol Oncol 20:190, 1985

24. Piver MS, Baker T: The potential for optimal (<2 cm) cytoreductive surgery in advanced ovarian carcinoma at a tertiary medical center: a prospective study. Gynecol Oncol 24:1, 1986

25. Heintz APM, Hacker NF, Berek JS et al: Cytoreductive surgery in ovarian carcinoma: feasibility and morbidity. Obstet Gynecol 67:783, 1986

26. Potter ME, Partridge EE, Hatch KD et al: Primary surgical therapy of ovarian cancer: how much and when. Gynecol Oncol 40:195, 1991

27. Luesley D, Finn C, Varma R: The role of surgery in epithelial ovarian cancer. p. 357. In Sharp F, Mason WP, Creasman W (eds): Ovarian Cancer. Biology, Diagnosis and Management. Chapman & Hall, London, 1992

28. Chen SS, Lee L: Incidence of para-aortic and pelvic lymph node metastases in epithelial carcinoma of the ovary. Gynecol Oncol 16:95, 1983

29. Burghardt E, Pickel H, Lahousen M, Stettner H: Pelvic lymphadenectomy in operative treatment of ovarian cancer. Am J Obstet Gynecol 155:315, 1986

30. di Re F, Fontanelli R, Raspagliesi F, di Re E: Pelvic and paraaortic lymphadenctomy in cancer of the ovary. Ballieres Clin Obstet Gynecol 3:131, 1989

31. Bridges JE, Leung Y, Hammond IG, McCartney AJ: En bloc resection of epithelial ovarian tumors with concomitant rectosigmoid colectomy: the KEMH experience. Int J Gynecol Cancer 3:199, 1993

32. O'Hanlon KA, Kargas S, Schreiber M et al: Ovarian cancer metastases to gastrointestinal tract appear to spread like colon carcinoma: implications for surgical resection. Gynecol Oncol 59:200, 1995

33. Nicklin JL, Copeland LJ, O'Toole RV et al: Splenectomy as part of cytoreductive surgery for ovarian carcinoma. Gynecol Oncol 58:244, 1995

34. Deppe G, Malviya VK, Boike G, Malone JM Jr: Use of Cavitron surgical aspirator for debulking of diaphragmatic metastases in patients with advanced ovarian carcinoma of the ovaries. Surg Gynecol Obstet 168:455, 1989

35. Brand E, Pearlman N: Electrosurgical debulking of ovarian cancer: a new technique using the argon beam coagulator. Gynecol Oncol 39:115, 1990

36. Fanning J, Hilgers RD: Loop electrosurgical excision procedure for intensified

cytoreduction of ovarian cancer. Gynecol Oncol 57:188, 1995

37. Hunter RW, Alexander NDE, Soutter WP: Meta-analysis of surgery in advanced ovarian carcinoma: is maximum cytoreductive surgery an independent determinant of prognosis? Am J Obstet Gynecol 166:504, 1992

38. Kehoe ST, Luesley DM, Ward K, Chan KK: In vivo evidence of increased malignant cell proliferation following surgery in ovarian cancer. Int J Gynecol Cancer 5:121, 1995

39. Hacker NF: Cytoreduction for advanced ovarian cancer in perspective. Int J Gynecol Cancer 6:159, 1996

CHAPTER 5

SECOND-LOOK SURGERY

James L. Nicklin
Larry J. Copeland
David M. Luesley
Sean Kehoe

EDITORS' INTRODUCTION

Since about 1960, second-look surgery has been employed extensively in the management of ovarian cancer. The procedure has gained popularity over the past two decades as more ovarian cancer patients have been treated with chemotherapy and fewer have received radiotherapy. Within the past few years, however, there has been increasing skepticism about the benefits of this procedure.

Interpretation of reports of experience with second-look surgery has been complicated by the fact that no standard definition of the procedure exists. Most experts agree that the term *second-look surgery* should be restricted to an operation performed on a patient with no clinical evidence of persistent tumor for the purpose of determining disease status after a planned interval of treatment with chemotherapy. The term should not be applied to a surgical procedure performed in patients with clinical evidence of persistent or progressive disease for the primary purpose of debulking or for the treatment of complications.

Findings at second-look surgery are classified as negative (grossly and pathologically negative), microscopically positive (grossly negative, pathologically positive), and macroscopically positive (grossly and pathologically positive). The clinical variables most consistently associated with findings at second-look surgery and subsequent survival are histologic grade, amount of residual disease, and stage. Patients with low-grade tumors, minimal residual disease, and early-stage disease have a greater probability of negative findings at second-look surgery than do those with high-grade tumors, bulky residual disease, or advanced-stage disease.

Alternatives to second-look surgery include imaging studies and serum CA 125. Computed tomography (CT) of the abdomen and pelvis has been evaluated as a substitute for second-look surgery, but available information confirms the fact that tumor implants smaller than 2 cm in diameter are not reliably imaged. Therefore, a negative CT scan does not obviate the need for second-look surgery. However, a positive study may avoid second-look surgery in approximately 20% of patients.

A negative serum CA 125 level at completion of chemotherapy also does not reliably predict lack of persistent disease. Second-look laparotomy has been negative in only 40 to 50% of patients with normal CA 125 levels. A positive CA 125 level, however, reliably predicts persistence of disease and avoids a surgical procedure.

The benefits of second-look surgery have been seriously questioned during the past few years. Advocates of the procedure state that it remains the most reliable method for detection of persistent cancer. Furthermore, they emphasize that the findings at second-look surgery are of prognostic value; patients with macroscopic tumor have a worse survival rate than that of patients with either microscopic tumor or negative findings. Proponents also point out that resection of macroscopic tumor found at second-look surgery improves survival. The issue of debulking at second-look surgery, however, remains highly controversial.

Critics state that, although second-look surgery is superior to other methods of detecting residual ovarian cancer, the procedure does not accurately predict the presence or absence of disease. In patients with advanced-stage disease, the recurrence rate after negative second-look surgery is approximately 50%. Another major criticism of second-look surgery is the lack of evidence of enhanced survival as a result of the procedure or of the therapeutic decisions made on the basis of the findings.

QUESTIONS

1. In which settings, if any, should second-look surgery be used and why?
2. What is the role, if any, of laparoscopy in second-look surgery?
3. How do the findings at second-look surgery govern further therapy?
4. What are future directions or strategies to elucidate the role of second-look surgery?

QUESTION 1

In which settings, if any, should second-look surgery be used and why?

JAMES L. NICKLIN
LARRY J. COPELAND

Second-look laparotomy is a comprehensive surgical staging procedure in a patient who is clinically free of disease, after completion of a planned primary program of treatment, usually surgery and chemotherapy. The term *clinically free of disease* is defined as a physical examination indicating no evidence of cancer, negative imaging studies, and normal tumor markers.

The case in favor of second-look laparotomy

As epithelial ovarian cancer is a disease that remains largely confined to the peritoneum and retroperitoneal lymphatics until late in the course of the disease, laparotomy is an obvious method with which to evaluate this site of potential disease. Most patients will have no clinically detectable disease at the completion of primary therapy and, because of the deficiencies of contemporary investigational modalities, there is no nonoperative method of accurately determining disease status. While second-look laparotomy provides the most accurate prognostic information at the completion of primary treatment, the strongest argument for reoperation is the belief that survival can be improved by the instigation of salvage treatment regimens at an earlier stage than waiting for disease to become clinically apparent. Furthermore, this information can be obtained with demonstrably low morbidity rates.

The case against second-look laparotomy

The case against second-look laparotomy is predicated on the belief that there is either no survival advantage or such compromise in quality of life by the procedure and its attendant therapeutic implications that performance of the procedure is not justified. Even the prognostic information obtained can be regarded as of limited value, as patients with *any* persistent disease have a poor long-term survival, and patients with a negative second-look laparotomy have a 50% likelihood of recurrence in the long term.[1] Furthermore, it can be argued that as bowel obstruction and further surgery are a common feature of this disease, it is desirable to avoid any procedures that may cause adhesion formation.

That the place of second-look laparotomy remains controversial is a reflection of the inadequacy of the literature in answering this question. No large, well-constructed randomized trial has been published that can be used to answer this complex question. Luesley et al[2] published the results of a randomized prospective multicenter trial in ovarian cancer patients who had completed primary therapy that addressed this issue. This trial demonstrated a trend toward improved median survival for patients treated with second-look laparotomy, followed by consolidation chlorambucil, compared with chlorambucil alone without prior surgery. However, the paper has several deficiencies. It was a small study that had sufficient power to detect only large differences in survival, that is, a 95% confidence interval (CI) for true difference in median survival between − 10 and + 18 months, with overall median survival of 17 months. There was a high rate of protocol violation with only 32 of 53 eligible patients having second-look laparotomy. While the preoperative workup is not described, 23 of the 53 patients eligible for second-look laparotomy showed evidence of disease, which by contemporary criteria would render them ineligible for second-look laparotomy. Finally, the value of chlorambucil as either second-line or consolidation chemotherapy has been challenged.[3]

Fiorentino et al[4] also reported the results of a prospective, multicenter randomized trial. This trial also failed to show a statistically significant improvement in survival for patients randomized to second-look following primary therapy and negative metastatic workup. This study was also methodologically flawed. It was a small study, with only 102 patients available for randomization of the 340 initially referred. Three different chemotherapy regimens were used as primary therapy: cisplatinum-cyclophosphamide, doxorubicin plus cyclophosphamide, and mitoxantrone plus carboplatin. All stages of disease were included for analysis, including 47 patients (46%) with stage I and II disease. The selectively good prognosis of these patients would dilute any beneficial effect of second-look laparotomy in patients with advanced disease. Finally laparoscopy was used as part of the metastatic workup and contravenes the definition of second-look laparotomy. This practice would identify a significant number of patients with disease who might have benefited from cytoreduction and early initiation of salvage therapies.

The place of second-look laparotomy outside clinical studies

Outside the context of clinical studies, there is no compelling evidence in the literature with which to support or refute the role of second-look laparotomy. Furthermore, issues such as psychological factors and response to surgery may have a greater effect on a patient's outcome than the weight of accumulated evidence in the literature. The decision to undergo second-look laparotomy is probably best made between the individual patient and her physician, taking into account the many variables that affect survival and quality of life. The absence of irrefutable randomized controlled trial evidence in favor of second-look laparotomy is not reason enough to withhold this potentially beneficial operation.

The place of second-look laparotomy in clinical trials

While doubt may remain as to the value of second-look laparotomy "off-study," we believe that the place for second-look laparotomy in clinical trials is more straightforward. Clinical end points to evaluate primary therapy of ovarian cancer therapy have, by convention, included negative second-look laparotomy rate, progression-free interval, and survival. Clearly, disease status at second-look laparotomy more accurately reflects response to therapy than the other clinical indices, which are influenced by secondary factors. Progression-free interval is affected by the aggressiveness of follow-up management, and survival is influenced by the variable management of recurrent and terminal ovarian cancer.

From an ethical perspective, this aspect of treatment should remain acceptable to all concerned parties. The morbidity associated with second-look laparotomy is acceptably low, and the information obtained not only serves as valuable research material but can be used to guide the future management of each individual patient. In summary, we believe that second-look laparotomy is of fundamental importance in clinical trials evaluating primary therapy regimens in epithelial ovarian cancer.

Alternatives to second-look surgery

The role of second-look laparotomy has not been usurped by nonoperative modalities because these do not have the diagnostic accuracy of exploratory laparotomy. The bulk of experience has been accumulated with CT. CT scanning has good sensitivity for the detection of parenchymal hepatic disease and retroperitoneal nodal disease but cannot be relied on to detect peritoneal tumors of less than 2-cm diameter.[5,6] Occasionally, disease up to 4 cm in diameter can be found after a negative CT scan.[7] The diagnostic accuracy of CT scanning has been found to be as low as 28 to 63%.[6,8,9] Ultrasound, magnetic resonance imaging (MRI), positron emission tomography (PET), and even radioimmunoscintigraphy offer similar or inferior diagnostic accuracy.[5,10–17]

These investigational modalities do have a high positive predictive value, however, particularly when used in conjunction with fine-needle aspiration cytology, highlighting the importance of preoperative imaging in patients under consideration for second-look surgery. Because of the extensive accumulated experience and the widespread availability of CT scanning, this is most widely accepted as the standard imaging component of the preoperative workup.

Serum tumor markers, particularly CA 125, are a useful clinical adjunct that can be used to monitor approximately 80 to 90% of patients who have serous ovarian carcinomas. When used to test for disease before second-look laparotomy, CA 125 has been found to have a sensitivity of 96% and a specificity of 44%.[8] With the exception of occasional false-positives results, elevated CA 125 levels are almost always associated with persistent tumor, while CA 125 levels within normal limits are associated with persistent disease in approximately one-half of patients undergoing second-look laparotomy.[18–25] Other tumor markers have been evaluated for epithelial ovarian carcinoma monitoring, but these do not appear to offer any advantage.

Peritoneal cytology has been used as a minimally invasive test for occult residual disease before second-look laparotomy.[26,27] There is insufficient diagnostic accuracy in this test to replace the role of second-look laparotomy. Even at open laparotomy, Rubin and colleagues found that of patients with gross intraperitoneal disease, only 34% had positive cytology, and in patients with microscopic disease, 28% had positive cytology.[28]

DAVID M. LUESLEY
SEAN KEHOE

Second-look surgery, or second-look laparatomy, was originally introduced by Wangensteen et al.[29] in the late 1940s as a method to assess disease status following primary therapy in colonic carcinoma, with the added potential of resecting any residual tumor. This became part of ovarian cancer management since the early 1970s—a time when the appropriate duration of chemotherapy was unknown, although the risks of iatrogenic malignancies were recognized with prolonged exposure to alkylating agents.[30] A case series, reported by Smith et al.[31] demonstrated not only the safety of second-look surgery but also that chemotherapy could be discontinued, should it prove negative. Therefore, at that time second-look surgery had an important role in determining the efficacy of therapy; it also prevented unnecessary prolonged use in some patients. This fulfills important criteria required for any investigative procedures, in that the information gleaned must be of value, acted upon, and, it is hoped, of benefit to the patient. Concerns regarding prolonged use of single-agent alkylating cytotoxics have been overcome with the advent of platinum-based therapy in the treatment of ovarian cancer. The optimum cycles and efficacy of platinum-based regimens are well recognized, which means that the role of second-look surgery must be reconsidered.

Second-look surgery is generally undertaken after completion of adjuvant therapy and therefore depends on the duration of chemotherapy. The reported literature on second-look surgery spans a time when a full course of chemotherapy could range from 6 to 12 months. For example, Luesley et al[2] performed second-look surgery within 32 weeks from initial diagnosis, whereas 90% of patients in a series reported by Podratz et al[32] underwent second-look surgery after 52 weeks from diagnosis. The former study incorporated patients early in the disease process and the latter those (self-selected by the later intervention) with a better prognosis. Thus, populations in published series will differ rendering direct comparisons impossible. This should also be remembered when interpreting any publications on this topic.

Second-look laparotomy can have two outcomes—positive or negative. The possible value of these findings is indicated in Table 5-1. Second-look surgery in all patients may be justified, as it has been the most accurate way to determine tumor status after treatment. How this information alters practice and, most importantly, patient outcome is a different matter. A balance between the value of second-look surgery and the inherent morbidity it entails for the patient has to be considered.

In early-stage disease, the balance seems in favour of avoiding routine second-look surgery. Walton et al[33] published the largest series on its use in stage I or II ovarian cancer. Patients were included in randomized studies assessing the efficacy of adjuvant therapy (melphalan or intraperitoneal P53) versus observation. As an aspect of the protocols, second-look surgery was planned for all patients who were asymptomatic at 18 months from trial entry. If symptoms suggestive of recurrence occurred before this, re-exploration was performed. A total of 95 asymptomatic patients had second-look surgery, in whom recurrent disease was detected in 5%. In 9 of 17 (53%) symptomatic patients, recurrent disease was present at laparotomy. The overall positive yield from second-look surgery was 12%. When compared to a further 89 patients (not exposed to surgery for a variety of reasons), the incidence of recurrent disease was similar at 13%. This indicated that second-look surgery per se did not influence the rate of disease relapse and, as all patients succumbed irrespective of the method of diagnosis, the use of second-look seemed inappropriate. More recent studies corroborate these original findings. In assessing 54 patients with stage I disease after surgery and chemotherapy, Rubin et al[34] found only 5% to have a positive second-look outcome. Another series (with an observational arm) had a lower positive rate of 1 of 56, probably due to the fact that second-look surgery was performed 12 months from primary surgery.[35] There are no studies reported in which second-line therapy in patients with recurrent disease influenced survival. Therefore, it is possible to predict, without resorting to routine second-look surgery, that at least 90% of patients with prop-

TABLE 5-1
Potential Value of Second-Look Surgery

Cessation of chemotherapy with negative findings
Continuation/consolidation therapy with positive findings
Prognostic information for patient
Excision of residual disease
Assessing the efficacy of novel therapeutic strategies

erly staged I/II disease will not develop recurrence by 18 months postdiagnosis. Such predictability is better than many investigations. As second-look surgery in early-stage disease results in exposure of 90% of patients to unnecessary morbidity, its routine use cannot be advocated. The study conducted by Walton et al[33] did indicate a possible use of second-look surgery in a small group of patients. In those with clinically symptomatic recurrences within 18 months, 8 of 17 had negative findings. Arguably, this avoided inappropriate therapy for some patients, but some required surgical intervention on clinical grounds (i.e., bowel obstruction) and, with present techniques of tumor markers and radiology, some would not have undergone surgery. The fact that survival was not enhanced with second-look surgery makes it difficult to find any indication for its routine use, although occasional situations will inevitably arise when second-look surgery is deemed clinically appropriate.

In advanced disease, more than 50% of patients will have a positive second-look evaluation. There are certain courses of action. For example, chemotherapy could be continued or changed. Sufficient information is available to indicate that patients exposed to platinum-based regimens receive no benefit from exceeding six cycles of therapy. Alternatively, salvage therapies could be introduced—unfortunately, the development of effective second-line treatment is awaited. One exception is paclitaxel, which is now included as first-line therapy. A patient with positive second-look therapy without prior exposure to paclitaxel could benefit from its use.[36] Whether the introduction of second-line therapy on finding a positive second-look outcome, rather than when the disease is clinically detectable, influences the efficacy of treatment remains to be properly assessed. For other agents, we do know that salvage therapy initiated when microscopic disease is detected at second-look surgery confers no survival advantage over patients treated at clinical recurrence who had a previous negative second-look outcome.[37] The case for a clinical trial to identify the optimum approach to therapy on positive second-look evaluation versus clinical recurrence is evident.

On the basis of the findings that tumor debulking to residual disease of less than 1-cm maximum diameter is associated with improved survival[38] and with the more recent evidence that interventional cytoreduction increases median survival,[39] a case may be forwarded for cytoreduction at second-look surgery. Reports in the literature[2,32,40–42] on the value of cytoreduction at second-look surgery are conflicting, and all suffer from small patient numbers (Table 5-2). In the series by Podratz et al[32] a survival advantage was noted in those cleared of macroscopic disease or reduced to less than 5-mm residuum compared to greater than 5-mm residuum. The Lippman[40] series also reported a significant improvement in survival, with tumor reduction to less than 2 cm, although whether some patients were rendered tumor free is not mentioned. Interestingly, the report by Lippman et al[40] noted that patients with microscopic disease had a longer survival compared to those cleared of all macroscopic tumor, contradicting the findings of Podratz et al.[32] One of the larger series, which, significantly, is the only prospective randomized series on second-look surgery, included 29 patients who underwent successful debulking.[2] Fifteen were macroscopically cleared and 14 to less than 2-cm residual disease. Survival of this group, compared to patients inoperable at second-look surgery, was significantly better, but comparisons of each arm (second look versus no second look) revealed that both groups had

TABLE 5-2
Cytoreductive Surgery at Second-Look Surgery and Survival

REFERENCE	NO. OPTIMALLY DEBULKED	SURVIVAL
Podratz et al (1985)[32]	9	Improved
Luesley et al (1988)[2]	29	No impact
Lippman et al (1988)[40]	14	Improved
Chambers et al (1988)[41]	16	No impact
Miller et al (1992)[42]	9	No impact

similar survival rates. As all other series are nonrandomized studies, the conclusion from the work of Luesley et al[2] must be considered most accurate. A specific trial on cytoreduction at second-look surgery is required.

Patients with a negative second-look outcome have a better prognosis than those with a positive result, an obvious conclusion. The value to the patient of a negative second-look outcome is in hearing some positive information. Also, chemotherapy can be ceased—although, as already alluded to, this is not an issue at the present time. A certain amount of caution is required regarding negative findings as a significant proportion of patients will develop recurrent disease. The relapse rate following negative second-look surgery ranges from 30% to 44%, any time from 2 to 70 months after surgery.[1,43,44] Recurrences in early-stage disease are uncommon (10% or less), whereas in advanced disease 50% or more patients eventually relapse. Recognized variables associated with an increased risk of relapse after negative second-look surgery include residual disease after primary surgery, tumor grade, stage and age, and positive lymph nodes at primary surgery.[1,43–46] It is possible to categorize patients using these parameters to identify a group at high risk of recurrence after a negative second-look outcome.[45,47]

The sensitivity and specificity of such formulas are poor, although potentially of use in considering patients for consolidation therapy—when effective treatment becomes available.

Noninvasive methods of assessment

Second-look laparotomy remains the most sensitive method to determine tumor response to adjuvant therapies. Other assessments have failed to supersede second-look surgery. Even in CA 125-producing tumors, the sensitivity of CA 125 in predicting the presence of disease ranges from 38% to 100%.[19,23,48] Levels above 35 U/ml are often associated with a positive second-look.[19,49] Radiologic tools are also limited in accuracy. CT and MRI scans suffer from false negative results and cannot reliably detect smaller lesions—a similar difficulty with clinical examination.[7,50] Although abnormal CA 125 levels, radiologic findings, and clinical examination mean a high probability of recurrent disease, normal results do not exclude the presence of disease. The combination of tumor markers or addition of monoclonal antibodies could enhance the predictability of these investigations and progress in this area is to be welcomed.[24,51] Until more sensitive and specific noninvasive tools are available, second-look surgery remains the gold standard of evaluation.

QUESTION 2

What is the role, if any, of laparoscopy in second-look surgery?

JAMES L. NICKLIN
LARRY J. COPELAND

The role of laparoscopy has been investigated by a number of investigators as an alternative to second-look laparotomy.[52,53] Initial experiences were reported as unsatisfactory due to false-negative rates from of 20 to 55%[52,53] and surgical completion rates of only 11 to 73%.[54] With the resurgence of interest in minimally invasive surgical procedures and the development of innovative instrumentation and techniques, a comprehensive laparoscopic second-look procedure has become more feasible.[55–57] A detailed evaluation is now possible, almost equivalent to open surgery, including retroperitoneal lymphadenectomy.[57]

Limitations to this approach include a potentially significant learning curve and, in patients in whom primary surgery consisted of extensive radical debulking, is likely to be associated with widespread adhesions. The safety and efficacy of laparoscopic staging for epithelial ovarian cancer are under evaluation.[57] It is likely that second-look laparoscopy will assume an increasingly important role in the management of patients with epithelial ovarian cancer after primary therapy.

DAVID M. LUESLEY
SEAN KEHOE

Role of laparoscopy

The inherent benefits of laparoscopy over laparotomy are self-evident. Its application as an alternative to laparotomy is not novel. There are no available randomized prospective series comparing second-look laparoscopy to laparotomy. The reports on second-look laparoscopy indicate that in approximately one-third of patients, disease will be present at laparoscopy, which obviates the need for laparotomy.[53] Unfortunately, the false-negative rate of laparoscopy is around 20%. Failures and morbidity must also considered. Berek et al[58] undertook 119 laparoscopies in 57 patients treated for ovarian cancer, with a failure rate of 26%. Complications associated with successful laparoscopy were reduced by using needle laparoscopy before introducing a 12-mm laparoscope. Even so, organ perforation or hemorrhage occurred in 10% of procedures, with 6.7% of patients requiring laparotomy. It would seem that even in the most experienced hands, the rate of complications persists today.[57] Therefore, laparoscopy can reduce the number of laparotomies when used where the primary objective is assessing tumor status. The pertinent question is why and not how second-look procedures are performed.

QUESTION 3

How do the findings at second-look surgery govern further therapy?

JAMES L. NICKLIN
LARRY J. COPELAND

Negative second-look findings

The results of second-look surgery are of considerable prognostic value and significantly influence further therapy. Numerous studies have confirmed that patients with negative second-look findings have a superior survival to patients with positive findings.[40,59] Many major centers would recommend close clinical follow-up evaluation in this setting. However, in an attempt to improve survival in this potentially curable group, a number of consolidation therapies have been suggested and pilot studies activated. At this stage there is no consensus recommendation.[60] Based on promising results from nonrandomized studies,[61,62] The Gynecologic Oncology Group (GOG) has completed accrual for a prospective trial evaluating the role of intraperitoneal ^{32}P following negative second-look laparotomy. Pilot studies using intraperitoneal chemotherapy (cisplatin with or without etoposide, cisplatin with or without mitoxantrone) following negative second-look have been promising, however, the follow-up on these studies is somewhat limited.[63–65] In a more radical approach, investigators at the Royal Hospital for Women, Sydney, Australia, have commenced a pilot study evaluating the role of high-dose chemotherapy and autologous bone marrow rescue in this setting.

Tamoxifen may prove useful as a consolidation agent following negative second-look laparotomy. This hormone has a response rate similar to other chemotherapy agents in the salvage setting[66] but may have superior activity following negative second-look laparotomy. This is by virtue of a higher incidence of estrogen receptor positivity and lower grade tumor in this prognostically select group. Of great importance is that it is almost devoid of side effects, has some beneficial metabolic effects,[67] and is less likely to compromise quality of life in this cohort likely to experience moderate longevity. This novel approach awaits clinical testing.

Microscopic positive second-look laparotomy

At second-look surgery, up to 20% of patients with advanced epithelial ovarian cancer will have no macroscopic evidence of disease but will demonstrate microscopic evidence of tumor.[68] This cohort of patients has been shown to have significantly better survival than those with macroscopic disease, but extended survival is probably limited.[40] This group may benefit from additional therapy. Promising results have been published using intraperitoneal chemotherapy.[69–71] Whole abdominal radiotherapy has also been suggested for this subgroup of patients.[72]

Macroscopic positive second-look laparotomy

Macroscopic tumor detected at second-look laparotomy is associated with a very poor prognosis, especially if the disease has shown evidence of progression following primary therapy or if the disease is multifocal, bulky, or unresectable. In a GOG review, even in patients optimally debulked at their primary surgery the 4-year survival was only 41% when persistent macroscopic tumor was present at second-look surgery.[73] For patients with persistent macroscopic disease at second-look laparotomy the median survival is probably 15 to 20 months.

If macroscopic disease is found at second-look laparotomy, a decision must be made whether to attempt debulking, or to terminate the operation and pursue a more palliative course. Secondary debulking of macroscopic tumor at second-look laparotomy is the subject of controversy. However, it is apparent that where macroscopic disease remains after secondary surgery, prognosis is poor.[40,74–76] Hoskins and colleagues,[76] Potter and colleagues,[75] and others[2,40,74,77–79] report a survival advantage for secondary debulking within this context. Raju and colleagues[80] report contradictory results. The relationship between resectability of tumor within this context, and survival, may be in part a reflection of tumor biology as well as the value of secondary cytoreduction. On the basis of the limited data available, if optimal resection can be easily or realistically achieved, this appears to prolong survival and should be attempted. Heroic surgical efforts are probably contraindicated, as morbidity may be considerable and survival improved minimally, if at all. Ultimately, the decision to proceed with secondary cytoreduction must be made on an individual judgment basis, taking into consideration the known tumor characteristics, the response to prior treatment, treatments still available, the patient's overall medical condition, and the surgical findings.[81]

When macroscopic chemoresistent disease is found at second-look laparotomy, the opportunity exists for tumor to be harvested for in vitro chemosensitivity testing. The information obtained in this manner potentially can predict chemoresistence and provide a guide to salvage regimens that may be offered. This approach is being prospectively evaluated.

While there is currently no consistently efficacious salvage chemotherapy regimen in this setting, the opportunity exists to instigate a change in chemotherapy, at the earliest possible time, with agents known to be active against epithelial ovarian cancer. The opportunity also exists for the patient to enrol in prospective clinical trials to evaluate experimental therapies.

DAVID M. LUESLEY
SEAN KEHOE

Throughout this review, the potential impact of second-look surgery has been discussed. It can affect the implimentation of consolidation therapy or use of cytoreductive surgery. Both strategies do need to be proved within the context of clinical trials. One area in which second-look surgery could directly govern therapies is in the assessment of novel agents. For example, results from the randomized study comparing paclitaxal and cisplatinum versus cisplatin and cyclophosphamide have shown that among those who underwent second-look surgery, 14% of patients on the paclitaxel arm had microscopic disease, compared to 4% in the cisplatin arm.[82] This information is of value in that by increasing dose or prolonging therapy it may be possible to render some of these 14% of patients disease free. Ongoing studies on dose intensification with these agents should identify the relevancy of basing dose or duration of treatment on findings at second-look surgery.

QUESTION 4

What are future directions or strategies to elucidate the role of second-look surgery?

JAMES L. NICKLIN
LARRY J. COPELAND

To clarify the role of second-look laparotomy, it would be ideal to instigate a large, prospective randomized multicenter trial of patients following primary therapy. Realistically, it is unlikely that this will be undertaken in the foreseeable future for several reasons. Differences in survival are likely to be modest; therefore, only a large study would have sufficient power to demonstrate the anticipated differences in survival. A study of 560 patients would be necessary to have an 85% chance of detecting a 15% difference in median survival. The most objective end points of such a study would include progression-free interval and, more importantly, survival. These are subject to considerable bias because of difficulty standardizing both follow-up evaluation and the management of recurrent and terminal ovarian cancer. The study would also have to control for the many variables that influence second-look findings, as discussed above. Finally, an important aspect of the study would be to evaluate quality-of-life indices prospectively. In this era of some skepticism regarding second-look laparotomy, it may prove difficult to initiate a study with these demanding requirements even within well organized multicenter organizations.

In summary, we believe there is an important place for second-look laparotomy in the management of patients with epithelial ovarian cancer. In the absence of definitive data, the decision to proceed to second-look laparotomy is appropriately made between the patient and the physician, after careful discussion of the many complex issues that involve an informed decision.

DAVID M. LUESLEY
SEAN KEHOE

Future strategies with second-look surgery

Many aspects of second-look surgery need to be addressed. The role of cytoreduction at second-look surgery has already been discussed, as was the need to assess the introduction of second-line treatments. Other evidence suggests that there may be a subgroup of patients in whom debulking at second-look surgery improves outcome. Segna et al[83] reported that patients optimally debulked at second-look surgery had a median survival of 27 months compared with 9 months in those with bulky tumor (greater than 2 cm). Analysis showed secondary cytoreduction more likely to succeed in those with less than 2 cm after primary surgery, at less than 55 years of age, with an interval from primary diagnosis to secondary surgery of 12 months or more. A smaller study, by Janicke et al[84] also revealed the preferable outcome in patients macroscopically cleared of disease at second-look surgery, who had a 12-month disease-free interval from diagnosis and no residual tumor after primary surgery. Vaccarello et al[85] have also shown improved survival with debulking recurrent tumor after a negative second look. An important point about these series is that second-look was undertaken when disease was clinically or symptomatically present. In view of the potential benefits to this subgroup of patients, we (West Midlands Ovarian Cancer Group) are undertaking a prospective randomized trial in patients with a disease-free interval of at least 12 months from completion of primary therapy.

Conclusions

Second-look surgery in its true definition is a diagnostic procedure. It may assist in guiding dosages of novel therapies and have a role in clinical trials comparing therapy at positive second-look against clinical recurrence, and indeed in trials assessing cytoreductive surgery. It has not been proved to benefit patient outcome when used routinely in practice. Anecdotal cases will occur when second-look surgery may have influenced outcome. Practice should be based on evidence. Efforts should be targeted toward developing better noninvasive methods to evaluate tumor response. Response is important, although arguably survival is a better end point. Confining second-look surgery to pertinent clinical trials would seem a prudent course of action.

EDITORS' COMMENTARY

In response to the question about the use of second-look surgery in the management of ovarian cancer, both sets of authors nicely articulate the potential advantages and disadvantages of the procedure, albeit from a somewhat different perspective. They agree that the current literature does not irrefutably support the use of this procedure on a routine basis. There is also general consensus among the authors that second-look surgery is the gold standard in terms of accuracy of predicting presence or absence of persistent ovarian cancer. No alternative to date matches the sensitivity of second-look surgery.

Drs. Nicklin and Copeland seem to be approaching the issue more positively than Drs. Kehoe and Luesley. They distinguish the use of second-look surgery based on whether it is within the context of a clinical trial but seem to favor its use even in the absence of a protocol setting. The British investigators discuss second-look surgery based on prognostic factors. They do not believe that there is sufficient evidence to support its general use in early-stage patients. We would agree with their conclusion, provided such patients have undergone comprehensive surgical staging initially. We also agree that available retrospective data on the benefits of secondary cytoreduction at second-look surgery are not totally convincing; a randomized trial to resolve this issue would be of considerable importance if it could successfully accrue patients.

As to the question regarding the role of laparoscopy for second-look surgery, there is no major disagreement. The consensus among experts is that this technique will be employed with increasing frequency, in view of the increasing interest in, and enhanced technology of, operative laparoscopy.

Most experts agree that if second-look surgery is performed, the findings govern decision making about further therapy. Two areas deserve emphasis. As mentioned by Drs. Kehoe and Luesley, the development of new, more promising second-line therapies will create some degree of resurgence in the use of second-look surgery, since criteria for enrollment on clinical trials involving these agents will be most commonly rather strictly defined. In addition, if any of the ongoing prospective trials involving consolidation therapy for patients with negative second-look findings succeed in demonstrating a survival advantage over observation, enthusiasm for second-look surgery will be rekindled.

Both investigative groups focus on the need for prospective randomized clinical trials to resolve some of the issues discussed in this chapter. Actually, with a large enough group of patients, two questions could be addressed in the same trial: (1) randomization of patients with advanced stage epithelial ovarian cancer after completion of primary surgery and chemotherapy to either second-look surgery or observation, and (2) a second-tier randomization of those patients with macroscopic disease at second-look surgery to either secondary debulking or no debulking. Although the biases in both directions in the United States may be too great to complete such a trial, cooperative groups in Europe or elsewhere may be able to be more successful.

Meantime, decisions about the use of second-look surgery will be made within the context of a clinical trial or as part of standard care as jointly decided by physician and patient. In the current managed-care environment of the United States, pressures will be great to avoid the procedure altogether.

References

1. Rubin SC, Hoskins WJ, Saigo PE et al: Prognostic factors for recurrence following negative second-look laparotomy

in ovarian cancer patients treated with platinum-based chemotherapy. Gynecol Oncol 42:137, 1991

2. Luesley D, Lawton F, Blackledge G et al: Failure of second-look laparotomy to influence survival in epithelial ovarian cancer. Lancet 2:599, 1988
3. Nicklin JL, Copeland LJ: The role of second-look laparotomy and secondary cytoreduction in ovarian carcinoma. In Rock JA, Faro S, Grant NF Jr, Horowitz IR, Murphy AA (eds): Advances in Obstetrics and Gynecology. Vol. 3. Mosby-Year Book, Chicago, 1996
4. Fiorentino MV, Nicoletta MO, Tumolo S et al: Uselessness of surgical second-look in epithelial ovarian cancer: a randomized study, abstracted. Proc Am Soc Clin Oncol 13:259, 1994
5. Lund B, Jacobson K, Rasch L et al: Correlation of abdominal ultrasound and computed tomography scans with second- or third-look laparotomy in patients with ovarian carcinoma. Gynecol Oncol 37:279, 1990
6. De Rosa V, Mangioni di Stefano ML, Brunetti A et al: Computed tomography and second-look surgery in ovarian cancer patients. Correlation, actual role and limitations of CT scan. Eur J Gynaecol Oncol 16:123, 1995
7. Clarke-Pearson D, Bandy LC, Dudzinski M et al: Computed tomography in evaluation of patients with ovarian carcinoma in complete clinical remission. Correlation with surgical-pathological findings. JAMA 255:627, 1986
8. Barter JF, Barnes WA: Second-look laparotomy. p. 269. In Rubin SC, Sutton GP (eds): Ovarian Cancer. McGraw-Hill, New York, 1993
9. Brenner DE, Shaff MI, Jones HW Jr et al: Abdominopelvic computed tomography: evaluation in patients undergoing second-look laparotomy for ovarian carcinoma. Obstet Gynecol 65:715, 1985
10. Khan O, Cosgrove DO, Fried AM, Savage PE: Ovarian carcinoma follow-up: US versus laparotomy. Radiology 159: 111, 1986
11. Murolo C, Constantini S, Foglia G et al: Ultrasound examination in ovarian cancer patients. A comparison with second look laparotomy. J Ultrasound Med 8:441, 1989
12. Nardelli GB, Onnis GL, Lamaina V, Petrillo MR: Ultrasound evaluation in the follow-up of ovarian cancer today. Clin Exp Obstet Gynecol 14:174, 1987
13. Fishman-Javitt M, Stein H, Lovecchio J: Imaging of the Pelvis: MRI With Correlations to CT and Ultrasound. Little Brown, Boston, 1990
14. Surwit EA, Childers JM, Krag DN et al: Clinical assessment of ^{111}In-Cyt-103 immunoscintigraphy in ovarian cancer. Gynecol Oncol 48:285, 1993
15. Barzen G, Friedmann W, Richter W et al: The place of radioimmunoscintigraphy in the diagnosis and follow-up of ovarian cancer in comparison with computed tomography and second-look surgery. Nuklearmedizin 31:15, 1992
16. Loboguerrero A, Perault C, Leihn JC: Volume rendering and binocular scale in double isotope studies: application to immunoscintigraphy and bone landmarking. Eur J Nucl Med 19:201, 1992
17. Forstner R, Hricak H, Powell CB et al: Ovarian cancer recurrence: value of MR imaging. Radiology 196:715, 1995
18. Niloff JM, Bast RJ, Schaetzl EM, Knapp RC: Predictive value of CA 125 antigen levels in second-look procedures for ovarian cancer. Am J Obstet Gynecol 151:981, 1985
19. Berek JS, Knapp RC, Malkasian GD et al: CA 125 serum levels correlated with second-look operations among ovarian cancer patients. Obstet Gynecol 67: 685, 1986
20. Atack DB, Nisker JA, Allen HH et al: CA 125 surveillance and second-look

laparotomy in ovarian carcinoma. Am J Obstet Gynecol 154:287, 1986

21. Potter ME, Moradi M, To AC et al: Value of serum CA-125 levels: does the result preclude second look? Gynecol Oncol, 33:201, 1989
22. Meier W, Stieber P, Eiermann W et al: Serum levels of CA 125 and histological findings at second-look laparotomy in ovarian carcinoma. Gynecol Oncol 35: 44, 1989
23. Rubin SC, Hoskins WJ, Hakes TB et al: Serum CA 125 levels and surgical findings in patients undergoing secondary operations for epithelial ovarian cancer. Am J Obstet Gynecol 160:667, 1989
24. Kierkegaard O, Mogensen O, Mogensen B, Jakobsen A: Predictive and prognostic values of Cancer-Associated Serum Antigen (CASA) and Cancer Antigen 125 (CA 125) levels prior to second-look laparotomy. Gynecol Oncol 59:251, 1995
25. Patsner B, Orr JW, Mann WJ et al: Does serum CA 125 level prior to second look laparotomy for invasive ovarian adenocarcinoma predict size of residual disease? Gynecol Oncol 38:373, 1990
26. McGowan L, Bunnag B: The evaluation of therapy for ovarian cancer. Gynecol Oncol 4:375, 1976
27. Goldberg G, Learmonth G, BlochB, Levin W: Role of cul-de-sac aspiration cytology in the management and follow-up of patients with ovarian carcinoma. A preliminary report. J Reprod Med 30:867, 1985
28. Rubin SC, Dulaney ED, Markman M et al: Peritoneal cytology as an indicator of disease in patients with residual ovarian carcinoma. Obstet Gynecol 71:851, 1988
29. Wangensteen PH, Lewis FJ, Tongen LA: Second look in cancer surgery. Lancet 71:303, 1951
30. Reimer RR, Hoover R, Fraumeni JF Jr, Young RC: Acute leukemia after alkylating agent therapy of ovarian cancer. N Engl J Med 297:177, 1977
31. Smith JP, Delgado G, Rutledge F: Second-look operation in ovarian carcinoma. Cancer 38:1438, 1976
32. Podratz KC, Malkasian GD, Hilton JF et al: Second-look laparotomy in ovarian cancer: evaluation of pathological variables. Am J Obstet Gynecol 152:230, 1985
33. Walton L, Ellenberg SS, Major F et al: Results of second-look laparotomy in patients with early-stage ovarian carcinoma. Obstet Gynecol 70:770, 1987
34. Rubin SC, Jones WB, Curtin JP et al: Second-look laparotomy in stage I ovarian cancer following comprehensive surgical staging. Obstet Gynecol 82:139, 1993
35. Schnider J, Centeno MM, Montoya F, Rodriguez-Escudero FJ: Negative second-look laparotomy does not preclude recurrence in stage I ovarian carcinoma of any histological variety. Eur J Gynaecol Oncol 14:36, 1993
36. McGuire WP: Ovarian cancer. p. 201. In McGuire WP, Rowinsky EK (eds): Paclitaxel in Cancer Treatment. Marcel Dekker, New York, 1995
37. Potter ME, Hatch KD, Partridge EE: Second-look laparotomy and salvage therapy: a research modality only? Gynecol Oncol 44:3, 1992
38. Griffiths CT, Fuller AF: Intensive surgical and chemotherapeutic management of advanced ovarian cancer. Surg Clin North Am 58:131, 1978
39. van de Berg MEL, van Lent M, Buyse M et al: The effect of debulking surgery after induction chemotherapy on the prognosis in advanced epithelial ovarian cancer N Engl J Med 332:629, 1995
40. Lippman SM, Alberts DS, Slymen DJ: Second-look laparotomy in epithelial ovarian carcinoma. Cancer 61:2571, 1988
41. Chambers S, Chambers JT, Kohorn EI et al: Evaluation of the role of second-look surgery in ovarian cancer. Obstet Gynecol 72:404, 1988

42. Miller DS, Spirtos NM, Ballon SC et al: Critical reassessment of second-look exploratory laparotomy for epithelial ovarian carcinoma. Cancer 69:502, 1992

43. Podratz KC, Malkasian GD, Wieland SW et al: Recurrent disease after negative second-look laparotomy in stages III and IV ovarian carcinoma. Gynecol Oncol 29:274, 1988

44. Luesley DM, Chan KK, Lawton FG et al: Survival after negative second-look laparotomy. Eur J Surg Oncol 15:205, 1989

45. Podratz KC, Cliby WA: Second-look surgery in the management of epithelial ovarian carcinoma. Gynecol Oncol suppl. 55:S128, 1994

46. Bolis G, Villa A, Guarnerio P et al: Survival of women with advanced ovarian cancer and complete pathological response at second-look laparotomy. Cancer 77:128, 1996

47. Morgan MA, Noumoff JS, King S, Mikuta JJ: A formula for predicting the risk of positive second-look laparotomy in epithelial ovarian cancer: implications for a randomised trial. Obstet Gynecol 80:944, 1992

48. Halila H, Lehtovirta P, Stenman U, Seppala M: CA125 in the follow-up of patients with ovarian cancer. Acta Obstet Gynecol Scand 67:53, 1988

49. Folk JJ, Botfords M, Musa AG: Monitoring cancer antigen 125 levels in induction chemotherapy for epithelial ovarian carcinoma and predicting outcomes at second-look procedures. Gynecol Oncol 178, 1995

50. Dershaw DD, Panicek DM: Radiologic evaluation of ovarian cancer. p. 133. In Markman M, Hoskins WJ (eds): Cancer of the Ovary. Raven Press New York, 1993

51. Muto MG, Kassis AI: Monclonal antibodies used in the detection and treatment of epithelial ovarian cancer. Cancer 76:2016, 1995

52. Ozols RF, Fisher RI, Anderson T et al: Peritoneoscopy in the management of ovarian cancer. Am J Obstet Gynecol 140:611, 1981

53. Piver MS, Lele SB, Barlow JJ, Gamarra M: Second-look laparoscopy prior to proposed second-look laparotomy. Obstet Gynecol 55:571, 1980

54. Berek JS, Hacker NF: Laparoscopy in the management of patients with ovarian carcinoma. Clin Obstet Gynaecol 10: 213, 1983

55. Krafft W, Konig EM, Schirmer A et al: Second-look operation oder second-look laparoskopie zur Sicherung der kompletten remission beim ovarialkarzinom. Zentralbl Gynakol 112:767, 1990

56. Marti VA, Sainz S, Soriano G et al: Utilidad de la laparoscopia como metodo do "second-look" en las neoplasias de ovario. Rev Esp Enf Dig 77:275, 1990

57. Childers JM, Lang J, Surwit EA, Hatch KD: Laparoscopic surgical staging of ovarian cancer. Gynecol Oncol 59:25, 1995

58. Berek JS, Griffiths CT, Leventhal JM: Laparoscopy for second-look evaluation in ovarian cancer. Obstet Gynecol 58: 192, 1981

59. Rubin SC: Second-look laparotomy. p. 175. In Markman M, Hoskins WJ (eds): Cancer of the Ovary. Raven Press, New York, 1993

60. NIH Consensus Conference: Ovarian cancer. Screening, treatment, and follow-up. JAMA 273:491, 1995

61. Varia M, Rosenman J, Venkatraman S et al: Intra peritoneal chromic phosphate therapy after second-look lapartomy for ovarian cancer. Cancer 61: 5919, 1988

62. Spencer TR, Marks RD, Fenn JO et al: Intraperitoneal P32 after negative second-look laparotomy in ovarian carcinoma. Cancer 63:2434, 1989

63. Menczer J, Baruch G, Rizel S et al: Intraperitoneal cisplatin chemotherapy in ovarian carcinoma patients who are clinically in complete remission. Gynecol Oncol 46:222, 1992

64. Schneider JG: Intraperitoneal chemotherapy. Obstet Gynecol Clin North Am 21:195, 1994

65. Tarraza HM, Boyce CR, Smith WG, Jones MA: Consolidation intraperitoneal chemotherapy in epithelial ovarian cancer patients following negative second-look laparotomy. Gynecol Oncol 50:287, 1993

66. Hatch KD, Beecham JB, Blessing JA, Creasman WT: Responsiveness of patients with advanced ovarian carcinoma to tamoxifen. A Gynecologic Oncology Group study of second-line therapy in 105 patients. Cancer 68:269, 1991

67. Powles TJ, Jones AL, Ashley SE et al: The Royal Marsden Hospital pilot tamoxifen chemoprevention trial. Breast Cancer Res Treat 31:73, 1994

68. Copeland LJ, Gershenson DM, Wharton JT et al: Microscopic disease at second-look laparotomy in advanced ovarian cancer. Cancer 55:472, 1985

69. Markman M, Reichman B, Hakes T et al: Responses to second-line cisplatin-based intraperitoneal therapy in ovarian cancer: influence of a prior response to systemic cisplatin. J Clin Oncol 9: 1801, 1991

70. Markman M, Hakes T, Reichman B et al: Intraperitoneal therapy in the management of ovarian carcinoma. Yale J Biol Med 62:393, 1989

71. Reichman B, Markman M, Hakes T et al: Phase I trial of concurrent intraperitoneal and continuous intravenous infusion of fluorouracil in patients with refractory cancer. J Clin Oncol 6:158, 1988

72. Thomas GM: Is there a role for consolidation or salvage radiotherapy after chemotherapy in advanced epithelial ovarian cancer? Gynecol Oncol 51:97, 1993

73. Creasman WT, Gall S, Bundy BN et al: Second-look laparotomy in the patient with minimal residual stage III ovarian cancer (A Gynecologic Oncology Group Study). Gynecol Oncol 35:378, 1989

74. Rome R, Fortune DW: The role of second-look laparotomy in the management of patients with ovarian carcinoma. Aust NZ J Obstet Gynaecol 28:318, 1988

75. Potter ME, Hatch KD, Soong S-J et al: Second-look laparotomy and salvage therapy: research modality only? Gynecol Oncol 44:3, 1992

76. Hoskins WJ, Rubin SC, Dulaney E et al: Influence of secondary cytoreduction at the time of second-look laparotomy on the survival of patients with epithelial ovarian carcinoma. Gynecol Oncol 34: 365, 1989

77. Ngan HY, Wong LC, Ma HK: Place of second-look laparotomy after 18 courses of chemotherapy in epithelial ovarian cancer. Aust NZ J Obstet Gynaecol 29: 52, 1989

78. Neijt J, ten Bokkel Huinink W, van der Berg M et al: Randomized trial comparing two combination chemotherapy regimens (Hexa-CAF vs CHAP-5) in advanced ovarian carcinoma. Lancet 2: 594, 1984

79. Janisch H, Schieder K, Koeble H: Diagnostic versus therapeutic second-look surgery in patients with ovarian cancer. Baillieres Clin Obstet Gynaecol 3:191, 1989

80. Raju KS, McKinna JA, Barker GH et al: Second-look operations in the planned management of advanced ovarian carcinoma. Am J Obstet Gynecol 144:650, 1982

81. Copeland LJ: Staging laparotomy. p. 3. In Greer BE, Berek JS (eds): Current Topics in Obstetrics and Gynecology. Elsevier, New York, 1991

82. McGuire WP, Hoskins WJ, Brady MF et al: Cyclophosphamide with cisplatin compared with paclitaxel and cisplatin in patients with stage III and stage IV ovarian cancer. N Eng J Med 334:1, 1996

83. Segna RA, Dottino PR, Mandeli JP et al: Secondary cytoreduction for ovarian cancer following cisplatin therapy. J Clin Oncol 11:434, 1993

84. Janick F, Holscher M, Kuhn W et al: Radical surgical procedures improves survival time in patients with recurrent ovarian cancer. Cancer 70:2129, 1992

85. Vaccarello L, Rubin SC, Vlamis V et al: Cytoreductive surgery in ovarian carcinoma patients with a documented previously complete surgical response. Gynecol Oncol 57:61, 1995

CHAPTER 6

SECONDARY CYTOREDUCTIVE SURGERY

Stephen C. Rubin
Ivor Benjamin
Jonathan S. Berek

EDITORS' INTRODUCTION

The role of secondary cytoreductive surgery in the management of epithelial ovarian cancer remains unclear. The term *secondary cytoreductive surgery* has no universal definition. It may denote cytoreductive surgery performed in one of several different clinical settings: (1) cytoreductive surgery for so-called "interval debulking" in patients whose primary surgery left suboptimal residual tumor and who have received a few (usually 3) cycles of chemotherapy; (2) cytoreductive surgery for recurrence after primary therapy (this group can be further subdivided by the duration of the disease-free interval [e.g., less than 6 months or more than 6 months]); and (3) cytoreductive surgery in patients who have persistent macroscopic tumor at second-look laparotomy. Most experts would agree that the term would not apply to cytoreductive surgery performed after neoadjuvant chemotherapy alone or after exploratory laparotomy/biopsy and chemotherapy, since there has not been a previous attempt at debulking. Likewise, the success or lack thereof of the attempt at cytoreduction should not influence the definition.

Tumors in these subgroups of ovarian cancer patients may have very different natural histories, principally defined by whether they are sensitive or resistant to subsequent treatment. Outcome may be influenced by both the biologic characteristics of the tumors and the surgical intervention. Therefore, it is extremely important for studies designed to assess the impact of these various secondary procedures on survival rates to define their study populations carefully. Because of the paucity of prospective randomized clinical trials in this area, it is difficult to draw many firm conclusions regarding the influence of secondary debulking in these settings.

In addition to addressing controversial issues surrounding the topic of secondary cytoreductive surgery, we have included a question regarding the role of surgery for gastrointestinal obstruction in patients with refractory ovarian cancer. Other questions on secondary cytoreductive surgery are addressed throughout the book.

QUESTIONS

1. What are the characteristics of an optimal candidate for secondary cytoreductive surgery and what intraoperative findings, if any, should lead to discontinuing a secondary cytoreductive procedure?
2. For patients who relapse 1 year or more after completion of primary therapy, what is the role, if any, of secondary cytoreductive surgery?
3. What is the role, if any, of secondary cytoreductive surgery at second-look surgery?
4. What is the evidence that interval debulking surgery is beneficial and should it be routine practice for any particular subset of patients?
5. What is the role of surgery for gastrointestinal obstruction in patients who have failed two or more chemotherapy regimens?

QUESTION 1

What are the characteristics of an optimal candidate for secondary cytoreductive surgery and what intraoperative findings, if any, should lead to discontinuing a secondary cytoreductive procedure?

STEPHEN C. RUBIN
IVOR BENJAMIN

Following the early reports by Griffiths et al in 1975[1] and 1979[2] demonstrating an inverse association between residual tumor and survival, a combined approach of cytoreductive surgery followed by chemotherapy has become the mainstay for the initial treatment of advanced-stage epithelial ovarian cancer. Although a prospective randomized clinical trial demonstrating the benefits of primary cytoreductive surgery has not been performed, there is significant indirect evidence in support of a survival benefit for patients who undergo a successful primary cytoreductive surgery.[3–9]

It is tempting to extrapolate the benefits of primary surgical cytoreduction to secondary surgical efforts. Effective secondary cytoreduction has proved technically feasible in nearly 60% of operations performed by skilled surgeons.[10–16] However, the benefits of secondary cytoreductive surgical procedures are more controversial and difficult to prove for a variety of reasons. Secondary surgical procedures have been attempted in a heterogeneous population of patients, making a consensus opinion of the approach difficult. In addition, patients offered secondary cytoreduction are often subjected to selection criteria that may alter outcome. Finally, the skill and aggressiveness of the surgeon affect the likelihood of successful secondary cytoreduction.

Secondary cytoreductive surgery has been attempted in four general clinical scenarios:

Group 1: Interval debulking procedure, with bulky intraperitoneal tumor deposits remaining at the conclusion of primary cytoreductive surgery, for which a brief course of chemotherapy is given before a planned second attempt at surgical cytoreduction

Group 2: Clinically occult but resectable bulky disease discovered at second-look laparotomy

Group 3: Clinically apparent recurrent disease after completing primary surgery and chemotherapy

Group 4: Progressive disease following primary cytoreduction during initial chemotherapy regimen

In our opinion, patients in groups 1 and 2 represent optimal candidates for secondary cytoreductive procedures. There is mounting evidence that an interval debulking procedure (group 1) may confer a tangible survival benefit, as discussed in detail later in this chapter. In the case of group 2 patients undergoing a second-look procedure, secondary debulking of occult disease is desirable, adds little morbidity, and may provide a survival benefit.[13,17–20] In selected cases, patients in group 3 may also be excellent candidates for secondary cytoreduction. The best group 3 candidates would be those who have had a long disease-free interval before relapse, as patients with long disease-free intervals have the highest likelihood of response to second-line chemotherapy. Markman et al[21] reported a 77% (17 of 22) clinical complete response rate and a 32% (7 of 22) surgically documented complete response rate to second-line treatment with platinum-based combination chemotherapy in patients previously treated with a similar regimen who had not received any treatment during the preceding 24 months. Therefore, secondary cytoreductive surgery is most appropriate in patients who have had a lengthy disease-free interval. In a recent report by Vaccarello et al[22] on patients experiencing recurrence after a negative second-look laparotomy, those patients secondarily debulked to small (less than 0.5-cm) disease had a significant survival advantage.

We believe there is no role for secondary cytoreductive surrey in patients who have progressive disease while receiving primary chemotherapy (group 4). These patients have a uniformly poor prognosis. Attempts at cytoreduction will contribute to morbidity without long-term benefit. Morris et al[14] reported a short-term survival benefit after optimal secondary cytoreduction among chemotherapy nonresponders. However, by 20 months after the secondary debulking procedure, the survival curves for the optimal and suboptimal groups overlapped. Morris and colleagues concluded that the lack of effective second-line chemotherapy for this group was the major factor accounting for the absence of apparent benefit for secondary cytoreduction in these patients. Therefore, it is critical that the surgeon be cognizant of the patient's likelihood of responding to additional chemotherapy when determining the appropriateness of embarking on a secondary cytoreductive effort.

Several intraoperative findings would lead us to discontinue or abort, a secondary cytoreductive procedure: (1) bulky disease at any of the following sites: intraparenchymal liver metastases, porta hepatis, renal pelvis, and para-aortic lymph nodes cephalad of the renal veins; (2) encasement and contraction of the root of the small bowel mesentery with a characteristic "cauliflower" appearance of the small bowel loops or diffuse carcinomatosis with sheeting of most peritoneal surfaces; and (3) bulky diaphragmatic disease. Kapnick et al[14a] reported that large diaphragmatic tumors (greater than 5 cm) tended to penetrate the thorax. These patients had a sobering median survival of 8 months. In addition, resection of these lesions often requires a synthetic patch such as Marlex mesh (Bard Vascular Cardiosurgical Division, Billerica, MA). The potential for major morbidity (e.g., pneumothorax, phrenic nerve injury) with these procedures probably outweighs any benefits.

JONATHAN S. BEREK

The role of secondary operations in patients with epithelial ovarian cancer has been difficult to define because there is considerable variation in the patterns of behavior of tumors among those with persistent or recurrent disease. Also, analyses of the subject have been based on heterogeneous therapies and on the application of numerous definitions of what constitutes "secondary debulking." However, in order to consider the operations within their appropriate context, the issues can be better understood by using some recently summarized definitions, which were presented at an international symposium to discuss the issue. The application of these criteria can help standardize the analysis of patient data and permit the more critical review of the subject. Secondary operations have been defined as follows:[23]

Secondary cytoreductive surgery—an operation performed on patients who either have persistent disease at the completion of a complete course of chemotherapy or who subsequently experience clinical relapse

Interval cytoreductive surgery—an operation performed in patients after a short course of induction chemotherapy, usually two or three cycles of chemotherapy, to remove as much primary and metastatic disease as possible to facilitate response to subsequent chemotherapy and to improve survival

Second-look surgery—an operation performed in patients who are clinically free of disease after the completion of a defined course of chemotherapy, typically six cycles

Palliative secondary surgery—an operation performed in patients who manifest symptoms and signs of progressive disease (e.g., gastrointestinal obstruction), in an effort to relieve the symptoms for a minimally acceptable period

We initially defined secondary cytoreductive surgery[11] and implied that these operations were performed in patients who had persistent or recurrent disease at the completion of a full-planned course of chemotherapy. This would exclude a set of patients who develop progressive disease during their initial therapy, that is, those patients whose tumors are probably resistant to the induction chemotherapy. The definition may or may not include "interval" operations. In these patients in whom a primary operation had been attempted and failed, the second operation is certainly a "second effort" at debulking, although it is potentially the first successful debulking of the patient's tumor. Clearly, these patients' operations must be stratified and analyzed separately.

In our experience, and in that of other researchers, patients with advanced ovarian cancer considered to be the most suitable candidates for a secondary debulking operation are those who had an initial response to chemotherapy, and those who had a long interval (i.e., longer than 12 months) before the development of clinically recurrent disease. Our initial report has generally been substantiated and refined by follow-up studies.[15,16,18] It has been shown that in patients whose recurrent disease after combination platinum-based chemotherapy can be completely resected at an attempted secondary debulking operation appear to be the only group who benefit significantly from this surgery.[18]

Patients in whom clinical evidence of recurrence develops, as determined by only a rising CA 125 or by clinical assessment either by physical examination or computed tomography (CT) may have tumors that behave differently from those found to have small occult disease at second-look laparotomy.[23] In the latter group of patients, the disease is likely to be smaller because it has been subclinical and potentially more readily resectable; and the outcome of these patients may be different than the patients with clinical recurrence.[10,13,19,24–26] Therefore, any analysis of patients whose disease is resected at second-look surgery must be stratified as well.

Table 6–1 presents a summary of secondary cytoreductive surgery reports.[27] Generally, the key findings of these reports substantiate that the longer the interval from completion of chemotherapy to clinical relapse, the more likely that a secondary resection will be associated with prolonged survival. Another important feature is the complete resectability of the distribution of the residual disease in the peritoneal cavity and whether the disease has metastasized to the parenchyma of the abdominal viscera (e.g., the liver). For example, patients whose disease is limited to the pelvis and whose lesion can be completely resected are more likely than those who have diffuse carcinomatosis to have any benefit from an attempted secondary debulking.[28] Prior response to chemotherapy is essential because those patients with progressive disease at chemotherapy are not likely to derive much benefit from the surgery. Performance status and

TABLE 6-1
Survival Impact of "Optimal" Secondary Cytoreduction

STUDY/YEAR	CLINICAL SITUATION	RESIDUAL DISEASE (cm)	SURVIVAL	SURVIVAL MEASURE	*P*
Schwartz and Smith[10] (1980)	SLL	Micro	47.5%	2 yr	NS
		≤2.0	29.5%		
		>2.0	9.0%		
Raju et al[24] (1982)	SLL	Micro	20%	3 yr	NS
		Macro	0%		
Berek et al[11] (1983)	SLL + RD	≤1.5	20 mo	Median	<0.01
		>1.5	5 mo		
Luesley et al[25] (1988)	SLL	Micro	50%	20 mo	>0.05
		≤2.0	28%		
		>2.0	0%		
Dauplat et al[26] (1986)	SLL	Micro	NS	2 yr	<0.05
		Macro			
Lippmann et al[13] (1988)	SLL	≤2.0	42%	4 yr	0.001
		>2.0	0%		
Morris et al[14] (1989)	RD	≤2.0	18.8 mo	Median	>0.05
		>2.0	13.3 mo		
Podratz et al[19] (1988)	SLL	Micro	55%	4 yr	<0.01
		≤0.5	21%		
		>0.5	14%		
Hoskins et al[18] (1989)	SLL	Micro	51%	5 yr	0.013
		Macro	<10%		
Michel et al[16] (1989)	SLL + PD	≤2.0	18 mo	Median	>0.05
		>2.0	13 mo		
Morris et al[15] (1989)	PRD	>2.0	12 mo	Median	<0.03
		<2.0	8 mo		

Abbreviations: SLL, second-look laparotomy; Micro, microscopic residual disease; NS, not stated; macro, macroscopic residual disease; RD, recurrent disease; PD, persistent disease; PRD, progressive disease. (Modified from Burke and Morris,[27] with permission.)

patient age also correlate with a positive outcome.[27]

In summary, the following variables have been found to make a patient an optimal candidate for secondary cytoreductive surgery:

1. Long interval from time of complete remission to evidence of relapse (12 months or longer)
2. Potential for the complete resection of residual or recurrent disease
3. Response to prior induction chemotherapy
4. High-performance status
5. Younger patient age

Intraoperative findings that might lead to discontinuing a secondary cytoreductive procedure would be obvious evidence of diffuse carcinomatosis that would preclude resection of most or all residual disease. Certainly for a patient found to have unresectable disease greater than 1 cm, especially if it is in the upper abdomen, resection of pelvic disease is likely to be merely palliative. In general, disease is unresectable if it is located in the porta hepatitis or if there are diffuse liver metastases. Occasionally patients with focal liver disease may undergo partial hepatic resection or experimental cryotherapy.

QUESTION 2

For patients who relapse 1 year or more after completion of primary therapy, what is the role, if any, of secondary cytoreductive surgery?

STEPHEN C. RUBIN
IVOR BENJAMIN

A long disease-free interval is a favorable prognostic factor. As mentioned previously, long disease-free intervals (greater than 24 months) after primary surgery and platinum-based chemotherapy are associated clinical response rates up to 77% to second-line retreatment with platinum-containing agents.[21] However, the results with patients having shorter disease-free intervals have been less encouraging. In another study, Morris et al[15] looked at 30 patients undergoing secondary cytoreduction after at least a 6-month disease-free interval after initial surgery and chemotherapy. The median survival was 18 months for patients cytoreduced to 2 cm or less and 13.3 months for patients with a residual tumor of greater than 2 cm. These differences were not statistically significant.

In a larger study, Segna et al[29] reported their experience with 100 cases of recurrent or progressive epithelial ovarian cancer who underwent secondary cytoreductive surgery. These investigators were able to cytoreduce 61% of these patients successfully to less than 2-cm residual tumor with an acceptable degree of perioperative morbidity and mortality. The median survival was 27.1 months in the group with 2-cm or less residual and was 9.0 months for patients with larger residual tumor ($P = 0.0001$).

Therefore, secondary cytoreductive surgery may be advantageous in patients who have tumors that are sensitive to first-line chemotherapy regimens. A longer disease-free and treatment-free interval improves the patient's candidacy for secondary surgical procedures. Two caveats must be kept in mind: (1) the 1-year cutoff for the treatment-free interval is arbitrary, and (2) the interval debulking studies in the literature have reported on platinum-based combination regimens that did not include paclitaxel, which has recently become a component of most first-line chemotherapy regimens for epithelial ovarian cancer. Paclitaxel in combination with cisplatin has been shown to provide a survival benefit when compared with cisplatin and cyclophosphamide in a phase III trial for patients with suboptimal stage III and stage IV ovarian cancer conducted by the Gynecologic Oncology Group (GOG).[30] The impact of paclitaxel on the efficacy of secondary cytoreductive procedures remains to be determined. This issue is currently under study by the GOG.

JONATHAN S. BEREK

Surgical exploration in an attempt to perform secondary cytoreductive surgery may be beneficial in selected patients.[11,16,18,19,26] Patients must be judged likely to benefit from the surgery and to be in sufficient medical condition to warrant exploration. An additional important feature would be the availability of appropriate second-line drugs or protocols, or both, with which the patient can be treated. Incomplete or limited secondary resections of disease may be palliative and can be justified within the context of relief of symptoms, rather than in an effort to prolong survival.

QUESTION 3

What is the role, if any, of secondary cytoreductive surgery at second-look surgery?

STEPHEN C. RUBIN
IVOR BENJAMIN

Since Wangensteen et al[31] first described the concept of reassessment laparotomy for carcinoma of the colon, the second-look laparotomy has been the subject of numerous retrospective studies on the management of advanced ovarian cancer. Unfortunately, the definition of second-look laparotomy has often been applied too broadly by the inclusion of patients with clinically apparent persistent disease. In 1988, Rubin and Lewis[32] defined second-look laparotomy "to indicate a systematic surgical reexploration in asymptomatic patients who have no clinical evidence of tumor following initial surgery and completion of a planned program of chemotherapy for ovarian cancer."

Patients undergoing second-look laparotomy are excellent candidates for secondary cytoreductive procedures. By definition, these patients are presumed chemotherapy responders who are clinically free of disease and are already undergoing an exploratory laparotomy. Therefore, the secondary debulking procedure is unlikely to incur significant additional morbidity. Most importantly, five retrospective studies reporting on a combined 358 secondary cytoreductive procedures performed at second-look laparotomy have shown a survival benefit for patients who were successfully cytoreduced.[13,17–20] Despite variations in the definition of "optimal" cytoreduction used by these investigators the evidence supporting a benefit for secondary cytoreduction at second-look laparotomy is significant.

Lippman et al[13] reported on 27 secondary debulking procedures performed during 70 consecutive second-look laparotomies. Their data revealed a survival benefit for patients who were able to be cytoreduced to less than 2 cm. In a Danish multicenter trial, Bertelsen[17] reported improved survival for patients who were able to be successfully cytoreduced at second-look surgery to less than 1-cm disease when compared to patients who were not (25% versus 4% at 4 years). Hoskins et al[18] published a series of 67 similar patients. These workers showed that the group of patients found to have microscopic disease at second-look laparotomy or those cytoreduced to no visible residual disease had significantly better 5-year survival than those who were left with gross residual tumor. Potter et al[20] showed a survival advantage for the 20 of 56 patients with macroscopic disease who were successfully cytoreduced to no gross residual disease during second-look laparotomy. In a large series of 250 patients who underwent second-look laparotomy, Podratz et al[19] reported a survival advantage for a group of 116 patients who were successfully cytoreduced.

JONATHAN S. BEREK

Patients who have persistent disease at second-look surgery should be viewed and analyzed separately from than those who develop subsequent clinical relapse. Often these patients have small residual disease that may or may not be focal or resectable. The same principles apply, however, in patients who have extensive disease, small carcinomatosis that was subclinical until second-look surgery or in those patients whose CA 125 levels were negative in whom the disease went undetected by physical examination and radiologic assessment. Except for palliative indications, resection should be performed only if most—if not all—persistent disease can be removed. As with the group who developed clinical recurrence, the patients who are most likely to benefit are those who are left with microscopic disease only at the completion of second-look laparotomy. Subsequent survival clearly correlates with the extent of residual disease, with the group that has microscopic residual only faring much better than those with any microscopic disease, even those with less than 1-cm maximum diameter residual disease.[18]

QUESTION 4

What is the evidence that interval debulking surgery is beneficial and should it be

routine practice for any particular subset of patients?

STEPHEN C. RUBIN
IVOR BENJAMIN

There is mounting evidence that interval cytoreductive surgery is effective at prolonging survival in patients with advanced epithelial ovarian cancer. Several reports attest to the feasibility of achieving optimal cytoreduction during an interval debulking procedure.[33–35] However, the most compelling evidence that interval debulking procedures are beneficial comes from the Gynecological Cancer Cooperative Group of the European Organization for Research and Treatment of Cancer (EORTC). These investigators reported the results of a prospective randomized trial of interval debulking surgery in patients with stage IIb through IV epithelial ovarian cancer.[36] In this trial, patients with ovarian cancer who underwent primary cytoreductive surgery with suboptimal residual were evaluated after three cycles of cisplatin (75 mg/m^2) and cyclophosphamide (750 mg/m^2) chemotherapy given every 3 weeks. Patients with a complete response, partial response, or stable disease were randomized (n = 319) either to undergo an exploratory laparotomy for interval debulking surgery (n = 140) or not to undergo surgery (n = 138) before receiving three additional cycles of cisplatin and cyclophosphamide. The EORTC reported a survival advantage for patients who underwent the interval debulking surgery. When stratified on the basis of the residual disease at interval cytoreductive surgery, patients found to have small volume (less than 1 cm) disease upon exploratory laparotomy (median survival 41.6 months); those patients who had large volume disease but were able to achieve optimal status (less than 1 cm) (median survival 26.6 months) as result of the interval cytoreductive surgery survived significantly longer than those with bulky disease (median survival 19.4 months) or the no interval surgery arm (median survival 20.0 months).

It is difficult to recommend interval debulking surgery as routine clinical practice for several reasons. While the results of the EORTC study are encouraging, this investigation was in its accrual phase during the dawn of the paclitaxel era. While we suspect that substituting paclitaxel for cyclophosphamide may further improve the benefit of interval debulking, the true impact of the integration of paclitaxel into an interval debulking scheme is unknown. In addition, front-line treatment plans that incorporate an interval debulking procedure would mandate at least two laparotomies in the primary treatment of advanced ovarian cancer, unless a neoadjuvant chemotherapy approach that is currently unproven is taken. How a second-look operation would fit into an interval debulking approach is unknown. Most experts presently advocate second-look procedures only in the context of a clinical trial or if effective salvage therapy is available.[37,38]

Outside the context of a clinical trial, we would recommend consideration of an interval debulking procedure for patients in whom the adequacy of the initial debulking effort is in question. All too often, a patient is referred to a gynecologic oncologist after recently undergoing an inadequate staging and debulking procedure for advanced ovarian cancer by a general obstetrician-gynecologist or a general surgeon. Often all that is known about the nature of the staging procedure is that the tumor was deemed unresectable with bulky residual tumor in the pelvis and elsewhere. These patients are often excellent candidates for an abbreviated course of chemotherapy, followed by an interval cytoreductive procedure by a gynecologic oncologist and additional chemotherapy.

JONATHAN S. BEREK

As demonstrated in a recent EORTC study,[36] interval debulking surgery plays a role in the treatment of advanced-stage ovarian cancer and appears to be associated with a prolonged survival of those patients who can successfully undergo an interval debulking compared to those who cannot. In this study, persons who underwent a successful interval debulking had a median subsequent survival of 37.5 months, compared to only 19 months in the group who did not ($P < 0.001$). This prospective randomized trial has been the only such study conducted on cytoreductive surgery. These patients underwent "open and close" operations as their primary debulking attempt and were then started on induction chemotherapy in an effort to make the disease resectable after several cycles of chemotherapy at an interval procedure.

Based on this positive trial for interval debulking, patients should undergo an attempt at optimal primary cytoreductive surgery whenever possible in an effort to minimize the need for resection at interval or secondary operation.[28] This interval debulking should probably not be "routine" in any group of patients, with the exception of those who could not have appropriate resection at initial surgery. Planned interval debulking is not warranted based on these data, as survival comparisons were not made between patients who underwent optimal primary cytoreductive surgery versus those who underwent optimal interval secondary cytoreductive surgery.

QUESTION 5

What is the role of surgery for gastrointestinal obstruction in patients who have failed two or more chemotherapy regimens?

STEPHEN C. RUBIN
IVOR BENJAMIN

The development of gastrointestinal obstruction in patients who have failed multiple chemotherapy regimens is an ominous sign. In the vast majority of patients with bowel obstruction, recurrence or progression tumor is the cause. With medical management, these patients can be expected to have a median survival of approximately 2 weeks.[39] However, in approximately 5 to 24% of cases, obstruction may be the result of adhesions from previous surgery or treatment with ^{32}P.[40–42] This group of cancer-free patients is most likely to derive long-term improvement in survival and quality of life from surgical relief of gastrointestinal obstruction.

For most patients with ovarian cancer who have obvious chemoresistant progressive disease, the relative benefit of gastrointestinal surgery depends on the outcome measures considered. Long-term survival is dismal in these patients. No known medical or surgical intervention, or both, will result in an improvement of this measure of outcome. If the end points of short-term survival, restoration of gastrointestinal function, and discharge from the hospital are used, surgical intervention appears to be beneficial. Castaldo et al[52] showed that short-term survival, arbitrarily defined as 2 months, is possible in up to 80% of patients.[43] Subsequently, Clarke-Pearson et al[53] devised an equation to estimate the probability for at least 60-day postoperative survival.[44]

In 1989, we reported on 54 operations performed on 52 patients at the Memorial Sloan-Kettering Cancer Center with gastrointestinal obstruction secondary to advanced ovarian cancer.[45] In 43 of 54 (79%) of operations, a definitive surgical procedure to correct the obstruction was possible. In 6 to 11 (54%) of the remaining patients, drainage tubes were successfully placed. Therefore, in 49 of 54 (91%) of laparotomies, a palliative surgical procedure was accomplished to afford decompression of the gastrointestinal tract. Restoration of gastrointestinal function was achieved in 79% of patients who underwent a definitive surgical procedure. The mean short-term survival was also reasonable for these patients (6.8 months).

In our series, we unable to identify clinical variables that correlated with operability or survival. Therefore, surgical approaches to the management of gastrointestinal obstruction in the setting of chemoresistant ovarian cancer must be individualized on the basis of sound clinical judgment. However, we believe that the likelihood for successful palliation of symptoms is significant and that exploratory laparotomy is a reasonable approach in most cases that do not respond to conservative management of the obstruction.

JONATHAN S. BEREK

Typically, patients who have failed two or more chemotherapeutic regimens would not be candidates for secondary cytoreductive surgery. In these women, disease is often diffuse and extensive, making, palliation of symptoms particularly those of intestinal obstruction paramount. Selection of candidates for surgery to relieve intestinal obstruction is often difficult and challenging for both the clinician and the patient. Even employing general guidelines, the decision must be individualized as every circumstance is unique.

Based on several earlier reviews of this subject,[39,44–47] it would appear that some adverse selection criteria would suggest that an attempted surgical correction is likely to be unsuccessful. Obviously patients who have had a prior history of a laparotomy at which the disease was found to be unresectable and bowel obstruction present would generally not be candidates for re-exploration. Patients with very poor performance status (e.g., low Karnofsky index), those with extensive ascites, and those with extensive mesenteric carcinomatosis often preclude surgical correction.

Several reports attempt to categorize the presumptive estimate of duration of survival as a relative indication or contraindication for exploratory surgery to correct intestinal obstruction. Most references suggest that those patients who would live no longer than 1 or 2 months after correction would generally not be candidates for exploration. Part of the problem with this suggestion is the presumption that these predictions are accurate. Indeed, estimates of duration of survival in terminal patients with ovarian cancer are often inaccurate, so the surgeon must be quite careful and take care not to overuse these prognostications.

Selection criteria for exploratory surgery in patients with an obstruction would be those who have overall good medical status with a good performance status, limited or no ascites, the will to live, prior laparotomy tended to have more focal disease, and a suspicion of focal obstruction where a bypass or local resection might be feasible. The distribution of disease might be predicted on the basis of the pattern of dissemination detected at prior laparotomies, that is, in patients with widespread carcinomatosis at second-look surgery; for example, correction of intestinal obstruction may be less likely to prove successful.

An alternative to surgical exploration for gastrointestinal obstruction is to use the approach recommended by St. Christopher's Hospice, London, in which the patient is given minimal intravenous fluids and frequent small feedings, with avoidance of nasogastric suctioning.[48] In patients who are otherwise terminally ill, this can be a compassionate means of managing terminal and intestinal obstruction.

EDITORS' COMMENTARY

As with primary cytoreductive surgery, sorting out the independent influences of tumor biology and surgical intervention is extremely difficult in patients with persistent or refractory ovarian cancer. Very few prospective randomized studies exist with which to make sound clinical decisions. Nevertheless, there is general agreement between the authors on most issues addressed, largely on the basis of their experience and clinical impressions.

On the topic of secondary cytoreductive surgery for recurrent disease, the authors agree that the procedure may be most appropriate for patients with a longer disease-free interval (e.g., more than 12 months). Although there are a few retrospective studies, this seems to be an excellent area for consideration of a prospective clinical trial in which patients are randomized between chemotherapy alone versus secondary debulking plus chemotherapy. We agree that other clinical features to be considered in selection of patients for secondary debulking are responsiveness to prior chemotherapy, good performance status, lack of other serious medical conditions, and younger age.

A survey of the literature indicates that there is no consensus on intraoperative findings that would lead to discontinuation of an attempt at secondary cytoreduction. As with primary cytoreductive surgery, there is a wide range of levels of aggressiveness in determining resectability. Nevertheless, the authors have delineated several features that would dissuade many gynecologic oncologists from proceeding with such an attempt, including bulky disease in the porta hepatis, hepatic parenchyma, diaphragmatic surfaces, or para-aortic lymph nodes cephalad of the renal veins. However, data are lacking.

Although the authors, particularly Drs. Benjamin and Rubin, view secondary debulking at second-look surgery favorably, other experts take a rather dim view of such procedures. They would argue that retrospective studies in this area are flawed by selection bias. As with recurrent disease, this would be a great setting for a prospective randomized clinical trial, but physician bias on both sides of the issue may well preclude adequate patient accrual to such a study.

In general, we agree with the comment of the authors regarding interval debulking. Despite the encouraging results from the EORTC study, we believe that this procedure should not be recommended for routine use until confirmatory data are available. A similar trial is currently being conducted by the Gynecologic Oncology Group. In this study, however, the combination of paclitaxel and cisplatin is being used instead of cyclophosphamide and cisplatin.

The authors appropriately outline the great difficulty associated with selection of patients with gastrointestinal obstruction for surgery. Clinical characteristics that allow the physician to select or rule out such surgery are not easily defined. In general, survival after such procedures is brief—on the order of 2 to 3 months. Although not mentioned above, we have found that percutaneous gastrostomy is an excellent alternative for palliation of patients with gastrointestinal obstruction deemed unlikely to benefit from surgery. It is hoped that future studies will provide information that will be more helpful in resolving this dilemma.

References

1. Griffiths CT: Surgical resection of tumor bulk in the primary treatment of ovarian carcinoma. Natl Cancer Inst Monogr 42:101–104, 1975
2. Griffiths CT, Parker LM, Fuller AJ: Role of cytoreductive surgical treatment in the management of advanced ovarian cancer. Cancer Treat Rep 63:235–240, 1979
3. Delgado G, Oram DH, Petrilli ES: Stage III epithelial ovarian cancer: the role of maximal surgical reduction. Gynecol Oncol 18:293–298, 1984
4. Vogl S, Pagano M, Kaplan B et al: Cisplatin based combination chemotherapy for advanced ovarian cancer: high overall response rate with curative potential only in women with small tumor burdens. Cancer 51:2024–2030, 1983
5. Pohl R, Dallenback-Hellweg G, Plugge T, Czernobilsky B: Prognostic parameters in patients with advanced ovarian malignant tumors. Eur J Gynaecol Oncol 3:160–169, 1984
6. Piver MS, Lele SB, Marchetti DL et al: The impact of aggressive debulking surgery and cisplatin-based chemotherapy on progression-free survival in stage III and IV ovarian carcinoma. J Clin Oncol 6:983–989, 1988
7. Hoskins WJ, Bundy BN, Thigpen JT, Omura GA: The influence of cytoreductive surgery on recurrence-free interval and survival in small-volume stage III epithelial ovarian cancer: a Gynecologic Oncology Group study. Gynecol Oncol 47:159–166, 1992
8. Hoskins W, Rubin S: Surgery in the treatment of patients with advanced ovarian cancer. Semin Oncol 18:213–221, 1991
9. Hoskins WJ, McGuire WP, Brady MF et al: The effect of diameter of largest

residual disease on survival after primary cytoreductive surgery in patients with suboptimal residual epithelial ovarian carcinoma. Am J Obstet Gynecol 170: 974–979, 1994

10. Schwartz PE, Smith JP: Second-look operations in ovarian cancer. Am J Obstet Gynecol 138:1124–1130, 1980
11. Berek JS, Hacker NF, Lagasse LD et al: Survival of patients following secondary cytoreductive surgery in ovarian cancer. Obstet Gynecol 61:189–193, 1983
12. Vogl SE, Seltzer V, Calanog A et al: "Second-effort" surgical resection for bulky ovarian cancer. Cancer 54:2220–2225, 1984
13. Lippman SM, Alberts DS, Slymen DJ et al: Second-look laparotomy in epithelial ovarian carcinoma. Prognostic factors associated with survival duration. Cancer 61:2571–2577, 1988
14. Morris M, Gershenson DM, Wharton JT: Secondary cytoreductive surgery in epithelial ovarian cancer: nonresponders to first-line therapy. Gynecol Oncol 33: 1–5, 1989

14a. Kapnick SJ, Griffiths CT, Finkler NJ: Occult pleural involvement in stage III ovarian carcinoma: role of diaphragm resection. Gynecol Oncol 39:135–138, 1990

15. Morris M, Gershenson DM, Wharton JT et al: Secondary cytoreductive surgery for recurrent epithelial ovarian cancer. Gynecol Oncol 34:334–338, 1989
16. Michel G, Zarca D, Castaigne D, Prade M: Secondary cytoreductive surgery in ovarian cancer. Eur J Surg Oncol 15: 201–204, 1989
17. Bertelsen K: Tumor reduction surgery and long-term survival in advanced ovarian cancer: a DACOVA study. Gynecol Oncol 38:203–209, 1990
18. Hoskins WJ, Rubin SC, Dulaney E et al: Influence of secondary cytoreduction at the time of second-look laparotomy on the survival of patients with epithelial ovarian carcinoma, Gynecol Oncol 34: 365–371, 1989
19. Podratz KC, Schray MF, Wieand HS et al: Evaluation of treatment and survival after positive second-look laparotomy. Gynecol Oncol 31:9–24, 1988
20. Potter ME, Hatch KD, Soong SJ et al: Second-look laparotomy and salvage therapy: a research modality only? Gynecol Oncol 44:3–9, 1992
21. Markman M, Rothman R, Hakes T et al: Second-line cisplatin therapy in patients with ovarian cancer previously treated with cisplatin. J Clin Oncol 9:389–393, 1991
22. Vaccarello L, Rubin SC, Vlamis V et al: Cytoreductive surgery in ovarian carcinoma patients with a documented previously complete surgical response. Gynecol Oncol 57: 61–65, 1995
23. Sharp F, Blackett AD, Leake RE, Berek JS: Conclusions and recommendations from the Helene Harris Memorial Trust Fifth Biennial International Forum on Ovarian Cancer, May 4–7, 1995, Glasgow, UK. Int J Gynecol Cancer 5:449–458, 1995
24. Raju KS, McKinna JA, Barker GH et al: Second-look operations in the planned management of advanced ovarian carcinoma. Am J Obstet Gynecol 144:650–654, 1982
25. Luesley D, Lawton F, Blackledge G, Kelly K et al: Failure of second-look laparotomy to influence survival in epithelial ovarian cancer. Lancet 2:599–603, 1988
26. Dauplat J, Ferriere JP, Gorbinet M et al: Second-look laparotomy in managing epithelial ovarian carcinoma. Cancer 57:1627, 1986
27. Burke JW, Morris M: Secondary cytoreductive operations. pp. 301–312. In Rubin SC, Sutton GP (eds): Ovarian Cancer. McGraw-Hill, New York 1993
28. Berek JS: Interval debulking of epithelial ovarian cancer: an interim measure. N Eng J Med 332:675–677, 1995

29. Segna RA, Dottino PR, Mandeli JP et al: Secondary cytoreduction for ovarian cancer following cisplatin therapy. J Clin Oncol 11:434–439, 1993

30. McGuire WP, Hoskins WJ, Brady MF et al: Cyclophosphamide and cisplatin compared with paclitaxel and cisplatin in patients with stage III and stage IV ovarian cancer. N Engl J Med 334: 1–6, 1996

31. Wangensteen O, Lewis F, Tongen L: The "second-look" in cancer surgery. Lancet 71:303, 1951

32. Rubin SC, Lewis JJ: Second-look surgery in ovarian carcinoma. Crit Rev Oncol Hematol 8:75–91, 1988

33. Ng LW, Rubin SC, Hoskins WJ et al: Aggressive chemosurgical debulking in patients with advanced ovarian cancer. Gynecol Oncol 38:358–363, 1990

34. Lawton F, Luesley D, Redman C et al: Feasibility and outcome of complete secondary tumor resection for patients with advanced ovarian cancer. J Surg Oncol 45:14–9, 1990

35. Wils J, Blijham G, Naus A et al: Primary or delayed debulking surgery and chemotherapy consisting of cisplatin, doxorubicin, and cyclophosphamide in stage III-IV epithelial ovarian carcinoma. J Clin Oncol 4:1068–1073, 1986

36. van der Burg ME, van Lent M, Buyse M et al: The effect of debulking surgery after induction chemotherapy on the prognosis in advanced epithelial ovarian cancer. Gynecological Cancer Cooperative Group of the European Organization for Research and Treatment of Cancer. N Engl J Med 332:629–634, 1995

37. Podratz KC, Kinney WK: Second-look operation in ovarian cancer. Cancer, suppl 4. 71:1551–1558, 1993

38. NIH Consensus Conference. Ovarian cancer. Screening, treatment, and follow-up. NIH Consensus Development Panel on Ovarian Cancer. JAMA 273:491–497, 1995

39. Krebs HB, Goplerud DR: The role of intestinal intubation in obstruction of the small intestine due to carcinoma of the ovary. Surg Gynecol Obstet 158: 467–471, 1984

40. Clarke-Pearson D, Chin NO, DeLong ER et al: Surgical management of intestinal obstruction in ovarian cancer. I. Clinical features, postoperative complications, and survival. Gynecol Oncol 26: 11–18, 1987

41. Lund B, Hansen M, Lundvall F et al: Intestinal obstruction in patients with advanced carcinoma of the ovaries treated with combination chemotherapy. Surg Gynecol Obstet 169:213–218, 1989

42. Tunca JC, Buchler DA, Mack EA et al: The management of ovarian-cancer-caused bowel obstruction. Gynecol Oncol 186–192, 1981

43. Castaldo TW, Petrilli ES, Ballon SC, Lagasse LD: Intestinal operations in patients with ovarian carcinoma. Am J Obstet Gynecol 139:80–84, 1981

44. Clarke-Pearson D, DeLong ER, Chin N et al: Intestinal obstruction in patients with ovarian cancer. Variables associated with surgical complications and survival. Arch Surg 123:42–45, 1988

45. Rubin SC, Hoskins WJ, Benjamin I, Lewis JJ: Palliative surgery for intestinal obstruction in advanced ovarian cancer. Gynecol Oncol 34:16–19, 1989

46. Fernandes JR, Seymour RJ, Suissa S: Bowel obstruction in patients with ovarian cancer: a search for prognostic factors. Am J Obstet Gynecol 158:244–249, 1988

47. Malone JJ, Koonce T, Larson DM et al: Palliation of small bowel obstruction by percutaneous gastrostomy in patient with progressive ovarian carcinoma. Obstet Gynecol 65:568–572, 1985

48. Baines M, Oliver DJ, Carter RL: Medical management of intestinal obstruction in patients with advanced malignant disease. Lancet 2:990–993, 1985

CHAPTER 7

PRIMARY CHEMOTHERAPY FOR ADVANCED-STAGE DISEASE

Jan P. Neijt
George A. Omura

EDITORS' INTRODUCTION

The management of advanced ovarian cancer has changed significantly over the past two decades with the introduction of cisplatin and carboplatin in the late 1970s and early 1980s and the introduction of paclitaxel in the early 1990s. It has become clear that response rates have increased with the addition of these two important new drug classes to the treatment of ovarian cancer. What is not clear, however, is whether either of these agents has improved survival. There are now 15 years of experience with the incorporation of platinum analogs into primary treatment. Many investigators appropriately feel that survival has not increased, particularly in patients with suboptimally debulked disease. There is some suggestion, however, that a modest survival benefit has accrued to patients with optimally debulked disease. The incorporation of paclitaxel into primary treatment has occurred only in the past few years. Thus, there is neither the magnitude nor the maturity of data available for this compound to make any categorical statements regarding its value in terms of survival advantage. Nevertheless, a single trial suggests an improvement in the median survival of patients when paclitaxel is added to cisplatin. Other trials are under way that may support or refute this impression. Probably another decade of Taxol-based therapy will be necessary before any effect of this new agent on long-term survival can be assessed.

We have posed several questions to our experts. We have specifically asked them to comment on the current standard postoperative chemotherapy for patients with advanced-stage disease. We have also asked that they discuss the number of cycles of therapy and whether maintenance therapy following a complete clinical or pathologic response is appropriate. We have asked these experts to comment on the need for cytokine support to allow more intense therapy. Additionally, we have asked them to discuss the value of neoadjuvant chemotherapy in patients with bulky disease, unresectable disease, or both. Finally, we have asked our experts to comment on what they feel should be the next generation of trials in this disease.

This is a period in the treatment of ovarian cancer in which a new and active agent—paclitaxel—is just being incorporated into primary therapy. Additionally, there are a large number of apparently active drugs, including gemcitabine, Doxil, topotecan, and possibly other compounds that are less advanced in terms of clinical development. An attempt to incorporate these new compounds into primary therapy presents a significant challenge, particularly when paclitaxel appears to be both sequence and schedule-dependent. Simply combining three or four agents may not be in the patient's best interest in terms of therapeutic index. New strategies for the 1990s may have to be developed in which patients are treated with two or more active doublets in a sequential manner.

Certainly the primary treatment of advanced ovarian cancer is changing and will continue to do so over the next decade or two. It is certainly feasible to consider the possibility that the therapeutic envelope may be expanded and even that there is a distant, though real, hope that cure may be a valid possibility for more women with this disease.

QUESTIONS

1. Based on current evidence, what is standard postoperative chemotherapy for patients with advanced-stage epithelial ovarian cancer?
2. What should be the next generation of primary chemotherapy trials in advanced-stage disease? Are there any investigational agents that are promising enough to be included in first-line regimens?
3. Which patients, if any, are candidates for neoadjuvant chemotherapy?
4. What is the optimal number of cycles of chemotherapy? Is there any role for "maintenance therapy"?

QUESTION 1

Based on current evidence, what is standard postoperative chemotherapy for patients with advanced-stage epithelial ovarian cancer?

JAN P. NEIJT

Systemic therapy is the treatment of choice for patients with epithelial ovarian cancer in an advanced stage. This includes women with stage II disease (growth involving one or both ovaries with pelvic extension) and with more advanced disease (stages III and IV). Even after surgical removal of all visible tumor, chemotherapy is the preferred treatment for these women.[1]

History

Single alkylating therapy (melphalan or cyclophosphamide) was the first treatment generally used for ovarian cancer. In the mid-1970s, cisplatin became available and rapidly became an accepted part of initial treatment. With cisplatin-based combinations, superior response rates and progression-free and overall survival were noted, as compared to results for combinations lacking this drug.[2,3] Studies designed to evaluate the addition of hexamethylmelamine or doxorubicin to cisplatin cyclophosphamide failed to show survival benefit.[4,5] In most countries, this led to acceptance of the combination of cisplatin and cyclophosphamide as a standard. Cisplatin 75 mg/m^2 intravenously over 4 hours with cyclophosphamide 750 mg/m^2 intravenously, both on day 1 and repeated after 3 weeks was the commonly used regimen.

The role of carboplatin, the less toxic analog of cisplatin, remained controversial. In the United States, carboplatin was accepted as effective therapy, but in Europe it was recommended only for patients with suboptimal stages III and IV and for palliative treatment. The reason for this difference is based on the criticism of studies that compared carboplatin and cisplatin. Although most trials suggest equivalent results for carboplatin- and cisplatin-based regimens, it is difficult to draw final conclusions because crossover, dose delivered, postponement of treatment, and follow-up flawed the results. Based on the currently available data, it was concluded that carboplatin should not replace cisplatin on a routine basis. For patients with potentially curable low-volume disease, CP appeared to be a better choice than carboplatin-based treatment.[6]

A number of physicians used doxorubicin as part of the combination for initial treatment. Their decision was based on the results of an overview analysis (or meta-analysis) that detected a small survival advantage for regimens using doxorubicin.[7] The advantage of meta-analysis is that the increased power may detect moderate treatment differences not revealed by individual trials. However, it remains whether the small survival benefit detected by this method is clinically relevant for future therapy.[8] Others argued that a regimen of CP with doxorubicin (CAP) 50 mg/m^2 offers a survival benefit at 6 years of 7% compared to CP.[9] For this reason, an international forum has accepted either CP or CAP as acceptable therapy.[10]

Results with cisplatin-based treatment

In most studies, the overall response rate achieved with cisplatin-based combinations is 70 to 80%. Forty to 50% of the women obtain a clinically complete response. In all studies, progression-free survival is longer for patients treated with the platinum regimen (the median for platinum regimens is about 19 months, and 25% are alive and progression free at 5 years).

Several investigators have published long-term survival results after platinum-based treatment. The Italian Gruppo Interregionale Cooperativo Oncologico Gynaecologia, reported on the long-term results of a randomized trial comparing three different regimens and in volving 529 cases. After treatment with a combination of cisplatin, cyclophosphamide, and Adriamycin, 22% of the patients survived 7 years. With the combination of cisplatin and cyclophosphamide, 17% survived and, with cisplatin alone, 12%.[11]

The Netherlands Joint Study Group for Ovarian Cancer updated their experience with cisplatin-based treatment. These studies were initiated in 1979 and 1981 and accrued 377 patients with advanced ovarian cancer. At 10 years, 9% patients initially treated with a non-cisplatin combination and 21% of patients assigned to a regimen including cisplatin were alive. Among the 10-year survivors treated without cisplatin, 50% had experienced progressive disease but were alive as a result of retreatment with cisplatin. The survival curves revealed that approximately 60% of patients who achieved complete remission at laparotomy were alive at 5 years and 40% at 10 years. These data show that relapses occur even after 5 years of follow-up, and in the most favorable group of patients with an incidence of about 5% each year. Patients with microscopic disease at second-look laparotomy had a less favorable outlook, with 35% surviving 5 years.[12]

Current standard of care

The results achieved with cisplatin have been further improved with the introduction of paclitaxel. Paclitaxel proved to have a unique mechanism of action and lack of cross-resistance with the platinum compounds.[13] After the first reports of its activity a large study was initiated in patients who had platinum-resistant tumors. The objective response rate in the first 1,000 patients was 22% (95% confidence interval 19 to 25%); the median survival duration was similar to the survival duration found in other phase II studies: 9 months.[14]

Because paclitaxel and cisplatin could be combined easily the Gynecologic Oncology Group (GOG) decided to move the combination to first line. Paclitaxel (135 mg/m^2/day), immediately followed by cisplatin, was compared with the "standard combination," CP.[15] A total of 386 patients were randomized between April 1990 and March 1992, all with suboptimal stage III (>1-cm residual disease) or stage IV disease. The paclitaxel combination resulted in a better response rate (73% of cisplatin/paclitaxel patients, as opposed to 60% of CP patients, $P = 0.01$) and more patients with microscopic disease or a surgically complete response. More important, a statistically significant improvement in progression-free interval was found (median 18 months 13 months). Median survival was 24 months for CP and 38 months for the paclitaxel combination ($P = 0.001$).

The deviation between prolongation of progression-free survival (5 months) and survival (13 months) is remarkable. This is due to early publication of the study, with the survival data for paclitaxel cisplatin not fully matured. The median duration of follow-up up for women alive was 37 months (range 5 to 56 months). This is less than the median survival of 38 months reported for patients who received the experimental treatment. It is to be expected that some patients will die before the current period of median survival is reached, with the effect of decreasing the median survival time. This shorter median survival duration will be obvious at the next study update. Another possible factor that may have influenced the period between progression and death is second-line treatment. At the start of the study, paclitaxel was unavailable for treatment of recurrence, but after December 1992 it was commercially available and retreatment occurred. One may assume that all patients with recurrent tumor after December 1992 may have benefited from treatment with paclitaxel.

Nevertheless, the survival prolongation obtained by the GOG is exceptional because it is uncommon to obtain improved results in patients with suboptimal disease. With the introduction of cisplatin, a survival advantage of such magnitude could not be achieved. For example, no difference were found in survival between patients treated with a cisplatin-based combination and a combination without cisplatin in tumours greater than 2 cm, whereas in other patients with small tumors, a significant advantage was seen for the cisplatin regimen.[16] This also applies to patients with tumors greater than 1 cm. These data show that studies intended to detect differences in survival are most likely to be successful in prognostically favorable patients (stages IIB-through III, small tumor residuals, and a good performance status).

Based on the data obtained by the GOG in women with large volumes of residual disease, it appears that the combination of paclitaxel and cisplatin is the most effective treatment available for patients with ovarian cancer. The results have led to acceptance of the combination of paclitaxel and cisplatin as the current standard of care for women with advanced epithelial ovarian cancer.[17]

GEORGE A. OMURA

The short answer in advanced ovarian cancer is six intravenous courses of cisplatin 75 mg/m^2, plus paclitaxel 135 mg/m^2 by 24-hour infusion given every 3 weeks without routine growth factor support.[15] Since the results of this study by the GOG are not universally accepted and since standard therapy ultimately leads to failure in most cases, it may be helpful to provide some background regarding the development of current chemotherapy for this disease.

Standard single agents

The main agents with demonstrated first-line activity in ovarian cancer include cisplatin (and carboplatin), paclitaxel, mustards, doxorubicin, and hexamethylmelamine. Cisplatin has been regarded as the most active agent in primary treatment of ovarian cancer, but its activity relative to that of paclitaxel is currently being studied by the GOG. In perhaps the largest trial conducted, chemotherapy-naive stage III and IV patients were treated with cisplatin 50 mg/m^2 every 4 weeks; a 20% (35 of 173) surgical complete response rate and 19.4-month median survival were observed.[18]

Cisplatin versus carboplatin

Carboplatin is another platinum coordination complex with a different toxicity profile compared to that of cisplatin. It has little or no nephrotoxicity or neurotoxicity and can be administered more easily since it does not require intravenous hydration. The dose-limiting toxicity of carboplatin is myelosuppression, primarily thrombocytopenia. Several prospective randomized trials comparing cisplatin to carboplatin (at about four times the dose) demonstrated equivalence in ovarian cancer; these results were supported by a Medical Research Council (MRC) overview of 11 randomized clinical trials involving 2,061 patients.[19] For single-agent therapy, carboplatin may be preferable, but in combination with marrow-toxic agents, cisplatin has some advantage since its marrow toxicity is limited. The neurotoxicity of cisplatin can be extremely troublesome, but severe neuropathy is not usually a problem if the total cumulative dose does not exceed 500 mg/m^2.

Paclitaxel (Taxol)

Paclitaxel is a natural product that stabilizes cellular microtubules, thereby interfering with cell replication. In the first trial in ovarian cancer, 11 partial responses and 1 pathologic complete response were noted in 40 patients, most of whom were heavily pretreated; in the subset considered platinum resistant, 24% (6 of 25) responded.[20] The results of this study were confirmed in other trials.[14,21] In a subsequent European and Canadian study, the dosing of paclitaxel was evaluated, comparing high dose (175 mg/m^2) with low dose (135 mg/m^2) and short (3-hour) versus long (24 hour) infusions in patients with relapsed ovarian cancer.[22] This report indicated that paclitaxel can be given safely over 3 hours with premedication and that responses are slightly more frequent in the 175-mg/m^2 group compared to the 135-mg/m^2 group (20% v 15% response). The response rates were similar in the 24-hour (19%) and 3-hour (16%) infusion groups, and with no survival difference. Another trial assessed a higher dose (250 mg/m^2) with growth factor support, yielding a 48% response rate (21 of 44) in platinum-resistant cases.[23] Whether there is a survival benefit for higher-dose paclitaxel has not been established but is being studied.

A preliminary report[24] on single-agent paclitaxel in previously untreated stage IV cases yielded one clinical complete response and eight partial responses in 28 evaluable patients. The results were somewhat disappointing, in view of the reproducible results with this drug in platinum-resistant cases and the possibility that as a consequence of its remarkable second-line activity, it might be more active than first-line platinum compounds.

Alkylating agents

The most commonly used mustards have included melphalan, cyclophosphamide, chlorambucil, and thiotepa. Recently, ifosfamide has shown second-line activity.[25] The GOG experience with oral melphalan in protocol 22 indicates an overall response rate of 37.5% (24 of 64) with a 20% clinical complete response rate in bulky stage III and IV disease.[26] Cyclophosphamide has been very popular in combination regimens, but evidence that it has contributed to combinations is limited.

It is possible that ifosfamide, usually given in divided doses, is more active than cyclophosphamide, which is usually a single dose per course, but a critical comparison has not been made, fractionating the administration of both drugs over multiple days. This bears mention since there is experimental evidence[27] that cyclophosphamide is more cytotoxic when fractionated than when given as a single dose.

Anthracyclines

Doxorubicin has an overall clinical response rate within a range of 30%[28] with one report of 3 clinical complete responses and 3 partial responses in 12 cases.[29] Much higher doses (120 mg/m^2 every 3 weeks for four doses) can be given, with considerably greater toxicity, but high-dose doxorubicin has not been systematically studied in ovarian cancer.[30] The experience with single-agent doxorubicin as primary treatment is not extensive since it was rapidly introduced into combination therapy.

Hexamethylmelamine

Hexamethylmelamine is a derivative of triethylene melamine used in various schedules by mouth. The single-agent experience has largely been with 8 mg/kg/day chronically or in 14-day courses. Using the former schedule in 22 previously untreated patients, there were seven clinical complete responses and three partial responses.[31] Although this agent is active, its current role in primary therapy is unclear.

Combination chemotherapy

Despite a compelling rationale for combination chemotherapy, it has been surprisingly difficult to show that drug combinations are superior to single agents in treating ovarian cancer. An MRC overview (meta-analysis) of 16 properly randomized trials, using raw data from 3,146 patients, compared single nonplatinum agents versus nonplatinum combination chemotherapy[19] and showed no survival difference whatsoever (this overview included some additional analyses to be described below).

Several clinical trials have addressed the value of cisplatin-based therapy compared to that of regimens not including cisplatin. A randomized GOG study compared the combination of doxorubicin and cyclophosphamide with or without cisplatin in 440 patients with bulky stage III and IV disease and demonstrated a significant improvement in clinical complete response rate, response duration, and overall survival with the addition of cisplatin.[32,33] The median survival was 16.4 months for cyclophosphamide plus cisplatin (CA) and 19.3 for CAP; the estimated benefit was a 20% decrease (P = 0.04) in the relative death rate among those who received CAP. These findings were challenged by one aspect of the MRC overview in which, evaluating 1,408 cases from eight randomized trials including the GOG study, there was no significant difference in overall survival between cisplatin- and non-cisplatin-treated groups. This discrepancy between the GOG trial and the overview might be explained by the fact that the other large trial[34] in the platinum-nonplatinum overview routinely crossed patients over to cisplatin, a practice that was not part of the design of the GOG trial. At any rate, the clinical impact of cisplatin in advanced ovarian cancer is obviously more modest than originally thought.

Since cyclophosphamide, hexamethylmelamine, doxorubicin, and cisplatin all exhibit activity in ovarian carcinoma and hexamethylmelamine and cisplatin are relatively nonmyelotoxic, it was reasonable to consider a combination of all four, variously known as CHAP, CHAD, or HEXA-CAP. Neijt et al[12] conducted a randomized trial of CHAP versus CP in 191 advanced-stage ovarian cancer patients; these investigators were unable to demonstrate any advantage for the CHAP regimen in either high- or low-volume disease groups.

Cisplatin alone or in combination

A revealing study, already alluded to,[18] randomly compared cisplatin 50 mg/m^2 every 4 weeks as a single agent to CP and to CAP. Despite greater dose intensity for the combinations, there was no significant difference in survival. The results, however, tended to slightly favor the combinations, especially CAP. Although this was a large (P = 173, CP = 181, CAP, 175 patients), well-done trial, it was not large enough to address the significance of small differences in outcome. By expanding the sample size to 838, the MRC overview was able to show a statistically significant advantage (P = 0.03) for cisplatin combinations over that of cisplatin alone, albeit a clinically small improvement. Since the results of the overview were, quite appropriately, not regarded as definitive, one outgrowth of that effort is an ongoing trial of moderately intensive carboplatin versus CAP being conducted by the MRC with a projected accrual of 2,000.

CAP Versus CP

Four randomized clinical trials comparing CP versus CAP individually failed to show a significant survival advantage with the addition of doxorubicin.[4,18,35,36] Because of these findings, the two-drug regimen of cisplatin and cyclophosphamide largely replaced the three-drug combination (CAP). However, a formal meta-analysis based on the raw data from the 1,194 patients in these trials demonstrated a 7% difference in the negative second-look rate (P = 0.01) and a 7% survival advantage at 6 years that is statistically significant in favor of the CAP regimen.[37] There was a 15% reduction in the odds of death in favor of CAP (P = 0.02). Because the dose intensity of CAP was greater than that of CP in three of the trials, the extent of the benefit of CAP obtained from greater dose intensity compared to that from the doxorubicin itself was uncertain. Long-term follow-up of the fourth trial suggests that the latter explanation is correct (Omura GA, Bundy BN: unpublished observations). Because the clinical impact of a 7% improvement in treatment outcome has been assumed to be very modest and because of its potential cardiac toxicity, doxorubicin has not been routinely reincorporated into the standard treatment regimen, but this agent warrants further study.[7]

Cisplatin plus paclitaxel

A GOG trial with 386 chemotherapy-naive suboptimal stage III and IV cases randomized cisplatin 75 mg/m^2 and cyclophosphamide 750 mg/m^2 versus cisplatin 75 mg/m^2 and paclitaxel 135 mg/m^2 given every 3 weeks for six courses. The clinical response rate in 216 evaluable patients with measurable disease was 60% for CP and 73% for paclitaxel/cisplatin (P = 0.01); the rates at negative second-look surgery were 20% and 26%, respectively (P = 0.08). The median durations of progression-free survival were 13 months and 18 months, respectively. There was a significant (median 24 months) vs 38 months, respectively, P <0.001) survival difference. The toxicity associated with paclitaxel/cisplatin was acceptable.[15] The only troublesome aspect of an otherwise very positive study is the modest difference in negative second-look rates (20% for CP and 26% for thiotepa). One would have expected a more dramatic difference in what is presumably a key intermediate end point on the way to an improvement in overall survival. It is also unclear to what extent the improvement in overall survival will translate into improved long-term survival and more cures.

Intraperitoneal chemotherapy

Intraperitoneal therapy is discussed elsewhere, but a few comments are appropriate here. There is a potential 10- to 20-fold increase in drug exposure of the peritoneal surface from intraperitoneal administration of cisplatin compared to systemic exposure.[38] However, direct penetration of tumor tissue is limited to a few millimeters from the surface, and so the common problem of relatively large tumor masses, even after debulking surgery, precludes the widespread application of this approach. Even in the most favorable cases, with microscopic to millimeter-size residual disease, it has been unclear whether the objective responses seen in as many as 30 to 50% of selected patients would translate into a survival benefit.

Recently, the use of intraperitoneal therapy as a component of initial management in ovarian cancer has been evaluated. Intergroup collaborators reported on a randomized trial comparing intraperitoneal cisplatin

100 mg/m^2 and intravenous cyclophosphamide 600 mg/m^2 versus intravenous cisplatin 100 mg/m^2 and intravenous cyclophosphamide 600 mg/m^2 each given every 21 days for six courses in small-volume stage III disease.[39] Patients were stratified by performance status and by residual disease after initial surgery ≤0.5 cm vs >0.5 to 2 cm). The extent of disease before surgery was not given. There were 654 patients accrued, of whom 17% were inevaluable. Patient characteristics were not extensively described. The intraperitoneal treatment arm was associated with a significant survical benefit (P = 0.02) overall, but not for the very small-volume cases ≤0.5 cm) (P = 0.10).

That the benefit was associated with the larger-volume subset is surprising since, as already noted, one assumes that local therapy would not effectively diffuse into tumors larger than a few millimeters and would have its effect largely through systemic absorption. Moreover, drug distribution within the peritoneal cavity might well be uneven, at least in some cases. It seems unlikely that this large trial would have a serious imbalance in prognostic factors, but that remains a possibility pending the reporting of patient characteristics such as substage at diagnosis and cell type. At any rate, this provocative study needs to be replicated, at least in principle. The challenge is to design a study that is acceptable to patients and investigators in the face of this very positive trial and to accommodate the importance of paclitaxel in combination with cisplatin.

One approach would be to repeat the trial with cisplatin (intravenous vs intraperitoneal) plus intravenous paclitaxel. Alternatively, one might restrict the study to larger-volume disease (0.5 to 2 cm) where there is, perhaps understandably, more skepticism about the initial report. One could also ask the intraperitoneal question in reference to paclitaxel, which has been given by that route second line as secondary therapy with acceptable toxicity.[40]

Another GOG trial recently completed accrual comparing intensive carboplatin (every 4 weeks for two courses), followed by intraperitoneal cisplatin 100 mg/m^2 and intravenous paclitaxel (135 mg/m^2) every 21 days for six courses versus cisplatin 75 mg/m^2 and paclitaxel 135 mg/m^2 every 21 days for six courses in small-volume stage III disease (<1 cm). This randomized study evaluates whether high-dose systemic chemotherapy (carboplatin) to debulk the tumor initially, followed by the regional (intraperitoneal) treatment strategy, has an advantage over systemic therapy alone. Since the experimental arm does not simply address the role of intraperitoneal therapy, the results do not take the place of a confirmatory trial but should be of great interest.

Dose intensity

This subject is discussed elsewhere in this volume, but a brief comment is indicated here as it applies to primary therapy. It has been assumed that higher drug doses and/or more drugs per unite of time will produce better results. However, the foregoing discussion has provided only limited support for the notion that more drugs are better. Only a few large-scale trials have examined this issue with respect to cisplatin dose intensity in a prospective randomized fashion. Kaye et al[41] gave ovarian cancer patients cyclophosphamide 750 mg/m^2 plus cisplatin 50 mg/m^2 or 100 mg/m^2, and six courses were to be given. Randomization was stopped early after accuring 159 evaluable patients because a significant survival advantage was observed for the double-dose cisplatin arm.

A larger trial (458 patients) compared 100 mg/m^2 cisplatin plus 1,000 mg/m^2 cyclophosphamide for four courses versus 50 mg/m^2 and 500 mg/m^2 of the same drugs for eight courses in large-volume stage III and IV cases. There was much more toxicity but no improvement in response rate or survival with the double-dose therapy.[42] It is difficult to reconcile these results with those of Kaye et al except that the latter study probably had relatively more patients with small-volume disease (almost one-third of the patients had stage IC or II disease). The effect of dose might be easier to demonstrate in that setting. A potentially serious criticism of Kaye's study concerns the presence of an imbalance in performance status favoring the high-dose arm; moreover, no information was provided about distribution of cell type, which some investigators consider another important prognostic factor.[32] As a practical matter Kaye et al concluded from their study that an intermediate dose of cisplatin, namely, 75 mg/m^2, was more realistic in view of cumulative neurotoxicity with the double dose, which reached 600 mg/m^2 in those receiving the full course.

A third trial compared cisplatin at a dose intensity of 25 mg/m^2 or 50 mg/m^2/wk to the same total dose of 450 mg/m^2 (75 mg/m^2 every 3 weeks for six courses or 50 mg/m^2/wk for nine courses). An interim report did not indicate significant improvement in 296 eligible patients.[43] A preliminary report on a fourth trial comparing 100 mg/m^2 versus 50 mg/m^2 of cisplatin, each in combination with epirubicin and cyclophosphamide, so far has not shown a big difference except in toxicity.[44] The weight of evidence does not suggest a consistent advantage for dose-intensive platinum therapy.

Duration of therapy

Retrospective analysis has suggested an advantage for longer treatment.[45] Two trials have prospectively addressed the duration of cisplatin-based combination chemotherapy; randomized comparisons of 5 versus 10 courses and 6 versus 12 courses have shown no survival difference.[46,47] The question of longer treatment was not entirely settled by these studies. Bertelsen et al[46] studied 202 patients, comparing 6 or 12 courses of CAP, but used an unbalanced randomization and had partial responders in the 6-course group receive an additional 6 courses. Moreover, only 52% of those in the 12-course group received all courses. As a consequence, there was only a 15% difference in received doses between the two groups. In spite of that, there was a slight improvement (not significant) in median survival with the longer treatment. Hakes et al[47] did a similar study comparing 5 versus 10 courses of CAP in 78 patients (five = 41, ten = 37) every 4 weeks, using 100 mg/m^2 of cisplatin. Partial responders to CAP 5 were to receive five more courses. Ninenty percent of the CAP 5 cases and 49% of the CAP 10 cases received all courses; the mean number of courses was 4.9 versus 8.4, respectively. As might be predicted, CAP 10 was more toxic because of cumulative effects. Survival favored CAP 10, but not significantly. It was noted that very few patients improved from partial response to complete response with additional courses. Both trials were relatively small and neither ultimately provided a clear separation of short versus long treatment. The question should be asked again in reference to paclitaxel, perhaps in combination with carboplatin, to reduce the problem of cumulative neurotoxicity. Such a trial should have a large sample size, since the difference in outcome may be small, and should not allow additional therapy, except perhaps at progression.

Any discussion of maintenance therapy (as opposed to a finite period of cytoreductive therapy, i.e., consolidation) requires consideration of the objective and the duration of such treatment. If the objective is to continue the current response status (ranging from stable response to partial or complete response) as long as possible, the answer to the second question should be indefinite therapy (until progression) despite the cumulative toxicities of such an approach. In regard to the first objective, however, if the mechanism of the treatment is cytotoxicity, that implies that a perfect or near-perfect balance has been achieved between tumor cell growth and tumor cell killing, which not only seems unlikely but also does not appear to have been demonstrated in controlled clinical trials. When other mechanisms of growth inhibition are brought into the clinical area, it would be reasonable to revisit the question of indefinite treatment, toxicity permitting.

When curative drug treatments have been identified in other adult cancers such as testicular cancer, Hodgkin's disease, and large-cell lymphoma, studies have demonstrated that therapy succeeds or fails within weeks to a few months. Why should epithelial ovarian cancer be any different?

To what extent does chemotherapy cure advanced disease? Prolonged follow-up is necessary to gain confidence about the outcome since recurrence and death may occasionally be observed even beyond 7 years. With a minimum follow-up of 10 years in a nonplatinum trial, 9 of 319 (2.8%) of women who began with bulky stage III or IV cancer were alive and progression-free at last contact; with at least 7 years of follow-up in a CAP trial in a similar population, at least 90% (178 of 198) of patients had already progressed[32]. Another CAP trial which included small- as well as large-volume stage III and IV cases had 7.1% disease-free patients at 10 years[80]. Similar results have been reported by others[81] using cisplatin-based therapy. Thus, the likelihood of cure in advanced disease remains low. Whether cisplatin paclitaxel regimens or other strategies reviewed here will improve the cure rate is to be hoped but has not been established.

QUESTION 2

What should be the next generation of primary chemotherapy trials in advanced-stage disease? Are there any investigational agents that are promising enough to be included in first-line regimens?

JAN P. NEIJT

With acceptance of the 24-hour paclitaxel/cisplatin combination as a new standard, new questions have emerged: What is the best dose and scheduling of paclitaxel together with cisplatin? Is carboplatin an acceptable substitute for cisplatin in the new combination? Are there any conventional agents that can be added to the current standard?

Dose-time schedule for paclitaxel

Although a steep dose-response relation in ovarian cancer has never been proved, there is a suggestion from phase II trials with paclitaxel that an increase in the dose above 135 mg/m^2 improves the response rate.[48] Furthermore, it is convenient to shorten the administration time for paclitaxel to a few hours because then the drug can be administered to outpatients.

In a European-Canadian study the question about the optimal dose-time schedule for paclitaxel was addressed in women previously treated with a cisplatin combination. The dose of paclitaxel was increased from 135 mg/m^2 to 175 mg/m^2 and the time of administration shortened from 24 hours to 3 hours. The higher dose was safe and even resulted in a modest prolongation of time to progression. Results with the 3-hour infusion were at least equivalent to those achieved with the 24-hour infusion and were associated with less neutropenia.[22] Unfortunately in these pretreated women a neuropathy was found in about 50% after treatment with the higher dose. Based on pharmacodynamic data, it is indeed likely that neurotoxicity becomes more severe when paclitaxel is given in a shorter period and a higher dose.[49]

In combination with cisplatin this neurotoxicity may become dose-limiting after a few cycles and preclude the delivery of an adequate total dose.[50] For ovarian cancer, this is of importance because it may be important to treat patients for more than six cycles to achieve further response. That neurotoxicity is becoming a problem with prolonged treatment was confirmed by the results obtained from a study in women who received paclitaxel/cisplatin as initial treatment. Paclitaxel (either 175 or 135 mg/m^2 in 3 hours) with cisplatin (75 mg/m^2) caused neurotoxicity after a mean of four cycles in 40% of the women.[51]

The 175 mg/m^2 over 3 hours was further evaluated in previously untreated patients by an intergroup study. They compared this dose-time schedule to that of CP. The study revealed that 175 mg/m^2 of paclitaxel over 3 hours with cisplatin improves progression-free and overall survival in comparison to the old standard. Unfortunately, severe sensory loss and paresthesias interfering with daily function (toxicity grade 3–4) developed in almost 20% of the patients.[52] Because of this toxicity, the conclusion can be drawn that this dose-time schedule of paclitaxel in combination with cisplatin appears not suitable as future standard treatment.

Paclitaxel in combination with carboplatin

One way to decrease the severity of the side effects of the combination of paclitaxel 175 mg/m^2 over 3 hours and cisplatin is to substitute the non-neurotoxic analog carboplatin for cisplatin. Although carboplatin in combination with cyclophosphamide is probably inferior to CP, this is uncertain in combination with the far more potent drug paclitaxel.[6] Several groups tested carboplatin and paclitaxel together.[53] In a dose-finding study of paclitaxel and carboplatin, previously untreated patients with ovarian cancer received escalating doses of either carboplatin or paclitaxel. Doses of carboplatin could be escalated to 450 mg/m^2 and of paclitaxel to 175 mg/m^2 without dose-limiting myelosuppression. Other side effects consisted of nausea and vomiting, peripheral neurotoxicity, and arthralgia, all mild. The results show that this treatment is well tolerated.[54]

From the present data it can be concluded that it is feasible to combine both drugs in adequate doses and with acceptable toxicity. The use of carboplatin in combination with paclitaxel would allow administration to outpatients and has financial advantages, and the combination may be better tolerated, allowing prolonged treatment. For this reason randomized trials have been initiated to explore the efficacy and side effects of the paclitaxel carboplatin combination in previously untreated patients. In the United Kingdom a comparison has been made between paclitaxel 175 mg/m^2 over 3-hours plus carboplatin and single-agent carboplatin or CAP (ICON-3 study). Dosing of carboplatin is based on calculation of a desired area under the plasma concentration versus time curve (AUC) according to the following formula. Dose (mg) = [AUC (mg/ml/min)] [GFR (ml/min) + 25 (ml/min)], where GFR is the glomerular filtration rate.[55] In the English study an AUC of 5 or greater is recommended. European University Hospitals initiated a comparison between paclitaxel 175 mg/m^2 over 3 hours plus cisplatin 75 mg^2/m versus paclitaxel 175 mg/m^2 over 3 hours plus carboplatin AUC 5. A higher dose is feasible, but it has not been proved that this is essential to achieve optimal results, and an AUC 5 dose is easy to administer for six to nine cycles of treatment without the use of growth factors. The dose-time schedule for cisplatin paclitaxel is similar to the one used by the EORTC. Preliminary results confirmed that the paclitaxel-carboplatin arm was better tolerated, as grade 2–3 neurotoxicity developed in 20% of women versus 34% of women treated with paclitaxel plus cisplatin. Response rates and time-to-progression were identical. The study was too small (211 patients randomized) to prove that the two treatments were identical in efficacy but if larger studies confirm the results, the carboplatin-paclitaxel combination could become the new standard of care for advanced ovarian cancer.

Paclitaxel combined with other agents

Paclitaxel can also be combined with other drugs active in ovarian cancer. Combinating it with cyclophosphamide and cisplatin is thought to be feasible. Cisplatin and cyclophosphamide damage DNA by two very different mechanisms, and paclitaxel appears to markedly slow the repair of DNA lesions caused by cisplatin adducts, and cyclophosphamide cross-links. Preliminary data show that these three agents are well tolerated and that this combination deserves further testing in ovarian cancer.[56]

The combination of doxorubicin and paclitaxel is also feasible. Doxorubicin (50 mg/m^2)

followed by paclitaxel 150 mg/m^2 is identified as the maximum tolerable dose. This combination is currently being used in patients with advanced breast cancer but is also an option for future use in ovarian cancer.[57]

Etoposide alone has shown activity in patients who develop progressive disease while on platinum. A combination of paclitaxel and cisplatin has been used in lung cancer, and in these patients the combination was well tolerated.[58] A phase III trial in ovarian cancer with a regimen including etoposide is being considered for study by Canadian investigators.

New investigational agents to be included in first-line regimens

Several new agents have recently become available with activity in patients with ovarian cancer that has progressed during platinum therapy: docetaxel, 2′,2′-difluorodeoxicytidine, and topoisomerase I inhibitors (topotecan and irinotecan). The results obtained with these new drugs will certainly encourage investigators to include them in first-line regimens.

Docetaxel (Taxotère)

Docetaxel is a semisynthetic compound structurally related to paclitaxel and derived from the needles of the European yew tree (*Taxus baccata*). An advantage of this agent is that it is easier to produce and is more water-soluble than paclitaxel. In vitro the drug is more potent than paclitaxel.[59] Renal excretion of docetaxel is very low, and so the drug appears to be suitable for patients with compromised renal function. The most commonly used dose is 100 mg/m^2 given over 1 hour every 3 weeks.

Compared to paclitaxel, docetaxel has a different spectrum of toxicity. More pronounced skin toxicity is encountered (palmar and plantar erythrodysesthesia), and many patients develop edema after prolonged treatment (including ascites and pleura effusion).[60] Alopecia is observed in nearly all patients, and neutropenia is dose-limiting. No neurotoxicity or cardiotoxicity has been observed, and very few hypersensitivity reactions have been reported. In four phase II trials with 327 evaluable patients, the response rate was between 17 and 37%.[61] The Early Clinical Trial Group of the EORTC reported their experience with 76 patients. Even in a group of patients progressing on cisplatin or with progressive disease within 4 months of treatment with a cisplatin-containing regimen, a response rate of 24% was found.[62] Efforts to ameliorate the development of fluid retention and skin toxicity with premedication look successful.[63] Clearly an assessment of the drug's activity in comparison to that of paclitaxel and its tolerance in combination schedules need to be determined.

2′,2′-Difluorodeoxicytidine (Gemcitabine)

2′,2′-Difluorodeoxicytidine (gemcitabine) is a primary antimetabolite with a close resemblance to cytosine-arabinoside. In a multicenter phase II study 42 patients who had received a maximum of two prior regimens were evaluated for response. Eight patients (19%, 95% confidence limits 9 to 34%) achieved a partial response. Seven out of eight had had progressive disease while on previous platinum treatment. Treatment with gemcitabine was very well tolerated. Nausea and vomiting (grade III) occurred in only six patients, and no hair loss was observed. Leuko- and thrombocytopenia were the main reasons for dose omissions and reductions.[64] These data indicate that gemcitabine may be non-cross-resistant to platinum, but more studies are needed to confirm the results.

Topoisomerase I Inhibitors

Topoisomerases are nuclear enzymes with important cellular activity during cell replication. Topoisomerase I induces single-strand breaks and repair of the DNA double-helix. Inhibition of this process represents a new target for the development of new cytotoxic agents. There are two topoisomerase I inhibitors currently in clinical trial: irinotecan (CPT11) and topotecan.

Topotecan has been explored using a variety of dosages and schedules. The dose-limiting toxicity in all studies is neutropenia. Other toxicities include diarrhea, alopecia, very mild nausea and vomiting, anemia, and occasional fever.[65] In a phase II study a dose of 1.5 mg/m^2 5 times a day every 3 weeks was used. In 28 evaluable patients four partial responses (14%) with a median duration of 9 months were noted. One-fourth of the patients were hospitalized with febrile neutropenia, and one-third developed a pruritic maculopapular rash requiring oral steroids.[66] A 21-day infusion of topotecan at 0.53 mg/m^2 is well tolerated with dose intensity exceeding that of other schedules for administration of this agent. The dose-limiting toxicity is hematologic, with thrombocytopenia more frequent than leukopenia.[67]

Topotecan is able to produce responses in patients with ovarian cancer refractory to cisplatin, carboplatin, or paclitaxel. In such patients with poor patient characteristics features (81% had relapsed within 6 months of their first-line therapy and 48% had tumors >5 cm in diameter), a response rate of 13% was found.[68] Of interest are the results of a randomized comparison of topotecan (1.5 mg/m^2 day over 30 minutes for 5 days) and paclitaxel (175 mg/m^2 over 3 hours) administered to patients who failed one platinum-based regimen. In evaluable patients who received topetecan (n = 96) 23% achieved a response, while 14% of patients treated with paclitaxel (n = 105) responded. Time to progression was 8 months after treatment with topotecan, and 4 months after treatment with paclitaxel ($P = 0.002$).[69] These data indicate for the first time in history of ovarian cancer that second-line treatment can prolong progression-free survival and indicate that topotecan is another new agent that deserves further evaluation in previously untreated patients.

GEORGE A. OMURA

More studies on paclitaxel are needed, beginning with a confirmation of the cisplatin paclitaxel trial[15]. The results of this trial are very convincing, but the reproducibility of the outcome should be demonstrated. The MRC is conducting a similar trial, randomizing patients to paclitaxel plus carboplatin versus CAP (or intensive carboplatin); the accrual goal is 1,000 patients. The assumption has been made that carboplatin can replace cisplatin, allowing simpler administration and resulting in less neurotoxicity. GOG 158 is comparing cisplatin/paclitaxel by 24-hour infusion versus carboplatin/paclitaxel by 3-hour infusion, the infusion time being another variable. The European-Canadian study on second-line paclitaxel in which a 3-hour infusion had comparable effectiveness and less neutropenia compared with a 24-hour infusion is the basis for this.[22] While shorter infusions may not be less effective, there is some evidence that longer exposure to paclitaxel (96 hours) is more cytotoxic, at least in breast cancer.[70] This issue is being addressed in ovarian cancer by GOG protocol 162.

Regarding dose intensity of paclitaxel, a GOG trial with relapsed or refractory patients showed an increase in response rate for 250 mg/m^2 plus granulocyte colony stimulating factor (GCSF) over 175 mg/m^2, but no survival benefit.[71] This should be explored in first-line therapy, seeking a survival benefit. This drug can be given at 250 mg/m^2 plus cisplatin 75 mg/m^2 and GCSF, but higher doses cause dose-limiting neuromuscular toxicity.[50] Additional paclitaxel studies may be generated by the results of GOG 132, which has recently completed accrual; if paclitaxel 200 mg/m^2 proves to be comparable to cisplatin 75 mg/m^2 plus paclitaxel 135 mg/m^2, this would imply that there is a dose response with first-line paclitaxel and that it is more active than cisplatin. Further intraperitoneal studies have already been discussed.

The possibility of adding a third drug such as doxorubicin, cyclophosphamide, or etoposide to paclitaxel/cisplatin is of interest but is not likely to produce a major improvement. A large trial would be needed, and the perennial problem of balancing more toxicity against possible small improvements would be an issue.

Postremission consolidation therapy

After initial chemotherapy, even patients with a negative second-look surgery are at substantial risk of fatal recurrence. In one large chemotherapy trial[4] in small-volume disease (<1 cm residual lesions), (40% 19 of 48) of women who began the study with residual disease, and (41%) (16 of 39) of those who began without residual disease and then had a negative second-look laparotomy, had already progressed after only 2 years of follow-up. Clearly there is a need to consider further treatment for women with negative second-look surgery, but no standard recommendation can be made at this time.

Three approaches to this important question will be considered, namely, longer treatment with the same regimen, changing the treatment, and increasing the drug doses. Regardless of the approach, randomized trials are essential, and a large group of patients is needed at the "front end" of such a study. For example, if one wished to ask of a consolidation question in patients with involving small-volume disease who had achieved a negative second look, assuming a 25% negative second-look rate and no loss from ineligibility, withdrawal of consent, and so on, 800 patients accrued would yield only 200 to be randomized. Nevertheless, this type of study should have a high priority over the next few years.

In regard to longer treatment, this issue has already been discussed in a different context: with regard to all patients, might longer treatment be better? This question is clearly different from asking whether patients already in remission might benefit from longer treatment. A consolidation study, randomizing, paclitaxel and carboplatin for several courses versus observation, would be important.

A change in treatment after remission induction is an attractive strategy. Since very small-volume disease is presumably being investigated, agents with only modest activity in treating gross disease but with a different mechanism of action might prove useful. Again, randomized trials are needed. The GOG is comparing intraperitoneal ^{32}P versus observation, and the Southwestern Oncology Group (SWOG) is randomizing α-interferon versus no further treatment.

Longer infusions of paclitaxel might be considered. A promising new drug like topotecan[72,73] would be of interest, especially if activity can be shown in patients resistant not only to platinum compounds but to paclitaxel as well.

There is increasing interest in megadose chemotherapy for cancer, including ovarian cancer, using agents with exclusively marrow toxicity (at more conventional doses), followed by hematopoietic reconstitution or "rescue" with autologous marrow or with peripheral blood stem cells harvested with a cell separator. Cyclophosphamide doses can be increased 7-fold, melphalan 6-fold, and thiotepa more than 30-fold before nonhematologic toxicities such as cardiac damage mucositis and/or central nervous system effects supervene. Carboplatin, etoposide, and mitoxantrone doses can also be dramatically escalated using this approach. A combination of cyclophosphamide, mitoxantrone, and carboplatin in doses of 120 mg/kg, 75 mg/m^2, and 1,500 mg/m^2, respectively, followed by autografting, was used in 30 relapsed ovarian cancer patients, resulting in an 89% response.[74] The median survival was 29 months. Similar studies are ongoing. Long-term follow-up is clearly needed, as well as appropriate randomized trials. The greatest impact could be on consolidation therapy.

Investigational agents for first-line regimens

In view of the substantial hematologic and nonhematologic toxicity of current paclitaxel/platinum combinations, a new agent added to such therapy would need to be highly active and have a very different toxicity profile; none is currently apparent. With regard to substitutions, however, it is appropriate to compare paclitaxel/platinum with docetaxel/platinum. Docetaxel is another taxane that is active in platinum-refractory ovarian cancer and has shown equal or greater cytotoxicity in preclinical studies.[62] Finally, there is interest in agents that may reverse drug resistance, such as PSC 833, an analog of cyclosporin D. This agent can potentially enhance the effect of drug like paclitaxel[75] and can be easily studied, but it seems unlikely that this particular approach (with PSC 833) will result in a major advance in ovarian cancer treatment.

QUESTION 3

Which patients, if any, are candidates for neoadjuvant chemotherapy?

JAN P. NEIJT

Almost all patients with ovarian cancer undergo a laparotomy to establish the diagnosis, and during this laparotomy maximum effort to remove as much tumor as possible is certainly recommended. In experienced hands, optimal cytoreduction is feasible in about 85% of patients, and serious morbidity is acceptably low. Tumor removal provides relief from symptoms, improved quality of life, and prolonged survival. It is not yet clear whether the optimum margin for providing a significant survival benefit is 1, 1.5, or even 2 cm. Presumably the optimum size is related to the induction chemotherapy subsequently used. Tumor residuals greater than 1 cm are considered suboptimal for induction with a cisplatin-based combination.

Neoadjuvant chemotherapy (primary chemotherapy) is the use of chemotherapy as the initial treatment for patients for whom the alternative is cytoreductive surgery. For most individuals this is an unattractive option: a surgeon removes the tumor in a few hours in 85% of the women, while response to chemotherapy in suboptimal disease is in the 60 to 70% range. Only in cases where the initial operation is too risky, or the tumor is judged unesectable, is primary chemotherapy an alternative. One retrospective study supports this strategy. A comparison of the survival of a group of women treated with neoadjuvant chemotherapy to that of a group of women with suboptimal debulking treated with the same chemotherapy demonstrated that the difference between the two approaches may be small. The progression-free survival for 11 women receiving neoadjuvant chemotherapy was 9.1 months, and for 18 women with suboptimally debulked stage IIIC or IV disease it was 8.5 months. Overall survival was similar. Neoadjuvant-treated patients tended to tolerate chemotherapy better than the other women.[76]

In patients in whom the tumor is deemed unesectable at the initial laparotomy, maximum cytoreduction is advised as soon as chemotherapeutic response renders the tumor masses respectable. This is called intervention, or interval, cytoreductive surgery and differs from the concept of neoadjuvant chemotherapy in that an attempt to remove the tumor is made prior to chemotherapy but did not succeed.[77,78] The benefits of this type of surgery are likely but have not been proved and are discussed elsewhere in this book.[79]

GEORGE A. OMURA

In neoadjuvant, protoadjuvant, induction, or anterior chemotherapy drug treatment is given before definitive local measures such as surgery or irradiation in order to enhance the outcome of local treatment and/or to convert inoperable cases to operable ones, ultimately increasing survival. In principle, this is an attractive strategy since the tumor blood supply is still intact, allowing better drug delivery, and since micrometastases can be treated before further growth occurs. In addition, the chemosensitivity of the tumor can be more readily assessed, and organ preservation may be possible. This approach has been studied in, for example, breast cancer, head and neck cancer, and cervix cancer, with mixed results.

In advanced ovarian cancer, chemotherapy is generally regarded as the definitive treatment; the question to be addressed concerns the possible benefit of giving chemotherapy before a maximal surgical effort when the value of the latter has not been rigorously established. In order to study the latter issue, a randomized trial was activated by the GOG comparing maximal surgery first, followed by chemotherapy, versus chemotherapy alone. Patients eligible for the study were those initially seen outside participating centers with only a limited initial operation. There was great interest in the study, and the trial design seemed appropriate, but almost no patients were accrued and the trial was abandoned. A different question concerns interval debulking, which has been shown by the EORTC to have significant survival benefit.[78] The GOG is attempting to confirm this finding.

There is no clear answer regarding neoadjuvant chemotherapy. It seems straightforward to propose a randomization to surgery followed by drugs versus drugs followed by surgery and more drugs, but how do patients enter such a study? The suggestion has been made that cases "not likely to be effectively cytoreduced surgically" be randomized.[76] That means that half the patients would be offered initial surgery that was assumed prospectively not to be useful (albeit not proven) for those patients. How would the consent form be worded? Alternatively, if eligible patients were individuals the gynecologic oncologist thought could be effectively cytoreduced surgically, would he or she be willing to randomly delay this intervention (even though its true value remains controversial)?

Some interesting ideas are not subject to rigorous study. Instead, it is likely that at some future date, advances in treatment will in one fashion or another make this neoadjuvant question moot. (If chemotherapy becomes extremely effective, debulking may not be needed at all.) Until chemotherapy becomes much more effective, the current practice of performing maximal debulking surgery first (with the added benefit of resolving any diagnostic uncertainty about tumor origin and substage) seems justified in most cases. Chemotherapy first (with the possibility of interval debulking for stage III partial responders) remains an option.

QUESTION 4

What is the optimal number of cycles of chemotherapy? Is there role for "maintenance therapy"?

JAN P. NEIJT

Cure is a reality after cytotoxic treatment of ovarian cancer. Some patients treated with a cisplatin-based combination in the first Dutch collaborative studies are still alive after 15 years without evidence of progressive disease and have an excellent quality of life. The choice of primary chemotherapy and probably total dose are among the many factors that determine long-term survival. Six cycles of chemotherapy is the suggested number of cycles for optimal results. Firm evidence that longer treatment prevents or delays recurrence is lacking. Very few studies examined the duration of treatment, but these studies were not conclusive.

In one study, 202 patients were randomized to 6 or 12 cycles of cyclophosphamide, doxorubicin, and cisplatin. Those randomized to 6 cycles and found to be in partial remission at second-look, surgery were to receive an additional 6 cycles. Median survival was 23 months for 6 cycles and 27 months for 12 cycles and 3-year survival was 29% for 6 cycles and 35% for 12. None of these differences were statistically significant, but they at least suggest that longer is better. This seems to be true especially because prolongation of treatment for patients in partial remission (randomized to 6 cycles) and early stopping of treatment in the 12-cycle group (because of toxicity) reduced the survival differences. Of interest is that 6 of 24 patients who received further treatment after tumor was found at second-look laporatomy had a complete pathological response at third-look surgery.[46]

The results of another trial that randomized between 5 and 10 cycles of chemotherapy suggested that 5 cycles are preferable to 10.[47] But this study was too small to draw any firm conclusions. Seventy-eight patients were randomized in total, and 12 women randomized to receive 5 cycles received a larger number because of remaining tumor. The conclusion may have been the reverse of that opined by the authors because the overall survival curve of patients with 10 cycles was better than that of patients who received 5 cycles. With more patients included in the study this difference may have become significant and in favor the patients who received prolonged treatment.

One retrospective study showed that progression-free survival for patients receiving 12 planned cycles of chemotherapy was 30 months versus 15 months for those receiving six planned cycles. Based on a Cox proportional hazard model, the use of prolonged therapy predicted increased progression-free survival.[45] Further suggestion that long treatment is justifiable comes from dose intensity studies in which differences in total dose rather than intensity were of importance for survival.

Certainly, prolonged treatment is toxic, and during chemotherapy the quality of live is miserable. The above-mentioned, studies do not prove that more courses of treatment improve survival, but the data are provocative. In chemosensitive tumors like testicular cancer, choriocarcinoma, and Hodgkin's disease, at least four to six courses are necessary to cure patients. Ovarian cancer is only a moderately sensitive tumor, and it is likely that more would be necessary to cure these patients. Randomized trials to prove this point are difficult to design and are of less importance than exploring the role of new drugs. Without evidence still to come, the best strategy is presumably to treat patients until a clinical complete remission is obtained (including normalization of the marker CA 125 and no further decrease during chemotherapy) and then to add another 3 cycles. In this way patients receive 6 and in most cases 9 to 12 cycles of treatment. Under no circumstances should patients receive fewer than 6 cycles.

The role of growth factors

For the major drugs used in the treatment of ovarian cancer (paclitaxel and carboplatin), myelosuppression is one of the dose-limiting side effects. Growth factors like GCSF can selectively stimulate production of granulocytes but cannot alleviate thrombocytopenic complications. A number of compounds showed promising activity in ameliorating thrombocytopenia, such as interleukin-1α[82] and interleukin-6 and -11. Even more interesting is thrombopoietin which was recently cloned and is now under clinical investigation.[83]

The key question is whether the use of growth factors can improve response rates and survival by an increase in dose intensity. The importance of dose intensity (defined as mg/m^2 per time period) in relation to clinical outcome has been analyzed by several investigators,[84,85] and the data suggest an association between outcome of treatment and dose intensity for platinum (alone or in multiagent regimens). For other drugs like cyclophosphamide and doxorubicin this association was of no significance.[86] Unfortunately clinical studies addressing the question of the importance of dose intensity did not confirm this hypothesis.[87] In one study performed by the University of Milan, patients were randomized to receive a double dose intensity (50 mg/m^2 vs 25 mg/m^2) per week with similar total dose of 450 mg/m^2. No differences were observed in complete remission rate, overall response rate, or survival.[43]. In another prospective study by the GOG increased toxicity was the only difference between the dose-intense regimen and standard treatment.[42] As in the Milan study the total dose of cisplatin received in the two groups was kept the same: 400 mg/m^2. Only one study reported initially improved results with a dose-intense treatment. In this study patients received cisplatin at 50 mg/m^2 (low dose) or 100 mg/m^2 (high dose) plus cyclophosphamide for a maximum of six cycles. In 1992 median survival was 17 months in the low-dose group and 28 months in the high-dose group.[41] At present, after a follow-up of 5 years, the survival differences have disappeared, with 4-year survival rates for high and low doses of 32% and 27%, respectively.[88] Because of the unacceptable side effects of the high dose (neurotoxicity, hearing loss, alopecia, vomiting, and anemia), the group did not adopt it for future use.

These trials suggest that a modest change in dose intensity does not result in improved survival. Further escalation of a cisplatin dose beyond standard levels does not appear to be clinically relevant because of the severe toxicity and because the effect on survival is limited. Therefore, arguments are lacking that support the use of expensive growth factors to maintain a dose-intense regimen for a longer period.

Another question is whether the use of hematopoietic support can prevent fever and hospitalization. Paclitaxel/cisplatin over 24 hours causes myelosuppression with febrile episodes in 20% of patients. In theory growth factors can prevent neutropenic morbidity but at considerable cost. Simple dose adjustment is easier, and there is no proof that this will influence treatment outcome negatively. Another useful approach seems to be chemoprophylaxis. In a retrospective review ciprofloxacin given through the granulocyte nadir was reported to be effective in preventing febrile morbidity for patients receiving Taxol. The estimated cost of prophylactic ciprofloxacin was $5,215 versus $104,000 for GCSF. A prospective trial is under way to evaluate this approach[89].

The use of cytokines to prevent hematologic toxicity and maintain dose intensity has not been established and remains experimental. This probably applies for all agents active in ovarian cancer, including carboplatin and paclitaxel. Dose adjustment according to general guidelines for hematological toxicity is the routine approach to preventing complications.

In conclusion, paclitaxel is currently accepted worldwide as a component of the initial treatment of ovarian cancer. Based on current results, the GOG regimen is the preferred dose-time schedule. Whether the schedule of administration of paclitaxel can be modified and whether cisplatin can be replaced by carboplatin without compromising the results is not known. Cure is the main objective of primary chemotherapy in women with advanced ovarian cancer. To reach this goal, at least six cycles of treatment are necessary, and in certain cases with a slowly responding tumor prolonged treatment beyond six cycles may be beneficial. Growth factors have no proven value in this setting and are expensive. Adjustment of the dose to prevent neutropenic complications is easier and has not been proved to compromise outcome. Cytoreductive surgery before chemotherapy is standard, but in patients where an operation cannot be performed, primary chemotherapy (neoadjuvant) is an alternative. Current trials are exploring the optimal dose-time schedule of paclitaxel and will establish the role of carboplatin. Further improvement is to be expected with the introduction of new drugs. The next generation of chemotherapy trials should focus on the role of new drugs such as docetaxel and topotecan in initial treatment schedules.

EDITORS' COMMENTARY

It is notable that both our authors agree that the current standard of care for chemotherapeutic management of advanced ovarian cancer is a combination of cisplatin and paclitaxel with the paclitaxel administered as a 24-hour infusion. They also agree that major issues concerning future development relate to whether carboplatin can be substituted for cisplatin and whether infusion duration of paclitaxel makes a difference in terms of outcome. It is quite clear that shorter paclitaxel infusion times lead to less hematologic toxicity but more neurotoxicity and myalgia. Ongoing studies performed both in the United States and abroad will help to better define these two issues over the next 5 years. We agree that the combination of cisplatin and paclitaxel as a 24-hour infusion should remain the standard of care based on the single GOG study. We anxiously await the results of a large European trial that utilized the same comparison as in the GOG trial with the exception of paclitaxel being administered as a 3-hour infusion at a higher dose. Should this study be concordant with the GOG study, then cisplatin and paclitaxel will become firmly established as primary therapy. The issues of which platinum analog should be used and which infusion duration of paclitaxel is the most effective will have to await the completion of ongoing studies and maturation of their data.

Both authors agree that six cycles of therapy represents the optimal treatment, however, Dr. Neijt gives some latitude for additional cycles of therapy if complete clinical response does not occur during the first three courses. Most data suggest that additional cycles of chemotherapy after six do not lead to an improved outcome and certainly has a real potential of increasing cumulative toxicity such as peripheral neuropathy. Both authors agree, and we concur, that cytokine support should not be used to maintain full dosing of chemotherapy or to allow further escalation of a chemotherapy dose. This is based on multiple studies that fail to show any outcome benefit with a doubling of total dose or dose intensity.

In regard to maintenance or consolidation therapy, both authors agree that there are currently no data that support this approach. Dr. Omura feels that the question is appropriate if it is put to the test of a rigorous randomized clinical trial. Such a study would have to involve a large number of patients on the front end to evaluate the effect of consolidation therapy in subgroups of patients: those with complete pathologic response, complete clinical response, and response without complete pathologic clearance of tumor. Consolidation therapy has been difficult in the past because of the development of cumulative toxicity: neuropathy with cisplatin and thrombocytopenia with carboplatin. There have been relatively few agents that could be used in a consolidation approach, however, paclitaxel offers a lack of known cumulative toxicity. Additionally, other new agents such as gemcitabine and topotecan offer the use of apparently non-cross-resistant therapy in patients with low-volume persistent disease or complete response with high risk of recurrence. Finally, each author proposes studies for the future that incorporate new or old drugs into primary therapy. Several drugs mentioned include topotecan, taxotere, etoposide, Cytoxan, doxorubicin, Doxil, and gemcitabine. Neither of our experts specifies how these agents should be incorporated into primary treatment. We feel that adding a third and fourth drug would be difficult and excessively toxic and propose the use of sequential doublet therapy in an attempt to incorporate non-cross-resistant drugs into these sequential doublets.

The next decade or two should be exciting for primary treatment of advanced ovarian cancer. Never have so many active agents been available. Several years of clinical investigation will be required to best determine how all these drugs should be used as part of a primary treatment regimen. Nevertheless, the future appears to have some "brightness around what has heretofore been a rather cloudy sky."

References

1. NIH consensus conference. Ovarian cancer. Screening, treatment, and follow up. JAMA 273:491–497, 1995
2. Neijt JP, ten Bokkel Huinink W, van der Burg MEL et al: Randomised trial comparing two combination chemotherapy regimens (Hexa-CAF vs CHAP-5) in advanced ovarian carcinoma. Lancet 2:594–600, 1984
3. Thigpen T, Vance R, Puneky L, Khansur T: Chemotherapy in advanced ovarian carcinoma: current standards of care based on randomized trials. Gynecol Oncol 55(3 pt 2):597–107, 1994
4. Omura GA, Bundy BN, Berek JS et al: A randomized trial of cyclophosphamide plus cisplatin with or without doxorubicin in ovarian carcinoma: a Gynecologic Oncology Group study. J Clin Oncol 7:457–465, 1989
5. Neijt JP, ten Bokkel Huinink W, van der Burg M et al: Randomized trial comparing two combination chemotherapy regimens (CHAP-5 vs CP) in advanced

ovarian carcinoma. J Clin Oncol 5:1157–1168, 1987

6. Vermorken JB, ten Bokkel Huinink WW, Eisenhauer EA et al: Carboplatin versus cisplatin. Ann Oncol, suppl 4. 4:41–48, 1993
7. A'Hern RP; Gore ME: Impact of doxorubicin on survival in advanced ovarian cancer. J Clin Oncol 13(3):726–732, 1995
8. McGuire WP: Primary treatment of epithelial malignancies. Cancer, suppl. 71: 1541–1550, 1993
9. Colombo N, Mangioni A, Vignali M et al: Options for primary chemotherapy in advanced ovarian cancer: the European perspective. Gynecol Oncol 55(3 pt 2): S108–113, 1994
10. Advanced epithelial ovarian cancer: 1993 consensus statements. Ann Oncol, suppl 4.4:83–89, 1993
11. Gruppo Interregionale Cooperativo Oncologico Ginecologia. Long-term results of a randomized trial comparing cisplatin with cisplatin and cyclophosphamide with cisplatin, cyclophosphamide, and Adriamycin in advanced ovarian cancer. Gynecol Oncol 45(2): 115–117, 1992
12. Neijt JP, ten Bokkel Huinink WW, van der Burg MEL et al: Long-term survival in ovarian cancer: matured data from the Netherlands Joints Study Group for Ovarian Cancer. Eur J Cancer 27:1367–1372, 1991
13. Gelmon K: The taxoids: paclitaxel and docetaxel. Lancet 344(8932):1267–1272, 1994
14. Trimble EL, Adams JD, Vena D: Paclitaxel for platinum refractory ovarian cancer: results from the first 1,000 patients registered to the National Cancer Institute Treatment Referral Center 9103. J Clin Oncol 11:2405–2410, 1993
15. McGuire WP, Hoskins WJ, Brady MF et al: Cyclophosphamide and cisplatin versus paclitaxel and cisplatin in patients with stage III and stage IV ovarian cancer. New Engl J Med 334:1–6, 1996
16. Neijt JP: Ovarian cancer: rethinking prognostic factors and chemotherapy. Educational book, 30th annual meeting. Am Soc Clin Oncol, 214–220, 1994
17. Neijt JP: New therapy for ovarian cancer. New Engl J Med 334:50–51, 1996
18. Gruppo Interegionale Cooperativo Oncologico Ginecologia: Randomised comparison of cisplatin with cyclophosphamide/cisplatin and with cyclophosphamide/doxorubicin/cisplatin in advanced ovarian cancer. Lancet 2:353–359, 1987
19. Advanced Ovarian Cancer Trialists Groups: Chemotherapy in advanced ovarian cancer: an overview of randomized clinical trials. 303:884–893, 1991
20. McGuire WP, Rowinsky EK, Rosenshein NB et al: Taxol: a unique antineoplastic agent with significant activity in advanced ovarian epithelial neoplasms. Ann Intern Med 111:273–279, 1989
21. Einzig AI, Wiernik PH, Sasloff J et al: Phase II study and long-term follow-up of patients treated with Taxol for advanced ovarian adenocarcinoma. J Clin Oncol 10:1748–1753, 1992
22. Eisenhauer EA, ten Bokkel Huinink WW, Swenerton KD et al: European-Canadian randomized trial of paclitaxel in relapsed ovarian cancer: high-dose versus low-dose and long versus short infusion. J Clin Oncol 12:2654–2666, 1994
23. Kohn EC, Sarosy G, Bicher A et al: Dose-intense Taxol: high response rate in patients with platinum-resistant recurrent ovarian cancer. J Natl Cancer Inst 86:18–24, 1994
24. Gore ME, Rustin G, Slevin M et al: Single agent paclitaxel in previously untreated patients with stage IV epithelial ovarian cancer. Proc ASCO 14:269, 1995

25. Sutton GP, Blessing JA, Homesley HD et al: Phase II trial of ifosfamide and mesna in advanced ovarian carcinoma: a gynecologic oncology group study. J Clin Oncol 7:1672–1676, 1989

26. Omura GA, Morrow CP, Blessing JA et al: A randomized comparison of melphalan versus melphalan plus hexamethylelamine versus Adriamycin plus cyclophosphamide in ovarian carcinoma. Cancer 51:783–789, 1983

27. Teicher BA, Holden SA, Eder JP et al: Influence of schedule on alkylating agent cytotoxicity in vitro and in vivo. Cancer Res 49:5994, 1989

28. Young RC, Ozols RF, Myers CE: The anthracycline antineoplastic drugs. N Engl J Med 305:139–153, 1981

29. Depalo GM, DeLena M, Bonadonna G: Adriamycin versus Adriamycin plus melphalan in advanced ovarian carcinoma. Cancer Treat Rep 61:355–357, 1977

30. Wheeler RH, Ensminger WD, Thrall JH, Anderson JL: High-dose doxorubicin: an exploration of the dose-response curve in human neoplasia. Cancer Treat Rep 66:493–498, 1982

31. Smith JP, Rutledge FN: Random study of hexamethylmelamine, 5-fluorouracil, and melphalan in treatment of advanced carcinoma of the ovary. Natl Cancer Inst Monogr 42:169–172, 1975

32. Omura GA, Brady MF, Homesley HD et al: Long-term follow-up and prognostic factor analysis in advanced ovarian carcinoma: the Gynecologic Oncology Group experience. J Clin Oncol 9:1138–1150, 1991

33. Omura G, Blessing JA, Ehrlich CE et al: A randomized trial of cyclophosphamide and doxorubicin with or without cisplatin in advanced ovarian carcinoma. Cancer 57:1725–1730, 1986

34. Gynecological Group, Clinical Oncological Society of Australia and Sydney Branch, Ludwig Institute for Cancer Research: Chemotherapy of advance ovarian adenocarcinoma: a randomized comparison of combination versus sequential therapy, using chlorambucil and cisplatin. Gynecol Oncol. 23:1–13, 1986

35. Bertelsen K, Jakobsen A, Andersen JE et al: A randomized study of cyclophosphamide and cis-platinum with or without doxorubicin in advanced ovarian carcinoma. Gynecol Oncol 28:161–169, 1987

36. Conte PF, Bruzzone M, Chiara S et al: A randomized trial comparing cisplatin plus cyclophosphamide versus cisplatin, doxorubicin, and cyclophosphamide in advanced ovarian cancer. J Clin Oncol 4:965–1071, 1986

37. Ovarian Cancer Meta-Analysis Project: Cyclophosphamide plus cisplatin versus cyclophosphamide, doxorubicin, and cisplatin chemotherapy of ovarian carcinoma: a meta-analysis. J Clin Oncol 9:1668–1674, 1991

38. Markman M, Reichman B, Hakes T et al: Intraperitoneal chemotherapy in the management of ovarian cancer. Cancer 71:1565–1570, 1993

39. Alberts DS, Liu PY, Hannigan EV et al: Intraperitoneal cisplatin plus intravenous cyclophosphamide vs intravenous cisplatin plus intravenous cyclophosphamide for patients with stage III ovarian cancer. N Eng J Med 335:1950–1955, 1996

40. Francis P, Rowinsky E, Schneider J et al: Phase I feasibility and pharmacologic study of weekly intraperitoneal paclitaxel: a Gynecologic Oncology Group pilot study. J Clin Oncol 13:2961, 1995

41. Kaye SB, Lewis CR, Paul J et al: Randomized study of two doses of cisplatin with cyclophosphamide in epithelial ovarian cancer. Lancet 340:329–333, 1992

42. McGuire WP, Hoskins WJ, Brady MF et al: Assessment of dose-intensive therapy in suboptimally debulked ovarian cancer: a Gynecologic Oncology Group study. J Clin Oncol 13(7):1589–1599, 1995

43. Colombo N, Pittelli MR, Parma G et al: Cisplatin (P) dose intensity in advanced ovarian cancer (AOC): a randomized study of conventinal dose (DC) vs dose-intense (DI) cisplatin chemotherapy. Proc ASCO 12(806):255, 1993

44. Conte PF, Bruzzone M, Gadducci A et al: High doses versus standard doses of cisplatin (P) in combination with epidoxorubicin (E) and cyclophosphamide (C) in advanced ovarian cancer (AOC) patients (PTS) with bulky residual disease: a randomized trial, abstract 880. ASCO 12:273, 1993

45. Gershenson DM, Mitchell MF, Atkinson N: The effect of prolonged cisplatin-based chemotherapy on progression-free survival in patients with optimal epithelial ovarian cancer: "maintenance" therapy reconsidered. Gynecol Oncol 47(1):7–13, 1992

46. Bertelsen K, Jakobsen A, Stroyer J et al: A prospective randomized comparison of 6 and 12 cycles of cyclophosphamide, Adriamycin, and cisplatin in advanced epithelial ovarian cancer: a Danish Ovarian Study Group trial (DACOVA). Gynecol Oncol 49(1):30–36, 1993

47. Hakes TB, Chalas E, Hoskins WJ et al: Randomized prospective trial of 5 versus 10 cycles of cyclophosphamide, doxorubicin, and cisplatin in advanced ovarian carcinoma. Gynecol Oncol 45(3):284–289, 1992

48. Arbuck SG, Canetta R, Onetto N, Christian MC: Current dosage and schedule issues in the development of paclitaxel. Semin Oncol, 20(4 suppl 3):31–39, 1993

49. Rowinsky EK, Wright M, Monsarrat B, Donehower RC: Clinical pharmacology and metabolism of taxol (paclitaxel): update 1993. Ann Oncol, suppl 6. 5:S7–S16, 1994

50. Rowinsky EK, Chaudhry V, Forastiere AA et al: Phase 1 and pharmacologic study of paclitaxel and cisplatin with granulocyte colony-stimulating factor: neuromuscular toxicity is dose-limiting. J Clin Oncol 11:2010–2020, 1993

51. Connelly E, Markman M, Webster K et al: Three hour infusional Taxol with cisplatin in patients with gynecological cancers, abstract. Proc ASCO 14:277, 1995

52. Piccart MJ, Bertelsen K, Stuart G et al: Is cisplatin-paclitaxel (P-T) the standard in first-line treatment of advanced ovarian cancer (ov ca)? The EORTC-GCCG, NOCOVA, NCI-C and Scottish intergroup experience. Proc ASCO 16:352a, 1997

53. Ozols RF: Carboplatin and Taxol (paclitaxel) in advanced ovarian carcinoma. Ann Oncol. suppl 6. 5:S39–43, 1994

54. ten Bokkel Huinink W, Veenhof C, Helmerhorst T et al: Paclitaxel plus carboplatin in the treatment of ovarian cancer. Semin Oncol 22(3 suppl 6):97–100, 1995

55. Calvert AH, Newell DR, Gumbrell LA et al: Carboplatin dosage: prospective evaluation of a simple formula based on renal function. J Clin Oncol 17(11): 1748–1756, 1989

56. Reed E, Kohn EC, Sarosy G et al: Paclitaxel, cisplatin, and cyclophosphamide in human ovarian cancer: molecular rationale and early clinical results. Semin Oncol 22(3 suppl 6):90–96, 1995

57. Sledge GW Jr, Robert N, Sparano JA et al: Paclitaxel (Taxol)/doxorubicin combinations in advanced breast cancer: the Eastern Cooperative Oncology Group experience. Semin Oncol 21(5 suppl 8):15–18, 1994

58. Greco FA, Stroup SL, Hainsworth JD: Paclitaxel by 1-hour infusion in combination chemotherapy of stage III non-small cell lung cancer. Semin Oncol 22(4 suppl 9):75–77, 1995

59. Braakhuis BJ, Hill BT, Dietel M et al: In vitro antiproliferative activity of docetaxel (Taxotere), paclitaxel (Taxol) and cisplatin against human tumor and nor-

mal bone marrow cells. Anticancer Res. 14(1A):205–208, 1994

60. Hurris H, Irvin R, Kuhn J et al: Phase I clinical trial of Taxotère administered as either a two hour or a six hour intravenous infusion. J Clin Oncol 11:950–958, 1993

61. Kaye SB: Docetaxel (Taxotère) in the treatment of solid tumors other than breast and lung cancer. Semin Oncol 22(2 suppl 4):30–33, 1995

62. Piccart M, Gore M, Ten Bokkel Huinink W et al: Docetaxel: An active new drug for treatment of advanced epithelial ovarian cancer. J Natl Cancer Inst 87(9):676–681, 1995

63. Piccart MJ, Klijn J, Paridaens R et al: Steroids do reduce the severity and delay the onset of docetaxel (dtx) induced fluid retention: final results of a randomized trial of the EORTC investigational drug branch for breast cancer (IDBBC), abstract. Eur J Cancer S75, 1995

64. Lund B, Hansen OP, Theilade K et al: Phase II study of gemcitabine (2′,2′-difluorodeoxycytidine) in previously treated ovarian cancer patients. J Natl Cancer Inst 86(20):1530–1533, 1994

65. Rowinsky EK, Grochow LB, Hendricks CB et al: Phase I and pharmacologic study of topotecan: a novel topoisomerase I inhibitor. J Clin Oncol 10(4):647–656, 1992

66. Kudelka A, Edwards C, Freeman R et al: A phase II study of topotecan administered intravenously as 5 daily infusions every 21 days to women with refractory epithelial ovarian carcinoma, ECCO-7. 7th Eur Conf on Clin Oncol and Cancer Nursing. Eur J Cancer 29a(6):132, 1993

67. Hochster H, Liebes L, Speyer J et al: Phase I trial of low-dose continuous topotecan infusion in patients with cancer: an active and well-tolerated regimen. J Clin Oncol 12(3):553–559, 1994

68. Gordon A, Bookman M, Malmstrom H et al: Efficacy of topotecan in advanced epithelial ovarian cancer after failure of platinum and paclitaxel: international topotecan study group trial. Proc ASCO 15:282, 1996

69. Carmichael J, Gordon A, Malfetano J et al: Topotecan, a new active drug, vs paclitaxel in advanced epithelial ovarian carcinoma: international topotecan study group trial. Proc ASCO 15:283, 1996

70. Wilson WH, Berg SL, Bryant G et al: Paclitaxel in doxorubicin refractory or mitoxantrone-refractory breast cancer: a phase I/II trial of 96-hour infusion. J Clin Oncol 12:1621, 1994

71. Omura GA, Brady MF, Delmore JE et al: A randomized trial of paclitaxel (T) at 2 dose levels and filgrastim (G; G-CSF) at 2 doses in platinum (P) pretreated epithelial ovarian cancer (OVCA): a Gynecologic Oncology Group, SWOG, NCCTG and ECOG study. Proc ASCO 15:000, 1996

72. Kudelka A, Edwards C, Freedman R et al: An open phase II study to evaluate the efficacy and toxicity of topotecan administered intravenously as 5 daily infusions every 21 days to women with advanced epithelial ovarian carcinoma. Proc ASCO 12:259, 1993

73. Armstrong D, Rowinsky E, Donehower R et al: A Phase II trial of topotecan as salvage therapy in epithelial ovarian cancer. Proc ASCO 14:275, 1995

74. Stiff P, Bayer R, Camarda M et al: A phase II trial of high-dose mitoxantrone, carboplatin, and cyclophosphamide with autologous bone marrow rescue for recurrent epithelial ovarian carcinoma: analysis of risk factors for clinical outcome. Gynecol Oncology 57:278, 1995

75. Jachez B, Nordmann R, Loor F: Restoration of taxol sensitivity of multidrug-resistant cells by the cyclosporine SDZ PSC 833 and the cyclopeptolide SDZ

280–446. J Natl Cancer Inst 85:478, 1993

76. Schwartz PE, Chambers JT, Makuch R: Neoadjuvant chemotherapy for advanced ovarian cancer. Gynecol Oncol. 53(1):33–37, 1994
77. Berek JS: Interval debulking of ovarian cancer—an interim measure. N Engl J Med 332:675–677, 1995
78. van der Burg MA van Lent M, Buyse M et al: The effect of debulking surgery after induction chemotherapy on the prognosis in advanced epithelial ovarian cancer. N Engl J Med 332:629–634, 1995
79. Neijt JP: Interval cytoreduction in ovarian cancer. N Engl J Med 333:254–255, 1995
80. Sutton GP, Stehman FB, Einhorn LH et al: Ten-year follow-up of patients receiving cisplatin, doxorubicin, and cyclophosphamide chemotherapy for advanced epithelial ovarian carcinoma. J Clin Oncol 7:223–229, 1989
81. Hoskins PJ, O'Reilly SE, Swenerton KD et al: Ten-year outcome of patients with advanced epithelial ovarian carcinoma treated with cisplatin-based multimodality therapy. J Clin Oncol 10:1561–1568, 1992

CHAPTER 8

IMPORTANCE OF DOSE INTENSITY IN OVARIAN CANCER

Paul A. Vasey
Stan B. Kaye
J. Tate Thigpen

EDITORS' INTRODUCTION

The relationship between the dose of chemotherapy and some outcome, either response or survival, has been discussed and more recently evaluated in multiple clinical trials. As long as 30 years ago, the group at the Southern Research Institute showed that higher doses of drug led to more cures in animal model systems. The suggestion at that time was that the relationship between dose and outcome was a linear one. Several assaults on this theory, however, have been promulgated during the past several years, the two most important being one proposed by Drs. Norton and Simon and a second proposed by Drs. Goldie and Coldman. Unfortunately these theories based on mathematical modeling have been difficult to either prove or disprove within the context of a randomized clinical trial.

More recently, retrospective meta-analysis of randomized clinical trials in breast cancer, ovarian cancer, and other tumors has suggested a relationship between dose intensity (dose of a given drug in mg/m^2/unit of time) and clinical outcome that has a linear shape. There have now been seven randomized studies of dose intensity in the treatment of ovarian cancer using systemically administered therapy, and two additional trials in which dose intensity was achieved by the use of intraperitoneal therapy. Clinically, dose intensity of 2- to 3-fold over standard chemotherapy is possible with cytokine support, and doses of 5-to 10-fold are possible with the use of autologous stem cell reconstitution. In vitro studies using ovarian cancer cell lines also suggest the possibility that increasing dose leads to increasing cell kill; however, for many currently available drugs, the in vitro dose capable of overcoming drug resistance is in a range currently achievable in a clinical trial setting. Additionally, significant questions remain about the true linearity of this dose-response relationship, with some suggestion that even a twofold increase in dose intensity does not lead to a significant improvement in outcome but to a significant increase in toxicity. The bulk of the clinical data relates to the dose intensity of platinum and outcome in ovarian cancer.

We have asked our experts in this area to address five key issues regarding the importance of dose intensity. We have asked the authors to discuss the current experimental and clinical evidence to either support or refute the importance of dose intensity in the treatment or ovarian cancer. We have also asked them to discuss future trials that may help resolve this issue. Similarly, we have asked them to discuss the issue of Taxol dose intensity and its relationship to outcome. In addition a we have asked the authors to discuss the role, if any, of high-dose chemotherapy and stem cell support for the treatment of either primary or recurrent ovarian cancer. Finally, we have asked the authors to comment on the relative importance of dose intensity versus total cumulative dose in outcome of ovarian cancer and to comment on what they believe to be the shape of the dose-response curve, linear or nonlinear.

QUESTIONS

1. What is the evidence, experimental or clinical, to support or refute the importance of platinum dose intensity in ovarian cancer?
2. What is the evidence, experimental or clinical, to support or refute the importance of Taxol dose intensity in ovarian cancer?
3. In what settings, if any, should we currently be studying high-dose chemotherapy (with autologous bone marrow transplant or peripheral stem cell support) for epithelial ovarian cancer?
4. What is the relative importance of dose intensity versus total dose?
5. What do you believe to be the shape of the dose-response curve in ovarian cancer?
6. What are your recommendations for future directions in this area?

QUESTION 1

What is the evidence, experimental or clinical, to support or refute the importance of platinum dose intensity in ovarian cancer?

PAUL A. VASEY
STAN B. KAYE

Up to 80% of patients with advanced ovarian cancer will eventually die from their disease[1] despite demonstrating encouraging initial response rates of 60 to 80% to platinum-based chemotherapeutic regimens.[2] Frequent relapses following therapy are due to the emergence of acquired cellular resistance to chemotherapy; the notion that increasing the amount of drug administered per unit time (dose intensity) could potentially overcome this emerging resistance is based on both preclinical observations in experimental model systems and retrospective analysis of studies correlating dose intensity with response rates or survival.

In 1985, Ozols et al[3] produced in vitro evidence of a dose-response relationship for both cisplatin and carboplatin, using a chemosensitive human ovarian cell line A2780 and a cisplatin-resistant cell line 2780.^{CP8} Clonogenic assay cytotoxicity studies demonstrated a steep dose-response curve for both cisplatin and carboplatin in the sensitive and resistant cell lines and revealed extensive cross-resistance between the two platinum analogs. Furthermore, studies in murine tumor models, including ovarian cancer, have demonstrated that a key factor underlying cure in chemosensitive tumors is dose intensity and that in animal models dose intensification is especially important to achieve complete cure of small tumors.[4] Moreover, further preclinical work has indicated that in order to overcome relative drug resistance in vitro, drug concentrations need to be in excess of fivefold higher than the usual cytotoxic range.[5] Extrapolation to the clinical situation suggests that it the benefit from dose intensification lies in circumventing drug resistance, dose escalations of this magnitude may be required as well.

The weight of evidence suggests a relationship between dose intensity and efficacy for certain cancers. From preclinical studies in ovarian cancer, it is reasonable to infer that increasing the dose of chemotherapy, and in particular platinum, could be curative in patients with small chemosensitive tumors but would probably not be curative in patients with tumors resistant to chemotherapy at standard doses or with bulky disease. A retrospective analysis of 33 trials of combination chemotherapy in advanced ovarian cancer (mainly FIGO stages III and IV with suboptimally debulked disease) was reported in 1987 by Levin and Hryniuk[6] and appeared to demonstrate a statistically significant correlation between the intensity of cisplatin and both response rate and overall survival. This seminal work was the impetus for several prospective clinical trials to be set up to examine dose intensity in advanced ovarian cancer; however, several important factors need to be considered when analyzing this overview. First, as pointed out by McGuire[7] in 1993, the correlation reported between outcome and average dose intensity (r^2 = 0.17–0.23) was a weak one. Second, analysis of the actual doses used in the comparison of the dose-response relationship indicated that what was actually being compared was *optimal* versus *suboptimal* dosing rather than high-dose versus standard-dose cisplatin therapy.[8] The dose intensity of cisplatin achieved was with in the range of 30 to 110% of a standard dose (which actually equates to a total lower dose of 36 mg/m^2 over 3 weeks, certainly lower than that which most clinicians would consider adequate). If the preclinical models are to be believed, and at least a fivefold increase in dose intensity is needed, this level of clinical dose intensification may be insufficient to overcome drug resistance.

The results of nine large randomized prospective trials of platinum dose intensification not requiring colony-stimulating factor support have been reported and are shown in Table 8-1.

The results of the Hong Kong Ovarian Carcinoma Study Group trial were published in 1989.[9] In this small study, 65 untreated patients with advanced ovarian cancer were randomized to receive postoperatively either a high-dose (HD) regimen of cisplatin 120 mg/m^2 plus cyclophosphamide 600 mg/m^2 or a low-dose (LD) regimen of 60 mg/m^2 with the same dose of cyclophosphamide, all on a 3-weekly cycle. Both dose intensity and cumulative dose of cisplatin were higher in the HD arm, and these patients achieved a statistically significant doubling of their 3-year survival rate (60% vs 30%). Myeloid and nonmyeloid toxicities were significantly more severe and common in the HD arm, but there were no episodes of sepsis or treatment-related deaths. However, no details are available on the target accrual for this study or on longer-term follow-up.

The West of Scotland Clinical Trials Group trial randomized untreated patients with FIGO stages IC to IV to receive six courses of either cisplatin 100 mg/m^2 plus cyclophosphamide 750 mg/m^2 (HD) or cisplatin 50 mg/m^2 with the same dose of cyclophosphamide (LD) on a 3-week cycle. There was therefore a twofold difference in both planned dose intensity and total dose of cisplatin. An interim analysis after the first 165 patients had been randomized showed a significant survival benefit for the HD arm (median survival 114 vs 69 weeks, P = 0.0008), and the trial was therefore closed.[18] However, a long-term follow-up, with a median observation period of 57 months, indicates that this survival benefit has been significantly reduced. Although there is still an overall benefit of HD versus LD (P = 0.043), there is clearly a difference between the first and second year periods of follow-up. Surprisingly, this is more apparent for patients with minimal (<2-cm) compared to bulky (>2-cm) residual disease at the time

TABLE 8-1

Prospective Trials of Platinum Dose Intensification Not Requiring Colony-Stimulating Factor Support

STUDY AND YEAR	DRUG INTENSIFIED	PATIENT SELECTION	NUMBER OF ELIGIBLE PATIENTS	REGIMEN	DOSE INTENSITY PLANNED	HIGHER CUMULATIVE DOSE OF PLATINUM IN INTENSIFIED ARM?	OVERALL RESPONSE (%)	MEDIAN SURVIVAL	COMMENTS
Ngan et al[9] (1989)	Cisplatin	Unclear	65	120 vs 60 mg/m^2 q3–4 wk	×2	Yes, ×2	55 vs 30	60 vs 30% 3YS	Significant improvement in 3YS but more severe myelosuppression in the HD arm
McGuire et al[10] (1995)	Cisplatin (+cyclophosphamide)	Bulky suboptimal	458	100 vs 50 mg/m^2 q3 wk	×2	No	55 vs 60	21.3 vs 19.5 mo	No difference; also increased dose intensity of cyclophosphamide
Kaye et al[11] (1996)	Cisplatin	IC–IV	165	100 vs 50 mg/m^2 q3 wk	×2	Yes, ×2	61 vs 34	28.5 vs 17.2 mo	Significant difference ($P = 0.0008$) in median survival, but overall survival 32 vs 27%
Columbo et al[12] (1993)	Cisplatin	III and IV	296	75 mg/m^2 q3 wk ×6 vs 50 mg/m^2 q1 wk ×8	×2	No	66 vs 61	36 vs 33 mo	No difference
Jakobsen[13] (1995)	Carboplatin	II–IV	222	AUC 8 vs 4	×2	Yes, ×2	16 vs 15 (complete response)	33 vs 30% 3YS	No difference
Gore et al[14] (1996)	Carboplatin	II–IV	241	AUC 12 vs 6	×2	Yes (×1.22)	63 vs 57	Not reported	No improvement in progression-free survival or overall survival
Ehrlich et al[15] (1983)	Cisplatin	III and IV	56	100 mg/m^2 q4 wk ×3 vs 50 mg/m^2 q3 wk ×6	×1.5	No	86 vs 75	27.5 vs 23.5 mo	Trend to increased survival, but not significant; combination with cyclophosphamide and doxorubicin
Bella et al[16] (1994)	Cisplatin	III and IV	99	100 mg/m^2 q3 wk ×6 vs 100 mg/m^2 q1 wk ×6 (5 wk between wk 3 and 4)	×2	No	69 vs 65	31 vs 13% 4YS	Significant difference in survival maintained at 8 yr
Conte et al[17] (1993)	Cisplatin	Bulky residual	122	50 mg/m^2 q4 wk vs 50 mg/m^2 d1 + 2q4 wk	×2	Yes, (×2)	44 vs 56	Not reported	No difference; combination with cyclophosphamide and epirubicin; progression-free survival 19 vs 15 mo

of initial surgery. Moreover, long-term toxicity, particularly neurotoxicity, is more evident in HD compared to LD patients.

The Gynecological Oncology Group (GOG) performed a similar prospective randomized study in 458 patients with suboptimally debulked (≥1 cm residual disease) stage III or IV ovarian cancer.[10] Here, patients were randomized to receive either four courses of a dose-intensified (HD) arm consisting of cisplatin 100 mg/m^2 and cyclophosphamide 1,000 mg/m^2 given 3-weekly, or eight cycles of a LD regimen with cisplatin 50 mg/m^2 and cyclophosphamide 500 mg/m^2 again given three weekly, following surgery. An increase in dose intensity of ×2 was therefore planned for both drugs in the HD arm, with no difference in the planned total dose. Analysis of this study revealed that there was no significant difference in the overall response rate (HD vs LD, 59% vs 65%) or median survival (21.3 vs 19.5 months, respectively). As in the Scottish study, toxicities were significantly more common and severe in the HD arm.

Columbo et al[12] reported the results of the University of Milano and Instituto "M. Negri" trial of conventional versus dose-intense platinum single-agent therapy in 1993. Untreated patients with stage III or IV ovarian tumors were randomly allocated to receive a dose-intense arm of 50 mg/m^2 cisplatin weekly for eight courses (HD) or a standard arm of 75 mg/m^2 every 3 weeks for six courses (LD). This trial was therefore designed to deliver a two fold increase in dose intensity in the HD arm while the total cumulative dose was similar in both the HD and LD arms. No significant difference was found in overall response rates (66% vs 61%) or median survival (36 vs 33 months) between the two patient groups.

Bella et al[16] reported mature results of a trial in which 101 untreated patients with stage III or IV disease were randomly allocated to receive 600 mg/m^2 cisplatin over either 9 weeks (100 mg/m^2/wk for six courses with a 5-week gap between courses 3 and 4) or a more conventional 18-week (100 mg/m^2 every 3 weeks for six courses) period. All patients received four cycles of Adriamycin and cyclophosphamide following their platinum treatment periods. Although there was no statistically significant difference in overall response rates between the HD and LD arms (65% vs 69%), there was a 4-year survival advantage for patients receiving the HD arm (31% vs 13% 4YS), which has persisted at 8 years).

The London Gynaecological Oncology Group trial randomized 241 untreated patients with advanced disease to receive either four courses of high-dose (HD) carboplatin (AUC 12) or six courses at a conventional (LD) dose (AUC 6), given at monthly intervals.[14] Dosage was determined according to the glomerular filtration rate as measured by chromium ^{51}EDTA clearance and using the Calvert[19] formula. Both delivered dose intensity, and total cumulative doses were higher in the HD arm by factors of 2 and 1.22, respectively. Response rates were similar for the two treatments (63% vs 57%), but the incidence of significant toxicities was higher in the HD arm. No significant difference between the two arms was observed in progression-free or overall survival.

Like the London group, the Danish Ovarian Cancer Study Group (DACOVA) randomized untreated ovarian cancer patients to receive different dose intensities of carboplatin. Here, postsurgical stage II–IV patients received six courses of carboplatin at either AUC 8 (HD) or AUC 4 (LD) with cyclophosphamide 500 mg/m^2 on a monthly cycle. This study was therefore designed to produce a twofold increase in both dose intensity and total cumulative dose for this platinum compound in patients receiving the HD arm. However, the results showed that increasing both these parameters did not improve either the response rate (16% vs 15% complete pathological responses) or survival (33% vs 30% 3YS). The incidence of side effects, particularly grade III and IV myelosuppression, was significantly increased in the HD patient group, although there were no treatment-related deaths.

Two other smaller prospective randomized studies have been reported that planned a dose-intensified cisplatin arm. Ehrlich et al[15] randomized patients to receive either cisplatin 100 mg/m^2 every 4 weeks for three cycles

(HD) or 50 mg/m^2 every 3 weeks for six cycles (LD) along with Adriamycin and cyclophosphamide the dose intensity differed by a factor of 1.5 without any change in total cumulative dose between the two study arms. High response rates were seen with both arms (80% vs 75%) which were not significantly different. The median survival was shown to be higher in the dose-intensified arm (27.5 vs 23.5 months), although this did not reach statistical significance. Conte et al[17] randomized 122 patients with bulky residual disease following laparotomy to receive either a dose-intensified arm (called PEC 100) consisting of cisplatin 50 mg/m^2 on d1 and d2 (plus epirubicin and cyclophosphamide on d1) on a monthly cycle or a standard dose arm (called PEC 50) with cisplatin 50 mg/m^2 on d1 only (again, with epirubicin and cyclophosphamide on d1). This design implemented a twofold dose intensification as well as a twofold increase in the total cumulative dose of administered cisplatin to patients randomized to the HD arm. Overall response rates were higher in the LD arm (56% vs 44%), however, progression-free survical was longer for the HD arm (19 vs 15 months), demonstrating a trend toward statistical significance.

This analysis of these published randomized prospective trials indicates that increasing the dose intensity of platinum by twofold—a level achievable without resort to hemopoeitic growth factor support or incurring unacceptable toxicities—is only of limited long-term benefit in the chemotherapy of advanced ovarian cancer. Indeed, within this range of dose intensity the total dose of platinum may be at least as important a factor in determining outcome. In the nine studies described in Table 8-1, eight had a planned twofold increase in dose intensity of cisplatin or carboplatin of two (Ehrlich et al, 1.5-fold), but only three demonstrated a beneficial outcome with this therapeutic maneuver. Interestingly, two of these three studies[9,18] had actually also administered a significantly, increased total cumulative dose of platinum to the patients randomized to the high-dose arm, suggesting that the relative dose intensity of platinum in itself may not be the major determinant of treatment response, but that the total dose actually received could be at least as important. This may not necessarily be the case if higher levels of dose intensification are achieved, and this should be the subject of further trials. It is now feasible to safely deliver four-fivefold increases in dose (of carboplatin) compared to conventional doses, using myeloprotective peripheral blood stem cells, and an important issue will therefore be the number of very high-dose treatments given. As mentioned, in vitro models predict that these are the levels of dose intensification that will be required for platinum compounds if a meaningful impact on drug resistance is to be made.

A further strategy for platinum dose intensification is the combination of carboplatin and cisplatin, an approach made practicable because of the different dose-limiting toxicities of these compounds. Increasing platinum dose intensity in this way to 45 mg/m^2/wk in a phase II study produced a response rate of about 60%,[20] which is not an improvement over that observed by McGuire[21] for the Taxol/standard dose platinum combination. An overall response rate (ORR) of 84% in patients receiving >50 mg/m^2/wk platinum (cisplatin/carboplatin) has been reported,[22] however, neurologic toxicity was prohibitive and the small number of patients and short follow-up reported prevented any absolute conclusions about efficacy. Another study using this intensification technique reported a high response rate in untreated stage III and IV patients, but a concurrent high degree of ototoxicity (undoubtably due to the cisplatin, despite limiting this drug to a conventionally acceptable dose of 75 mg/m^2).[23] The median progression-free survival observed was 14 months, and the overall median survival was 32.5 months, again less than the 38 months median survival observed for the Taxol/cisplatin combination by McGuire.[21]

Decreasing the observed high incidence of significant neurotoxicity would mean reducing the dose of cisplatin, and on balance this approach seems to carry few advantages over combination regimens of platinum and Taxol. In summary, we therefore recommend a standard dose intensity for cisplatin of 25 mg/m^2/

wk (as used in the current GOG studies, i.e., cisplatin 75 mg/m^2 plus paclitaxel 135/175 mg/m^2 every 3 weeks). We believe that escalations above this level for cisplatin clearly lead to increased toxicity, with a limited prospect of long-term benefit.

J. TATE THIGPEN

The use of the platinum compounds in the treatment of ovarian carcinoma started with a demonstration of the activity of cisplatin in patients previously treated with alkylating agents.[24] Shortly thereafter, randomized trials proved the superiority of platinum-based combination chemotherapy over non-platinum-containing regimens.[25] The subsequent introduction of carboplatin prompted seven randomized trials which demonstrated that carboplatin could be substituted for cisplatin with no decrement in clinical benefit and substantial reduction in toxicity.[26–30] By 1990, the standard of care for the management of advanced ovarian carcinoma was a combination of a platinum compound and an alkylating agent. Because the platinum compounds were the most active agents, attention turned to determining the optimal dose and schedule.

Evidence from preclinical studies and meta-analyses

In vitro data suggested a steep dose-response relationship for cisplatin.[31] The first widely accepted clinical demonstration of the importance of the dose intensity of platinum compounds, however, was a meta-analysis of over 60 randomized trials in ovarian carcinoma.[6] The key observation in this report noted that there was a correlation between response to chemotherapy and dose intensity of cisplatin over a range of dose intensity from 0.4 to 0.8 and that cisplatin was the only drug for which such a correlation was present. This translates to a dose range of 6 mg/m^2/wk to 12 mg/m^2/wk (18 to 36 mg/m^2 every 3 weeks), a range below the lowest commonly used dose of 50 mg/m^2. There were insufficient data at higher dose levels to document a correlation between dose and response.

An extended meta-analysis by the same investigators[32] included more studies in the higher dose range. This study demonstrated the superiority of combination chemotherapy over single agents and also noted a correlation between response and cisplatin dose up to a level of 25 mg/m^2/wk (or 75 mg/m^2 every 3 weeks). In this analysis, the investigators also suggested that total dose delivered might be as important as dose intensity. Neither meta-analysis, however, offered any evidence supporting the importance of total dose or of a correlation between response and dose intensity for any drug other than cisplatin; and neither was able to support the importance of cisplatin dose intensity beyond 25 mg/m^2/wk.

Evidence from uncontrolled trials

Evidence from uncontrolled observations is often cited to support the clinical importance of dose intensity. However, such citations ignore important considerations. One such observation cites the fact that at least some patients refractory to first-line therapy with platinum-based combinations respond to second-line treatment with higher doses of a platinum compound. One example is a report on a series of 30 patients deemed refractory to initial platinum-based therapy by virtue of either recurrence or progression after initial treatment.[33] Eight of the 30 responded to second-line treatment with carboplatin 800 mg/m^2 every 35 days. Closer examination of these data, however, shows that all eight responses occurred among the 21 patients who responded to initial platinum-based therapy and hence could still be considered platinum-sensitive. Among the nine patients who progressed while receiving initial platinum-based treatment, no responses occurred. This observation holds true for virtually every series in which the distinction between platinum-sensitive and platinum-resistant patients based on initial response to a platinum compound is reported.

A second observation from phase II trials notes that patients who have failed initial platinum-based therapy respond to intraperitoneal administration of a platinum compound.[34] The responses are presumably due to greater exposure of malignant cells in the peritoneal cavity to drug and hence to greater effective dose intensity. Closer examination of these phase II data, however, reveals the same phenomenon seen with higher intravenous doses of the platinum compound in the salvage setting. Responses occur almost exclusively in patients who respond to initial platinum-based therapy and relapse more than 4 months after completion of front-line therapy.[35]

A third observation from phase II trials concerns studies employing very high intravenous doses of cisplatin of 200 mg/m^2 per course in combination with hypertonic saline to protect the kidneys.[36] This cisplatin regimen in combination with cyclophosphamide 1,000 mg/m^2 per course repeated every 4 weeks reportedly yields very high response rates. The total number of patients included in the study is relatively small (46), and the population is a mix of patients with small-volume (21) and large-volume (25) disease. Although not a randomized comparison, it is instructive to look at the results of GOG studies with regimens using 50 mg/m^2 of cisplatin in the combination regimen as compared to the results using high-dose cisplatin. In patients with small-volume stage III disease (no nodule larger than 2 cm remaining), the high-dose regimen yields a pathologic complete response rate of 38%,[36] the GOG regimen (cisplatin 50 mg/m^2 plus cyclophosphamide 1,000 mg/m^2 every 3 weeks) a pathologic complete response rate of 30%.[37] In patients with bulky stage III or IV disease, the high-dose regimen yields a pathologic complete response rate of 12%,[36] and the GOG regimen (cisplatin 50 mg/m^2 plus doxorubicin 50 mg/m^2 plus cyclophosphamide 500 mg/m^2 repeated every 3 weeks) a pathologic complete response rate of 11%.[25] There is therefore no evidence that the high-dose cisplatin regimen yields a superior result even though the dose intensity of the platinum compound as a function of dose and time is three times as high (50 mg/m^2/wk versus 16.7 mg/m^2/wk).

In conclusion, when carefully examined, data from uncontrolled trials provide little support for benefit from dose intensity over a clinically relevant range of doses.

Evidence from randomized trials

Evidence for the value of greater dose intensity, if it is to be credible, must ultimately come from randomized trials. Seven such trials have been reported (Table 8-2).

GOG Protocol 97

This trial[12] randomized patients with large-volume disease to receive either eight cycles of cisplatin 50 mg/m^2 plus cyclophosphamide 500 mg/m^2 every 3 weeks or four cycles of cisplatin 100 mg/m^2 plus cyclophosphamide 1,000 mg/m^2 every 3 weeks. A total of 458 eligible patients, 130 with clinically measurable disease, entered the trial. Progostic features were evenly distributed between the two treatment arms. If the prescribed low dose is assigned a dose intensity of 1.0, the actual received dose intensity for the low-dose regimen was 0.95, and for the high dose regimen, 1.90. No difference in total dose received was noted between the two arms as planned.

Among the 130 patients with clinically measurable disease, 60 received the high-dose regimen. Of these, 19 achieved a clinical complete response (32%), 16 a partial response (27%), 18 stable disease (30%), and 7 increasing disease (12%). The overall response rate for the high-dose arm was thus 59%. Seventy patients received the low-dose regimen. Of these, 27 (39%) achieved a clinical complete response, 18 a partial response (26%), 24 stable disease (34%), and 1 increasing disease (1%). The overall response rate for the low-dose arm was thus 65%. The median progression-free intervals for the low- and high-dose regimens, respectively, were 12 and 13 months, whereas the median survivals were 24 and 21 months, respectively.

TABLE 8-2
Seven Randomized Trials of Platinum Dose Intensity in Advanced Ovarian Carcinoma

TRIAL	PLATINUM DOSE INTENSITY (PRESCRIBED)	RESPONSE RATE (%)	SURVIVAL
Trials showing no difference			
GOG[10]	Cisplatin 16.7 mg/m^2/wk	65	21 mo median
	Cisplatin 33.3 mg/m^2/wk	59	24 mo median
GICOG[12]	Cisplatin 25 mg/m^2/wk	61	33 mo median
	Cisplatin 50 mg/m^2/wk	66	36 mo median
GONO[38]	Cisplatin 12.5 mg/m^2/wk	61	24 mo median
	Cisplatin 25 mg/m^2/wk	58	29 mo median
London GOG[15]	Carboplatin AUC 6 per 4 wk	57	Hazard ratio 0.91
	Carboplatin AUC 12 per 4 wk	63	
Austrian trial[39]	Cisplatin 25 mg/m^2/wk	42	38 mo median
	Cisplatin 25 mg/m^2 plus carboplatin 75 mg/m^2/wk[a]	39	42 mo median
Trials showing a difference			
Scottish trial[11]	Cisplatin 16.7 mg/m^2/wk	34	27% at 4 yr
	Cisplatin 33.3 mg/m^2/wk	61	32% at 4 yr
Hong Kong trial[9]	Cisplatin 15–20 mg/m^2/wk	30	30% at 3 yr
	Cisplatin 30–40 mg/m^2/wk	55	60% at 3 yr

[a] *Platinum dose intensity advantage for the cisplatin/carboplatin regimen 1.6.*

In summary, this study was designed as a pure dose intensity study. There is no evidence that a twofold increase in dose intensity yields any greater patient benefit over the range of doses used in this trial (16.7 mg/m^2/wk to 33.3 mg/m^2/wk) for patients with large-volume disease. The higher-dose regimen was clearly more toxic.

Gruppo Interregionale Cooperativo Oncologico Gynecologie (GICOG) Trial

This study[12] randomized 306 patients with advanced disease to either cisplatin 75 mg/m^2 every 3 weeks for six cycles or cisplatin 50 mg/m^2 weekly for 9 weeks. The actual received dose intensity of the high-dose regimen was twice that of the low-dose regimen, and there were no differences in the total dose delivered in either arm of the trial. In contrast to the GOG study, 45% of the patients in this study had small-volume advanced disease. No significant differences were observed between the arms with regard to pathologic complete response (24% high dose vs 28% low dose), progression-free interval (21 vs 18 months), and survival (36 vs 33 months). Like the GOG study, this was a trial of pure dose intensity since each regimen delivered the same total dose of drug. Also like the GOG trial, this study provides no support for the importance of dose intensity over the range of cisplation dose intensity from 25 mg/m^2/wk to 50 mg/m^2/wk.

Gruppo Oncologico Nord-Ovest (GONO) Trial

This trial[38] randomized 145 patients with large-volume advanced disease to receive cyclophosphamide 600 mg/m^2 plus epirubicin 60 mg/m^2 plus either cisplation 50 mg/m^2 or cisplatin 100 mg/m^2 every 4 weeks for six cycles. In contrast to the GOG and GICOG trials, this study called for the delivery of a total dose of cisplatin twice as large as that in the high-dose regimen. The actual received dose intensity achieved a 2:1 ratio between the high- and low-dose regimens and evaluated the range of cisplatin dose intensity from 12.5 mg/m^2/wk to 25 mg/m^2/wk. No significant differences were noted with regard to clinical response (57.5% high dose vs 61.1% low dose), pathologic complete response (9.6% high dose vs 18.1% low dose), progression-free interval (18 months high dose vs 13 months low dose), and survival (29 months high dose vs 24 months low dose). The high-dose regimen was clearly more toxic. The trial provides no support for the importance of either dose intensity or total dose over the range of cisplatin dose intensity tested (12.5 mg/m^2/wk to 25 mg/m^2/wk).

London GOG Trial

This study[14] randomized 241 patients with either small- or large-volume advanced disease to single-agent carboplatin dosed to an AUC of either 6 for six courses or 12 for four courses at 4-week intervals. In the high-dose arm, dose intensity was doubled and total dose increased by 22%. No significant differences were noted with respect to response (63% high dose vs 57% low dose), progression-free interval (hazard ratio 0.98), and survival (hazard ratio 0.91). This trial also provides no support for the importance of dose intensity or total dose over the range tested.

Austrian Trial

This trial[39] approached the problem of platinum dose intensity by combining cisplatin and carboplatin. A total of 253 patients with stage IC to IV disease were randomized either to cisplatin 100 mg/m^2 plus carboplatin 300 mg/m^2 or to cisplatin 100 mg/m^2 plus cyclophosphamide 600 mg/m^2 monthly for six cycles. The actual received dose intensity for platinum was 1.6-fold greater with the cisplatin/carboplatin regimen. The platinum-intensified regimen produced more myelosuppression, ototoxicity, and gastrointestinal toxicity. The cisplatin/carboplatin regimen produced a response rate of 39%, a complete response rate of 26%, a progression-free median survival of 22 months, and an overall median survival of 42 months. These results were not significantly different from those seen with the cisplatin/cyclophosphamide regimen: 42% response rate, 26% complete response rate, 25-month median progression-free survival, and 38-month median overall survival. This trial thus fails to confirm an advantage for a 1.6-fold increase in platinum dose intensity.

Scottish Trial

This study[11] from the Scottish Gynaecology Cancer Trials Group randomized 159 patients with stage IC to IV disease to cyclophosphamide 750 mg/m^2 plus either cisplatin 50 mg/m^2 or cisplatin 100 mg/m^2 every 3 weeks. The actual received dose intensity for the higher-dose versus the lower-dose regimen was 1.8 to 1. The lower-dose regimen produced significantly less neurotoxicity. At 4 years of follow-up, 32% of those receiving the higher-dose regimen were alive as compared to 27% of those on the lower-dose regimen. The ratio of deaths among those receiving the higher-dose regimen versus those receiving the lower-dose regimen was 0.52 at 2 years and 0.68 at 4.75 years. These results suggest that, in contrast to results from the previous five studies, there was an advantage for the higher-dose regimen which diminished with time. The investigators' conclusion was that the optimal dose of cisplatin is 75 mg/m^2 every 3 weeks.

This trial has major problems. First, 49 of the 159 (31%) patients had stage IC or II disease. The heterogeneous patient population resulting from the inclusion of these limited-disease patients makes interpretation of the results very difficult, especially when one considers the relatively small total number of patients in the study. Second, the actual difference in 4-year survival of less than 6% is not impressive; and the relative death rate of the higher-dose versus the lower-dose regimen after the first 2 years is 1.30. The overall advantage of the higher-dose regimen is significant only at $P = 0.061$. Finally, the choice of 75 mg/m^2 every 3 weeks as the optimal dose of cisplatin does not follow from the results of the study which did not deal with the rommended dose.

Hong Kong Trial

This trial[9] is the smallest of the randomized studies, with only 50 patients entered, and the patient population is not well characterized. Cisplatin doses on the two regimens were 60 mg/m^2 and 120 mg/m^2, respectively. The higher-dose regimen yielded a response rate of 55% and a 3-year survival of 60% as compared to the lower-dose regimen results of a response rate of 30% and a 3-year survival of 30%. Even though these results suggest that the higher-dose regimen offered an advantage, the size of the trial and the poor characterization of the patient population make the conclusions less convincing.

Summary

On balance, the results of the seven randomized trials favour the conclusion that a doubling of dose intensity over a clinically relevant range offers increased toxicity without therapeutic gain. Five of the seven studies show no difference in response rate or survival; and three of these five studies include not only a difference in dose intensity but also a difference in total dose of the platinum compound. The two trials that show an advantage for a doubling of dose intensity of the platinum compound have major flaws which make interpretation difficult. These flaws relate to the total number and nature of the patient populations in the two trials. All seven trials show the higher-dose regimen to be more toxic.

QUESTION 2

What is the evidence, experimental or clinical, to support or refute the importance of Taxol dose intensity in ovarian cancer?

PAUL A. VASEY
STAN B. KAYE

Taxol has been shown to be active as monotherapy in previously treated patients with ovarian cancer[40,41] and has demonstrated an overall response rate of 30% (24% for patients with true platinum-resistant disease). However, data for activity in untreated patients are scarce, although Gore et al[42] recently reported a response rate of 46% in 30 untreated stage IV patients using a 3-hour infusion of 225 mg/m^2 every 3 weeks, a figure that compares favorably with that for single-agent platinum compounds.

Preclinical studies suggest that although there may be a dose-response relationship for Taxol, the duration of infusion (scheduling) may be a more important factor than the dose itself. Taxol is a phase-specific drug and is cytotoxic to cells in the S phase (DNA synthesis) of the cell cycle.[43] It is therefore theoretically more advantageous to expose solid tumors with long doubling times to a continuous cytotoxic concentration in order to increase the chances of cells progressing through the cell cycle during the treatment period. In vitro experiments support this, demonstrating the fact that prolongation of cell exposure time to Taxol increases the cytotoxicity in many different tumor lines to a greater degree than merely increasing the dose intensity.[44] Taxol also exhibits nonlinear pharmacokinetics, with saturable parameters of distribution and elimination.[45] This means that increasing the dose of the drug does not subsequently result in a proportional increase in maximum plasma concentrations (C_{max}) or drug exposure (AUC). The importance of this feature for any cytotoxic agent is that dose escalations may lead to excessive toxicities, and also that dose reductions may lead to an unacceptable decrease in efficacy. Furthermore, Gianni and colleagues[45] demonstrated that the nonlinearity of Taxol pharmacokinetics becomes more evident as the duration of infusion is shortened.

Dose escalation of Taxol is clinically achievable but requires the coadministration of hemopoietic growth factors, as the conventional dose-limiting toxicity at standard doses is myelosuppression. For high-dose Taxol, the next form of dose-limiting toxicity (at a dose of 300 mg/m^2, given over 24 hours with coadministration of G-CSF), is peripheral neuropathy.[46] Nevertheless, with G-CSF support, a dose of 250 mg/m^2 was shown to be feasible every 3 weeks at this schedule. This represents almost a two-fold increase over the conventional maximum tolerated dose when the drug is given over 24 hours. A phase II study using this regimen in 44 platinum-resistant ovarian cancer patients was reported in 1994 and demonstrated an overall response rate of 48% with 14% radiologic complete responses.[47] This is a higher response rate than that reported using conventional doses, and it implied a potential dose-response relationship for this drug, although clearly such nonrandomized comparisons of different studies should be interpreted with caution.

A randomized prospective study was set up by a European-Canadian group in order to examine in a bifactorial design the issues of both dose and infusion duration of Taxol in advanced ovarian cancer.[48] A total of 382 eligible patients previously treated with platinum compounds were randomized to receive single-agent Taxol at doses of either 135 or 175 mg/m^2 administered over either 3 or 24 hours. Response was found to be slightly higher with the 175-mg/m^2 dose (20%) than with the 135-mg/m^2 dose (15%), but this was not statistically significant ($P = 0.2$). Progression-free survival was, however, significantly longer in the high-dose group (19 vs 14 weeks, ($P = 0.02$), indicating a modest dose effect. More interesting perhaps, was the fact that no difference was observed in tumor response or survival between the 24- and 3-hour infusion times (19% vs 16%, ($P = 0.6$) but that significantly more grade IV neutropenia was seen in patients given the longer infusion (71% vs 18%, ($P < 0.0001$).

Studies in other tumor types, such as breast cancer, have indicated that the maximum tolerated dose of Taxol at longer infusions (96 to 120 hours) is significantly *lower* than that of either 3- or 24-hour infusions[49,50] and that these longer infusion times may be more effective. Seidman and colleagues[51] treated 25 women with metastatic breast cancer who had progressed on a 3-hour infusion of Taxol with a 96-hour infusion of the same drug. A response rate of 28% was noted (seven partial responses), demonstrating that clinically acquired resistance to Taxol could be circumvented using a prolonged infusion schedule. A possible explanation for these various results is therefore that the clinical effects of Taxol a solid tumor require a duration of exposure above a certain threshold concentration, a parameter that relies as much upon the schedule of administration as on the dose received (or dose intensity). Moreover, it is possible that this threshold concentration differs for the disparate cellular targets responsible for toxicity and antitumor efficacy.

Another method of delivering higher cumulative doses of Taxol per cycle (and therefore simulating to some extent prolonged continuous infusion techniques) is to use a multiday fractionated administration schedule. Lokich et al[52] recently reported the results of a feasibility study in which 47 patients with resistant cancers were treated with daily 1-hour infusions of Taxol for 3 to 5 days on a 3-week cycle. Objective partial responses were observed in four patients, including two ovarian cancer patients. The optimal dose of Taxol was 40 to 50 mg/m^2/day over 4 days, delivering a cumulative dose per cycle of 200 to 250 mg/m^2 without requiring cytokine support. While 96-hour infusion schedules seem to require a significant dose reduction, this fractionated scheduling allows an increased cumulative dose to be given per cycle. Whether there is any advantage to be gained with either 96-hour infusions or fractionated schedules over shorter, more clinically convenient, infusion times will be determined by the results of randomized prospective clinical trials currently in progress.

From this discussion, it is evident that although there may be a dose-response relationship for Taxol (within an achievable two-fold increase in dose intensity), it is likely that the duration of infusion (or tumor cell exposure) is at least as important a factor in defining the outcome in ovarian cancer. This is in contrast to cisplatin/carboplatin where infusion duration is of no apparent relevance as regards efficacy. On the other hand, the *total dose* of Taxol (or number of courses) may be of considerable importance in determining the outcome. However, a recent meta-analyses of three phase II studies in previously-tested ovarian cancer patients has indicated that there may in fact be a weak negative effect of total dose of Taxol.[54] Clearly, such a finding warrants investigation, and this is also the subject of current trials.

J. TATE THIGPEN

As already described, the addition of pacilitaxel to combination chemotherapy with a platinum compound produces significantly better survival. Even in the absence of evidence that further dose enhancement of the platinum compound results in greater therapeutic benefit, the possibility that increased paclitaxel dose intensity will yield better results must be considered. Three studies provide information on this topic. The first is a meta-analysis of phase II data from studies on previously treated ovarian carcinoma.[53] A total of 191 patients who initially had stage III or IV ovarian carcinoma were included. Of the 157 of these for whom platinum sensitivity could be assessed based on definitions cited earlier in this article, 121 (77%) were judged to be platinum-resistant. Paclitaxel dosing ranged from 110 mg/m^2 to 312 mg/m^2 with a mean dose of 195 mg/m^2 and a mean dose intensity of 61 mg/m^2/wk. The overall response rate was 27%, and neither dose nor dose intensity correlated with response. More strikingly, when maximum percentage reduction in tumor size is correlated, a strong negative effect of dose intensity and a weak negative effect of total dose were observed. These data provide no support whatsoever for, escalating doses of paclitaxel above the range of 135 to 175 mg/m^2 every 3 weeks.

The second study that examined the value of enhanced paclitaxel dose intensity randomized 338 patients previously treated with first-line platinum-based combination chemotherapy to either 175 mg/m^2 over 24 hours every 3 weeks or 250 mg/m^2 over 24 hours plus G-CSF support.[54] The higher dose produced a higher response rate (36% vs 28%), but no differences in progression-free survival (5.3 vs 4.8 months median) or overall survival (11.9 months vs 12.5 months median) were observed. The higher dose caused significantly more anemia, thrombocytopenia, gastrointestinal toxicity, neurotoxicity, and myalgia.

The third study that assessed the efficacy of increased dose compared paclitaxel 135 mg/m^2 over 24 hours every 3 weeks to 175 mg/m^2 every 3 weeks in a bifactorial design that also randomized all patients to either a 3-hour infusion or a 24-hour infusion.[55] No differences were observed between the two dose levels in regard to response rate, progression-free interval, or overall survival. The higher dose was more toxic, as was the longer infusion.

In summary, the results of trials to date provide evidence of at best only a modest dose-response effect for paclitaxel. This modest gain in response rate is not accompanied by a gain in progression-free or overall survival and is purchased at the cost of greater toxicity as well as greater drug expense because of the requirement for G-CSF support of the higher dose. These facts do not support use of the higher-dose schedule.

QUESTION 3

In what settings, if any, should we currently be studying high-dose chemotherapy (with autologous bone marrow transplant or peripheral stem cell support) for epithelial ovarian cancer?

PAUL A. VASEY
STAN B. KAYE

As outlined in previous sections, a key factor in the failure to cure patients with advanced ovarian cancer using conventional dose chemotherapy is the development of drug resistance. Extrapolation from in vitro data suggests that dose intensification to levels that can circumvent this emergent drug resistance would require patients to receive hematopoietic progenitor cell support—either as autologous bone marrow transplantation (ABMT) or peripheral blood stem cell (PBSC) reinfusion—as these doses are myeloablative and otherwise fatal. Development and refinement of the techniques involved (harvesting stem cells or bone marrow, subsequent hematopoietic reconstitution, and patient care during this high-risk phase) proceeded in the 1980s and early 1990s, and many pilot and phase I and II studies have been published for a variety of tumor types during this period. Encouraging results from nonrandomized trials in terms of long disease-free survival (and therefore possibly cure) have been reported in patients with refractory lymphomas[56] and germ cell tumors,[57] and a recently reported randomized trial in patients with relapsed intermediate and high-grade lymphoma has confirmed this survival advantage for high-dose chemotherapy.[58] Furthermore, a prospective randomized trial of high-dose (with ABMT/PBSCT) versus conventional dose chemotherapy in metastatic breast cancer patients has recently been reported to show significantly higher response rates and longer survival for patients receiving the high-dose arm.[59] However, this study is flawed in that only *responding* patients were given maintenance therapy with tamoxifen, a distinction that will undoubtably exaggerate the difference in survival between responders (predominantly in the HD arm) and nonresponders.

In ovarian cancer, a number of small studies have revealed that myeloablative chemotherapy with ABMT or PBSCT support is technically feasible in this (usually) heavily pretreated patient population and is capable of producing extremely high response rates (reviewed by Schilder.[60] However, most responses observed were of short duration (i.e., less than 6 months), and there was significant mortality associated with the chemotherapy, which approached 10% in the earlier studies.

Alkylating agents (e.g., thiotepa, melphalan, and cyclophosphamide) are particularly suitable for use in a dose intensification regimen because (1) myelosuppression is their dose-limiting toxicity and (2) they have non-overlapping nonmyeloid toxicities. Carboplatin is also an appropriate choice, as doses up to five-fold higher than standard can be reached before serious nonmyeloid toxicities develop. Theoretically, ovarian cancer is therefore an attractive candidate for high-dose chemotherapy because of its sensitivity to these drugs. The agents with the highest demonstrated efficacy against ovarian cancer, Taxol (neuropathy) and cisplatin (neuropathy and renal toxicity), are unfortunately less well suited to dose escalations of this magnitude.

Patients with refractory disease are an appropriate group in which to evaluate the feasibility of high-dose regimens, even though this may not be the optimal situation in which to prove their benefit. Various regimens have been tested in this patient group (e.g., cyclophosphamide/etoposide/carboplatin), and although high response rates are obtainable (over 50%), including complete responses, they are not durable to any significant degree (reviewed by Viens and Maranichi[61]).

One would predict that high-dose chemotherapy regimens might be more effective if administered to patients with small residual volumes of tumor and/or chemosensitive disease at the time of treatment. Categories of patients with ovarian cancer for which this approach is considered suitable are patients who have completed initial conventional dose chemotherapy and have (1) clinical complete or good response or good partial response, (2) microscopic disease at second-look laparotomy (SLL), (3) significant debulking (interval surgery or SLL), (4) negative SLL but high risk (e.g., stage IV), or patients who have relapsed after a long initial remission (>12 months) and have a further partial response or complete response to conventional dose chemotherapy.

There is evidence accumulating from individual centers that these patient groups may derive significant benefit from high-dose chemotherapy, although patient numbers are small. Most importantly, there are as yet no prospective randomized trials comparing standard dose therapy with the individual high-dose regimens. Lotz et al[62] reported the results of a tandem transplantation protocol carried out on seven patients with "sensitive" disease (defined as a partial response to platinum-based therapy. There was a 100% overall response rate in these patients, as compared to a 70% response rate when the same protocol therapy was administered to patients with refractory disease. Mulder et al[63] treated

11 patients with residual disease following induction therapy with high-dose chemotherapy and ABMT. These patients were classified after SLL as having microscopic disease (three patients), minimal disease ≤2 cm (five patients), or bulky disease (three patients). Following high-dose chemotherapy, a further laparotomy was performed, which demonstrated five pathological complete responses one clinical complete response, two stable disease, and three progressive disease. One interesting feature of this study is that all three patients with progressive disease had presented with bulky residual disease following induction therapy. Viens and Maraninchi[61] treated 12 "chemosensitive" patients (eight partial responses and four clinical complete responses) following induction with platinum-based chemotherapy with a single cycle of high-dose chemotherapy (different regimens) and ABMT. The resulting 3-year progression-free survival was 50%, however, it is possible that some of the patients with clinical complete response would have done just as well without further chemotherapy. Finally, Stiff et al[64] treated 30 patients with a single course of a high-dose regimen consisting of mitoxantrone, carboplatin, and cyclophosphamide with ABMT support. Of these, 20 were "platinum resistant" (defined as progression or relapse within 6 months of platinum-based therapy), and 22 had >1-cm disease. The overall response rate was 89%, but more complete responses were observed in the platinum-sensitive patients than in the platinum-resistant group (88% vs 47% $P = 0.06$). Also, at a median follow-up of 12 months, 80% of the platinum-sensitive patients were alive, whereas the median overall survival was only 10.4 months in the patients with platinum-resistant disease.

Another subgroup with a poor prognosis consists of patients with large-volume disease following initial debulking surgery, and perhaps these patients would benefit from more intensive front-line chemotherapy. In 1990, Viens et al[65] performed a retrospective analysis of 35 patients initially treated with platinum-based chemotherapy followed by a single cycle of high-dose melphalan and ABMT. Patients underwent a SLL prior to transplant to document disease status, and in 12 evaluable patients the overall response rate was 75% with an actuarial survival of 47% at 54 months. There were three deaths related to the high-dose treatment phase. In a further study by Juttner et al,[65] 13 patients were treated with three cycles of cisplatin/cyclophosphamide followed by a single high-dose chemotherapy regimen consisting of carboplatin, etoposide, and melphalan supported by PBSCT. Despite three toxic deaths, the remaining 10 patients achieved a complete clinical response after the transplant phase of the protocol. These studies demonstrate that high-dose protocols can be used as up-front therapy with conventional induction regimens but involve significant toxicity. Clearly randomized trials involving conventional dose therapy would be neccessary before such an approach could be recommended, but the strategy is an intriguing one.

In summary, the use of high-dose chemotherapy is clearly feasible in patients with ovarian cancer, but in the patient populations studied it generally did not produce long-duration remissions or prolong survival when compared with historical controls using conventional doses of chemotherapy. It appears that the ideal situation for researching high-dose chemotherapy is in patients with *minimal tumor burden and chemosensitive disease*. Randomized controlled trials are obviously required in order to define the appropriate patient population likely to benefit from this approach. One such trial is the SWOG 9106 protocol which is planning to use the least toxic of two high-dose chemotherapy regimens (with PBSCT support) in a randomized study in patients with stage III or IV disease and ≤3-cm residual disease at SLL, with standard doses of cisplatin/taxol as the control arm. It will be important in such studies to examine both progression-free survival and overall survival since it is quite conceivable that high-dose chemotherapy might substantially delay the emergence of drug-resistant cells—resulting in prolonged progression-free survival—yet might not be capable of eradicating a tumor cell population completely. The impact on overall survival might therefore be less evident. In addition, and for the reasons described previously, randomized studies involving this approach will need to consider the issue of total dose administered. The availability of PBSCT means that repeated high-dose chemotherapy treatments are feasible and safe, and the number of treatments given could ultimately be a determining factor.

J. TATE THIGPEN

The data cited to this point concern increasing dose intensity over a range achievable with standard approaches to intravenous chemotherapy. Ovarian carcinoma affords an opportunity to enhance dose intensity to 10-fold or greater by two methods: intraperitoneal administration of drugs and support of very high-dose regimens with stem cells.

Intraperitoneal therapy

Ovarian carcinoma spreads primarily by intraperitoneal seeding. The most common stage at diagnosis is stage III which is defined as involvement of the peritoneal cavity outside the pelvis and/or involvement of retroperitoneal or inguinal lymph nodes. Since the disease remains at least grossly confined to the peritoneal cavity for a significant portion of its course, the administration of chemotherapy via the intraperitoneal route is logical. A number of cytotoxic drugs have been successfully given intraperitoneally with peak peritoneal to plasma concentration ratios of 18 to over 1,000.[67] Included among these are the platinum compounds, cisplatin and carboplatin. The intraperitoneal approach is thus reasonable and feasible.

Uncontrolled trials of intraperitoneal platinum compounds in patients with small-volume persistent or recurrent disease show that 25 to 35% of patients achieve a PCR.[68–71] This suggests an advantage for the intraperitoneal route of administration thought to be a consequence of the enhanced exposure of cancer cells to drug. Such an approach effectively increases the dose intensity. The obvious limitation of intraperitoneal therapy is the depth of drug penetration, which dictates that only patients with small-volume disease, the smaller the better, can be considered.

Subsequent results of phase II trials in persistent or recurrent disease showed that the case for intraperitoneal therapy was not as straightforward as it seemed.[72] Responses occurred almost exclusively in patients who had responded to initial platinum-based therapy and relapsed after a treatment-free interval of at least 6 months (platinum-sensitive disease). Those whose disease had progressed while they were receiving initial platinum-based therapy, whose best response to initial therapy was stable disease, or whose disease recurred less than 6 months after completion of initial therapy (platinum-resistant disease) responded less than 10% of the time. The response rates for platinum-sensitive disease to intraperitoneal therapy (40 to 60%) were in fact similar to those reported with the same therapy given intravenously.[73] At least in the salvage setting, therefore, no advantage for the intraperitoneal approach was observed.

Despite these rather discouraging results from phase II salvage trials, the ultimate answer as to the value of intraperitoneal therapy must come from randomized trials. Two such trials have been completed to date. The first of these[74] randomized 654 newly diagnosed patients with small-volume volume (nodules ≤2 cm) stage III disease to cyclophosphamide 600 mg/m^2 intravenously plus cisplatin 100 mg/m^2 either intravenously or intraperitoneally every 3 weeks for six cycles. Originally designed to randomize 400 patients and detect a hazard ratio of 0.67, the study accrual was extended to those with no nodules larger than 0.5 cm because it was believed that this subset stood the greatest chance to benefit from the intraperitoneal approach. The final analysis showed no statistically significant differences in surgically determined complete responses but a significant difference in overall survival ($P = 0.02$), favoring the intraperitoneal regimen (hazard ratio 0.77). This seems to establish the case for front-line intraperitoneal therapy for small-volume ovarian carcinoma.

Unfortunately, certain design aspects of the randomized trial cast doubt on the conclusions. The extension of the accrual derived its basis from the thesis that patients with the smallest residual (<0.5 cm) would benefit most because the intraperitoneal drug would penetrate more of the nodule. When analyzed separately (as was the intent when the accrual was extended), this subset showed no statistically significant improvement in survival (51 vs 46 months). In other words, the rationale for extension of accrual turned out to be in error. On the other hand, the overall population showed a statistically significant improvement in survival for the intraperitoneal regimen (49 vs 41 months) with a hazard ratio of 0.77, less than the original goal of the trial (a hazard ratio of 0.67). In short, the study did not reach its original goal of a hazard ratio of 0.67 despite extension of accrual to include larger numbers of the most favorable group. This leaves serious questions about the conclusions of the trial.

This still leaves the question whether intraperitoneal therapy is of value in the front-line treatment of small-volume residual stage III ovarian carcinoma. The second randomized trial will hopefully decide this issue. This study randomized over 400 newly diagnosed patients with small-volume residual disease (no nodule >1.0 cm) to either paclitaxel 135 mg/m^2 over 24 hours intravenously followed by cisplatin 75 mg/m^2 intravenously every 3 weeks for six cycles, or two courses of carboplatin intravenously dosed to an AUC of 9 every 4 weeks followed by six cycles at 3-4 week intervals of paclitaxel 135 mg/m^2 over 24 hours followed by cisplatin 100 mg/m^2 intraperitoneally. Although this trial has completed accrual, an additional 1 to 2 years of follow-up will be required before answers are forthcoming. If the study is positive, then further investigation of intraperitoneal approaches will be mandatory. If, on the other hand, the study is negative, it seems unlikely that intraperitoneal therapy can offer patients added benefit.

In short, available data on intraperitoneal therapy do not establish that major enhancement in effective dose intensity (18- to 20-fold for the platinum compounds in theory) offers an advantage. A definitive answer concerning the value of intraperitoneal therapy awaits the results of the last of the two randomized trials.

Stem cell–supported high-dose chemotherapy

Recent reviews of available phase I and II trials of stem cell–supported high-dose chemotherapy[75,76] demonstrate the feasibility of administering active regimens in very high doses (8- to 10-fold increase in dose intensity) together with stem cell support. Although response rates are high, the patient populations are poorly characterized as to whether the disease is platinum-sensitive or platinum-resistant, and the response durations are brief. These results are bought at the cost of significant toxicity and expense. On the basis of these data, no case can be made for the use of these approaches outside clinical trials.

A randomized trial of high-dose chemotherapy with stem cell support as front-line therapy is under consideration as a national effort and will be required to establish a role for such an approach. In theory, there are two possible ways to execute such treatment. First, newly diagnosed patients can be randomized to either standard chemotherapy or high-dose chemotherapy plus stem cell support as the initial treatment. Second, newly diagnosed patients can first be treated with standard chemotherapy and then subjected to a SLL. Those with residual disease that is clearly chemosensitive (i.e., disease that has decreased in size with the initial treatment) and small in volume (i.e., no nodule larger than 1 cm in diameter) can then be randomized to either continued standard chemotherapy or high-dose chemotherapy plus stem cell support. The latter approach has the advantage of selecting those patients who in theory have the greatest chance to benefit from high-dose chemotherapy (i.e., those with the least chance of having chemoresistance clones of cells) and avoiding the cost and toxicity of such an approach for those least likely to benefit (i.e., those with true cellular resistance).

Since studies on intraperitoneal chemotherapy as second-line treatment suggest that clinically platinum-resistant patients do not respond to greater dose intensity,[35] the combined efforts of the Gynecologic Oncology Group, Southwest Oncology Group, Eastern Cooperative Oncology Group, and Cancer and Leukemia Group B recently initiated a randomized trial based on the second design. Patients receive initial therapy with paclitaxel plus cisplatin, undergo SLL, and, if they meet the criteria discussed above, receive either paclitaxel plus carboplatin for additional cycles or one course of high-dose carboplatin plus mitoxantrone plus cyclophosphamide supported by peripheral blood stem cells.

Conclusion

Efforts to increase greatly the dose intensity of platinum-based regimens have failed to establish a therapeutic advantage for 8- to 20-fold dose enhancement. Until randomized trials establish conclusively the therapeutic value of toxic and expensive approaches such as intraperitoneal therapy and high-dose chemotherapy plus stem cell support, these treatments should be confined to clinical trials.

QUESTION 4

What is the relative importance of dose intensity versus total dose?

J. TATE THIGPEN

The question of the relative importance of total dose as opposed to dose intensity has not been addressed directly. Some of the randomized trials already cited, however, provide data that allow an estimate of the relative importance. Of the seven studies evaluating platinum dose intensity, five compare regimens with a difference not only in dose intensity but also in total dose of the platinum compound.[9,11,14,38,39] Three of the five show no difference.[14,38,39] Two show an advantage for the higher-dose regimen which confers not only greater total dose but also greater dose intensity.[9,11] These two studies, however, have major design flaws which have been described earlier.

The three studies of paclitaxel all evaluate not only increased dose intensity but also total dose.[53–55] These studies show no advantage for the high-dose regimens and hence do not favor the value of either greater dose intensity or greater total dose.

The weight of evidence from randomized trials thus dose not support any advantage for either dose intensity or total dose, at least over a clinically relevant range.

QUESTION 5

What do you believe to be the shape of the dose-response curve in ovarian cancer?

PAUL A. VASEY
STAN B. KAYE

As stated earlier, there is clearly a dose-response relationship in vitro for ovarian cancer cell lines, and studies using these cells suggest that dose escalations of greater than 5-fold would be required before clinical drug resistance is likely to be abrogated. Jodrell et al[77] analyzed the clinical relationship between the first cycle dosage of carboplatin based on AUC and response in ovarian cancer and concluded that although there was a dose-response relationship for this compound up to AUC 7, at lower levels of AUC the slope was fairly shallow and further dose escalation merely increased toxicity without producing higher response rates. However, survival data were not available for analysis, and therefore it was not possible to determine whether relating AUC to survival (or progression-free interval) would produce a similar result.

In the treatment of chemonaive ovarian cancer, the overall response rate to single-agent cisplatin at a dose intensity averaging 25 mg/m²/wk is about 40%.[78] Combination chemotherapy has been clearly shown to increase response rates, either at a lower platinum dose intensity in the cisplatin/Adriamycin/cyclophosphamide regimen (ORR 55%, platinum dose intensity 16 to 20 mg/m²/wk)[79] or at the same intensity when used with Taxol (ORR 73%, platinum dose intensity 25mg/m²/wk).[21]

Clearly, higher dose intensities of platinum-based chemotherapy regimens are associated with more myeloid, neurologic, and renal toxicities, and within the conventional dose range there is no conclusive evidence of a major survival benefit for the more dose-intense schedules even though response rates may be higher. A possible dose-response curve for ovarian cancer based largely on the overall response rates observed in randomized studies is shown in Figure 8-1. This notional dose-response curve for platinum is clearly speculative at its upper extreme, and extrapolation from available phase II data has been incorporated, suggesting that the curve is relatively shallow. Nevertheless, this does not preclude significant benefit from accruing at the highest levels of dose intensity, and this is likely to be the key issue.

J. TATE THIGPEN

While current results in patients with advanced ovarian carcinoma reflect clear progress, all agree that not enough responses are produced by standard therapy. Studies, particularly meta-analyses, suggest that the frequency of response can be enhanced over a low-dose range by an escalation of dose intensity. Beyond a threshhold dose, no further therapeutic benefit is observed with further dose escalation. At least for cisplatin, this threshhold appears to fall in the range from 15 to 25 mg/m²/wk (45 to 75 mg/m² every 3 weeks). Hints of a second threshhold at very high-dose intensities beyond which further benefit ensues come from studies of intraperitoneal therapy and very high-dose regimens supported by stem cells; but confirmation of

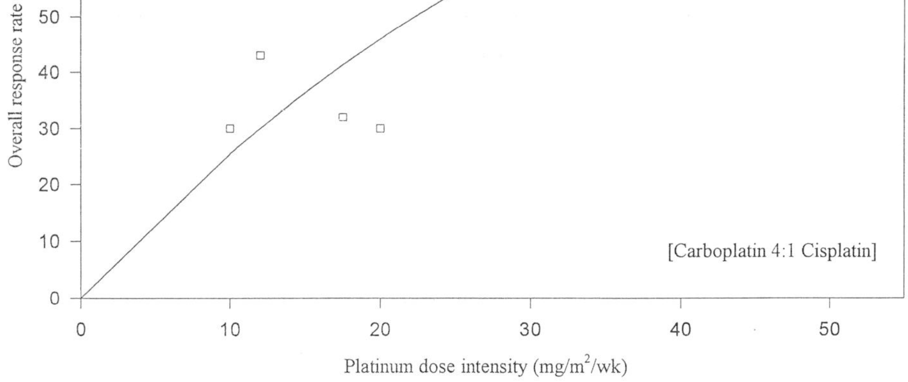

FIGURE 8-1. Putative dose-response curve in ovarian cancer patients.

such a second threshhold awaits further randomized trials which are either ongoing or planned for the near future.

These facts produce a dose-intensity curve (Figure 8-2) that reflects a confirmed dose-response relationship over low dose ranges and a plateau beyond a threshhold dose intensity. The second part of the proposed curve postulates a second threshhold at very high-dose intensities, but this part remains unconfirmed at the present time.

From a practical clinical perspective, the physician should seek to attain adequate dose intensity to reach the first threshhold. For the platinum compounds, a dose of cisplatin of 75 mg/m^2 every 3 weeks or an equivalent amount of carboplatin should more than suffice. For paclitaxel, a dose in the range of 135 to 175 mg/m^2 over 24 hours appears to be adequate.

The use of intraperitoneal therapy or of very high-dose regimens supported by stem cells should await further trials to establish the value of such approaches. In the case of intraperitoneal therapy, additional randomized trials should await analysis of the completed trial of Taxol plus either intravenous or intraperitoneal cisplatin. If this trial shows no advantage for intraperitoneal over intravenous cisplatin, then further studies of intraperitoneal chemotherapy are unlikely to produce positive results.

In the case of very high-dose chemotherapy supported by stem cells, potential approaches

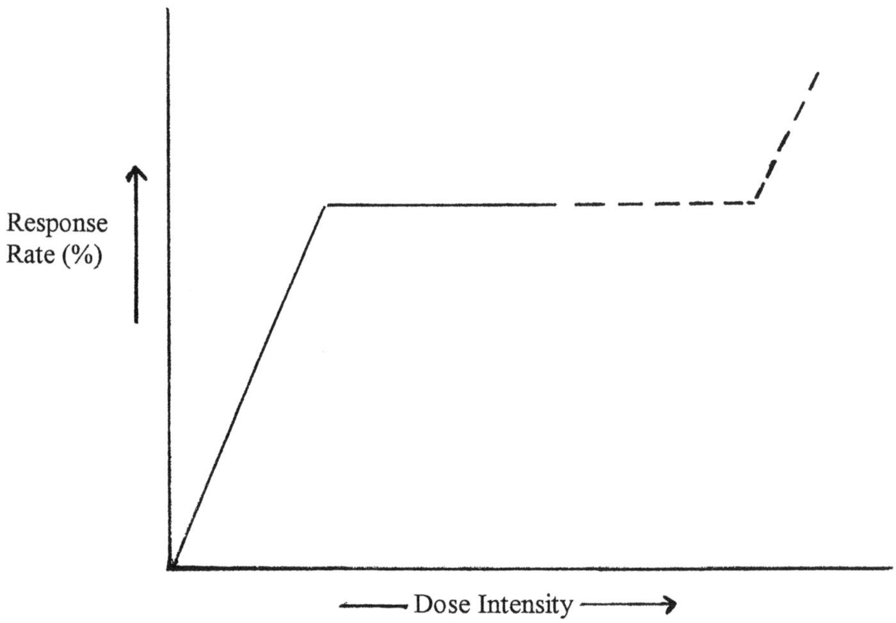

FIGURE 8-2. Based on available data for the platinum compounds and, to a lesser extent, paclitaxel, the dose intensity is probably as depicted. Over a low-dose range up to a cisplatin dose intensity of 15 to 25 mg/m^2/wk, response occurs more frequently as dose intensity is increased. When this threshold is reached, no further increase in benefit is observed as the dose intensity is increased further. This portion of the curve (solid portion) is supported by available data. Whether the second (dotted) portion of the curve is correct is speculative. Regimens involving intraperitoneal therapy and high-dose chemotherapy supported by stem cells have the potential to reach eight-fold or greater increases in dose intensity and may, as suggested by the one randomized trial of intraperitoneal therapy, reach a second threshhold beyond which further benefit is seen with further increases in dose intensity. Confirmation awaits further study.

include use as first-line therapy, use restricted to patients who have been shown to be chemosensitive with initial intravenous chemotherapy, and use in the salvage setting after failure of initial standard therapy. Phase II trials in the salvage setting cited earlier yield responses that are not durable; hence such an approach seems to be less likely to produce better results. Each of the other choices is a rational approach which should be tested in randomized trials, although no current data are available to support the use of either outside a clinical trial.

QUESTION 6

What are your recommendations for future directions in this area?

PAUL A. VASEY
STAN B. KAYE

The question of dose intensity as an important factor in the efficacy of chemotherapy for ovarian cancer was brought to the forefront of oncologists' thinking by retrospective analysis of studies that seemed to correlate dose intensity with higher response rates and increased survival. Further analysis of these trials allows us to outline future areas of research that may help to resolve this crucial issue.

The majority of individual phase II trials of high-dose (myeloablative) chemotherapy with ABMT or PBSC support have consistently demonstrated very high response rates in women with refractory advanced ovarian cancer. The implication from this is that treating patients early in the course of their disease (i.e., when the tumors are both small and chemosensitive) will potentially produce longer remissions and consequently increase the number of long-term survivors. The most appropriate way to investigate this is by conducting a prospective randomized clinical trial in patients with minimal residual disease following initial surgery. The control arm should be the currently accepted "gold standard" regimen consisting of multiple cycles of cisplatin 75 mg/m^2 plus Taxol 135 mg/m^2 over 24 hours (or 175 mg/m^2 over 3 hours), and in many centers this regimen would indeed, be considered the standard arm in any prospective phase III study in ovarian cancer.

In potentially curable solid malignancies, multiple cycles of conventionally dosed chemotherapy are required to achieve cure; it is perhaps reasonable therefore to assume that to cure malignancies like ovarian cancer—a tumor that readily acquires resistance to standard chemotherapy doses—multiple cycles of *high-dose* chemotherapy may be required. It has been shown that the use of PBSC support for multiple cycles of high-dose chemotherapy is feasible[80] and that this approach increases both the dose intensity and dose rate of the administered drugs (e.g., up to a sixfold increase in dose intensity for carboplatin in the 1992 study by Crown et al[81]).

A key issue in the chemotherapy of ovarian cancer is the choice of doses to be administered when myelosuppressive drugs are given together in combination schedules. Clearly the optimal schedule (in terms of dose intensity) is that which permits full doses of both or all agents to be given. Remarkably, and for reasons that are not yet clear, it appears that such is indeed the case for Taxol (at least when administered over 3 hours) when given together with carboplatin. Both agents have myelotoxicity as their dose-limiting toxicity, and therefore augmentation with hematopoeitic growth factors should maintain a dose-intensive schedule. Furthermore, this combination of agents could be administered completely in the outpatient setting, thus increasing convenience and decreasing overall costs. A GOG pilot study has demonstrated that both agents can be administered at full doses without G-CSF administration on a 3-week schedule[82] and that this combination produced response rates of 80 to 85% with an increased dose intensity over the Taxol/cisplatin regimen of nearly 50% (the 145 mg/m^2/wk carboplatin delivered by this schedule approximating 36 mg/m^2/wk cisplatin at 4:1 equivalence). Clearly this merits further study and needs to be compared with the 24-hour infusional Taxol/cisplatin combination.

The controversy concerning the best therapeutic schedule for Taxol in ovarian cancer has been discussed in more detail earlier. Many oncologists now consider the 3-hour infusion to be more convenient than, less than, toxic and equally efficacious as the 24-hour infusion following the publication of results from a large randomized European study[48] in 1994. However, the most important prospective trial to date[21] uses a 24-hour infusion for Taxol in combination with cisplatin, and some argue that this represents the standard by which other schedules should be judged. To complicate the issue, evidence is emerging the increased cytotoxicity of longer infusions of Taxol, and there is therefore clearly a need for more clinical trials to address the issue of intensification by dose scheduling. Whichever Taxol schedule is used, a further unresolved issue is the optimal number of cycles (or total dose) needed to give maximal benefit. The general recommendation of six cycles for most forms of therapy may not necessarily be appropriate for this drug, and further trials addressing this issue are ongoing.

Finally, intraperitoneal (IP) therapy merits renewed discussion in the context of a discussion on dose intensity. Pharmacokinetic data indicate that when given IP compared to IV there is a potential 20-fold increase in tumor cell exposure to cisplatin, comparing peak peritoneal cavity and plasma concentrations.[83] In 1995, Alberts et al[74] reported the mature results of the SWOG-GOG-ECOG phase III study which compared IP cisplatin and intravenous (IV) cisplatin (both in combination with IV cyclophosphamide). In this multicenter study, 539 eligible patients with untreated, optimally cytoreduced, stage III ovarian cancer were randomized (between 1986 and 1992) to receive six courses of IP or IV cisplatin (100 mg/m^2) plus IV cyclophosphamide (600 mg/m^2) every 3 weeks. A significant survival advantage was found for patients receiving the IP therapy (median survival 49 months vs 41 months, $P = 0.03$) and a trend toward an increased overall response rate and pathological complete response. Also, significantly more hearing loss and neutropenia were experienced by patients receiving the IV cisplatin. This survival benefit for IP over IV cisplatin in optimally debulked stage III ovarian cancer is certainly of interest and justifies further investigation in this subgroup with minimal residual disease, as the majority of cases (390) actually had less than 0.5-cm residual disease. The GOG trial comparing the standard six cycles of Taxol/cisplatin regimen with a dose-intensive regimen consisting of two cycles of carboplatin (AUC 9) followed by IP cisplatin and IV Taxol in untreated small-volume stage III patients is almost complete, and the results are eagerly awaited.

J. TATE THIGPEN

Future studies on the issue of drug dose in ovarian carcinoma should focus on determining whether there is a second threshold beyond which dose escalation will yield better results. In ovarian carcinoma, there are two ways to achieve this: intraperitoneal chemotherapy and stem cell–supported high-dose chemotherapy. In the case of intraperitoneal chemotherapy, studies demonstrating the feasibility of such an approach have been completed successfully. Both the platinum compounds and paclitaxel can be given intraperitoneally. Both drugs can also produce responses in the salvage setting in chemosensitive patients. In newly diagnosed patients, two randomized trials have been conducted. The first[74] has been completed and analyzed and suggests that a second threshhold may exist, but design flaws as discussed earlier prevent this trial from being definitive. The second has been completed and awaits data maturation prior to analysis. Whether further studies of intraperitoneal chemotherapy should be conducted depends on the results of the follow-up randomized trial. Current efforts are directed toward determining whether paclitaxel and a platinum compound can be given intraperitoneally concurrently and what the best strategy is for combining the two most active agents intraperitoneally.

In the case of high-dose chemotherapy supported by stem cells, phase I and II trials in the salvage setting demonstrate the feasibility and activity of such an approach.[75,76] The first randomized trial of front-line therapy is underway in the United States. If this is study is found to be negative, further interest in such approaches will lag because of the major expense and toxicity.

EDITORS' COMMENTARY

What is notable about the comment regarding dose intensity is that the contributors are not particularly divergent in their opinions. Dr. Thigpen has long been a critic of dose intensity, opining that it has never been proved, while Drs. Kaye and Vasey have been strong proponents of dose-intense therapy.

Drs. Kaye, Vasey, and Thigpen both reviewed the uncontrolled and controlled trials evaluating the effect of dose intensity on outcome in ovarian cancer. The authors conclude that there are hints of a dose-response relationship, but this rarely if ever is reflected in improved survival and is always at the cost of additional toxicity. We agree with the contributors in recommending that a dose of cisplatin 75 mg/m^2 every 3 weeks or of carboplatin 350 to 500 mg/m^2 every 3 to 4 weeks is an appropriate dose and that doses above this are associated with unacceptable side effects without improved efficacy.

Similarly, the contributors agree that there is little data to support dose-intense Taxol therapy. Taxol doses can be increased only twofold without the development of significant neurotoxicity, and although there is a hint of a higher response rate with doses in excess of 200 mg/m^2, there has not been a simultaneous improvement in either progression-free interval or survival. Thus, Taxol doses in the range of 135 to 175 mg/m^2 seem appropriate, and we agree with this recommendation.

Probably more important than the dose of Taxol is duration of infusion. The contributors address this issue, and we concur that ongoing clinical trials evaluating duration of Taxol infusion are important in terms of deciding whether the more facile 3-hour infusion or the more complex 24-hour infusion gives a superior therapeutic index.

Another way of administering high-dose chemotherapy is through intraperitoneal therapy. Although this was not a specific question, Dr. Thigpen feels that the "jury is out" in terms of the value of intraperitoneal therapy as part of primary therapy. He cites a single intergroup study as suggesting a difference but notes that there are some potential problems with this trial and awaits the outcome of a recently completed GOG trial currently undergoing data maturity before agreeing to treat patients initially with intraperitoneal therapy. One thing that remains clear is that intraperitoneal therapy is not indicated for patients with bulky disease.

With regard to high-dose chemotherapy and stem cell support, the contributors agree that there are no data verifying it as an appropriate form of therapy either as part of primary therapy or in a salvage setting. The contributors point out the difficulty in interpretating the existing data from several small phase II studies in which a very heterogeneous population of patients was treated. It is impossible from these studies to draw any conclusions about the relative value of this therapy over standard forms of salvage chemotherapy. This is in large part due to the small size of the studies, the variable preparative regimens, the inclusion of patients with bulky disease (unlikely to respond to any form of therapy), and the inclusion of patients with drug-resistant disease (very unlikely to respond to any form of therapy).

We asked each contributor to describe the shape of the dose-response curve. Interestingly, they have developed similar curves in which there is a relatively steep dose-response relationship from homeopathic to standard doses but a significant flattening of the slope of the curve at doses above what is now considered standard therapy. There is much speculation as to whether or not there will be a further increase in the slope of this curve at higher doses, however, such doses are not currently achievable clinically and thus it seems to be a moot question at this point in time.

No contributor specifically comments on the relative values of dose intensity and total dose. There are conflicting reports in the literature about the value of total dose, and attempting to design protocols that simultaneously address these two issues is problematic. What seems clear, however, from the currently available literature is that, with currently achievable approaches to the chemotherapy of ovarian cancer, neither dose intensity, dose density, or total dose leads to a significant impact on outcome.

Finally, Drs. Kaye, Thigpen, and Vasey outline recommendations for future studies. They agree, as do the editors, that intraperitoneal therapy in carefully selected patients with drug-sensitive, low-volume disease deserves further evaluation. We also feel that, with the advent of new active single agents for the treatment of this disease, during the next decade attention should be paid to how best to incorporate these new agents in as high a dose as is feasible for primary treatment. We may have to abandon the approach of adding additional drugs to existing doublets or triplets and take the approach popularized by Norton in which single agents are given in very high doses at frequent intervals for short numbers of cycles followed by a similar approach with other active and non-cross-resistant drugs. Probably only another decade of clinical research will begin to "tease out" these important questions.

References

1. Silverberg E, Boring C, Squires TS: Cancer Statistics 1990. CA Cancer J Clin 40:9–26, 1990
2. Ozols RF, Young RC: Chemotherapy of ovarian cancer. Semin Oncol 11:251–263, 1984
3. Ozols RF, Behrens BC, Ostchega Y, Young RC: High dose cisplatin and high dose carboplatin in refractory ovarian cancer. Cancer Treat Rev, suppl A. 12:59–65, 1985
4. Skipper HE: Dose intensity versus total dose of chemotherapy: an experimental basis. pp. 43–64. In DeVita VT, Hellman S, Rosenberg SA (eds): Important Advances in Oncology. JB Lippincott, Philadelphia, 1990
5. Behrens BC, Hamilton TC, Masuda H et al: Characteristics of cisdiammine-dichloroplatinum(II)-resistant human ovarian cancer cell line and the evaluation of platinum analogues. Cancer Res 47:414–418, 1987
6. Levin L, Hryniuk WM: Dose intensity analysis of chemotherapy regimens in ovarian carcinoma. J Clin Oncol 5:756, 1987
7. McGuire WP: Dose Intensity in Ovarian Cancer. American Society of Clinical Oncology Educational Book, 1993 pp 31–36
8. Fennelly D: Dose intensity in advanced ovarian cancer: have we answered the question? Clin Cancer Res 1:575–582, 1995
9. Ngan HYS, Choo YC, Cheung M et al: A randomized study of high-dose versus low-dose cisplatin combined with cyclophosphamide in the treatment of advanced ovarian cancer. Chemotherapy 35:221–227, 1989
10. McGuire WP, Hoskins WJ, Brady MF et al: Assessment of dose-intensive therapy in suboptimally debulked ovarian cancer: a Gynaecologic Oncology Group Study. J Clin Oncol 13:1589–1599, 1995
11. Kaye SB, Paul J, Cassidy J et al: Mature results of a randomized trial of two doses of cisplatin for the treatment of ovarian cancer. J Clin Oncol 14:2113–2119, 1996
12. Columbo N, Pittelli MR, Parma G: Cisplatin (P) dose intensity in advanced ovarian cancer (AOC): a randomized study of conventional dose (DC) vs dose-intense (DI) cisplatin monochemotherapy. Proc Am Soc Clin Oncol 12:255, 1993
13. Jakobsen A, on behalf of DACOVA: A dose intensity study of carboplatin in

ovarian cancer. Int J Gynaecol Cancer, suppl 5. 5:11, 1995

14. Gore ME, Mainwaring PN, Macfarlane V: A randomized study of high versus standard dose carboplatin in patients (pts) with advanced epithelial ovarian cancer (EOC). Proc Am Soc Clin Oncol 15:284, 1996
15. Ehrlich CE, Einhorn L, Stehman FB, Blessing J: Treatment of advanced epithelial ovarian cancer using cisplatin, Adriamycin and cytoxan—the Indiana University experience. Clin Obstet Gynecol 10:325–335, 1983
16. Bella M, Cocconi G, Lotticci R et al: Mature results of a prospective randomized trial comparing two different dose-intensity regimens of cisplatin in advanced ovarian carcinoma. Ann Oncol, 5 suppl 8. 5:2, 1994
17. Conte PF, Bruzzone M, Gadducci A et al: High doses versus standard doses of cisplatin in combination with epidoxorubicin and cyclophosphamide in advanced ovarian cancer patients with bulky residual disease: a randomized trial. Proc Am Soc Clin Oncol 12:273, 1993
18. Kaye SB, Lewis C, Paul J et al: Randomized study of two doses of cisplatin and cyclophosphamide in epithelial ovarian cancer. Lancet 340:329–333, 1992
19. Calvert AH, Newall DR, Gumbrell LA et al: Carbopatin dosage: prospective evaluation of a simple formula based on renal function. J Clin Oncol 7:1748–1756, 1989
20. Bertelsen K, Bastholt L: High-dose platinum chemotherapy in advanced ovarian cancer: a phase II study. Gynecol Oncol 44:79–82, 1992
21. McGuire WP, Hoskins WJ, Brady MF et al: Cyclophosphamide and cisplatin compared with paclitaxel and cisplatin in patients with stage III and stage IV ovarian cancer. N Engl J Med 334: 1–6, 1996
22. Fanning J, Hilgers RD: High-dose cisplatin carboplatin chemotherapy in primary advanced epithelial ovarian cancer. Gynecol Oncol 51:182–186, 1993
23. Gershenson MD, Morris M, Burke TW et al: Combined cisplatin and carboplatin chemotherapy for treatment of advanced epithelial ovarian cancer. Gynecol Oncol 58:349–355, 1995
24. Thigpen T, Lagasse L, Homesley H et al: Cisplatinum in the treatment of advanced or recurrent adenocarcinoma of the ovary: a phase II study of the Gynecologic Oncology Group. Am J Clin Oncol 6:431–435, 1983 support for patients with epithelial ovarian cancer. Semin Oncol 22:250–262, 1995
25. Omura GA, Blessing JA, Ehrlich CE et al: A randomized trial of cyclophosphamide and doxorubicin with or without cisplatin in advanced ovarian cancer. Cancer 57:1725–1730, 1986
26. Pecorelli S, Bolis G, Vassena L et al: Randomized comparison of cisplatin and carboplatin in advanced ovarian cancer. Proc ASCO 7:136, 1988
27. Alberts DS, Green SJ, Hannigan EV et al: Improved therapeutic index of carboplatin plus cyclophosphamide versus cisplatin plus cyclophosphamide: final report by the Southwest Oncology Group of a phase III randomized trial in stages III and IV ovarian cancer. J Clin Oncol 10:706–717, 1992
28. ten Bokkel Huinink WW, van der Burg MEL, van Oosterom AT et al: Carboplatin in combination therapy for ovarian cancer. Cancer Treat Rev, suppl B. 15:9–15, 1988
29. Swenerton K, Jeffrey J, Stuart G et al: Cisplatin-cyclophosphamide versus carboplatin-cyclophosphamide in advanced ovarian cancer: a randomized phase III study of the National Cancer Institute of Canada Clinical Trials Group. J Clin Oncol 10:718–726, 1992
30. Edmondson JH, McCormack GM, Wieand HS et al: Cyclophosphamide-cisplatin versus cyclophosphamide-carboplatin in stage III-IV ovarian carci-

noma: a comparison of equally myelosuppressive regimens. J Natl Cancer Inst 81:1500–1504, 1989

31. Frei E, Canellos G: Dose: a critical factor in cancer chemotherapy. Am J Med 69:585–594, 1980
32. Levin L, Simon R, Hryniuk W: Importance of multiagent chemotherapy regimens in ovarian carcinoma: dose intensity analysis. J Natl Cancer Inst 85: 1732–1742, 1993
33. Ozols RF, Ostchega Y, Curt G, Young RC: High-dose carboplatin in refractory ovarian cancer patients. J Clin Oncol 5:197–201, 1987
34. Howell S, Zimm S, Markman M et al: Long-term survival of advanced refractory ovarian carcinoma patients with small-volume disease treated with intraperitoneal chemotherapy. J Clin Oncol 5:1607–1612, 1987
35. Markman M, Reichman B, Hakes T et al: Intraperitoneal chemotherapy in the management of ovarian cancer. Cancer 71:1565–1570, 1993
36. Ozols R: High dose therapy with cisplatin and its analogs in ovarian cancer: current status and future studies. Educ Booklet ASCO 1987, pp 69–70
37. Omura G, Bundy B, Berek J et al: Randomized trial of cyclophosphamide plus cisplatin with or without doxorubicin in ovarian carcinoma: a Gynecologic Oncology Group study. J Clin Oncol 7:457–465, 1989
38. Conte P, Bruzzone M, Carnino F et al: High-dose versus low-dose cisplatin in combination with cyclophosphamide and epidoxorubicin in suboptimal ovarian cancer: a randomized study of the Gruppo Oncologico Nord-Ovest. J Clin Oncol 14:351–356, 1996
39. Dittrich C, Obermair A, Kurz C et al: Prospective randomized trial of cisplatin/carboplatin versus conventional cisplatin/cyclophosphamide in epithelial ovarian cancer: first results of the impact of platinum dose intensity on patient outcome. Proc Am Soc Clin Oncol 15:279, 1996
40. McGuire WP, Rowinsky EK, Rosenshein NB: Taxol, a unique antineoplastic agent with significant activity in advanced ovarian epithelial neoplasms. Ann Int Med 111:273–279, 1989
41. Thigpen T, Blessing J, Ball H et al: Phase II trial of Taxol as second-line therapy for ovarian carcinoma: a gynaecologic oncology group study. Proc Am Soc Clin Oncol 9:604, 1990
42. Gore ME, Slevin M, Gallagher C: Single agenţ paclitaxel in previously untreated patients with stage IV epithelial ovarian cancer. Int J Gynaecol Cancer, suppl 1. 5:11, 1995
43. Liebmann J, Cook JA, Lipshultz C et al: The influence of Cremophor EL on the cell cycle effects of paclitaxel (Taxol) in human tumour cell lines. Cancer Chemother Pharmacol 33:331–339, 1994
44. Leibmann JE, Cook JA, Lipschultz C et al: Cytotoxic studies of paclitaxel (Taxol) human tumour cell lines. Br J Cancer 68:1104–1109, 1993
45. Gianni L, Kearns CM, Giani A et al: Nonlinear pharmacokinetics and metabolism of paclitaxel and its pharmacokinetic/pharmacodymamic relationships in humans. J Clin Oncol 13:180–190, 1995
46. Sarosy G, Kohn E, Stone DA et al: Phase I study of Taxol and granulocyte colony-stimulating factor in patients with refractory ovarian cancer. J Clin Oncol. 10:1165–1170, 1992
47. Kohn EC, Sarosy G, Bicher A et al: Dose-intense Taxol: High response rate in patients with platinum-resistant recurrent ovarian cancer. J Natl Cancer Inst 86:18–24, 1994
48. Eisenhauer EA, ten Bokkel Huinink, Swenerton KD et al: European-Canadian randomized trial of Taxol in relapsed ovarian cancer: High vs low-

dose and long vs short infusion. J Clin Oncol 12:2654–2666, 1994

49. Spriggs DR, Tondini C: Taxol administered as a 120 hour infusion. Invest New Drugs 10:275–278, 1992
50. Wilson WH, Berg SL, Bryant G et al: Paclitaxel in doxorubicin-refractory or mitoxantrone-refractory breast cancer: a phase I/II trial of 96-hour infusion. J Clin Oncol 12:1621–1629, 1994
51. Seidman AD, Hochhauser D, Yao T-J: 96 hour paclitaxel after short taxane infusion: Phase II pharmacokinetic and pharmacodynamic study in metastatic breast cancer. Proc Ann (Mtg) Am Soc Clin Oncol 14:113, 1995
52. Lokich J, Anderson N, Bern M et al: Multi-day fractionated administration schedule for paclitaxel. Ann Oncol 6:883–885, 1985
53. Rowinsky E, Mackey M and Goodman S: Metaanalysis of paclitaxel dose-response and dose-intensity in recurrent or refractory ovarian cancer. Proc ASCO 15:284, 1996
54. Omura G, Brady M, Delmore J et al: A randomized trial of paciltaxel at 2 dose levels and filgastrim at 2 doses in platinum pretreated epithelial ovarian cancer: a Gynecologic Oncology Group, SWOG, NCCTG and ECOG study. Proc ASCO 15:280, 1996
55. Swenerton K, Eisenhauer E, ten Bokkel Huinink W et al: Taxol in relapsed ovarian cancer: high vs low dose and short vs long infusion: a European-Canadian study coordinated by the NCI Canada Clinical Trials Group. Proc ASCO 12:810, 1993
56. Gulati S, Yahalom Y, Acaba L et al: Treatment of patients with relapsed and resistant non-Hodgkin's lymphoma using total body irradiation, etoposide, cyclophosphamide and autologous bone marrow transplantation. J Clin Oncol 10:936–941, 1992
57. Motzer R, Gulati S, Crown J et al: High dose chemotherapy and autologous bone marrow rescue for patients with refractory germ cell tumours. Cancer 69:550–556, 1992
58. Philip T, Guglielmi C, Chauvin et al: Autologous bone marrow transplantation (ABMT) versus conventional chemotherapy (DHAP) in relapsed non-Hodgkin's lymphoma (NHL): Final analysis of the Parma randomised study (216 patients). Proc Ann (Mtg) Am Soc Clin Oncol 14:A1220, 1995
59. Bezwoda WR, Seymour L, Dansey RD: High-dose chemotherapy with haematopoietic rescue as primary treatment for metastatic breast cancer: a randomized trial. J Clin Oncol 13:2483–2489, 1995
60. Schilder RJ: High-dose chemotherapy with autologous haematopoietic cell support in gynaecologic malignancies. pp. 1–14. In Hoskins WJ, Perez CA, Young RC (eds): Principles and Practice of Gynaecologic Oncology Updates. JB Lippincott, Philadelphia, 1993
61. Viens P, Maraninchi D: High-dose chemotherapy and autologous marrow transplantation for common epithelial ovarian carcinoma. pp. 729–734. In Armitage JO, Antman KH (eds): High-Dose Cancer Therapy: Pharmacology, Haematopoietins, Stem Cells. Williams & Wilkins, Baltimore, 1992
62. Lotz JP, Machover D, Malassagne B et al: Phase I-II study of two consecutive courses of high-dose epipodophyllotoxin, ifosfamide and carboplatin with autologous bone marrow transplantation for treatment of adult patients with solid tumours. J Clin Oncol 9:1860–1870, 1991
63. Mulder PO, Willemse B, Aalders JG et al: High-dose chemotherapy with autologous bone marrow transplantation in patients with refractory ovarian cancer. Eur J Clin Oncol 25:645–649, 1989
64. Stiff PJ, McKenzie RS, Alberts DS: Phase I clinical and pharmacokinetic study of high-dose mitoxantrone combined with carboplatin, cyclophospha-

mide and autologous bone marrow rescue: high response rate for refractory ovarian corcinoma. J Clin Oncol 12:176–183, 1994

65. Viens P, Maraninch D, Legros M et al: High-dose melphalan and autologous marrow rescue in advanced epithelial ovarian carcinomas: a retrospective analysis of 35 patients treated in France. Bone Marrow Transplant 5:227–233, 1990
66. Juttner CA, Davy MLJ, To LB et al: Autologous PBSC transplantation in stage 3 and 4 ovarian cancer. Int J Cell Clon, suppl 1. 10:145, 1992
67. Markman M: Intraperitoneal chemotherapy. In Markman M, Hoskins W eds, *Cancer of the Ovary*, Raven Press, New York, 1993, pp 317–325.
68. Hacker N, Berek J, Pretorium R et al: Intraperitoneal cis-platinum as salvage therapy for refractory epithelial ovarian cancer. Obstet Gynecol 70:759–764, 1987
69. Reichman B, Markman M, Hakes T et al: Intraperitoneal cisplatin and etoposide in the treatment of refractory/recurrent ovarian carcinoma. J Clin Oncol 7:1327–1332, 1989
70. Markman M, Hakes T, Reichman B et al: Intraperitoneal cisplatin and cytarabine in the treatment of refractory ovarian carcinoma. J Clin Oncol 9:204–210, 1991
71. Piver MS, Lele S, Marchetti D et al: Surgically documented response to intraperitoneal cisplatin, cytarabine, and bleomycin after intravenous cisplatin-based chemotherapy in advanced ovarian carcinoma. J Clin Oncol 6:1679–1684, 1988
72. Markman M, Reichman B, Hakes T et al: Responses to second-line cisplatin-based intraperitoneal therapy in ovarian cancer: influence of a prior response to intravenous cisplatin. J Clin Oncol 9:1801–1805, 1991
73. Thigpen T, Vance R, Khansur T: Second-line chemotherapy for recurrent carcinoma of the ovary. Cancer 71:1559–1564, 1993
74. Alberts DS, Liu PY, Hannigan E et al: Phase III study of intraperitoneal cisplatin/intravenous cyclophosphamide vs intravenous cisplatin/intravenous cyclophosphamide in patients with optimal disease stage III ovarian cancer: a SWOG-GOG-ECOG intergroup study. Proc ASCO 14:273, 1995
75. Fennelly D, Schneider J: Role of chemotherapy dose intensification in the treatment of advanced ovarian cancer. Oncology 9:911–921, 1995
76. Kotz K, Schilder R: High-dose chemotherapy and hematopoietic progenitor cell
77. Jodrell DI, Egorin MJ, Canetta RM et al: Relationships between carboplatin exposure and tumour response and toxicity in patients with ovarian cancer. J Clin Oncol 10:520–528, 1992
78. Young RC, Van Hoff DD, Gormley P et al: (is-dichlorodiamine platinum/II) for the treatment of advanced ovarian cancer. Cancer Treat Rep 63:1539–1544, 1979
79. Conte PF, Bruzzone M, Chiara S et al: A randomized trial comparing cisplatin plus cyclophosphamide versus cisplatin, doxorubin and cyclophosphamide in advanced ovarian cancer. J Clin Oncol 4:965–971, 1986
80. Shea T, Mason J, Storniolo Am et al: Sequential cycles of high-dose carboplatin administered with recombinant human granulocyte-macrophage colony-stimulating factor and repeated infusions of autologous peripheral blood progenitor cells: A novel and effective method for delivering multiple courses of dose-intensive therapy. J Clin Oncol 10:464–473, 1992
81. Crown J, Wasserheit C, Hakes T et al: Rapid delivery of multiple high-dose

chemotherapy courses with granulocyte colony-stimulating factor and peripheral blood-derived haematopoietic progenitor cells. J Natl Cancer Inst 84:1935–1936, 1992

82. Bookman MA, McGuire WP, Kilpatrick D et al: Carboplatin and paclitaxel in ovarian cancer: a phase I study of the Gynecology Oncology Group. J Clin Oncol 14(6):1895–1902, 1996

83. Lopez JA, Krikorian JG, Reich SD et al: Clinical pharmacology of intraperitoneal cisplatin. Gynecol Oncol 20:1–9, 1985

CHAPTER 9

SALVAGE CHEMOTHERAPY FOR REFRACTORY DISEASE

Kenneth Swenerton
Hyman Bernard Muss
Emily G. Robinson

EDITORS' INTRODUCTION

Primary treatment of epithelial ovarian cancer leads to response rates as high as 90%, clinical complete response rates as high as 60%, and pathologic complete response rates ranging from 20% to 50%, depending on the bulk of the primary tumor after initial laparotomy. Unfortunately, the vast majority of these responders eventually develop recurrent disease and become candidates for salvage chemotherapy.

Since salvage chemotherapy is not curative, the treating physician must also consider the risk benefit ratio of such therapy, as well as the impact of the chemotherapy on quality of life. Quality of life (dealt with in Ch. 13) is notoriously difficult to measure reliably.

It has become clear over the past several years that there are several prognostic groups in which salvage chemotherapy can be used. Patients primarily refractory to initial therapy, with tumor growth *while* receiving this therapy, have the worst prognosis and the least chance of responding to salvage therapy. A second group of patients who respond briefly to primary chemotherapy, but develop a recurrence within 6 months of discontinuation of primary therapy, have an intermediate prognosis. Patients who have a significant response to primary therapy and a long treatment-free interval ($\geq$ 6 months) have the best prognosis and the best chance of responding to salvage therapy. This latter group of patients also frequently responds a second time to application of the same drugs used in primary treatment. Thus, it has become important to differentiate these three groups of patients when looking at the value of salvage agents. A significant response rate in the former group may identify a drug that deserves incorporation into primary therapy while a drug that is apparently active in drug-sensitive relapse may have less effect when moved into primary therapy. It is also unclear whether drug combinations are appropriate in the salvage setting, as it is quite clear that these combinations increase toxicity and very few data suggest that they improve response or survival.

We have asked our experts to comment on several areas. We have asked them to provide options with specific examples for both platinum-sensitive and platinum-resistant ovarian cancer in relapse. We have asked the authors to comment on the potential value of high-dose chemotherapy and stem cell support. We have specifically asked that they comment on which patients should be considered for such therapy. We have also asked about the role, if any, of chemoresistance assays and the use of molecular markers in the selection of salvage chemotherapy. Finally, we have asked our experts to comment on when, in the course of recurrent ovarian cancer, either investigational therapy or discontinuation of therapy is appropriate.

It is certainly the anticipation of the medical community that, as new chemotherapeutic drugs are identified for salvage therapy of ovarian cancer and moved into primary therapy, the cure rate of this disease will improve. Whether this anticipation can be met will depend on careful study of new compounds, particularly those with new mechanisms of action, in patients with recurrent ovarian cancer. Thus, salvage therapy with or without investigational agents will remain important in future attempts to improve survival in this disease.

QUESTIONS

1. What are the options for salvage treatment of a patient with platinum-sensitive epithelial ovarian cancer who has (1) partial response at second-look laparotomy or (2) relapse 6 or more months after completion of primary therapy? What is your preference?
2. What are the options for salvage treatment of a patient with platinum-resistant epithelial ovarian cancer (progression on Taxol/platinum therapy or relapse less than 6 months after completion of primary therapy)? What is your preference for second-line therapy?
3. What are the potential salvage settings, if any, for high-dose chemotherapy with either autologous bone marrow transplantation or peripheral stem cell support?
4. Is there currently any role for chemoresistance assays or molecular markers in the selection of salvage chemotherapy?
5. At what point in the course of refractory ovarian cancer should one consider (1) investigational therapy and (2) discontinuation of all therapy?
6. Please discuss future directions in this area, including any other major issues, new promising drugs, and so on.

QUESTION 1

What are the options for salvage treatment of a patient with platinum-sensitive epithelial ovarian cancer who has (1) partial response at second-look laparotomy or (2) relapse 6 or more months after completion of primary therapy? What is your preference?

KENNETH SWENERTON

Introduction

The intermediate-term prognosis of women with ovarian cancer has improved, but in most patients the disease either persists or recurs following primary therapy. Thus, a large proportion of patients have a need for retreatment, and the subject of salvage chemotherapy is of considerable clinical and research importance.

Disease biology and the diagnosis of treatment failure

Just as epithelial ovarian cancer is not a single entity at diagnosis, persistent or relapsed disease has a remarkably variable spectrum of behavior. The extent and virulence of the primary tumor dominate the subsequent natural history of women with ovarian cancer[1] and affect not only the likelihood of relapse and the tempo of events (duration of the failure-free and postfailure survivals) but also the difficulty of establishing a diagnosis of relapse. The diagnosis of recurrence is usually easier in patients with previously treated high-grade residual-positive tumors. In contrast, recurrence is less common in those having had complete surgery for low-grade lesions—the tempo is slower and the clinical findings may be less definitive, features which extend the differential diagnosis.

Follow-up and the timing of retreatment

Diligent clinical follow-up augmented by biomarker monitoring can detect treatment failure earlier.[2–4] Is this diligence justified? One group has adopted a policy of restarting treatment at the first sign of failure,[5] reporting that survival measured *from the time of retreatment* is better in patients treated earlier than in those treated later. The "lead time" flaw in this argument is obvious. Neijt has suggested that since smaller tumors respond more often, he too favors prompt detection of relapse and early retreatment.[6] However, this argument is also flawed. Delay is not the only, nor even the most important, reason large lesions are less responsive. Larger size may result from an inferior primary response (greater resistance) and more rapid regrowth (greater virulence).

A strategy that permits the earliest possible institution of retreatment is reasonable if *cure* is a possibility, but haste is of very doubtful benefit in a *palliative* setting. Vogel has eloquently argued that reintervention with chemotherapy during an asymptomatic remission "will produce immediate symptoms . . . in the undocumented hope of future gain".[7] Whether benefit accrues to a policy of earlier intervention may be shown by the European Organization for Research on Treatment of Cancer–Medical Research Council (EORTC-MRC) randomized trial involving early versus delayed chemotherapy in patients with raised CA 125 levels and no other evidence of disease. Data on breast cancer suggest it does not.[8]

However, the problem is not so much delay in the diagnosis of failure after primary therapy but rather inadequacy of available secondary therapies. We cannot monitor often enough or accurately enough to detect relapse with more than a minimal lead time in rapidly evolving disease. Ironically, earlier recognition of such treatment-resistant disease increases neither the range nor the effectiveness of treatment opportunities. In conclusion, exhaustive monitoring of patients who have completed primary treatment is unwarranted.

There is no convincing evidence that early introduction of second-line chemotherapy is beneficial, and it just might intrude into the patient's symptom and treatment-free survival.

The practice of rigoris monitoring inappropriately suggests that available second-line therapy is very valuable. As this often is not so, we may create unfulfillable expectations.

Estimating drug resistance

Prognostic factors predict the behavior of disease. They can be used to group patients according to risk and thereby permit more selective treatment. Prognostic factors are not well characterized in the setting of previously treated disease, which is not surprising, as few studies have sufficient patient numbers to allow meaningful multifactorial analysis. With failed disease, patient factors are often more important determinants of outcome than the treatment under investigation.[9] This is shown by Vermorken et al[10] who examined the response rates to several drugs in platin-pretreated ovarian cancer (Table 9-1). The length of the chemotherapy-free interval is confirmed to be a predictor of outcome, but it may not be the best—simply the most examined—reflecting more fundamental factors associated with disease extent, virulence, and resistance. Nonanemic patients with serous tumors of smaller size have better outcomes. It is provocative that the variability of response rates between prognostic categories seems greater than the variability of response rates between different drugs (and from this selected group of agents, no clear "winner" emerges).

Known factors are insufficient to allow the design of individualized care. For the moment, it seems appropriate to separate patients with failed disease into two broad groups according

TABLE 9-1
Response Rates (%) in Phase II Studies of 1,103 Patients with Platin-Pretreated Ovarian Cancer

	HISTOLOGY		ANEMIA		TUMOR SIZE		CHEMOTHERAPY-FREE INTERVAL	
DRUG	*SEROUS*	*OTHER*	*NO*	*YES*	*<5 CM*	*>5 CM*	*<6 MO*	*>6 MO*
Taxol $n = 382$ 66 responses	21	12	21	10	24	21	13	22
Epirubicin $n = 105$ 22 responses	23	17	24	19	23	19	16	29
CPT-111 $n = 55$ 13 responses	32	15						
Gemcitabine $n = 153$ 21 responses			14	7	13	14	11	17
Carboplatin $n = 273$ 52 responses	22	15	22	14	24	15	13	32
Docetaxel $n = 135$ 35 responses	29	22	22	28	21	31	18	38
P value	0.001		0.006		0.019		0.000	

(Modified from Vermorken,[10] with permission.)

to their likelihood of responding to the reuse of a platin analog: *more-resistant disease*, encompassing absolute platin resistance as well as relative platin resistance and *potentially platin sensitive disease* (see Appendix 9-1).

The characteristics of primary treatment may influence resistance. It seems at first glance that disease recurring after treatment with a single platin analog would be less resistant than disease recurring after multiagent treatment. However, "complex," more effective primary treatment might suppress the development of resistance or, alternatively, lead to reduced virulence (growth rate) of persisting disease. If either or both effects are in operation, the likelihood and quality of a secondary response will be improved. That this may be so, and that primary treatment can produce important and persisting effects, are suggested by the results of the Gynecologic Oncology Group (GOG) 111 study,[11] in which the *postfailure* survival of who received Taxol/cisplatin is substantially greater than that of the controls. It remains uncertain what effects primary platin/taxane treatment will have on resistance, or how this might alter our definitions of resistance, but disease relapsing after such a combination may be *less* difficult to retreat.[12]

Treating less-resistant disease

Persisting tumor

A definition of platin resistance based on a nonuniversal pattern of practice (second-look surgery) is problematic. It may not be possible to estimate the responsiveness of disease remaining at the completion of primary treatment. If disease persists that has continued to respond *throughout* primary Taxol/cisplatin for six cycles, we occasionally extend treatment with three additional cycles of carboplatin every four weeks if it proves to be well tolerated, and response improves. The initial carboplatin dose is determined by the Calvert formula [total dos(mg) = AUC (GFR + 25)], employing an AUC of 5 or 6, and adjusting subsequent doses to achieve a platelet nadir of 50 to 100 × 10^9 liter. GFR (glomerular filtration rate) is estimated by a nuclear renogram. Such patients are also candidates for secondary trials looking at ways to improve on the quality of the initial remission.

Relapsing tumor

The treatment of choice in this circumstance includes a platinum analog.[13] In patients with progressive symptomatic disease we usually reintroduce carboplatin as a single agent (dose as outlined in the previous paragraph) to a total of six cycles if an ongoing response is seen. Carboplatin is the preferred agent except in circumstances of allergy to platin compounds, intractable treatment-related nausea, or problematic myelosuppression (particularly thrombocytopenia). The role of surgery should be assessed. We tend not to intervene in the case of asymptomatic or "marker-only" relapse.

HYMAN BERNARD MUSS
EMILY G. ROBINSON

Only 15 to 25% of women with stage III or IV ovarian cancer are likely to be disease-free at 5 years; most ultimately become candidates for salvage treatment.[14,15] Salvage chemotherapy for refractory ovarian cancer remains palliative, and strategies for salvage treatment have recently been reviewed.[16–18] When available, all such patients should be considered for clinical trials. Although few would question the observation that platinum-based chemotherapy has substantially improved the frequency of remission in such individuals, it has added little to improving overall survival.[14] In one meta-analysis that included a group of 670 women treated with platinum based combination chemotherapy, the median survival was about 18 months for all patients. The recent observation that a combination of paclitaxel and cisplatin may improve median survival by about 1 year compared to a combination of cyclophosphamide and cisplatin represents a major improvement in treatment.[11] The majority of patients receiving taxane/platinum regimens eventually still progress, however, and careful selection of salvage therapy remains a crucial decision.

The major determinant relating to the probability of responding to salvage therapy is whether the patient is "platinum resistant".[19] We prefer to employ the definition of "platinum resistance" used by the GOG (Table 9-2). For patients who are not platinum resistant, the likelihood of responding to cisplatin or carboplatin alone or in combinatiois directly related to the length of time between completion of the initial platinum regimen and the time of progression. On average, about 25%, 33% and 60% of patients respond to salvage platinum regimens whose platinum-free interval is 6 to 12 months, 12 to 24 months, and greater than 24 months, respec-

TABLE 9-2
Gynecologic Oncology Group Criteria for Platinum Resistance[a]

1. Disease progression while on a first-line platinum-based regimen
2. Tumor progression within 6 months of completion of platinum-based therapy
3. Persistent clinically measurable disease with best response as stable disease at the *completion of planned* first-line therapy
4. Persistent clinically measurable disease with best response as stable disease with rising CA 125 while receiving first-line nonprotocol therapy. Rise must be documented by *two* CA 125 examinations, the last one being greater than or equal to 100.

[a] *Resistance is defined by* any *of the criteria listed.*

tively.[19,20] This time interval is also related to whether the patient is likely to respond to non-platinum-containing phase II regimens. In one study, the likelihood of responding to a phase II regimen was only 10% in 50 patients who had failed prior chemotherapy (in most cases a platinum regimen) within 6 months, compared to greater than 90% of patients whose treatment-free interval exceeded 18 months.[20] The exception to this rule is paclitaxel, for which the response rates are similar in both platinum-resistant and platinum-sensitive patients.[16]

Salvage chemotherapy after a partial response at second-look surgery

The role of second-look surgery in the management of ovarian cancer has been discussed elsewhere in this volume. Options for salvage therapy in these patients depends on the volume of residual disease at completion of second-look surgery (i.e., whether the size of the largest residual mass exceeds 0.5 cm), the initial volume of disease prior to chemotherapy, and for all treatment decisions, the preferences of the patient. Such women are unlikely to benefit from further systemic platinum-containing chemotherapy and should be considered for other treatment.

Women with minimal residual disease (largest mass $\leq$ 0.5 cm) are the most likely to derive benefit from intraperitoneal chemotherapy[21] or radiotherapy,[22,23] although there is no convincing evidence that these approaches are superior to other routes of systemic therapy. The role of intraperitoneal chemotherapy and radiotherapy in this setting is discussed in detail elsewhere in this volume. Also, such patients are prime candidates for clinical trials of high-dose chemotherapy with bone marrow and/or peripheral blood progenitor(stem) cell (PBPC) support. It is difficult to asses the value of any therapy in this population. First, almost all patients having second-look surgery have normal CA 125 levels prior to surgery. Second, these small lesions are not measurable or evaluable clinically; only disease progression can be detected. Last, the natural history of these patients is not well defined and is likely to be quite variable. Currently, the most effective systemic agent for these women is paclitaxel. At present, there is no evidence that combination regimens are superior to single-agent paclitaxel, and we recommend using paclitaxel as a single agent in this circumstance. The optimal duration and schedule for paclitaxel treatment are yet to be determined, but preliminary evidence from a large randomized trial comparing doses of 135 mg/m^2 and 175 mg/m^2 given over 3 or 24 hours suggests that a dosage of 175 mg/m^2 over 3 hours is as effective as longer, more costly, treatment. Since such patients are not likely to have elevated CA 125 levels or measurable or evaluable disease, the number of courses to administer is problematic. We recommend giving a total of six courses at 3-week intervals, and then stopping therapy and observing the patient for relapse. Some investigators might recommend staging with laparoscopy or third-look surgery for such patients (provided they maintain normal CA 125 levels and have no clinical evidence of disease), but we believe such procedures are not appropriate unless a specific investigational therapy is based on such findings. In addition to paclitaxel, several other agents might be considered in this setting (Table 9-3). As in the case of paclitaxel, we suggest giving these therapies for a finite period of time (six courses) and then observing the patient off treatment.

Salvage chemotherapy for relapse six or more months after primary treatment

Patients who relapse six or more months after primary treatment should be considered for salvage chemotherapy with a platinum-containing regimen. Since recent data suggest that the combination of paclitaxel and cisplatin given as primary treatment increases median survival by about 1 year when compared to standard platinum-containing regimens,[11] paclitaxeand either cisplatin or carboplatin should be considered in this setting.

TABLE 9-3
Salvage Regimens for Patients Refractory to Platinum and Taxanes

AGENT	DOSE AND SCHEDULE	TOXICITY
Hexamethylmelamine	260 mg/m^2 for 14 of 28 days	Nausea, vomiting, neuropathy
Topotecan	1.5 mg/m^2 daily for 5 days every 3 wk	Myelosuppression
5-FU plus leucovorin	200 mg/m^2 leucovorin followed by 370 mg/m^2 of 5-FU daily for 5 consecutive days every 4 or 5 wk, or 20 mg/m^2 of leucovorin followed by 425 mg/m^2 of 5-FU as above every 5 wk	Leukopenia, diarrhea
Ifosfamide	1.0-1, 2 gm/m^2 daily for 5 consecutive days every 3 wk with mesna, or 5 gm/m^2 single dose every 4 wk with mesna	Myelosuppression, central nervous system toxicity, nausea, vomiting, nephrotoxicity
Etoposide	50 mg/m^2 daily for 21 consecutive days every 4 wk	Myelosuppression

The paclitaxel and cisplatin doses used in this trial were 135 mg/m^2 and 75 mg/m^2, respectively,administered every 3 weeks for six courses, with the paclitaxel given before the cisplatin. A substantial body of data suggests that carboplatin is as effective as cisplatin in advanced ovarian cancer,[14] and it would be reasonable to substitute carboplatin for cisplatin in this setting. Also, paclitaxel infusions over 3 hours, together with carboplatin, are preferable for administration in the outpatient setting. The GOG is currently conducting a trial in patients with optimal stage III disease comparing paclitaxel 135 mg/m^2 over 24 hours followed by casplatin 75 mg/m^2, with paclitaxel (175 mg/m^2 over 3 hours) followed by carboplatin (AUC 7.5). This trial will define any major differences between these regimens. For patients who relapse after receiving a taxane/platinum regimen given as first-line therapy, single-agent chemotherapy with a platinum compound is appropriate. There is no convincing evidence that combination regimens are associated with a better outcome in this setting and such regimens are associated with higher costs and an increased risk of toxicity. Again we recommend that patients be treated with a finite number of courses. This entails two additional courses following complete response (as defined by clinical and CA 125 studies) or a maximum of eight courses. Patients who fail to achieve a complete response after eight courses are unlikely to do so and should be considered for a drug holiday or other salvage therapy.

QUESTION 2

What are the options for salvage treatment of a patient with platinum-resistant epithelial ovarian cancer (progression on Taxol/platinum therapy or relapse less than 6 months after completion of primary therapy)? What is your preference for second-line therapy?

KENNETH SWENERTON

Treating more-resistant disease

Patients with *absolute* or *relative resistance* to platin-based chemotherapy have a more dire prognosis and urgent needs. In fact, no agents have been identified that are substantially useful in the setting of absolute platin resistance, even if they have apparently differing mechanisms of antitumor action. Modest changes in dose schedule or the composition of combinations are very unlikely to be helpful. Resistance is not reversed by clinically achievable increases in dose-intensity: McGuire[79] believes that this would require a multifold increase in dose intensity, and Thigpen[80] feels that dose response may be linearly related over a limited range only (for example, Jodrell[81] showed no response rate benefit when the AUC of carboplatin was more than 7) The strategy of high-dose therapy with hematogenous stem cell support has no role here.[69]

Patients with disease resistant to *both* platin analogs *and* Taxol are offered phase II agents in a trial setting. Those with progressive symptomatic disease who are ineligible for or decline trial therapy are offered oral etoposide in a fixed dose of 75 mg daily (50 mg daily alternating with 100 mg daily) for 10 days out of every 21, gradually increasing to 100 mg daily for 14 days if dose-limiting myelosuppression and mucositis are not encountered. Importantly, etoposide has produced responses in individuals previously treated with both platin and Taxol.[24,25] Topotecan has a degree of effectiveness in patients pretreated with Taxol/platin[26–28] and will soon be more widely available.

Women with platin-resistant disease and no prior exposure to taxanes are offered Taxol. Although the overall response rate is modest, a proportion of patients treated with this drug have improvement insufficient to qualify as a response but nonetheless achieve a relief of symptoms that is occasionally durable. The lack of nausea makes Taxol more acceptable than other agents. Collected data[29] suggest that 1- or 3-hour schedules are no less effective than the 24-hour one. In fact, 96-hour infusions are inactive in patients not responding to 3- or 24-hour infusions.[30] A potentially useful dose effect is apparent, but 3-hour schedules using doses of more than 210 mg/m^2 produce prohibitive toxicity. Cytokines "buy"an increased dose of about 20%, but this produces no survival benefit.[31] We therefore employ a dose of 170 to 200 mg/m^2 over 3 hours every three weeks without colony stimulating factors (CSFs), reducing the dose to 135 mg/m^2 in patients who have demonstrated an unusual degree of marrow toxicity with previous treatment. Patients are treated in an ambulatory care facility by staff trained to recognize and manage the occasional hypersensitivity reaction. Active electrocardiogram monitoring is not required inindividuals free of significant cardiac pathology. Premedication including steroids and H1 and H2 blockers is employed. If patients tolerate the first two cycles without hypersensitivity and are troubled by the steroid premedication (e.g., aggravated diabetes, marked restlessness, or insomnia), the doses of steroid may be reduced cautiously. Arthromyalgia may respond to anti-inflammatory medication, and narcotics are occasionally required (or the dose of Taxol can be reduced).

Topotecan may be more active than taxol in patients with platinum-pretreated disease.[32] Although altretamine seems to have little activity in disease that is absolutely platin resistant, it may have some activity in circumstances of relative platin resistance.[33] Navelbine[34] and liposomal doxorubicin[35] may also be useful.

HYMAN BERNARD MUSS
EMILY G. ROBINSON

Salvage treatment for platinum-resistant patients

For platinum-resistant patients who have not received prior taxane therapy, paclitaxel is the treatment of choice for salvage.[36–40] An overall response rate of 25% can be anticipated. Even when used in platinum-refractory patients treated with at least three prior chemotherapy regimens, an overall response rate of 22% (4% complete and 18% partial) was noted in 652 patients receiving 135 mg/m^2 over 24 hours every 3 weeks.[40] In latter trial the median response duration was 4.9 months, the median time to progression 7.2 months, and the median survival 9 months. The major toxicity was a 78% frequency of grade 3 or 4 leukopenia, resulting in 12 patients (1.3%) dying of neutropenic sepsis. It appears prudent to consider growth factor support for patients who have been heavily pretreated, have poor performance status, or are older (age >70 years) during the first course of paclitaxel, with subsequent use based on patient tolerance.

The optimal dose and schedule for paclitaxel are yet to be defined. The GOG has recently completed accrual to a randomized trial comparing paclitaxel doses of 175 mg/m^2 and 250mg/m^2 [plus granulocyte colony stimulating factor (GCSF)] given as 24-hour infusions in patients with platinum-resistant disease. In that study,[31] response rate was higher with 250 mg/m^2 (36% vs 27%) but no significant difference in progression-free or overall survival was noted. Additionally, thrombocytopenia, anemia, gastrointestinal toxicity, neurotoxicity, and myalgia were significantly more common with 250 mg/m^2. Preliminary evidence from a large randomized trial comparing doses of 135 mg/m^2 and 175 mg/m^2 given over 3 or 24 hours suggests that a dosage of 175 mg/m^2 over 3 hours is as effective as longer, more costly, treatment. Moreover, myelosuppression was lower with the 3-hour regimen. At present, we recommend that a dose of 175 mg/m^2 over 3 hours repeated every 3 weeks be used. Shorter infusion durations (1 hour) are well tolerated and probably as effective, but more data are needed.[41] Of interest is the observation that patients refractory to shorter infusions of paclitaxel may respond to infusions of longer duration,[42] and a randomized trial comparing a 3-hour with a 96-hour infusion is now in progress. More recently, docetaxel (Taxotere) has shown activity in ovarian cancer similar to that of paclitaxel (Taxol).[43,44]

Following tumor progression on paclitaxel, patients may beconsidered for therapy with several other agents (Table 9-3). None of these regimens convincingly improves survival, and at best response rates may approach 20%. Treatment selection should be based on patient preferences as well as toxicity.

Only two agents, altretamine and topotecan, have been approved for salvage therapy by the Food and Drug Administration (FDA).[50–53] Altretamine (hexamethylmelamine) is associated with maximum response rates of 10 to 15% in platinum-refractory patients.[45–49] The major toxicity associated with this agent is nausea and vomiting which can be difficult to manage and is compounded by the treatment schedule which requires at least daily dosing for 2 weeks of every 4 week cycle.

Topotecan (Hycamtin) was recently approved by the FDA for salvage therapy in ovarian cancer based on a large study where it was compared to paclitaxel in patients with platinum-resistant disease.[32] Topotecan was administered at 1.5 mg/m^2 daily for 5 days every 3 weeks, and paclitaxel was administered at 175 mg/m^2 over 3 hours every 3 weeks. Patients receiving topotecan had a response rate of 20%, and those receiving paclitaxel a response rate of 13%. Toxicity was primarily hematologic and noncumulative. Nevertheless, it causes suppression of all three lineages and is more easily tolerated when used early in salvage therapy. Major toxicites include nausea, vomiting, peripheral neuropathy, and depression. Another regimen worthy of consideration in this setting is fluorouracil (5-FU) and leucovorin.[50–53] Several doses and schedules have been used, but a five consecutive day regimen using bolus administration of both leucovorin followed b5-FU is preferred. Look and colleagues noted a 17% response ratein platinum-refractory patients using a schedule of leucovorin 200 mg/m^2 followed by 5-FU 370 mg/m^2 daily for five consecutive days every 4 to 5 weeks.[52] Long and others noted a similar response rate using leucovorin 20 mg/m^2 followed by 5-FU 425 mg/m^2 daily for five consecutive days every 5 weeks.[51] The major toxicity of this regimen is grade 4 leukopenia in about one-third of individuals treated and severe diarrhea in about 15%. Overall this regimen is well tolerated by most patients.

Other salvage agents include ifosfamide and oral etoposide. Ifosfamide has been associated with response rates of 10 to 20% in patients with platinum-refractory ovarian cancer.[54–56] Schedules using five consecutive days of ifosfamide with mesna have been used In two trials[54,55] and produced response rates of 10 to 20%. A third trial[56] using a single dose of 5.0 gm/m^2 administered over 24 hours every 4 weeks produced with an 11% response rate. Myelosuppression is the major toxicity, but renal failure, confusion, and other major central nervous system toxicities also occur. Etoposide is given orally with minimal toxicity.[57–59] Two trials utilizing a 50-mg oral daily dose for 21 days of a 28-day period had response rates of 6% and 8% in 18 and 17 patients, respectively,[57,58] while a third trial using 50 mg/m^2 daily with the same schedule had a response rate of 16% in 25 patients.[59] Toxicity was modest and consisted mainly of myelosuppression. A recent study by the GOG using 50 mg/m^2 daily for 21 days led to a response rate of 27% in platinum-resistant disease and 34% in platinum-sensitive disease. Response duration was not reported. Hematologic toxicity was manageable.[25] Further, a study of 100 mg daily for 14 days every 3 weeks led to a response rate of 26% (21% in platinum-sensitive disease)[24] Thus oral, etoposide is a valid salvage therapy.

QUESTION 3

What are the potential salvage settings, if any, for high-dose chemotherapy with either autologous bone marrow transplantation or peripheral stem cell support?

KENNETH SWENERTON

With the agents currently available, there appears to be no role for such procedures in treating patients with failed disease.

HYMAN BERNARD MUSS
EMILY G. ROBINSON

High-dose chemotherapy with autologous cellular support

High-dose chemotherapy with autologous cellular support, including autologous bone marrow transplantation (ABMT) and/or peripheral blood progenitor cell (PBPC) transplantation has been shown to produce high response rates in patients in whom conventional salvage treatment regimens have failed. In one retrospective analysis, both improved response and longer survival of ovarian cancer patients correlated with increased dose intensity of chemotherapy.[60] There is a good rationale for the use of high-dose chemotherapy with autologous cellular support in the treatment of advanced ovarian cancer. First, ovarian cancer is a highly chemosensitive solid tumor with first-line therapy response rates of 70 to 80%.[17] Second, dose-response relationships have been demonstrated for cisplatin[61] and carboplatin,[62] as well as for several other agents active against ovarian cancer.[15,63] Third, ovarian cancer rarely metastasizes to the bone or bone marrow, decreasing the concern regarding marrow contamination. In a retrospective review of distant metastases in 255 patients, 4 patients (1.6%) developed bone metastasis, and only 1 of 18 patients was found to have bone marrow involvement at autopsy.[64] Fourth, cytoreductive surgery can often place patients in a low tumor burden state, which has been shown in other diseases such as lymphoma and leukemia to result in a greater likelihood response following ABMT. Last, the dosage of many active agents in ovarian cancer, such as cyclophosphamide, carboplatin, thiotepa, etoposide, and melphalan, can be significantly escalated in the setting of autologous cellular support.

Results of clinical trials

There have been multiple studies on high-dose chemotherapy with autologous cellular support in the treatment of refractory ovarian cancer (Table 9-4). Although most have small numbers of patients with short follow-up, results have been similar. High-dose chemotherapy has been shown to result in high overall response rates of 70 to 82% in heavily pretreated patients and in patients with disease refractory to conventional dose salvage therapy.[73] However, the duration of response is short, often less than 9 months, and the benefit in terms of overall survival is unclear. The longest response durations have been in patients with platinum-sensitive disease and in those with minimal residual disease at the time of transplant.

Several studies have highlighted the importance of optimal debulking prior to high-dose

TABLE 9-4
Selected Trials of High-Dose Chemotherapy with Autologous Stem Cell Support in Refractory Ovarian Cancer

REFERENCE	REGIMEN	NO. OF EVALUABLE PATIENTS	CR + PR	RR (%)	CR (%)	MEDIAN DURATION OF RESPONSE (MO)	COMMENT
Dauplat[65]	L-PAM	14	NA	NA	NA	NA	33% 3-yr PFS
Mulder[66]	VP16 + CTX	11	6 + 0	55	55	15	5 CR 2 sustained CR at 43 and 75 mo
Broun[67]	CBDCA + IFF	8	5 + 2	88	63	6	All patients relapsed 4–23 mo
Shpall[68]	CTX + TT + IP-CDDP	8	0 + 6[a]	75	0	6	All patients had bulky disease
Stiff[69]	MX + CBDCA + CTX	27	16 + 8	89	59	7	23% 3-yr DFS
Viens[70]	L-PAM	12	4 + 5	75	33	5	Overall actuarial survival 47% at 4.5 yr
Fennelly[71]	CTX + CBDCA	27	5 + 16	78	19	NA	CTX mobilization with PBPC support
Fennelly[72]	CTX + TX + CBDCA	13	5 + 8	100	38	NA	TX/CTX mobilization regimen for PBPC 62% suboptimally debulked disease

Abbreviations: L-PAM, melphalan; VP16, etoposide; CTX, cyclophosphamide; CBDCA, carboplatin; IFF, ifosfamide; TT, thiotepa; IP-CDDP, intraperitoneal cisplatin; MX, mitoxantrone; TX, paclitaxel; CR, complete response; pCR, pathologic complete response; PR, partial response; RR, response rate; DFS, disease-free survival; PFS, progression-free survival; PBPC, peripheral blood progenitor cell; NA, not available.
[a] *Pathologically documented PR (>75% tumor reduction).*

therapy. In a pilot study, Dauplat et al[65] evaluated high-dose melphalan with ABMT in patients with minimal residual disease after a cisplatin-based regimen. Five of 14 patients (37.5%) remained progression-free at a median of 43 months, with an actuarial 3-year survival of 64%. Similarly, Mulder et al[66] reported the use of high-dose etoposide and cyclophosphamide with ABMT in 11 patients with refractory ovarian cancer after standard therapy. Six of eight patients (75%) achieved a complete response, with five pathological complete responses. Only patients with minimal or microscopic disease responded, whereas all three patients with bulky disease did not. The median duration of response was 15 months, and two patients had a sustained complete response at 43 and 75 months.[66]

A GOG pilot study on nine patients with recurrent or refractory ovarian cancer after standard chemotherapy investigated a regimen consisting of high-dose carboplatin and ifosfamide given intravenously for 5 days, followed by ABMT. Of eight patients with evaluable disease, five (63%) achieved a complete response. Four of the five had minimal residual disease (<1 cm). Two patients (25%) who achieved a partial response had bulky disease. However, all patients relapsed with a median duration of remission of 6 months.[67]

Shpall et al,[68] in a phase I trial of high-dose cyclophosphamide, thiotepa, and intraperitoneal cisplatin and ABMT, reported an overall response rate of 75% in patients with advanced ovarian cancer with platinum-resistant progressive disease. All 12 women had gross disease (>1 cm) at the time of transplant, and the median duration of response was 6 months.[68] Viens et al, using a melphalan-based regimen, observed a 75% response rate in patients with persistent disease following cisplatin-based therapy. The duration of response was inversely related to the bulk of residual disease at the time of second-look operation.[70]

Platinum-sensitive disease is also a predictor of response to high-dose therapy. In a phase II trial involving 30 patients treated with mitoxantrone, carboplatin, and cyclophosphamide followed by ABMT, Stiff et al[69] reported an overall response rate of 89%. Twenty patients had platinum-resistant disease, and 22 had bulky residual disease (>1 cm). The platinum-sensitive patients achieved a significantly higher clinical complete response of 88% compared with 47% complete response in platinum-resistant patients. The median survival for all patients was 29 months, and the 3-year disease-free survival was 23%.[69] Similarly, a survey of ABMT centers across the United States, revealed a significantly higher complete response rate in patients with platinum-sensitive disease when compared to platinum-resistant disease (73% and 34%, respectively) (Table 9-5).[74]

The Southwest Oncology Group (SWOG) is currently conducting a randomized phase II trial for patients with residual ovarian cancer following first-line chemotherapy (SWOG 9106). Patients are randomized to one of two high-dose regimens (cyclophosphamide/mitoxantrone/carboplatin or thiotepa/cyclophosphamide, cisplatin) followed by ABMT. The primary goal of this trial is to evaluate the response rate, progression-free survival, overall survival, and toxicity of each regimen.

Although the number of patients in each of these studies is small, the results are consistent. When the data are compiled, over 200 women with advanced-stage ovarian cancer will have received high-dose chemotherapy supported by autologous progenitor cells.[73] In the majority of the studies, the response rate was quite high after a single course of high-dose chemotherapy, however, the responses were usually of short duration.

The inability of chemotherapy to eradicate all tumor is likely a result of drug resistance. Relative drug resistance can be overcome not only by increasing the dose of a chemotherapeutic agent but also by decreasing the time between doses. With repeated doses a greater tumor log kill can possibly be achieved, resulting in more durable responses. Fennelly et al[71] used multiple cycles of high-dose chemotherapy given at short intervals and supported by peripheral blood progenitor cells in 27 patients with ovarian cancer. An overall response rate of 78% was reported, with 5 patients achieving a pathologic complete response.[71] The same investigators, in a recently reported phase I study incorporating escalating-dose paclitaxel into the induction-mobilization regimen, found an overall response rate of 100% in 13 patients. Sixty-two percent of the women enrolled in this study had suboptimally debulked disease. Five patients (38%) achieved a pathologic complete response.[72] Other investigators are currently exploring this strategy, using PBPC to support the delivery of repetitive cycles of chemotherapy.

The majority of studies suggest that high-dose chemotherapy with autologous stem cell support will be most effective in producing high response rates and improved long-term survival in patients with minimal residual disease and in tumors that are still relatively sensitive to cytotoxic therapy. It is clear that pa-

TABLE 9-5
Survey of High-Dose Chemotherapy with Autologous Bone Marrow in Transplant Programs in the United States for Ovarian Cancer

153 patients from 11 ABMT centers
95% treated for relapsed or refractory disease
20 different preparative regimens
71% overall response rate
73% complete response in platinum-sensitive disease
34% complete response in platinum-resistant disease
Median time to progression 6 months
14% disease-free at 1 year

(Adapted from Stiff,[69] with permission.)

tients who have suboptimally debulked disease with ovarian derive little benefit from dose-intensive therapy. Patients with optimally debulked (<1 cm) residual disease, however, may have improved response to dose-intensive therapy, suggesting that both tumor volume and dose intensity are critical. The above findings suggest that trials of high-dose chemotherapy are most appropriate for patients with minimal residual disease following first-line therapy. Only randomized trials are likely to resolve the question of whether increased dose is superior to other salvage treatments. Therefore, this approach can be considered only investigational for patients with refractory disease.

The authors of a recent review of drug resistance markers in ovarian cancer[77] conclude that many mechanisms of resistance are likely to be involved, only some of which are known, but their clinical relevance is unestablished. Resistance modulators are likely to be of most benefit at diagnosis, not later when mechanisms of resistance become multiple and established (unless tests accurately predict treatment failure, saving the cost of ineffective therapy).

Nonetheless, the concept of predictive testing remains attractive and the underlying principles important. What can be done? Mechanisms identified in tissue culture or animals must be explored in patients, where the problems are much more complex.[78]

QUESTION 4

Is there currently any role for chemoresistance assays or molecular markers in the selection of salvage chemotherapy?

KENNETH SWENERTON

Predictive tests

Clinicians are willing to embrace tests with alleged prognostic merit (especially those with a quantitative facade and a biologic rationale) to guide treatment decisions. However, the ultimate worth of such tests is whether or not they contribute to an improved outcome.[75] An obvious example is the usefulness of the estrogen receptor assay to guide treatment of breast cancer. By this measure, techniques such as in vitro chemosensitivity testing, estimating clonogenic tumor growth, genotyping, and so on, cannot yet be recommended for nonstudy use. Durand[76] has shown that the actions of chemotherapeutic agents differ in single-cell versus multicell systems,[76] which questions the utility of any predictive assay based on the in vitro response of tumor cells.

HYMAN BERNARD MUSS
EMILY G. ROBINSON

The role of chemosensitivity testing in patient management

The development of drug resistance is a major clinical problem that limits the overall effectiveness of chemotherapy. Salvage chemotherapy in platinum/taxane-resistant patients typically results in response rates of only 10 to 20%. The choice of chemotherapy is usually based on reported response rates in clinical trials rather than on individualized in vitro sensitivity studies. Clinical trials, however, do not take into account individual patient differences. Chemosensitivity assays have been developed in an attempt to predict clinical responses to therapy, while avoiding unnecessary therapy and its associated costs and toxicity. The ideal chemosensitivity test for clinical use should be one with a high success rate and predictive accuracy. It should also be simple, relatively rapid to perform, and easily standardized.

Five major types of chemosensitivity assays have been studied in ovarian cancer (Table 9-6). The human tumor clonogenic assay (HTCA), one of the most widely studied techniques, evaluates the ability of chemotherapeutic agents to inhibit tumor stem cell prolif-

TABLE 9-6
Major Types of Chemosensitivity Assays in Ovarian Cancer

ASSAY	COMMENT
Human tumor clonogenic assay (HTCA)	Requires tumor cell growth and colony formation Low plating efficiency and evaluability rate
Radiolabeled DNA precursor uptake assay	Requires active DNA/RNA synthesis Low sensitivity
3-[4,5-dimethylthiazol-2-yl]-2,5-diphenyl tetrazolium bromide (MTT) dye reduction assay	Stromal cells may interfere with results
Fluorescent cytoprint assay (FCA)	No separate untreated control
Adenosine triphosphate–cell viability assay (ATP-CVA)	High evaluability rate High sensitivity and specificity Total cell kill assay

eration in agar. It is based on the hypothesis that the cells that proliferate in agar are identical to the stem cells of a given tumor. A major disadvantage of this assay is that only 40 to 70% of tumor samples grow in this system.[82] Several studies have attempted to correlate in vitro chemosensitivity by HTCA with clinical response.[83,84] A prospective study by the SWOG reported a response rate of 28% when patients with refractory ovarian cancer were treated according to HTCA results, compared with 11% in patients treated according to the clinician's choice.[85] However, there was no difference in survival between the two groups (6.25 months vs 7.0 months).

Radiolabeled DNA precursor uptake methods such as the thymidine incorporation assay detect cellular radioactive nucleotide incorporation into DNA after drug exposure. This method measures the effect of cytotoxic drugs only in cells that are actively synthesizing DNA or RNA. Tumors in vivo often have only a small fraction of cells undergoing DNA synthesis, and these tests select a small specific tumor population for evaluation and provide little information regarding the effect of drugs on cells in the resting (G_0/G_1) phase of the cell cycle.[82] One study on 58 patients with stage I through IV ovarian cancer revealed a significantly longer median relapse-free interval in patients with chemosensitive tumors when compared with that in patients with chemoresistant tumors (30.3 months vs 22.6 months, respectively; $P < 0.05$).[86]

The 3-[4,5-dimethylthiazol-2-yl]-2,5-diphenyltetrazolium bromide (MTT) dye reduction assay, used primarily with hematologic malignancies, has also been used with ovarian cancer. After drug exposure, disaggregated tumor cells are pulsed with MTT. Viable cells produce a blue color, and greater color density is associated with a lesser effect of the drug on the cells. A major disadvantage of this assay is that stromal cells, which are often present in solid tumor specimens, may interfere with assay results. Correlation between in vitro results and clinical outcome has been evaluated in several studies.[87,88] In one trial with 37 patients, the survival at 1 year was 89% for those with drug-sensitive tumors compared with 66% for those with drug-resistant tumors, but long-term survival rates were similar.[88]

A number of drug-sensitivity assays use the conversion of nonfluorescent fluorescein monoacetate to fluorescein by nonspecific cell esterases to determine cell survival. The fluorescent cytoprint assay (FCA) measures cytotoxicity by comparing photographs of fluorescent cytoprints before, during, and after drug exposure. Evaluability rates of 73 to 95% have been reported.[89] There are no separate untreated controls, as the cytoprint prior to drug exposure is used as the internal control. It is therefore difficult to determine whether tumor cells are dying in response to drug treatment or because they are not viable in culture.

Particle concentration fluorescence immunoassay technology has been used to develop a unique chemosensitivity assay.[90] Fluorophores pass through cell membranes of viable cells and are hydrolyzed to fluorescent molecules. In a small study of six ovarian cancer cell lines, the assay detected cell lysis in all six after incubation with cisplatin. Advantages of this assay include high plating efficiency, speed, and simplicity. Further studies on human ovarian tumors will help determine the clinical relevance of this technique.

A newer assay, the ATP–cell viability assay (ATP-CVA) measures changes in tumor cell ATP levels after drug exposure. The assay measures light production as cellular ATP interacts with the luciferin/luciferase complex. The level of cellular ATP is one of the most sensitive end points of cell survival because ATP levels decrease immediately with cell death. This is a total cell kill assay rather than a proliferation-inhibition assay like the clonogenic and thymidine incorporation assays. In addition, the assay has been adapted to evaluate radiation effects on ovarian cancer in vitro.[91] The overall evaluability of the ATP-CVA has been reported to be 88%.[92] There is good correlation when compared with in vivo chemosensitivity in tumor-bearing nude mice, suggesting that this method provides an approach approximating a clinical situation.[93] Prospective trials are under way to evaluate whether drugs selected by this assay provide superior outcomes when compared with conventional treatment.

Molecular markers that might predict drug resistance in ovarian cancer are also under investigation. A great deal of research has been undertaken to identify specific mechanisms of drug resistance markers, including steroid receptors, HER-2/*neu*, bcl-2, MDR-1, and glutathione S-transferase. Overexpression of P-glycoprotein has been associated with multidrug resistance in a small series of ovarian cancer patients.[94] Determination of levels of MDR-1 mRNA as a measure of multidrug resistance could be used to identify tumors that may fail to respond to a given regimen and might direct the use of more specific therapy. There are preliminary data on ovarian cancer evaluating MDR-1 expression and paclitaxel resistance. Evaluation of a series of 94 ovarian tumors suggests that prior therapy affects in vitro paclitaxel resistance and MDR-1 expression.[95] An analysis of in vitro paclitaxel response and MDR-1 expression illustrated that MDR-1 overexpression was related to a twofold decrease in paclitaxel activity. Whether this carries over to the clinical setting is yet to be determined.

Clinical attempts have been made to modulate MDR-mediated resistance using calcium channel antagonists. In one small study, eight patients with refractory disease were treated with doxorubicin and infused verapamil.[96] No objective responses occurred, and most patients had some degree of heart block or hypotension. Other MDR modulators are currently under investigation. A cyclosporin derivative, PJC 833, that is not immunosuppressive and blocks multidrug resistance in vitro is currently being evaluated in conjunction with paclitaxel in the treatment of ovarian cancer.

Elevated glutathione levels have also been associated with increased drug resistance to both cisplatin and alkylating agents. Buthionine sulfoximine (BSO) is a compound that inhibits the enzyme involved in thiol production, depleting intracellular glutathione levels. This subsequently leads to enhanced cytotoxicity in ovarian cancer cell lines treated with melphalan or cisplatin.[97] Clinical trials are underway in patients with advanced malignancies to further study this effect. Results of a phase I trial of BSO followed by melphalan show that marked depletion of glutathione levels may be achieved without significant toxicity.[98]

Platinum-DNA adduct levels have been associated with response to chemotherapy. In a small cohort of patients with platinum-resistant ovarian cancer, the adduct level in white blood cell DNA was more closely related to disease response than other previously identified prognostic variables.[99] A GOG trial (GOG 9303) is currently investigating cisplatin-DNA adducts as a predictor of response to platinum-based chemotherapy.

QUESTION 5

At what point in the course of refractory ovarian cancer should one consider (1) investigational therapy and (2) discontinuation of all therapy?

KENNETH SWENERTON

Enrollment of patients in well-designed clinical trials is always to be encouraged and may be the only appropriate option when available treatments will predictably be of no help.

We do not institute secondary chemotherapy in a patient who cannot maintain oral nutrition or who has a substantially impaired performance status, nor do we continue chemotherapy unless the quality of life is improved or stabilized.

HYMAN BERNARD MUSS
EMILY G. ROBINSON

When to consider investigational therapy

In our opinion, investigational therapy is almost always appropriate in the salvage setting. The only major exception is the patient with major symptoms and organ dysfunction who is platinum-resistant but has not had taxane therapy. This type of patient should be treated with a taxane or considered only for investigational therapy that includes a taxane combination regimen, as failure to achieve an immediate response in this setting is likely to result in life-threatening disease. All other patients who have good performance status should be offered the opportunity to participate in clinical trials involving investigational therapy when available.

When should chemotherapy be discontinued?

The decision to discontinue chemotherapy should always rest with the patient, but the guidance of the physician in this situation is always sought. Since salvage therapy is almost always palliative, how such treatment affects the patient's quality of life is of major consideration. For some patients the hope that comes with treatment, even if the chance of a meaningful response is small, far outweighs the risk of toxicity. Slevin has shown that patients are much more likely than their physicians to accept potentially toxic therapy that has only a small chance of success. For other patients, chemotherapy should be declined unless major benefit is likely. Agents such as tamoxifen, which have reported response rates similar to those of other salvage regimens in platinum/taxane-refractory patients are worthy of consideration in this situation.[100] When discontinuing chemotherapy, it is always important to assure the patient that care will be given to ensure maximum comfort and that "there is always something that can be done."

QUESTION 6

Please discuss future directions in this area, including any other major issues, new promising drugs, and so on.

KENNETH SWENERTON

We must strive to identify more efficient trial designs, employing improved response criteria (especially serologic criteria, dropping the prerequisite of measurability). The use of randomized trials should be encouraged to decide *important* issues, employing quality of life and survival end points as well as response end points, enlarging the pool of patients, and thereby increasing the generalizability of results. We suggest that those who are functionally well with a prolonged failure-free survival be considered "new" patients, allowing their enrollment in *primary* treatment studies.

It is important to provide the patient with options, recognizing the reality of differing preferences. For example, trials might be designed to offer both a "higher-risk" and "lower-risk" randomization, as well as the choice of a "nontrial option." The "higher-risk" option could be open to those with a particularly short prognosis; their need for innovative treatment is immediate, whether upon failure or at diagnosis. Trials exploring dose intensification (in all its guises) in patients with resistant disease should be abandoned—they don't work.

Conclusion

The challenges for those treating failed carcinoma of the ovary are great, greater than those faced at diagnosis. Hope lies in the direction of innovative strategies that may activate the "self-destruct" apoptosis sequences in tumor cells.[101,102]

HYMAN BERNARD MUSS
EMILY G. ROBINSON

Future directions

New approaches being evaluated for patients with refractory disease include the use of new chemotherapeutic agents with different mechanisms of action and/or non-cross-resistance with platinum or paclitaxel. Agents currently in phase II clinical trials include the topoisomerase I inhibitors, irinotecan (CPT-11), and aminocamptothecin, as well as vinorelbine doxil and suramin. In addition, studies on paclitaxel dose intensification and identification of more effective paclitaxel-based combination regimens are in progress. Attempts to overcome drug resistance by high-dose chemotherapy with autologous cellular support, or by modulating cellular mechanisms of drug resistance, are also a priority in clinical research.

EDITORS' COMMENTARY

This is a controversial area and, as reflected by these comments from the authors, there are significant differences of opinion as to how such patients should be treated. All authors agree, however, that multiple issues are involved in selecting salvage therapy. First, response to primary therapy has a significant impact on response to subsequent salvage therapy, with patients responding to primary therapy having a significantly greater chance of responding to salvage agents. Second, the treatment-free interval also appears to be important for patients responding to initial therapy. Patients with an interval in excess of 6 months between discontinuation of primary therapy and development of recurrence have better outcomes than those with shorter intervals. Third, patients with poor performance status, comorbid illnesses, and more advanced-stage disease generally do more poorly with salvage treatment. Finally, less easily defined issues such as therapeutic index of the proposed treatment, quality-of-life issues, and patient preference are important. Primary treatment of ovarian cancer is now in transition, with most patients in the United States receiving a taxane/platinum compound as part of primary therapy. Nevertheless, in other countries taxanes may be reserved for salvage therapy and so the type of primary therapy may also be important in the selection of salvage treatment.

Of the numerous specific questions put to our authors, there are several areas of general agreement but many areas where selection of specific therapies differs. In patients with platinum-sensitive persistent disease at second look, Dr. Swenerton administers additional cycles of carboplatin, while Drs. Robinson and Muss consider intraperitoneal therapy or ABMT in women with low-volume disease (to 5 mm) or possibly Taxol if she has not had prior exposure to this agent. To date, randomized studies have not shown a benefit for additional cycles when the agent(s) are the same as used in primary therapy. Additionally, cumulative toxicities often supervene in such situations. This has been particularly true of cisplatin, with peripheral neuropathy, and carboplatin, with thrombocytopenia. Although we agree that intraperitoneal therapy or bone marrow transplantation may be appropriate in selected patients, only a small population of such individuals are eligible, and assessment of response requires long-term follow-up since the volume of disease at the initiation of salvage therapy is, by definition, small. In patients with recurrent disease six or more months after completion of primary therapy, the authors are in agreement that treatment with a platinum analog or potentially a platinum analog with a taxane constitutes appropriate therapy. All authors, however, comment that there are few data supporting the general use of combination therapy in a recurrent disease setting. We agree with this. Dr. Swenerton also rarely treats patients based on elevation of a tumor marker only, and we agree with this in theory, however, it is very difficult to convince most patients that institution of salvage therapy at the time of marker elevation is not in their best interest.

In patients with platinum-resistant ovarian cancer, the authors are in reasonable agreement. Taxol is utilized if the patient has not been exposed to this agent previously. Other agents include oral etoposide, topotecan, Doxil, altretamine, 5-FU, and ifosfamide, or the use of investigational drugs in phase II studies.

Regarding the use of ABMT in a salvage setting, Dr. Swenerton feels that there is no defined role for this modality at the current time, and we agree with this. Drs. Muss and Robinson basically concur with this approach but suggest that clinical trials are urgently needed to compare high-dose chemotherapy and some form of standard salvage chemotherapy. They recommend that such trials be conducted in patients with drug-sensitive, low-volume, persistent disease following primary therapy. We agree with the authors and strongly support the recently activated intergroup study.

With regard to the use of chemoresistance, assays, or molecular markers in the selection of salvage chemotherapy, no author makes specific recommendations. This likely reflects a lack of knowledge about the value of such assays in guiding salvage therapy. Dr. Swenerton feels that this is an area appropriate for investigation, and with this we strongly agree. At the current time many investigators utilize chemoresistance assays to exclude salvage agents to which the patient's tumor demonstrates extreme drug resistance. Nevertheless, there are situations in which patients have responded, albeit it briefly, to drugs falling into the extreme drug resistance category.

The authors agree that investigational therapy is often appropriate in patients with recurrent and refractory ovarian cancer. It is certainly our feeling that any patient with platinum-resistant ovarian cancer should be a candidate for investigational therapy. It seems most appropriate to evaluate investigational agents in patients who have had the smallest amount of previous therapy. This allows utilization of adequate doses with as little toxicity as possible. As to when therapy should be discontinued, all authors agree that multiple factors have an impact on this decision. Importantly, quality of life becomes a major factor. Additionally, patients with dysfunctional bowel secondary to tumor implants, nutritional deprivation, and decreased performance status predict a poor outcome to any therapy, and these patients are appropriate candidates for hospice care.

In regard to future directions there are also a large number of approaches promulgated.

Dr. Swenerton feels that defining additional criteria for response, including quality of life and change in a marker, would generate more patients for clinical trials. He also believes that patients with long treatment-free intervals can be considered "new" patients for primary treatment protocols. We agree with this approach but feel that including such patients in primary treatment protocols would require stratification based on how "new" is defined. Drs. Muss and Robinson feel, as do we, that new agents should continue to be developed and that more appropriate usage of current agents by the use of resistance modulators should be explored.

In any event, recurrent and persistent ovarian cancer will remain a major problem. Well-designed studies in good performance status patients will continue to be a priority, hopefully allowing us to generate better primary therapies. It is important to remember that paclitaxel was originally evaluated in good performance status patients with recurrent ovarian cancer. It was activity of this compound in these patients that led to trials that have now firmly established it as part of primary therapy. It is our hope that other current salvage agents will soon be incorporated into primary therapy, leading to improved quality and quantity of life in these patients.

APPENDIX 9-1

COMMENTS ON TERMINOLOGY

KENNETH SWENERTON

The adoption of accurate terminology has become increasingly important, particularly for terms that can imply sensitivity or resistance of disease to treatment.

Salvage

Implies saving from destruction. Given the prognosis of persistent or relapsed ovarian cancer, a presumptive and misleading descriptive, creating unrealistic expectations.

Refractory

Difficult to manage. A term used inconsistently to describe pretreated disease or to imply an uncertain degree of drug resistance.

Failure

The point in the natural history when either persistent disease first progresses or fully responsive disease first recurs.

The point of failure divides the natural history of disease into two major phases:

Failure-free survival, the interval from diagnosis until failure,

Postfailure survival, the interval from failure until death

Importantly, treatment failure is not synonymous with *resistance* or *refractoriness* to treatment.

Failure-free survival

Equivalent to *progression-free survival* and *relapse-free survival* and preferred to measurements of *remission duration* (which are inconsistently measured from either the start of treatment or the time that remission is first achieved).

The length of failure-free survival may be a useful clinical indicator of drug resistance at retreatment. It avoids the potentially confounding need to assess the quality of the response to prior treatment (this is often not possible, e.g., in patients with initially unevaluable tumors) or the need to rely upon other intervals of variable duration. In one group of patients, no responses to secondary platin treatment were seen when the failure-free survival was less than 24 months, while nearly two-thirds responded when it was longer than 24 months.[103]

Chemotherapy-free interval

The usefulness of the chemotherapy-free interval is confounded by variations in the duration of primary treatment and practices governing the timing of the start of secondary treatment. Despite these shortcomings it is increasingly being used to classify patients into categories of differing resistance to treatment.[104]

A variation of this, the *posttreatment* failure-free interval (from the end of initial treatment until failure) predicts secondary responsiveness. If less than 18 months, 17% respond, and if greater than 18 months, 53% respond.[105]

Platin resistance

Increasingly used are clinical definitions such as these, modified from those proposed by Cannistra[104]:

Absolute platin resistance. Tumors that progress through platin treatment; coincides with *primary resistance.*[106]

Relative platin resistance. Characterized by a initial response to this agent, with a post treatment failure-free interval less than 6 months.

Potentially platin sensitive. With a posttreatment failure-free interval greater than 6 months.

References

1. Swenerton KD: Prognostic indices in ovarian cancer—their significance in treatment planning. Acta Obstet Gynecol Scand 71 S155:67, 1992
2. Rustin GJS, Nelstrop A, McLean P: Definitions for progression of ovarian carcinoma according to serum CA 125 levels, abstract. Int J Gynecol Cancer, suppl 3:58, 1993
3. Isioka S, Sagae S, Terasawa K et al: Serum CA 125 monitoring of ovarian cancer patients during primary therapy. Int J Gynecol J Cancer, suppl. 3:61, 1993
4. van der Burg MEL, Lammes FB, Verweij J: The role of CA 125 in the early diagnosis of progressive disease in ovarian cancer. Ann Oncol 1:301, 1990
5. Lahousen M: Treatment options at relapse. p. 180. In Lawton FG, Neijt JP, Swenerton KD (eds): Epithelial Cancer of the Ovary. BMJ Publishing, London, 1995
6. Neijt JP: New therapy for ovarian cancer. N Eng J Med 334:50, 1996
7. Vogel SE: Ovarian cancer: diagnostic second laparotomy and salvage intraperitoneal chemotherapy fail again. Eur J Cancer 31A:651, 1995
8. Peters WP, Jones RB, Vrendenburgh J et al: A large, prospective, randomized trial of high-dose combination alkylating agents with autologous cellular support as consolidation for patients with metastatic breast cancer achieving complete remission after intensive doxorubicin-based induction therapy, abstract. 18th Annual San Antonio Breast Cancer Symposium, San Antonio, Texas, 1995
9. Beale PJ, Friedlander ML: Prognostic variables in ovarian cancer. p. 96. In Lawton FG, Neijt JP, Swenerton KD (eds): Epithelial Cancer of the Ovary. BMJ Publishing, London, 1995
10. Vermorken JB, Eisenhauer EA, Lu F et al: Prognostic features of importance for phase II studies in platinum-pretreated ovarian cancer patients, abstract. p. 130. Proceedings of the 6th International Congress on Anticancer Treatment, Paris, 1996
11. McGuire WP, Hoskins WJ, Brady MF et al: Cyclophosphamide and cisplatin compared with paclitaxel and cisplatin in patients with stage III and stage IV ovarian cancer. N Eng J Med 334:1, 1996
12. Kavanagh J, Tresukusol D, Edwards C et al: Carboplatin reinduction after taxane in patients with platinum-refractory epithelial ovarian cancer. J Clin Oncol 13:1584, 1995

13. Colombo N, Marzola M, Parma G et al: Paclitaxel versus CAP in recurrent platinum sensitive ovarian cancer: A randomized phase II study, abstract. Proc ASCO 15:279, 1996

14. Advanced Ovarian Cancer Trialists Group Chemotherapy in advanced ovarian cancer: an overview of randomized clinical trials. BMJ 303:884, 1991

15. Torri V, Korn EL, Simon R: Dose intensity analysis for advanced ovarian cancer patients. Br J Cancer 67:190, 1993

16. Thigpen JT, Vance RB, Khansur T: Second-line chemotherapy for recurrent carcinoma of the ovary, review Cancer 71:1559, 1993

17. Christian MC, Trimble EL: Salvage chemotherapy for epithelial ovarian carcinoma, review. Gynecol Oncol 55:S143, 1994

18. Caldas C, Morris LE, McGuire WP III: Salvage therapy in epithelial ovarian. Obstet Gynecol Clin North America 21:179, 1994

19. Markman M, Rothman R, Hakes T et al: Second-line platinum therapy in patients with ovarian cancer previously treated with cisplatin. J Clin Oncol 9:389, 1991

20. Blackledge G, Lawton F, Redman C, Kelly K: Response of patients in phase II studies of chemotherapy in ovarian cancer. implications for patient treatment and the design of phase II trials. Br J Cancer 59:650, 1989

21. Markman M: Second-line chemotherapy for refractory cancer: intraperitoneal chemotherapy, review. Semin Surgi Oncol 10:299, 1994

22. Schray MF, Martinez A, Howes AE et al: Advanced epithelial ovarian cancer: salvage whole abdominal irradiation for patients with recurrent or persistent disease after combination chemotherapy. J Clin Oncol 6:1433, 1988

23. Reddy S, Lee MS, Yordan E et al: Salvage whole abdomen radiation therapy: its role in ovarian cancer. Int J Radiation Oncol Biol Phys 27:879, 1993

24. Hoskins PJ, Swenerton KD: Oral etoposide is active against platinum-resistant epithelial ovarian cancer. J Clin Oncol 12:60, 1994

25. Rose PG, Blessing JA, Mayer AR, Homesley HD: Prolonged oral etoposide as second line therapy for platinum resistant and platinum sensitive ovarian carcinoma: Gynecologic Oncology Group Study, abstract. Proc ASCO 15:282, 1996

26. Gordon A, Bookman M, Malmstrom H et al: Efficacy of topotecan in advanced epithelial ovarian cancer after failure of platinum and paclitaxel: International Topotecan Study Group trial, abstract. Proc ASCO 15:282, 1996

27. ten Bokkel Huinink W, Gore M, Bolis G et al: A phase II trial of topotecan for the treatment of relapsed advanced ovarian carcinoma, abstracted. Proc ASCO 15:284, 1996

28. Hochster H, Speyer J, Wadler C et al: Phase II study of topotecan 21-day infusion in platinum-treated ovarian cancer, abstract. Proc ASCO 15:285, 1996

29. Swenerton KD: The emerging role for paclitaxel in the treatment of ovarian cancer. Indian J Med Paediatr Oncol 15:20, 1994

30. Markman M, Rose P, Kennedy A et al: A phase II study of 96 hour paclitaxel as salvage therapy in ovarian carcinoma, abstract. Proc ASCO 15:283, 1996

31. Omura GA, Brady MF, Delmore JE et al: A randomized trial of paclitaxel at 2 dose levels and filgrastim at 2 doses in platinum pretreated epithelial ovarian cancer (OVCA): a Gynecologic Oncology Group, SWOG, NCCTG and ECOG study, abstract. Proc ASCO 15:280, 1996

32. Carmichael J, Gordon A, Malfetano J et al: Topotecan, a new active drug, vs paclitaxel in advanced epithelia ovarian carcinoma: International Topotecan Study Group trial, abstract. Proc ASCO 15:283, 1996

33. Lee CR, Faulds D: Altretamine: a review of its pharmacodynamic and pharmacokinetic properties, and therapeutic potential in cancer chemotherapy. Drugs 49:932, 1995

34. Burger RA, Burman S, White R, DiSaia PJ: Phase II trial of navelbine in advanced epithelial ovarian cancer, abstract. Proc ASCO 15:286, 1996

35. Muggia F, Hainsworth J, Jeffers S et al: Liposomal doxorubicin is active against refractory ovarian cancer, abstract. Proc ASCO 15:287, 1996

36. Ozols RF: USA update on paclitaxel in ovarian cancer, review. Ann Med 27:127, 1995

37. Swenerton K, Eisenhauer E, Ten Bokkel Huinink W et al: Taxol in relapsed ovarian cancer: high vs low dose and short vs long infusion, abstract. Proc ASCOncol 12:256, 1993

38. Einzig AI: Review of phase II trials of Taxol (paclitaxel) in patients with advanced ovarian cancer, review. Ann Oncol suppl 6, 5:S29, 1994

39. Thigpen JT, Blessing JA, Ball H et al: Phase II trial of paclitaxel in patients with progressive ovarian carcinoma after platinum-based chemotherapy: a Gynecologic Oncology Group study. J Clin Oncol 12:1748, 1994

40. Trimble EL, Adams JD, Vena D et al: Paclitaxel for platinum-refractory ovarian cancer: results from the first 1,000 patients registered to National Cancer Institute Treatment Referral Center 9103. J Clin Oncol 11:2405, 1993

41. Greco FA, Hainsworth JD: One-hour paclitaxel infusion schedules: a phase I/II comparative trial. Semin Oncol 22:118, 1995

42. Chang AY, Boros L, Garrow G, Asbury R: Paclitaxel by 3-hour infusion followed by 96-hour infusion on failure in patients with refractory malignant disease. Semin Oncol 22:124, 1995

43. Piccart MJ, Gore M, Ten Bokkel Huinink W et al: Docetaxel: an active new drug for treatment of advanced epithelial ovarian cancer. J Nat Cancer Inst. 87:676, 1995

44. Francis P, Schneider J, Hann L et al: Phase II trial of docetaxel in patients with platinum-refractory advanced ovarian cancer. J Clin Oncol 12:2301, 1994

45. Rosen GF, Lurain JR, Newton M: Hexamethylmelamine in ovarian cancer after failure of cisplatin-based multiple-agent chemotherapy. Gynecol Oncol 27:173, 1987

46. Stehman FB, Ehrlich CE, Callangan MF: Failure of hexamethylmelamine as salvage therapy in ovarian epithelial adenocarcinoma resistant to combination chemotherapy. Gynecol Oncol 17:189, 1984

47. Manetta A, MacNeill C, Lyter JA et al: Hexamethylmelamine as a single second-line agent in ovarian cancer. Gynecol Oncol 36:93, 1990

48. Vergote I, Himmelmann A, Frankendal B et al: Hexamethylmelamine as second-line therapy in platin-resistant ovarian cancer. Gynecol Oncol 47: 282, 1992

49. Moore DH, Valea F, Crumpler LS, Fowler WC Jr: Hexamethylmelamine/altretamine as second-line therapy for epithelial ovarian carcinoma. Gynecol Oncol 51:109, 1993

50. Reed E, Jacob J, Ozols RF, Young RC, Allegra C: 5-Fluorouracil (5-FU) and leucovorin in platinum-refractory advanced stage ovarian carcinoma. Gynecol Oncol 46:326, 1992

51. Long HJ III, Nelimark RA, Su JQ et al: Phase II evaluation of 5-fluorouracil

and low-dose leucovorin in cisplatin-refractory advanced ovarian carcinoma. Gynecol Oncol 54:180, 1994

52. Look KY, Muss HB, Blessing JA, Morris M: A phase II trial of 5-fluorouracil and high-dose leucovorin in recurrent epithelial ovarian carcinoma: a Gynecologic Oncology Group study. Am J Clin Oncol 18:19, 1995
53. Morgan RJ Jr, Speyer J, Doroshow JH et al: Modulation of 5-fluorouracil with high-dose leucovorin calcium: activity in ovarian cancer and correlation with CA 125 levels. Gynecol Oncol 58:79, 1995
54. Sutton GP, Blessing JA, Homesley HD et al: Phase II trial of ifosfamide and mesna in advanced ovarian carcinoma: a Gynecologic Oncology Group study. Clin Oncol 7:1672, 1989
55. Eckhardt S, Hernadi Z, Thurzo L et al: Phase II clinical evaluation of etoposide (VP-16-213, Vepesid) as a second-line treatment in ovarian cancer: results of the South-East European Oncology Group (SEEOG) study Oncology 47:289, 1990
56. Sorensen P, Pfeiffer P, Bertelsen K: A phase 2 trial of ifosfamide/mesna as salvage therapy in patients with ovarian cancer refractory to or relapsing after prior platinum-containing chemotherapy. Gynecol Oncol 56:75, 1995
57. Markman M, Hakes T, Reichman B et al: Phase 2 trial of chronic low-dose oral etoposide as salvage therapy of platinum-refractory ovarian cancer. J Cancer Res Clin Oncol 119:55, 1992
58. Marzola M, Zucchetti M, Colombo N et al: Low-dose oral etoposide in epithelial cancer of the ovary. Ann Oncol 4:517, 1993
59. de Wit R, van der Burg ME, van den Gaast A et al: Phase II study of prolonged oral etoposide in patients with ovarian cancer refractory to or relapsing within 12 months after platinum-containing chemotherapy. Ann Oncol 5:656, 1994
60. Levin L, Hryniuk WM: Dose intensity analysis of chemotherapy regimens in ovarian carcinoma. J Clin Oncol 5:756, 1987
61. Ozols RF, Ostchega Y, Myers CE, Young RC: High-dose cisplatin in hypertonic saline in refractory ovarian cancer. J Clin Oncol 3:1246, 1985
62. Ozols RF, Ostchega Y, Curt G, Young RC: High-dose carboplatin in refractory ovarian cancer patients. J Clin Oncol 5:197, 1987
63. Kohn EC, Sarosy G, Bicher A et al: Dose-intense Taxol: high response rate in patients with platinum-resistant recurrent ovarian cancer. J Nat Cancer Inst 86:18, 1994
64. Dauplat J, Hacker NF, Nieberg RK et al: Distant metastases in epithelial ovarian cancer. Cancer 60:1561, 1987
65. Dauplat J, Legros M, Condat P et al: High-dose melphalan and autologous bone marrow support for treatment of ovarian carcinoma with positive second-look operation. Gynecol Oncol 34:294, 1989
66. Mulder PO, Willemse PH, Aalders JG et al: High-dose chemotherapy with autologous bone marrow transplantation in patients with refractory ovarian cancer. Eur J Cancer Clin Oncol 25:645, 1989
67. Broun ER, Belinson JL, Berek JS et al: Salvage therapy for recurrent and refractory ovarian cancer with high-dose chemotherapy and autologous bone marrow support: a Gynecologic Oncology Group pilot study. Gynecol Oncol 54:142, 1994
68. Shpall EJ, Clarke-Pearson D, Soper JT et al: High-dose alkylating agent chemotherapy with autologous bone marrow support in patients with stage III/IV epithelial ovarian cancer. Gynecol Oncol 38:386, 1990

69. Stiff P, Bayer R, Camarda M et al: A phase II trial of high-dose mitoxantrone, carboplatin and cyclophosphamide with autologous bone marrow rescue for recurrent epithelial ovarian carcinoma: analysis of risk factors for clinical outcome. Gynecol Oncol 57:278, 1995
70. Viens P, Maraninchi D, Legros M et al: High dose melphalan and autologous marrow rescue in advanced epithelial ovarian carcinomas: a retrospective analysis of 35 patients treated in France. Bone Marrow Transplant 5:227, 1990
71. Fennelly D, Wasserheit C, Schneider J et al: Simultaneous dose escalation and schedule intensification of carboplatin-based chemotherapy using peripheral blood progenitor cells and filgrastim: a phase I trial. Cancer Res 54:6137, 1994
72. Fennelly D, Schneider J, Spriggs D et al: Dose escalation of paclitaxel with high-dose cyclophosphamide, with analysis of progenitor-cell mobilization and hematologic support of advanced ovarian cancer patients receiving rapidly sequenced high-dose carboplatin/cyclophosphamide courses. J Clin Oncol 13:1160, 1995
73. Shpall EJ, Jones RB, Bearman SI, Purdy MP: Future strategies for the treatment of advanced epithelial ovarian cancer using high-dose chemotherapy and autologous bone marrow support. Gynecol Oncol 54:357, 1994
74. Stiff P, Antman K, Brown ER et al: Bone marrow transplantation for ovarian carcinoma in the US: a survey of active programs, review Proceedings of the 6th International Autologous Bone Marrow Transplant Symposium, 1992
75. Cannistra SA: Why should the clonogenic cell assay be prognostically important in ovarian cancer? J Clin Oncol 9:368, 1991
76. Durand RE: Contributions of flow cytometry to studies with multicell spheroids. Methods Cell Biol 42:405, 1994
77. van der Zee AGJ, Hollema HH, de Bruijn HWA et al: Cell biological markers of drug resistance in ovarian carcinoma. Gynecol Oncol 58:165, 1995
78. Olive PL, Banath JP, Durand RE: Detection of subpopulations resistant to DNA damaging agents in spheroids and murine tumors. Mutat Res 375:157, 1997
79. McGuire WP, Hoskins WJ, Brady MF et al: Assessment of dose-intensive therapy in suboptimally debulked ovarian cancer: a Gynecologic Oncology Group study. J Clin Oncol 13:1589, 1995
80. Thigpen T: High-dose chemotherapy with autologous bone marrow support in ovarian carcinoma: the bottom line, more or less. Gynecol Oncol 57:275, 1995
81. Jodrell DI, Egorin MJ, Canetta RM et al: Relationships between carboplatin exposure and tumor response and toxicity in patients with ovarian cancer. J Clin Oncol 10:520, 1992
82. Sevin BU, Perras JP, Averette HE et al: Chemosensitivity testing in ovarian cancer, review. Cancer 71:1613, 1993
83. Federico M, Alberts DS, Garcia DJ et al: In vitro drug testing of ovarian cancer using the human tumor colony-forming assay: comparison of in vitro response and clinical outcome. Gynecol Oncol 55:S156, 1994
84. Carenza L, Villani C, Rulli G et al: Ovarian cancer: relationship between in vitro chemosensitivity and clinical response. Gynecol Oncol 36:13, 1990
85. Von Hoff DD, Kronmal R, Salmon SE et al: A Southwest Oncology Group study on the use of a human tumor cloning assay for predicting response

in patients with ovarian cancer. Cancer 67:20, 1991

86. Auner H, Petru E, Hofmann HM et al: In vitro chemosensitivity testing in the treatment of ovarian carcinoma. Arch Gynecol Obstet 246:227, 1989
87. Wilson JK, Sargent JM, Elgie AW et al: A feasibility study of the MTT assay for chemosensitivity testing in ovarian malignancy. Br J Cancer 62:189, 1990
88. Sargent J, Elgie A, Taylor CG et al: The identification of drug resistance in ovarian cancer and breast cancer: application of the MTT assay. Contrib Gynecol Obstet 19:64, 1994
89. Meitner PA: The fluorescent cytoprint assay: a new approach to in vitro chemosensitivity testing. Oncology 5:75, 1991
90. Fanning J, Chapman L, Meyers W, Hilgers RD: Particle concentration fluorescence immunoassay chemosensitivity assay for human epithelial ovarian cancer. Obstet Gynecol 84:314, 1994
91. Rodriguez M, Steren AJ: Application of the ATP-cell viability assay for assessment of in vitro radiation treatment response in gynecologic cancer cell lines. Contrib Gynecol Obstet 19: 156, 1994
92. Sevin BU, Perras JP, Kochli OR: Current status and future directions of chemosensitivity testing. p. 179. In: Kochli OR, Sevin BU, Haller U (eds): Chemosensitivity testing in gynecologic malignancies and breast cancer. Karger, Basel, 1994.
93. Perras JP, Hurst J: In vivo/in vitro correlation of xenografts in nude mice and the ATP-cell viability assay. Contrib Gynecol Obstet 19:122, 1994
94. Bell DR, Gerlach JH, Kartner N et al: Detection of P-glycoprotein in ovarian cancer: a molecular marker associated with multidrug resistance. J Clin Oncol 3:311, 1985
95. Fruehauf JP, Manetta A: Use of the extreme drug resistance assay to evaluate mechanisms of resistance in ovarian cancer: Taxol resistance and MDR-1 expression. Contrib Gynecol Obstet 19:39, 1994
96. Ozols RF, Cunnion RE, Klecker RW Jr et al: Verapamil and Adriamycin in the treatment of drug-resistant ovarian cancer patients. J Clin Oncol 5:641, 1987
97. Fojo A, Hamilton TC, Young RC, Ozols RF: Multidrug resistance in ovarian cancer, review, Cancer 60: 2075, 1987
98. O'Dwyer PJ, Hamilton TC, LaCreta FP et al: Phase I trial of buthionine sulfoximine in combination with melphalan in patients with cancer. J Clin Oncol 14:249, 1996
99. Reed E, Ostchega Y, Steinberg SM et al: Evaluation of platinum-DNA adduct levels relative to known prognostic variables in a cohort of ovarian cancer patients. Cancer Res 50:2256, 1990
100. Hatch KD, Beecham JB, Blessing JA, Creasman WT: Responsiveness of patients with advanced ovarian carcinoma to tamoxifen: a Gynecologic Oncology Group study of second-line therapy in 105 patients. Cancer 68:269, 1991
101. Lowe SW, Ruley HE, Jacks T, Housman DE: p53-dependent apoptosis modulates the cytotoxicity of anticancer agents. Cell 74:957, 1993
102. Martin SJ, Green DR: Apoptosis and cancer: the failure of controls on cell death and cell survival. Artical Rev Oncol Hematol 18:137, 1995
103. Hoskins PJ, O'Reilly SE, Swenerton KD: The "failure-free interval" defines the likelihood of resistance in patients with advanced epithelial ovarian cancer previously treated with cisplatin: relevance to therapy and new drug testing. Int J Gynecol Cancer 1:205, 1991
104. Cannistra SA: Paclitaxel in ovarian cancer: how can we make it better? J Clin Oncol 12:1743, 1994

105. Gore ME, Fryatt I, Wiltshaw E, Dawson T: Treatment of relapsed carcinoma of the ovary with cisplatin or carboplatin following initial treatment with these compounds. Gynecol Oncol 36:207, 1990

106. Markman M, Hakes T, Reichman B et al: Ifosfamide and mesna in previously treated advanced epithelial ovarian cancer: activity in platinum-resistant disease. J Clin Oncol 10:243, 1992

CHAPTER 10

MANAGEMENT OF BORDERLINE TUMORS OF THE OVARY

Edward L. Trimble
Janne Kaern
Claes Tropé

EDITORS' INTRODUCTION

Although borderline tumors of the ovary were first described almost 70 years ago, it has been only about 25 years since this group of tumors was first recognized officially by international sanctioning organizations. Furthermore, only within the last decade have we begun to fully appreciate their natural history and biologic behavior.

Borderline tumors represent approximately 10 to 15% of all epithelial ovarian malignancies. In contradistinction to invasive epithelial tumors, most borderline tumors are confined to the ovary(ies) (stage I). Currently, controversy exists regarding the classification of these tumors. Because the prognosis of stage I serous borderline tumors is excellent, with 5-year survival rates of almost 100%, some experts are advocating that this subset be classified as benign. But this concept has met with stiff resistance from the gynecology and pathology communities (see Ch. 20).

Although the standard treatment for older patients is abdominal hysterectomy and bilateral salpingo-oophorectomy, many young patients who have not completed childbearing can be safely treated with unilateral salpingo-oophorectomy coupled with comprehensive surgical staging, thereby preserving fertility potential. Even ovarian cystectomy has been reported, but the recurrence rate in the ovary approximates 15%. Despite the fact that experts have recommended comprehensive surgical staging for several years, most patients referred to university or comprehensive cancer centers after primary surgery have had incomplete surgery.

Another major controversy associated with these tumors is the clinical management of patients with advanced-stage disease or peritoneal implants. Many experts strongly believe that surgery is the only effective treatment for borderline tumors. Others routinely employ postoperative chemotherapy for at least some subsets of patients with peritoneal implants. Currently, insufficient information is available to make a definitive statement regarding the efficacy of postoperative therapy. Nevertheless, clinicians are faced with the difficult task of making treatment recommendations to anxious patients.

Over the past few years, there has been increasing interest in the pathogenesis of borderline tumors of the ovary. Several investigators have focused on DNA ploidy as a predictor of recurrence and survival, but the findings are conflicting. Early studies suggest that p53 mutation does not appear to play a role in the pathogenesis of these tumors. Studies on other molecular markers have not yet uncovered a reliable predictor of biologic behavior. However, it is hoped that future studies of the genetics and molecular biology of these tumors will lead to useful laboratory tests.

QUESTIONS

1. What are the management options for a patient referred after surgery for an ovarian borderline tumor seemingly confined to the ovary, but without surgical staging or appendectomy? What is your recommendation?
2. What is the role, if any, of postoperative therapy in the treatment of patients with advanced-stage borderline tumors? Are prospective randomized clinical trials recommended?
3. What is the role, if any, of secondary cytoreductive surgery in the management of recurrent borderline tumors?
4. Are there any laboratory or molecular markers that may assist in the management of borderline tumors?
5. What are the future directions in this area?

QUESTION 1

What are the management options for a patient referred after surgery for an ovarian borderline tumor seemingly confined to the ovary, but without surgical staging or appendectomy? What is your recommendation?

EDWARD L. TRIMBLE

Before management options for this scenario can be outlined, the clinician must make every effort to gather additional data. Not only is it unreliable to diagnose an ovarian tumor as borderline on frozen section, but the accuracy of the final diagnosis depends in part on the adequacy of tissue sampling.[1,2] The clinician may need to work with the pathologist at the primary hospital to make sure that this is accomplished. In addition, the diagnosis of an ovarian tumor as borderline or of low malignant potential should be confirmed by a pathologist who is familiar with this entity and in whom the clinician has confidence. Ideally, the pathologist and clinician should review the histologic slides together.[3,4]

The clinician should also work to define the extent of abdominal exploration performed at initial surgery. A review of the operative note may indicate whether the diaphragms were visualized, whether the liver, gallbladder, spleen, stomach, and large and small bowel were palpated, and whether the uterus and contralateral adnexa were evaluated. Discussion of the operative findings with the surgeon who performed the initial operation may also be helpful. The size and location of the scars on the patient's abdomen may also shed light on the extent of visualization possible at initial surgery.

The purpose of these inquiries is to establish whether the tumor really is borderline, a diagnosis that generally conveys a benign prognosis, as well as to determine the stage of the tumor. Other diagnoses that convey a worse prognosis, such as ovarian carcinoma and primary peritoneal carcinoma, should be excluded. In most cases, patients who undergo surgical resection of a borderline ovarian tumor experience the same mortality as their age-matched peers without ovarian disease. Some patients experience tumor recurrence, almost entirely confined to the abdominal cavity. The risk of tumor progression, although small, is greater in patients with more advanced-stage disease. A large prospective study of patients with stage I disease who received no adjuvant therapy after surgical staging and resection has recently been published by the Gynecologic Oncology Group (GOG).[5] Of the 146 study patients, none developed recurrent disease, with a mean follow-up interval of 45.7 months. This finding is consistent with other prospective and retrospective studies. In Kurman and Trimble's meta-analysis of 22 series, totaling 953 patients with serous borderline tumors, survival was 99% for patients with stage I disease and 92% for patients with advanced-stage disease, with a mean follow-up of 7 years.[6] Reporting a large retrospective series from the Norwegian Radium Hospital (NRH), Aure et al[7] noted 95% 10-year survival and 80% 20-year survival for patients with mucinous borderline tumors. One subset of patients, those with mucinous borderline tumors with pseudomyxoma peritonei, are at high risk of tumor progression and death. When these women are excluded, survival for patients with borderline mucinous tumors is comparable to that observed in those with serous borderline tumors.

Management options for the patient in the clinical scenario described include (1) observation; (2) surgical staging with preservation of the contralateral ovary, tube, and uterus; and (3) surgical staging with total hysterectomy and bilateral salpingo-oophorectomy.

Surgical staging should be conducted in accordance with FIGO guidelines, including four quadrant cytologic washings; pelvic and para-aortic lymph node sampling; partial omentectomy; biopsies of any suspicious lesions in the pelvis or abdomen; and random biopsies from both abdominal gutters, anterior and posterior cul-de-sacs, pelvic sidewalls, and right diaphragm.[8] Patients with mucinous borderline tumors should also undergo an appendectomy. Issues that may influence the choice among the three options outlined include the histologic cell type of the tumor, the patient's interest in future fertility, and her options for hormone replacement therapy.

More than 95% of borderline tumors are serous or mucinous, and we have the most information about the clinical behavior of these two subtypes. Less is known about endometrioid, clear-cell, and Brenner borderline tumors.[3] Of 468 patients with serous borderline tumors in 10 retrospective studies, 65% had stage I disease, 14% stage II, 20% stage III, and 1% stage IV. For mucinous tumors, the distribution for 236 patients in eight studies was 89% stage I, 1% stage II, 9% stage III, and 0.4% stage IV.[9] Mucinous tumors grossly confined to one ovary are therefore probably unlikely to be upstaged at a restaging procedure. In the event of evidence of extraovarian disease, complete surgical staging and appendectomy are indicated. Several recent reports suggest that mucinous tumors with abdominal spread may arise in the appendix, or simultaneously in the appendix and in one or both ovaries.[10–13] Patients with serous borderline tumors are more likely to be upstaged at a second procedure. It may be reasonable to offer a staging operation patient with a serous borderline tumor grossly confined to the ovary, particularly if the first surgery failed to provide a thorough evaluation of the upper abdomen and pelvis. When the patient has had a thorough evaluation, however, with no abnormalities appreciated, tumor grossly confined to one ovary, and a desire to preserve fertility, observation alone is a reasonable option.

The recent GOG report suggests that retention of reproductive tissue, including uterus, tubes, and contralateral ovary, is safe.[5] There have been reports of patients who underwent conservative surgery initially and were later found to have persistent or recurrent disease on subsequent hysterectomy.[3] In almost all cases, however, the disease was not symptomatic. In the limited reports available, therefore, diagnosis of a borderline tumor in pregnancy or pregnancy subsequent to the diagnosis does not appear to increase the risk of recurrent progressive disease.

The patient's need for estrogen replacement therapy must also be considered. Mean age at diagnosis for these tumors ranges from 40 to 45 years.[3] Bilateral oophorectomy may place a young patient in need of estrogen replacement therapy for many years. Compliance rates for such regimens have been estimated at 50%.[14] In addition, a personal or family history of breast cancer may preclude estrogen replacement therapy. Bilateral oophorectomy in a patient unwilling or unable to take estrogen replacement therapy may substantially increase her risk of osteoporosis, heart disease, and sexual dysfunction.

Surgical staging should be performed if evaluation of the abdomen or pelvis, has not been adequate, with the reservations discussed above. Several studies have documented borderline disease in retroperitoneal lymph nodes.[15–17] In some cases, this may represent endosalpingiosis rather than metastatic disease. Lymph node involvement does not appear to convey a worse prognosis. Total hysterectomy and bilateral salpingo-oophorectomy should be performed if the patient desires definitive surgical therapy for her disease.

JANNE KAERN
CLAES TROPÉ

Recommended standard primary surgery for borderline ovarian tumor patients follows the guidelines for invasive ovarian carcinomas: total abdominal hysterectomy, bilateral salpingo-oophorectomy, omentectomy, peritoneal washing, multiple biopsies (including pelvic and periaortic lymph node sampling), and tumor debulking. For mucinous tumors, appendectomy is recommended. Removal of potential tumor-infiltrated organs is important. In advanced stages, tumor debulking surgery has been performed, but lymph node sampling has not been part of the standard procedure.

Limited surgery with preservation of fertility has been performed in young fertile women with early-stage disease. The surgical approach is now directed toward less aggressive surgery in early-stage tumors, assuming a proper staging procedure. Unfortunately, frozen-section diagnosis is not always accurate. Frozen sections may be useful for discrimination between borderline ovarian tumor–ovarian carcinoma and benign tumor but not for discrimination between borderline ovarian tumor and ovarian carcinoma.[18]

Generally accepted parameters affecting recurrence and survival include extent of residual disease after primary surgery, FIGO stage, histologic type, and age. The only reports including more than 100 patients are those by Russell and Merkur[19] (n = 144), Bostwick et al[20] (n = 109) and Kaern et al[21] (n = 370). The only disagreements among these three studies are that serous tumors were more common than mucinous tumors in the study by Bostwick et al[20] compared to those by Russel and Merkur[19] and Kaern et al[21] 67%, 49%, and 47% serous tumors, respectively. In all three studies, 15 to 20% had stage II to III disease, but none of those with mucinous tumors in the study by Bostwick et al[20] had advanced disease. In the retrospective Norwegian Radium Hospital (NRH) study,[21] 370 borderline ovarian tumors were treated between 1970 and 1982. Follow-up was complete, with a median follow-up time of 152.5 months (range 6.5 to 354.6 months). By multivariate analysis, the independent prognostic factors for disease-free and long-term survival were FIGO stage (Fig. 10-1A), histologic type (Fig. 10-2A), and age. Serous (n = 174) and mucinous (n = 178) tumors were found with equal frequency. Eighteen tumors were non-serous-mucinous types: eight mixed, seven endometrioid, two clear cell, and one unclassified. Most patients had stage I disease (n = 311, 89%), and only 11% (n = 59) had advanced disease (20 stage II, 39 stage III). After primary surgery, only six patients had residual disease. Four of these relapsed within 7 to 35 months and survived a median of 44 months. By univariate analysis, histologic type, FIGO stage, presence of residual tumor, surgical procedure, tumor growth on ovarian surfaces and pseudomyxoma peritonei had a prognostic impact on survival. Age was significant only for long-term survival.

Grade of atypia was not significant. Within the group of 364 tumor-free patients, the extent of surgery and addition of adjuvant treat-

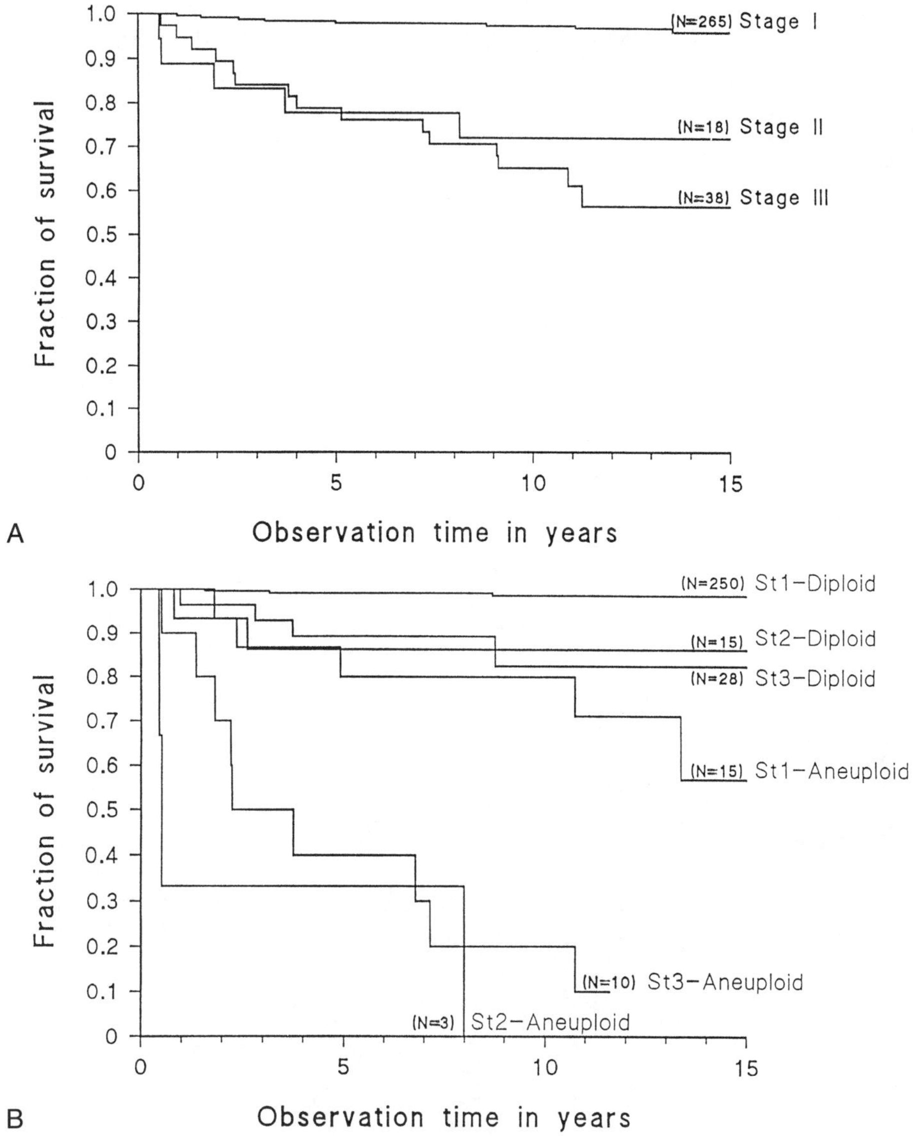

FIGURE 10–1. Borderline ovarian tumors 1970–1982: (A) 15 years corrected survival in relation to stage; (B) Corrected survival in relation to stage and ploidy.

ment had no influence on disease-free and long-term survival. In the tumor-free operated group, 287 patients had undergone hysterectomy, bilaterall salpingo-oophorectomy, and omentectomy; 77 patients had less extended surgery. Concerning adjuvant treatment, 87 of the 364 patients had no postoperative treatment. Of these, 85 had stage I disease. Adjuvant treatment consisted of radiotherapy or chemotherapy or a combination of these two treatment modalities. Within stage I patients (n = 311), there were no survival differences between the different treatment arms and no difference between the treated and untreated (n = 85) patients. From this study, we were able to identify risk groups. The low-low risk group (100% disease-free survival) was characterized by stage I disease, serous tumor, and age below 40 years. The high-risk group (75% or higher risk of dying of disease)

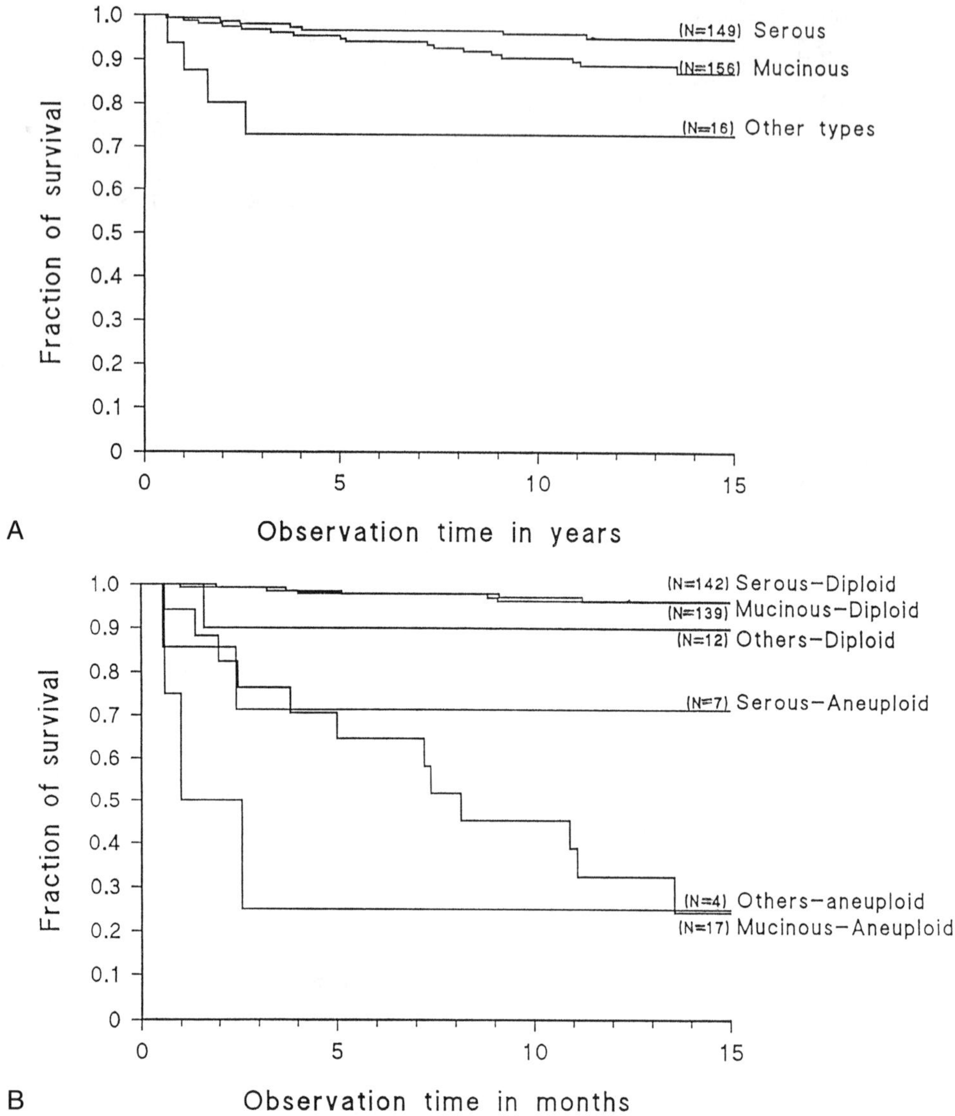

FIGURE 10-2. Borderline ovarian tumors 1970–1982: (A) 15 years corrected survival in relation to histologic type; (B) 15 years corrected survival in relation to ploidy and histologic type.

had serous or mucinous tumor, stage II or III disease, and age above 70 years or had non serous-mucinous tumor and stage II or III disease, independent of age.

Correct staging of borderline ovarian tumor follows the same principles used for ovarian carcinoma and is based on the findings at primary laparotomy. The accuracy of the first exploratory surgery varies a great deal. Thus, many tumors could be understaged. The degree of understaging is unknown. Few reports on borderline tumors give information about lymph node status and whether peritoneal washing and diaphragmatic biopsy have been done.[15,21] In serous tumors, the reported lymph node involvement is about 20% in apparent stage I tumors and even higher in more advanced stages.[15] By contrast, retroperitoneal lymph node involvement has not been reported in mucinous tumors. However, lymph node status does not seem to have a significant effect on survival. In the NRH study,[21] none of the patients with serous stage I tumors (n = 148) died of disease. None of these tumors had been properly staged, as lymph node biopsies had not been performed. Furthermore, none of the patients with recurrent disease had lymph node metastasis.

Patients with borderline ovarian tumor seemingly confined to the ovary have excellent survival (95%), even without proper staging. Conservative surgery is safe in young women with early-stage disease under conditions of careful staging with thorough exploration of the abdomen. In the NRH study,[21,22] no omentectomy was performed in 5 of 20 patients classified as stage II, and 3 of these patients relapsed (all three were DNA aneuploid). Careful inspection of a macroscopic normal contralateral ovary should be sufficient in young women with stage I disease who wish to remain fertile. As wedge biopsy could lead to reduced fertility, this approach should be avoided. The risk of bilaterality is about 5%. In the NRH study,[21,22] only 4 of 51 patients with stage IB tumors did not have macroscopic disease in both ovaries, and none of these stage IB patients relapsed. The frequency of persistence or recurrence in 35 patients with serous borderline ovarian tumor treated by unilateral cystectomy, bilateral cystectomy, or unilateral cystectomy with contralateral oophorectomy or salpingo-oophorectomy were retrospectively investigated by Lim-Tan et al.[23] Conservative surgical treatment was performed either because the patient was young and wanted to preserve her fertility or because the nature of the tumor was not determined at the time of surgery. Thirty-three had stage I disease (19 stage IA, 10 stage IB, and 4 stage Ic), and two had stage III disease. Four patients with stage I (2 stage IA, 1 stage IB and 1 stage IC) tumors and both patients with stage III tumors had persistent or recurrent disease. Almost three-fifths of patients had additional and, in some cases definitive, operations within relative short periods after initial cystectomy or cystectomies but 21 had conservation of ovarian tissue and were followed on average for 7.5 years. All stage I patients are alive without evidence of disease after surgical treatment alone. Both stage III patients were treated with second-look relaparotomy and cisplatin combination chemotherapy and were alive 4 years later. The presence of persistent or recurrent disease correlated with multiplicity and involvement of resection margins. Multifocality may be a strong predictor of failure of cystectomy to control the disease. No recurrence of disease was seen in ovaries from which a single cyst with negative resection margins had been removed. Generous sampling of the resection margins of ovarian cysts is very important. To allow conservative surgery, careful evaluation of the extent of disease by the gynecologist at the time of operation and meticulous examination of the cystectomy specimen by the gynecologist and pathologist are desirable to determine the prognosis after cystectomy. Eight of the 16 stage I patients treated with conservation of ovarian tissue subsequently had normal pregnancies; another three chose not to become pregnant.

More individualized treatment will be possible through the use of modern prognostic parameters. Conservative surgery is justifiable for some patients with a good prognostic index. Unilateral oophorectomy and omentectomy in stage I mucinous tumors are indicated in young women who wish to preserve fertility. In stage I serous tumors, the same procedure is safe if the contralateral ovary is macroscopically normal. The recurrence rate for conservatively operated stage IA patients is reportedly 0 to 30%.[21,24–26] Survival is not affected if the patient again undergoes surgery at recurrence. The corresponding recurrence rate is below 5% for patients with borderline serous tumors who have received treatment.[23,27] Conservatively treated patients need close follow-up.

QUESTION 2

What is the role, if any, of postoperative therapy in the treatment of patients with advanced-stage borderline tumors? Are prospective

randomized clinical trials recommended?

EDWARD L. TRIMBLE

There is no role for postoperative therapy in the treatment patients with advanced stage borderline tumors, as the recent National Institutes of Health (NIH) Consensus Conference on Ovarian Cancer has concluded.[28] Few randomized prospective trials of postoperative adjuvant therapy for this patient population have been reported. Thirty-two patients with stage III optimally debulked borderline tumors were included in the GOG trial of cisplatin/cyclophosphamide with or without doxorubicin.[29] After a median follow-up up of 32 months, 31 were alive and free of disease. The remaining patient died of sepsis after developing bone marrow failure following chemotherapy and radiotherapy. The GOG concluded that the role of chemotherapy in treating this patient population is unclear. Four retrospective institutional reports from Yale University, the University of Texas M.D. Anderson Cancer Center, Massachusetts General Hospital, and the NRH, which included a total of 712 patients, were unable to identify a survival benefit associated with adjuvant therapy, whether chemotherapy or radiotherapy.[21,26,30,31] The meta-analysis conducted by Kurman and Trimble[6] of 953 patients with serous borderline tumors found that more patients died of treatment-related complications (12) than of progressive disease (8). Current oncologic practice might be able to avoid such a complication rate with the abandonment of intraperitoneal ^{32}P and the substitution of cisplatin or carboplatin/paclitaxel for melphalan. Investigators at Memorial Sloan–Kettering Cancer Center have reported success in surgically documenting responses to chemotherapy in patients with advanced borderline tumors.[32,33] Even the conclude, however, that "the benefit [of adjuvant chemotherapy] in improving survival is unproven." In the absence of proven survival benefit, post surgical observation, rather than adjuvant treatment, appears prudent.

The GOG experience with its protocol for borderline ovarian tumors highlights the difficulty in conducting randomized clinical trials with this patient population. This study included both an observation arm and a treatment arm. In the treatment arm, patients with progressive disease were to be treated with melphalan for six cycles. At second-look surgery, those progressing with melphalan therapy were to receive cisplatin. So few patients experienced progressive disease that it was not possible to reach the accrual goals necessary to complete that portion of the study. After remaining open for 9 years, the treatment arm was eventually closed for lack of accrual.

Several studies on hormonal therapy have been proposed for this patient population. They have included evaluation of an antiprogestational agent, megestrol acetate (Megace), or an antiestrogenic agent, tamoxifen (Nolvadex), in decreasing the risk of recurrent progressive disease, as well as evaluation of the safety of estrogen replacement therapy. As the incidence of recurrent progressive disease is so low, the number of patients required in such studies is high. In an era of limited financial support for clinical research, such trials do not appear practical. Prospective phase II studies might be appropriate for patients with progressive recurrent disease. It is likely that intergroup studies, perhaps even with international cooperation, will be needed to complete patient accrual in a timely fashion.

JANNE KAERN
CLAES TROPÉ

Adjuvant treatment for borderline ovarian tumor is questionable. Most patients have stage I disease and a very low risk of recurrence. Prospective randomized studies with ovarian carcinoma have included borderline ovarian tumor, but the number of patients has been small. Most studies have not included a control arm (a no-treatment arm). The GOG[34] randomized 55 stage I patients in a three-arm study: control, pelvic irradiation, and melphalan. Only one patient died of disease, and it was concluded that surgery alone was the treatment of choice. In the first trial, patients with stage IA and IB, grade 1 and 2, epithelial ovarian carcinoma were randomized between melphalan and observation.[35] In this trial, 27 tumors were reclassified as borderline ovarian tumor: 12 in the melphalan arm and 15 in the control arm. In the second trial patients with stage IA–ii, IB-ii, IC, IIA through IIC, or stage IA and IB, grade 3 carcinomas were randomized between ^{32}P and melphalan. In this trial, 24 tumors were reclassified, as borderline ovarian 14 in the ^{32}P arm and 10 in the melphalan arm. Only two patients with borderline ovarian tumor relapsed and died of disease, one from each trial. In a retrospective trial, Chambers et al.[26] analyzed the efficacy of adjuvant treatment in 73 patients with stage I borderline ovarian tumor. Of these, 56 did not receive adjuvant treatment, 15 were treated with melphalan, and 2 had radiotherapy. Five year survival was 80% for treated patients and 85% for the untreated patients. Thus, no benefit from adjuvant therapy could be demonstrated. We have studied the efficacy of adjuvant therapy in four prospective randomized trials in epithelial invasive carcinoma treated between 1970 and 1988. The borderline ovarian tumor included were equally distributed between the randomization arms in all four trials.[36] The overall corrected and crude survivals for stage I patients were 99% and 94%, respectively. The four trials were randomized as follows: (1) external irradiation combined with intraperitoneal instillation of ^{198}Au or external irradiation, (2) isotope interperitoneally followed by thiotepa or observation, (3) thiotepa or observation, and (4) cisplatin or ^{32}P intraperitoneally. No differences between either treatment arm and the observation arm could be demonstrated. Barnhill et al.[5] studied the effect of adjuvant melphalan in 146 patient with stage I ovarian serous borderline tumor treated between 1983 to 1992, in a trial conducted by the GOG. No patient had recurrent disease after a median follow-up time of 42.4 months (range 1.6 to 108). It is concluded from all trials that there is no need for adjuvant therapy in stage I borderline ovarian tumor.[5,34–36] All treatment cause acute or chronic toxicity that may then lead to death in cured patients. It is impossible to demonstrate a statistically significant improved survival benefit conferred by adjuvant therapy for early-stage borderline ovarian tumor patients, as the survival following surgery alone is close to 100%.

Few patients have advanced borderline ovarian tumor, and the possible positive effect of adjuvant chemotherapy or radiotherapy in these patients has not been demonstrated. No randomized trials have been performed for this group of patients, either between different treatment arms or between a treatment arm and a control arm.

Only a few patients with advanced borderline ovarian tumor are left with residual disease. These individuals have been treated identically to members of the comparative group with ovarian carcinoma. No randomized studies have evaluated the effect of chemotherapy on disease-free survival in advanced-borderline ovarian tumor patients with residual disease, although for women with advanced-stage and residual disease, cisplatin-based chemotherapy has proved effective.[32,33] Seven of eight patients with microscopic disease and two of seven patients with macroscopic disease had pathologic complete remission at second-look surgery.[33] In a study by Fort et al[32] 12 of 19 patients with residual disease after initial surgery were free of disease at second-look laparotomy. The adjunctive therapy was either a single alkylating agent, a cisplatin combination regimen, or a combination of alkylating agent and pelvic irradiation. Sutton et al[29] demonstrated a more modest activity of cisplatin-based chemotherapy, as only 2 of 8 patients with residual disease at the completion of initial surgery had pathologic complete remission at second-look surgery. Gershenson et al[30] found a complete response to chemotherapy at second-look laparotomy in 8 of 20 patients with metastatic serous borderline ovarian tumor with macroscopic residual disease after initial surgery and in 5 of 12 patients with microscopic residual disease after initial surgery. Of the responding patients with microscopic disease 4 had invasive implants and 1 had noninvasive implants, while only 1 of the responding patients with macroscopic disease had invasive implants and 7 had noninvasive implants. The type of implant did not influence survival, in contrast to the results reported by Russel et al[37] and Bell et al.[31] This might be due to differences in the definition of noninvasive and invasive implants, inadequate follow-up times, and variations in the type of postoperative treatment. The patients with residual disease at second-look surgery seem to be at high risk of dying of disease.[32,33]

Probably, cisplatin (intravenously or intraperitoneally) and paclitaxel combination therapy should be tested in a prospective multinational randomized study with standard pathologic criteria and surgical staging procedures in advanced borderline ovarian tumor stratified for amount of residual disease (microscopic, $\leq$1 cm and $>$1 cm). An important study should randomize between highly active therapy (platinum/paclitacel) and observation after optimal surgery, although the expected efficacy of chemotherapy is minor, as most tumor cells in borderline ovarian tumor are in the quiescent phase of the cell cycle and therefore theoretically resistant to chemotherapy.

QUESTION 3

What is the role, if any, of secondary cytoreductive surgery in the management of recurrent borderline tumors?

EDWARD L. TRIMBLE

Secondary cytoreductive surgery appears to be the only effective treatment for patients with recurrent disease. Although responses to chemotherapy have been documented, these tumors appear to lack sufficient mitotic activity for current chemotherapeutic agents to work effectively. Sugarbaker[38] has advocated a complete stripping of the visceral and parietal peritoneum, followed by intraperitoneal chemotherapy with 5-fluorouracil and mitomycin C for patients with peritoneal carcinomatosis from colorectal and appendiceal cancer. He recently reported a series of 181 patients treated in this fashion. Among 76 patients with grade 1 histology, no lymph node metastases, and complete cytoreduction, 3-year survival was 99%.[39] These techniques may have promise for patients with widespread ovarian borderline tumors, although it is unclear whether Sugarbaker's painstaking surgical techniques for peritoneal stripping can be replicated widely.

Extensive intra-abdominal disease, however, together with adhesions from prior surgery, may increase the risk of intraoperative and postoperative complications, including the need for extensive bowel resection, infection, and the development of fistulas. If the patient is not symptomatic, then surgery does not seem warranted. Should surgery fail to restore integrity to the gastrointestinal tract, then these patients may require total parenteral nutrition.

JANNE KAERN
CLAES TROPÉ

Surgical resection is the preferred treatment for recurrent disease. Nearly all patients with recurrent borderline ovarian tumor have recurrent disease inside the abdominal cavity. Distant metastasis are an exception. In some patients borderline ovarian tumor recurs as borderline ovarian tumor but in some it progresses to invasive carcinoma. Invasive recurrences should be treated identically to recurrences of ovarian carcinoma. The question is whether the tumor has indeed progressed or an invasive component of the primary tumor has been overlooked. In an attempt to clarify this problem, extended sampling should be done during the primary laparotomy and new molecular approaches should be analyzed. At the moment surgery is the recommended treatment for recurrences of borderline ovarian tumor.

Patients with pseudomyxoma peritonei have recurrences with bowel obstruction, leading to death. The treatment is surgery; even repeated laparotomies with removal of the mucinous material should be performed.

Repeated surgical intervention can contribute to long-term survival for individual patients. Neither intravenous nor intraperitoneal chemotherapy appears to be effective. Total peritoneiectomy has been attempted in a few patients with this condition, but it is too early to draw any conclusions regarding its effect on survival. Experimental cases have been done in our institution (unpublished data).

Patients with advanced disease, residual disease after initial surgery, pseudomyxoma peritonei, or invasive implants are considered at high risk of recurrent disease. The recurrent disease is localized within the abdominal cavity, distant metastases being unusual, and it is managed by surgical debulking. Chemotherapy might also be successful, as occasional responses have been reported.

QUESTION 4

Are there any laboratory or molecular markers that may assist in the management of borderline tumors?

EDWARD L. TRIMBLE

Tumor markers might be useful in the management of borderline tumors in the following settings:

1. To determine which patients are at high risk for developing recurrent disease and might potentially benefit from adjuvant therapy. As noted above, no adjuvant therapy has been shown to prolong survival. It is possible, however, that a tumor marker might be able to identify a high-risk group appropriate for trials involving adjuvant therapy.
2. To monitor patients for the development of recurrent disease. Patients with surgically resected borderline tumors are at low risk for recurrence. It seems more cost-effective to evaluate patients with imaging studies and physical examinations only if they develop symptoms. Otherwise, they should be followed with yearly clinical visits.
3. To evaluate response to chemotherapy or hormonal therapy in patients with progressive disease. To date, neither chemotherapy nor hormonal therapy has been consistently shown to halt or reverse progressive symptomatic disease.

Elevations of serum CA 125 have been noted in some serous borderline tumors. CA 125 may be potentially useful in the clinical management of certain patients with serous borderline tumors. As expected, serum CA 125 has not been observed in patients with mucinous borderline tumor.[3]

Investigators have examined a variety of cellular and molecular markers in borderline tumors. A few of these investigations have had a clinical focus, primarily to determine whether a subset of borderline tumors at high risk of progression can be identified. Most have been exploratory, in an effort to define a continuum for benign ovarian cysts, borderline ovarian tumors, and ovarian carcinomas. Most of these exploratory studies appear to confirm clinical observations that borderline ovarian tumors comprise a benign entity rather than a midway point on the progression to cancer. Many are limited by the small sample size and infrequency of recurrence in patients with borderline tumors.

Baak et al[40] have used computer-assisted quantitative microscopic analysis to discriminate among benign ovarian tumors, borderline tumors, and ovarian carcinoma. In a retrospective study of 20 benign mucinous tumors, 19 borderline tumors, and 1 carcinoma, their techniques identified the carcinoma and the 2 borderline tumors that progressed.[41] They have subsequently reported the use of these techniques in the clinical management of a patient with a borderline ovarian tumor.[42]

Several investigators have examined the role of flow cytometry in borderline tumors. Unfortunately, the heterogeneity in DNA content in different parts of a tumor may compromise the effectiveness of DNA ploidy in predicting recurrence. Erhardt et al[43] found no aneuploidy in 26 serous borderline tumors. Friedlander et al[44] reported 42 of 44 borderline tumors to be diploid. One of the two patients with aneuploid tumors experienced tumor progression and death, while none of those with diploid tumors had a recurrence. Klemi et al[45] reported aneuploidy in 3 of 27 (11%) benign lesions, 7 of 43 (17%) borderline tumors, and 56 of 90 (66%) serous carcinomas. They were unable to find any association between aneuploidy and aggressive behavior in benign or borderline tumors. Kaern et al[46] have reported a pilot study on tumor ploidy in 64 patients abstracted from 370 patients with borderline ovarian tumor treated at the NRH between 1970 and 1982. They found a 47% (18 of 38) incidence of aneuploidy in mucinous borderline tumors, compared to 15% (4 of 26) in serous borderline tumors. In this study, however, patients with mucinous tumors were more likely to present with later-stage disease than those with serous tumors. Aneuploidy was also associated with shorter survival compared to diploidy. They have subsequently expanded this study to 335 patients, including 178 with mucinous borderline tumors and 174 with serous borderline tumors.[47] In this study 293 (91%) were diploid, while 28 (9%) were aneuploid. Aneuploidy was associated with older age, more advanced disease, and nonserous histologic types. In Cox analysis ploidy was the most important indicator of survival, followed by stage. Seidman et al[48] examined ploidy in 40 serous borderline tumors and 26 serous carcinomas.[54] Sixteen (40%) of the borderline tumors were aneuploid compared to 14 (54%) of the carcinomas. These investigators were unable to correlate aneuploidy with risk of progression. Harlow et al[49] reported aneuploidy in 5 of 20 (25%) women who died with a diagnosis of borderline ovarian tumor compared to 9 of 38 (24%) in controls, women matched for age at diagnosis, histologic subtype, and stage of disease, who were still alive after 5 years of follow-up. Griffiths et al[50] reported aneuploidy in 1 of 56 cystadenomas, 0 of 21 borderline tumors, 11% of mucinous carcinomas, and 46% of serous carcinomas. Ploidy was not predictive of survival in borderline tumors or carcinomas. Drescher et al[51] found aneuploidy in 9 of 21 (43%) ovarian borderline tumors, which was associated with a higher risk of recurrence. Esposito and Fuchs[52] examined ploidy in 15 serous and 9 mucinous borderline ovarian tumors. Twenty-three were diploid and one aneuploid. Among the 17 women with clinical follow-up, 2 patients with diploid tumors had experienced recurrence, while the patient with an aneuploid tumor had no evidence of disease. Guerrieri et al[53] have examined DNA flow cytometry and clinical outcome among 60 patients with borderline ovarian tumors and 32 with mucinous carcinomas. Of the 57 patients they classified as having intestinal mucinous borderline tumors, 44 had diploid tumors. Of the three "endocervical-like mucinous tumors," two were diploid.

Malignant cells have been shown to display a high-resolution protein magnetic resonance (MR) spectrum, thought to be explained by a high plasma membrane content of triglyceride molecules. Mountford et al[54] found MR signals indicating metastatic potential in zero of three benign ovarian tumors, five of six borderline tumors, and all ten ovarian carcinomas examined.

Vaccarello et al[55] examined tumor-infiltrating lymphocytes (TIL) derived from borderline ovarian tumors and ovarian carcinoma. They noted that borderline tumors contained fewer TIL than carcinomas and that borderline TIL lacked the selective enrichment in CD3+CD8+ T lymphocytes generally seen in TIL derived from ovarian carcinomas.

Several investigators have examined the association between a score given the silver-stained nucleolar organizer region (AgNOR), which has been related to cell growth rate, and ovarian tumors. Criscuolo et al[56] found no difference in AgNOR score between 13 benign ovarian tumors and 10 borderline tumors, while 56 carcinomas had higher mean AgNOR scores. In the study by Griffiths et al[50] involving 56 cystadenomas, 21 borderline tumors, and 40 carcinomas, borderline tumors had elevated AgNOR numbers despite low proliferative indices and universal diploidy. Trabucco et al[57] have reported intermediate

AgNOR counts for six borderline serous tumors, compared to 6 benign serous tumors and six malignant serous carcinomas.

Thomas et al[58] have investigated proliferating cell nuclear antigen (PCNA) as a measurement of tumor cell proliferation in six borderline ovarian tumors and 92 ovarian carcinomas. The six stage I borderline tumors had significantly lower PCNA labeling indices than 13 stage I carcinomas.

Henriksen et al[59] examined the expression of Ki-67 in normal ovarian epithelium, benign ovarian tumors, borderline ovarian tumors, and ovarian carcinomas. Staining for Ki-67 was noted in none of the normal ovaries, two of 11 (18%) benign tumors, seven of nine (78%) borderline lesions, and 36 of 45 (80%) ovarian carcinomas. Garzetti et al[60] found a significantly higher expression of Ki-67 antigen in 28 serous ovarian carcinomas than in 10 benign serous cystadenomas or 16 serous borderline tumors. Expression of Ki-67 antigen in borderline tumors was intermediate between that in benign lesions and carcinomas.

Stromberg et al[61] examined 8 normal ovaries, 20 ovarian cystadenomas, 10 borderline ovarian tumors, and 17 ovarian carcinomas for the epidermal growth factor (EGF) family of ligands and receptors, including EGF, transforming-growth factor-alpha, amphiregulin, cripto, and the receptors EGF receptor and c-erb-2. Amphiregulin was detected almost exclusively in borderline tumors, leading these investigators to conclude that borderline tumors "may not arise as a pathological continuum between benign cystadenomas and invasive cystadenocarcinomas." Cripto was found in 86% of normal ovaries, 29% of cystadenomas, 100% of borderline tumors, and 53% of carcinomas. Simpson et al[62] have studied c-erbB-3 protein expression in 71 patients with ovarian tumors: 13 benign tumors, 7 borderline tumors, and 51 carcinomas. The majority of all tumors studied were positive for c-erbB-3 regardless of whether they were malignant (89%), borderline (100%), or benign (61%). Significantly more intense staining with c-erbB-3 was noted in borderline tumors compared to carcinomas. From a study of 13 benign ovarian tumors, 8 borderline tumors, and 46 carcinomas, these investigators have also reported that coexpression of EGF receptor and c-erbB-2, and c-erbB-2 and c-erbB-3, was significantly greater in carcinomas than in benign or borderline tumors.[63]

Kacinski et al[64] reported increased expression of *c-myc* in 1 of 3 borderline tumors. Polacarz et al,[65] who examined cellular distribution of the *c-myc* oncogene product $p62^{c\text{-}myc}$ in 60 mucinous tumors, found that borderline tumors had staining intermediate between that of benign and invasive tumors. Six of the 17 borderline tumors had the same staining pattern as invasive carcinoma, but these patients had the same benign course as the other 11 borderline patients.

Mok et al[66] noted k-*ras* mutations in 12 of 19 (63%) mucinous borderline tumors and 9 of 25 (36%) serous borderline tumors, compared to 3 of 4 mucinous carcinomas and 3 of 10 serous ovarian carcinomas. Among the serous borderline tumors, increased expression of k-*ras* mutations was associated with increased stage at diagnosis. Teneriello et al[67] found an activated k-*ras* gene in 1 of 20 ovarian cystadenomas, 6 of 20 borderline tumors, and 1 of 23 ovarian carcinomas. Ichikawa et al[68] reported k-*ras* mutations in 4 of 30 (13%) mucinous cystadenomas, 4 of 12 (75%) mucinous borderline tumors, and 7 of 15 mucinous carcinomas (46%). Fujita et al[69] discovered k-*ras* mutations in 12 of 17 (71%) mucinous ovarian carcinomas and 4 of 5 (80%) mucinous borderline ovarian tumors.

Most studies have failed to find abnormal expression of p53 in borderline tumors. Teneriello et al[67] observed no p53 mutations in 20 ovarian cystadenomas or 20 borderline tumors, compared to 11 of 23 (48%) ovarian carcinomas. Kupryjanczyk et al[70] studied 70 borderline tumors and 75 ovarian carcinomas for p53 protein accumulation. They detected it in 14% of borderline tumors, 36% of stage I carcinomas, and 64% of higher-stage carcinomas. Berchuck et al[71] found overexpression of p53 in 0 of 17 benign ovarian tumors and in only 2 of 49 (4%) borderline tumors. Overexpression was seen in 2 of 8 (25%) of the patients with stage III borderline tumors, but not in any of the stage I or II cases. Fujita et al[69] have reported a p53 mutation in 1 of 5 mucinous borderline ovarian carcinomas. Kappes et al[72] detected no somatic p53 mutations in 18 borderline ovarian tumors, compared to p53 mutations noted in 15% of 39 (38%) carcinomas. Zheng et al[73] have reported p53 mutations in 0 of 16 ovarian cystadenomas and 0 of 21 borderline ovarian tumors, but in 24 of 46 (52%) ovarian carcinomas. Kiyokawa et al[74] studied p53 mutations in 50 ovarian carcinomas, 7 borderline tumors, and 2 adenomas. Although they detected nuclear accumulation of p53 protein in 60% of the carcinomas, they found none in the borderline tumors or adenomas. Koshiyama et al[75] found p53 expression in 2 of 6 (33%) borderline ovarian tumors and 15 of 32 (47%) ovarian carcinomas. Klemi et al[76] detected p53 suppresser gene expression in 0 of 6 benign serous ovarian tumors, 1 of 10 borderline tumors, and 24 of 45 (53%) serous ovarian carcinomas.

Eccles et al[77] examined 30 benign ovarian tumors, 22 borderline tumors, and 94 carcinomas for evidence of allele loss on chromosome 17q. They observed no difference in the incidence of allele loss (13%) between benign and borderline ovarian tumors, compared to a much higher rate of allele loss (70%) in carcinomas. Dodson et al,[78] who studied loss of heterozygosity in 54 patients with ovarian carcinomas and 4 with borderline tumors, found no common event between carcinomas and borderline tumors. Rodabaugh et al[79] investigated the pattern of allelic loss at chromosome 6q in 46 borderline tumors and 20 ovarian carcinomas. They noted loss of heterozygosity in 29% of carcinomas and in only 11% of borderline tumors.

Taylor et al[80] examined expression of the retinoblastoma gene (Rb) in 18 ovarian cystadenomas, 19 borderline tumors, and 22 ovarian carcinomas. All the benign cystadenomas and borderline tumors had normal expression of Rb protein, while 3 of the 22 carcinomas had altered Rb gene expression.

In summary, no laboratory or molecular marker that consistently delineates borderline ovarian tumors from benign ovarian lesions or ovarian carcinomas has been identified. Similarly, no marker that can reliably predict which borderline tumor is at high risk of recurrence has been found. Most published studies have been hampered by small sample size. Future investigations might benefit from the use of large ovarian tumor banks, such as that run jointly by the Cooperative Human Tissue Network and the GOG.

JANNE KAERN
CLAES TROPÉ

DNA content

In an attempt to improve the prognostic classification of borderline ovarian tumor, we have looked for parameters more objective than the classic prognostic factors with the intention of minimizing overtreatment. For borderline ovarian tumor, it has been difficult to identify risk factors, as the recurrent rate is low (about 10%) and the tumors show a tendency toward late recurrence. The possible prognostic value of DNA ploidy in epithelial ovarian borderline tumors has been investigated. In the NRH study,[22] evaluable DNA histograms were obtained for 321 tumors, while no material was left for DNA analysis in 35 tumors and the DNA histograms were too poor in quality to be evaluated in 14 cases. No statistical differences existed between patients with and without DNA ploidy measurements in terms of the classic prognostic factors. Except for one stage IA patient who died of disease, all 31 patients with recurrent disease had evaluable DNA histograms, including 6 patients with residual disease. Only 9% (n = 28) had DNA aneuploid tumors. Aneuploidy correlated with advanced stage of disease, older age, nonserous tumors, severe atypia, and pseudomyxoma peritonei. Complete surgery was performed on 79% of diploid (228 of 293) and on 79% of aneuploid (22 of 28) tumors. However, within stage I all patients with aneuploid tumors had complete surgery compared to 61% of those with diploid tumors. Only 2 (7%) of the 28 women with aneuploid tumors did not receive postoperative treatment compared to 77 (41%) of the 187 with diploid tumors. Of the patients with recurrent disease, only two are still alive, both of whom had diploid tumors. Only 9% (n = 29) of the patients died of disease. By univariate analysis, the following parameters had prognostic significance: DNA ploidy, FIGO stage, age, histologic type, grade of atypia, pseudomyxoma peritonei, and residual tumor. Based on multivariate analysis in the group of patients (n = 321) without residual tumor and with ploidy measurements, DNA ploidy, FIGO stage, histologic type, and age were the only independent prognostic factors. DNA ploidy was the strongest parameter (Fig. 10–1B and 10–2B). Patients with aneuploid tumors had 19 times the risk of dying of disease compared to patients with diploid tumors. Stage of disease was the second strongest variable (Fig. 10–1B). Based on a combination of the different independent prognostic factors, a prognostic index could be calculated for individual patients. The lowest-risk patient (100% long-term survival) had DNA diploid stage I serous or mucinous tumor and was below the age of 40 years. The highest-risk patient (less than 35% long-term survival) had DNA aneuploid stage III clear-cell tumor and was older than 70 years.

DNA aneuploidy has been reported in several studies[43,44,49,51] to indicate poor prognosis in borderline ovarian tumor. The DNA content of tumor cells can be measured by flow cytometry (FCM) and imagecytometry (ICM). Friedlander et al[44] analyzed 44 borderline ovarian tumors using FCM; and Erhardt et al[43] and Drescher et al[51] used ICM to analyze 26 and 21 borderline ovarian tumors, respectively. In these studies DNA ploidy was a very important prognostic factor. In a retrospective case-control study Harlow et al[49] used FCM to analyze 74 borderline ovarian tumor treated between 1975 and 1986. Twenty-five women with serous or mucinous borderline ovarian tumor died of disease (cases). These tumors were compared to age and histologic stage-matched tumors from women (with the same diagnosis) still living after at least 5 years of follow-up (49 controls). In 20% of the tumors the DNA histograms may have been too poor in quality for DNA ploidy classification, as the final results include only 20 cases and 58 controls. In this study 25% of the tumors were aneuploid, which is a very high frequency. Aneuploidy was equally distributed between cases and controls, and DNA aneuploidy was not associated with mortality. In a Danish study[81] of 121 borderline ovarian tumors, DNA ploidy was measured by FCM. The same frequency of aneuploidy was found as in the NRH study,[22] but DNA ploidy was not associated with prognosis. Thus, there is some disagreement concerning the prognostic value of DNA ploidy. This could partly be explained by the small number of borderline ovarian tumors analyzed in most studies, the relatively short follow-up time, and the difficulty of the histopathologic diagnosis. Different methods for DNA ploidy analysis may produce different results. When FCM is used, a large number of cells are measured with high resolution but without morphologic control. Small aneuploid stem lines, in particular those with high DNA content (DI > 2.5), may be overlooked and the tumor falsely classified as diploid. The sensitivity for detecting aneuploid cells is higher with ICM than with FCM. The advantage of ICM is the morphologic control, but this method is time-consuming. Only a few cells are measured, and the estimation of S phase is practically impossible, although the technique is under development. We currently recommend FCM as the routine screening procedure and examine the FCM diploid tumors by ICM also. A tumor is considered diploid only if found to be diploid by both methods. Other reasons for differences in results may be associated with nuclei suspension preparation technique (selective cell loss), fixation, staining, measuring devices, and gating, as well as subjective assessments of the DNA histogram. Tumor heterogeneity may also contribute to different results. To overcome this problem two or more different biopsies from each tumor should be analyzed. The few studies on borderline ovarian tumor that include estimation of S-phase fraction (SPF)[82] have demonstrated low values. This probably reflects, the slow progression rate of these tumors which contain few replicating stem lines. Measuring SPF from paraffin-embedded tissue is subject to many sources of error and is not reliable. No standard of reference for SFP estimation has been adopted by different laboratories. SPF should be estimated using fresh tumor tissue only. Future studies of modern ICM may clarify the possible prognostic value of S-phase estimations. It is very important that the cell suspension used for DNA analysis be examined by the cytologist to make sure that it is representative. DNA ploidy assessments improve the possibility of dividing patients into risk groups but is not sufficient. Other unknown factors (genetic, tumor-host relationship) may influence the evolution of neoplasia.

Morphometry

Baak et al[83] used a computer-assisted quantitative microscopic analysis to differentiate among benign, borderline, and malignant tumors. They found more than 30 mitosis per 25 high-power fields, an increased ratio of epithelial volume to stromal volume, and more irregular nuclei correlate with poor prognosis. Thus, mitotic activity index (MAI) and volume percentage of epithelium give important prognostic information.[83] Three more morphometric parameters seems important: mean nuclear area, mean nuclear perimeter, and mean of the short axis of the nucleus. The prognostic value of adding morphometric parameters and DNA cytometric measurements to well-known prognostic factors in borderline ovarian tumor have been studied by JPA Baak and CG Tropé (unpublished data). Morphometric measurements were performed on 303 tumors of the 321 borderline tumors (279 diploid and 24 aneuploid tumors) with DNA ploidy assessments in the study by Kaern et al.[22] Based on multivariate analysis, DNA ploidy was the strongest independent prognostic parameter. The mean nuclear area and FIGO stage were strong factors too, while histologic type was of minor importance. Using ICM, geometric, optical, and structural differences among epithelial and stromal cell nuclei of benign tumors, borderline ovarian tumor, and ovarian carcinoma could be analyzed. Differences in chromatin condensation have been found to exist between benign and malignant nuclei.[84] This might be an important step for improved classification of ovarian tumors.

Serum markers, receptors, oncogenes, and loss of heterozygosity

The prognostic value of CA 125, carcinogen embryonal antigen (CEA), estrogen and progesterone receptors, and platelet-derived grow factor (PDGF) receptors does not seem as important in borderline ovarian tumors as in ovarian carcinoma.[9,27,85,86] CA 125 can be used in follow-up of individual patients if increased before primary surgery. Especially in serous advanced-stage borderline ovarian tumor CA 125 may be useful. By immunohistochemical analysis borderline ovarian tumor generally seems to stain weaker compared to ovarian carcinoma and stronger compared to benign tissue. This may be useful in differentiating among benign, substitute borderline, and malignant tumors but hardly in identifying an aggressive borderline ovarian tumor. Henriksen et al[86] found a correlation of Ki-67 expression, FCM SPF, and DNA ploidy, but only 9 borderline ovarian tumor were analyzed. Ki-67 antibody and the monoclonal antibody MIB1 have been used as markers for cell proliferation in fresh frozen and fixed tissue, respectively. The antigens detect an antigen expressed in G-1, S and G-2 phase, but not in the G-0 phase. Borderline ovarian tumor shows a proliferative index intermediate between that of benign and invasive tumors. In a study of 17 serous borderline ovarian tumors, benign and borderline areas were examined for MIB1 and p53 expression.[87] Increased proliferation (MIB1) was observed in borderline areas compared to benign areas, and the expression of p53 was highest in a borderline area. No correlation was found between p53 and MIBI expression, indicating that other factors in addition to p53 are involved in determining the proliferative rate.

The expression of mutated p53 tumor suppressor gene has been demonstrated in a few borderline ovarian tumors,[85] but with different results.[67,76] Genetic alterations with loss of heterozygosity have been demonstrated in high-grade ovarian carcinoma while low-grade ovarian carcinoma shows a low rate of allelic loss, and no such loss was found in borderline ovarian tumors.[9,88,89] The role of oncogenes in the evolution of ovarian tumors is under investigation.[66] K-*ras* mutations were found in 48% of borderline ovarian tumors. This mutation was seen in higher frequency in mucinous borderline ovarian tumor (63%) compared to serous borderline ovarian tumor (36%). In serous borderline ovarian tumor, the mutation correlated with advanced stages of disease. Except for one, all the mutations were identified on codon 12. K-*ras* mutations may play a role in maintaining the mucinous differentiation pathways of the epithelial cells and in serous borderline ovarian tumor may be a late event in tumor progression. More information is needed to determine the role of k-*ras* mutations in ovarian carcinogenesis. The cell surface enzyme gamma-glutamyl transpeptidase (GGT) is expressed in many ovarian tumors. This enzyme cleaves extracellular glutathione, and some ovarian tumors express high levels of GGT prior to treatment, suggesting an inhererent resistance to chemotherapeutic drugs that are detoxified by glutathione.[90] Serous borderline ovarian tumors were GGT-positive in six of nine cases, while the one mucinous borderline ovarian tumor examined was negative. Future studies should concentrate on GGT expression as a marker for identifying tumors with enhanced resistance to platinum-based therapy.

The characterization of genetic alterations in borderline ovarian tumors may give insight into early tumorigenic events.[91] To improve prognostication and identification of the aggressive borderline ovarian tumors, useful markers should either predict genetic instability or preprogrammed progression toward an invasive phenotype.

QUESTION 5

What are the future directions in this area?

EDWARD L. TRIMBLE

An important future direction must be greater understanding of the clinical behavior of this subset of ovarian tumors. As discussed above, the vast majority of these tumors convey a benign prognosis. They are not carcinomas, nor do they turn into carcinomas. Kurman and Trimble found the incidence of malignant transformation to be less than 1%, comparable to the risk of uterine leiomyoma developing into leiomyosarcoma. Borderline tumors are not found more frequently in families with hereditary ovarian cancer syndromes, as might be expected if they were "precancerous"[92] It may be more appropriate to consider them a benign gynecologic entity, like leiomyomata or endometriosis, that can on occasion spread throughout the abdomen and cause bowel obstruction. Here nomenclature may convey a worse prognosis than the tumors themselves. Perhaps the terms *borderline* and *of low malignant potential* should be abandoned in favor of "proliferating ovarian tumors" as Russell, Kurman, CL Trimble, and EL Trimble have argued.[93] With a greater understanding of these tumors by pathologists and clinicians, more women might be treated conservatively, retaining reproductive potential if they wish and spared adjuvant therapy.

Further investigation into the pathogenesis of ovarian tumors may help us learn how to prevent borderline tumors. We know, for example, that oral contraceptives, pregnancy, and lactation all protect against the development of these tumors. An association between the use of fertility drugs and the development of borderline tumors has been reported.[94,95] Information on the molecular and cellular changes promoting these tumors may help us identify effective therapy for patients with progressive disease. As these tumors are indolent, perhaps cytostatic agents would be more effective than cytotoxic agents. And one day we may even to able to identify patients who are truly at high risk for tumor progression and prolong their survival with effective adjuvant therapy.

JANNE KAERN
CLAES TROPÉ

In epithelial ovarian borderline tumors without residual tumor, independent prognostic factors after initial surgery are DNA ploidy, morphometric parameters (MNA), FIGO stage, histologic type, and age. The presence of residual tumor indicates poor prognosis. High-risk patients are characterized by DNA aneuploidy, advanced stage of disease, nonserous tumor, and older than 70 years.[22]

One, preferable two, surgical biopsies from the primary ovarian tumor and one from suspect intra-abdominal lesions should be taken for DNA ploidy and morphometric analysis and studies of molecular alterations. From each biopsy one portion should be examined by the pathologist and/or cytologist. In retrospective studies the pathologist should select tissue for DNA ploidy assessments from the part of the tumor demonstrating the highest degree of nuclear atypia and avoid areas with necrotic cells and stromal tissue. The portion for DNA ploidy assessment should be divided for flow cytometric and image cytometric analysis.

Standard primary surgery includes bilateral salpingo-oophorectomy, omentectomy, peritoneal washing, and multiple biopsies. Hysterectomy is optional. A correct staging procedure is essential. In advanced cases total abdominal hysterectomy and tumor debulking should be performed, and with mucinous tumors appendectomy should be included. Lymphadenectomy is recommended only for DNA aneuploid and high-risk tumors. The follow-up is too short to evaluate if lymphadenectomy will improve survival for DNA aneuploid tumor patients.

Conservative surgery is indicated in young, fertile women with stage I DNA diploid tumors and consists of unilateral oophorectomy, omentectomy, and peritoneal washing. In young patients with a single ovarian cyst, cystectomy is sufficient if the gynecologist and the pathologist meticulously examine the resection margins. With multifocality and/or involvement of resection margins, reoperation with unilateral salpingo-oophorectomy is recommended. Biopsy from the contralateral ovary is not indicated if it appears normal to an experienced surgeon. Second-look laparotomy is recommended if histologic examination reveals disseminated disease or invasive carcinoma and/or DNA aneuploidy. Frozen sections are not reliable in discriminating between borderline tumor and carcinoma. Conservatively treated patients need close follow-up, including physical examination, ultrasound (transvaginal), and serum markers (CA 125).

Adjuvant postoperative therapy is not indicated in stage I DNA diploid tumors.

A large prospective randomized trial is needed for evaluation of the survival benefits of adjuvant chemotherapy (cisplatin/paclitaxel-based regimens) in advanced disease and/or DNA aneuploid tumors. The trial may be difficult to handle because of the relatively few high-risk patients and the tendency toward late recurrence. Also important is the difficult histopathologic diagnosis.

Occasional responses to chemotherapy have been reported, but no study has shown improved survival.

Secondary cytoreductive surgery is recommended for patients with recurrent disease; even repeated laparotomies are indicated in patients with pseudomyxoma peritonei. The importance of peritonectomy is speculative.

Estrogen replacement treatment should be given to prevent cardiovascular disease, osteoporosis, and climacteric disorders.

Follow-up should be lifelong, with a 3- to 4-month interval the first 2 years and every half year thereafter. Surveillance should include gynecologic examination, ultrasound, and CA 125 measurement. Although CA 125 is not as important an indicator of prognosis as in ovarian carcinoma, it is currently the best tumor marker in borderline ovarian tumor.

In the future an improved ability to discriminate among benign, borderline, and malignant tumors and an increased knowledge of ovarian carcinogenesis may be able to identify the few borderline tumors with aggressive malignant potential.

EDITORS' COMMENTARY

Incomplete surgical staging remains a very common feature of patients referred to a university or comprehensive cancer center following resection of a borderline ovarian tumor seemingly confined to the ovary(ies). Not infrequently, a low transverse abdominal incision has been employed. In our experience, a typical scenario is for the operating surgeon to have palpated and visualized the upper abdomen and retroperitoneum but not to have performed any staging biopsies. In response to our question, the authors emphasize the importance of the desirability and safety of conservative surgery in young patients who have not completed childbearing. Preservation of a normal uterus and a contralateral ovary is usually possible. The incidence of bilaterality of mucinous borderline tumors is only about 5%, and the incidence of bilaterality of serous borderline tumors is approximately 50%. Even in the latter case, however, an ovarian cystectomy (or even bilateral ovarian cystectomies) may be performed to accomplish the goal of preserving fertility potential. In addition, appendectomy in patients with mucinous borderline tumors is advisable to clearly rule out the possibility of a primary appendiceal carcinoma metastatic to the ovaries.

For patients, referred after incomplete surgical staging, the authors correctly outline the possible options for clinical management: (1) observation or (2) reoperation with comprehensive surgical staging, but still preserving fertility in young patients. As noted from the discussions, however, there is no standard in this setting. As Dr. Trimble points out, restaging makes somewhat more sense for a patient with a serous borderline tumor since the chances of extraovarian disease or contralateral ovarian involvement are higher than in mucinous borderline tumors. If the physician believes that restaging is preferable, operative laparoscopy should be considered an alternative to laparotomy. However, our usual management of such a problem is to perform a computerized tomography scan of the abdomen and pelvis and serum tumor markers. If these tests are normal, observation is generally our preference.

On the question of postoperative treatment for patients with borderline tumors of advanced stage, the authors correctly state that there is no convincing evidence that postoperative therapy is indicated in this patient population. The impact of either radiotherapy or chemotherapy for these patients, as outlined in retrospective studies, remains unknown. And, because of the relative rarity of this phenomenon, no prospective randomized studies exist. Although the authors believe that prospective studies are indicated, Dr. Trimble underscores the difficulties with such studies in this population. In our experience, approximately 25 to 30% of patients with serous borderline tumors with peritoneal implants have recurrent disease and only about one-third to one-half of those who do ultimately die of their tumor. Moreover, the average time to recurrence may be several years. We agree with Dr. Trimble that the likelihood of prospective randomized studies being performed in this area is not high. It is hoped that information derived from molecular and genetic studies and long-term retrospective studies will some day provide better clues to the identification of patients with advanced disease who will develop recurrent disease.

On the issue of secondary cytoreductive surgery, the authors agree that this procedure is the preferred treatment for those few patients who develop recurrent disease. As Drs. Kaern and Tropé indicate, recurrent tumor in these patients is not infrequently invasive tumor and not recurrent borderline tumor. Of course, we really don't know whether so-called recurrent tumor in these case represents a true recurrence or a new primary tumor. It is hoped that future clonality studies will elucidate this condition.

The authors accurately summarize the current status of our knowledge regarding laboratory and molecular markers of borderline tumors. DNA ploidy has been the most widely studied, but the findings are conflicting. As Drs. Tropé and Kaern points out, however, the difference in results may be related to a difference in methodology. Currently, we agree with Dr. Trimble's statement that "no marker that will reliably predict which borderline tumor is at high risk for recurrence has been found."

And finally, as the authors conclude, future directions should include studies that provide a better understanding of the pathogenesis and biologic behavior of borderline tumors of the ovary. Such information will in turn allow us to resolve the controversy regarding the classification of these tumors.

References

1. Spann CO, Kennedy JE, Musoke E: Intraoperative consultation of ovarian neoplasms. J Natl Med Assoc 86:141, 1994
2. Rose PG, Rubin RB, Nelson BE et al: Accuracy of frozen section (intraoperative consultation) diagnosis of ovarian tumors. Am J Obstet Gynecol 171:823, 1994
3. Trimble EL, Trimble CL: Epithelial ovarian tumors of low malignant potential. p. 415. In Markman M, Hoskins WJ (eds): Cancer of the Ovary. Raven Press, New York, 1993
4. Sakamoto A, Sasaki H, Furusato M et al: Observer disagreement in histological classification of ovarian tumors in Japan. Gynecol Oncol 54:54, 1994
5. Barnhill DR, Kurman RJ, Brady MF et al: Preliminary analysis of the behavior of stage I ovarian serious tumors of low malignant potential: a Gynecologic Oncology Group study. J Clin Oncol 13:2752, 1995
6. Kurman RJ, Trimble CL: The behavior of serous tumors of low malignant potential: are they ever malignant? Int J Gynecol Pathol 12:120, 1993
7. Aure JC, Hoeg K, Kolstad P: Clinical and histological studies of ovarian cancer. Obstet Gynecol 37:1, 1971
8. International Federation of Gynecology and Obstetrics. Annual report and results of treatment in gynecologic cancer. Int J Gynecol Obstet 28:189, 1989
9. Trimble CL, Trimble EL: Management of epithelial ovarian tumors of low malignant potential. Gynecol Oncol 55: S52, 1994
10. Ronnett BM, Kurman RJ, Shmookler BM et al: Pseudomyxoma peritonei in women: a clinicopathologic analysis of 30 cases with emphasis on site of origin, prognosis, and relationship to ovarian mucinous tumors of low malignant potenital. Hum Pathol 26:509, 1995
11. Seidman JD, Elsayed AM, Sobin LH et al: Association of mucinous tumors of the ovary and appendix. A clinicopathologic study of 25 cases. Am J Surg Pathol 17:22, 1993
12. Prayson RA, Hart WR, Petras RE: Pseudomyoma peritonei. A clinicopathologic study of 19 cases with emphasis on site of origin and nature of associated ovarian tumors. Am J Surg Pathol 18:591, 1994
13. Wertheim I, Fleischhacker D, McLachlin CM et al: Pseudomyxoma peritonei: a review of 23 cases. Obstet Gynecol 84:17, 1994
14. Mishell DR Jr: Menopause. p. 1245. In: Herbst AL, Mishell DR Jr, Stenchever MA, Droegemueller W (eds): Comprehensive Gynecology. 2nd Ed. Mosby-Yearbook, St. Louis, 1991
15. Leake JF, Rader JS, Woodruff JD et al: Retroperitoneal lymphatic involvement with epithelial ovarian tumors of low malignant potential. Gynecol Oncol 42;124, 1991
16. Maassen V: Ovarian tumors of malignant potential: an intra- and retroperitoneal disease? Geburtshilfe Frauenheilk 53:163, 1993
17. Tan LK, Flynn SD, Carcangiu ML: Ovarian serous borderline tumors with lymph node involvement. Clinicopathologic and DNA content study of seven cases and review of the literature. Am J Surg Pathol 18:904, 1994
18. Menzin AW, Rubin SC, Noumoff JS, LiVolsi VA: The accuracy of a frozen section diagnosis of borderline ovarian malignancy. Gynecol Oncol 59:183, 1995
19. Russell P, Merkur H: Proliferating ovarian "epithelial" tumors: clinicopathologic analysis of 144 cases. Aust NZ J Obstet Gynaecol 9:45, 1979

20. Bostwick DG, Tazelaar HD, Ballon SC et al: Ovarian epithelial tumors of borderline malignancy. A clinical and pathologic study of 109 cases. Cancer 58:2052, 1986

21. Kaern J, Tropé CG, Abeler VM: A retrospective study of 370 borderline tumors of the ovary treated at the Norwegian Radium Hospital from 1979 to 1982. A review of clinicopathologic features and treatment modalities. Cancer 71:1810, 1993

22. Kaern J, Tropé CG, Kristensen GB et al: DNA ploidy; the most important prognostic factor in patients with borderline tumors of the ovary. Int J Gynecol Cancer 3:349, 1993

23. Lim-Tan SK, Cajigas HE, Scully RE: Ovarian cystectomy for serous borderline tumors: a follow-up study of 35 cases. Obstet Gynecol 72:775, 1988

24. Kliman L, Rome RM, Fortune DW: Low malignant potential tumors of the ovary: a study of 76 cases. Obstet Gynecol 68:338, 1986

25. Tazelaar HD, Bostwick DG, Ballon SC et al: Conservative treatment of borderline ovarian tumors. Obstet Gynecol 66:417, 1985

26. Chambers JT, Merino MJ, Kohorn EI, Schwartz PE: Borderline ovarian tumors. Am J Obstet Gynecol 159:1088, 1988

27. Hoskins PJ: Ovarian tumours of low malignant potential: borderline epithelial ovarian carcinoma. p. 112. In Lawton FG, Neijt JP, Swenerton KD (eds): Epithelial cancer of the ovary. BMJ Publishing Group, BMA House, London, 1995

28. NIH Consensus Development Panel on Ovarian Cancer: Ovarian cancer: screening, treatment, and follow-up. JAMA 273:491, 1995

29. Sutton GP, Bundy GN, Omura GA et al: Stage III ovarian tumors of low malignant potential treated with cisplatin combination therapy (a Gynecologic Oncology Group study). Gynecol Oncol 41:230, 1991

30 Gershenson DM, Silva EG: Serous ovarian tumors of low malignant potential with peritoneal implants. Cancer 65: 578, 1990

31. Bell DA, Weinstock MA, Scully RE: Peritoneal implants of ovarian serous borderline tumors. Cancer 62:2212, 1988

32. Fort MG, Pierce VK, Saigo PE et al: Evidence of the efficacy of adjuvant therapy in epithelial ovarian tumors of low malignant potential. Gynecol Oncol 32:269, 1989

33. Barakat RR, Benjamin IB, Lewis JL Jr et al: Platinum-based chemotherapy for advanced-stage serous ovarian cancers of low malignant potential. Gynecol Oncol 59:390, 1995

34. Creasman WT, Park R, Norris H et al: Stage I borderline ovarian tumors. Obstet Gynecol 59:93, 1982

35. Young RC, Walton LA, Ellenberg SS et al: Adjuvant therapy in stage I and II epithelial ovarian cancer: Results of two randomized trials. N Engl J Med 322:1021, 1990

36. Tropé C, Kaern J, Vergote IB et al: Are borderline tumors of the ovary overtreated both surgically and systemically? A review of four prospective randomized trials including 253 patients with borderline tumors. Gynecol Oncol 51:236, 1993

37. Russell P: Borderline epithelial tumours of the ovary: a conceptual dilemma. Clin. Obstet Gynecol 11:259, 1984

38. Sugarbaker PH: Patient selection and treatment of peritoneal carcinomatosis from colorectal and appendiceal cancer. World J Surg 9:235, 1995

39. Sugarbaker PH, Jablonski KA: Prognostic features of 51 colorectal and 130 appendiceal cancer patients with peritoneal carcinomatosis treated by cytoreductive

surgery and intraperitoneal chemotherapy. Ann Surg 221:124, 1995

40. Baak JPA, Agrafolo-Blanco A, Kurva PHJ et al: Quantitation of borderline and malignant mucinous ovarian tumors. Histopathology 5:353, 1981
41. Baak JPA, Fox H, Langley FA et al: The prognostic value of morphometry in ovarian epithelial tumors of borderline malignancy. Int J Gynecol Pathol 4: 186, 1985
42. Baak JPA, Van der Ley G: Borderline or malignant ovarian tumour: a case report of decision making with morphometry. J Clin Pathol 37:1110, 1984
43. Erhardt K, Auer G, Bjorkholm E et al: Prognostic significance of nuclear DNA content in serous ovarian tumors. Cancer Res 44:2198, 1984
44. Friedlander, ML, Russell P, Taylor I et al: Flow cytometric analysis of cellular DNA content as an adjunct to the diagnosis of ovarian tumors of borderline malignancy. Pathology 16:301, 1984
45. Klemi PJ, Joensuu H, IIholma P et al: Clinical significance of abnormal DNA content in serous ovarian tumors. Cancer 62:2005, 1988
46. Kaern J, Trope C, Kjorstad KE et al: Cellular DNA content as a new prognostic tool in patients with borderline tumors of the ovary. Gynecol Oncol 38:452, 1990
47. Trope C, Kaern J, Abeler V et al: Borderline ovarian tumors: diagnosis, prognosis, and treatment. The Norwegian Radium Hospital experiences, (abstracted) Gynaecological Oncology, Eight International Meeting of the European Society of Gynaecoloigcal Oncology, June 9–12, 1993, Barcelona
48. Seidman JD, Norris HJ, Griffin JL, Hitchcok CL: DNA flow cytometric analysis of serous ovarian tumors of low malignant potential. Cancer 71:3947, 1993
49. Harlow BL, Fuhr JE, McDonald TW et al: Flow cytometry as a prognostic indicator in women with borderline epithelial ovarian tumors. Gynecol Oncol 50;305, 1993
50. Griffiths AP, Cross D, Kingston RE et al: Flow cytometry and AgNORS in benign, borderline, and malignant mucinous and serous tumours of the ovary. Int J Gynecol Oncol 12:307, 1993
51. Drescher CW, Flint A, Hopkins MP et al: Prognostic significance of DNA content and nuclear morphology in borderline ovarian tumors. Gynecol Oncol 48:242, 1993
52. Esposito MJ, Fuchs A: Computerized image analysis and flow cytometric evaluation of ovarian borderline tumors: a study of 24 cases. Cytometry 18:218, 1994
53. Guerrieri C, Hogberg T, Wingren S et al: Mucinous borderline and malignant tumors of the ovary. A clinicopathologic and DNA ploidy study of 92 cases. Cancer 74:2329, 1994
54. Mountford CE, May GL, William PG, et al: Classification of tumors by high-resolution magnetic resonance spectroscopy. Lancet 1:1573, 1986
55. Vaccarello L, Kanbour A, Kanbour-Shakir A et al: Tumor-infiltrating lymphocytes from ovarian tumors of low malignant potential. Int J. Gynecol Pathol 12:41, 1993
56. Criscuolo M, Martinelli AM, Migladi M et al: Prognostic significance of nucleolar organizer regions in ovarian epithelial tumors. Int J Gynecol Pathol 12;259, 1993
57. Trabucco S, Varcaccio-Garofalo G, Botticella MA et al: Expression of AgNORs in serous ovarian tumors. Eur J Gynaecol Oncol 15:222, 1994
58. Thomas H, Nasim MM, Sarraf CE et al: Proliferating cell nuclear antigen (PCNA) immunostaining — a prognos-

tic factor in ovarian cancer? Br J Cancer 71:357, 1995

59. Henriksen R, Strang P, Backstrom T et al: Ki-67 immunostaining and DNA flow cytometry as prosgnostic factors in epithelial ovarian cancers. Anticancer Res 14:603, 1994
60. Garzetti GG, Ciavattini A, Goteri G: Ki-67 antigen immunostaining (MIB monoclonal antibody) in serous ovarian tumors: index of proliferative activity with prognostic signficance. Gynecol Oncol 56:169, 1995
61. Stromberg K, Johnson GR, O'Connor DM et al: Frequent immunohistochemical detection of EGF supergene family members in ovarian carcinogenesis. Int J Gynecol Pathol 13:342, 1994
62. Simpson BJ, Weatherill J, Miler EP: c-erbB-3 protein expression in ovarian tumors. Br J Cancer 71:758, 1995
63. Simpson BJ, Phillips HA, Lessells AM et al: c-ErbB growth factor-receptor proteins in ovarian tumors. Int J Cancer 64:202, 1995
64. Kacinski BM, Carter D, Kohorn EI et al: Oncogene expression in vivo by ovarian adenocarcinomas and mixed-Mullerian tumors. Yale J Biol Med 62:379, 1989
65. Polacarz SV, Hey NA, Stephenson TJ et al: c-*myc* oncogene product P62 in ovarian mucinous neoplasms: immunohistochemical study correlated with malignancy. J Clin Pathol 42:148, 1989
66. Mok SC-H, Bell DA, Knapp RC et al: Mutation of k-ras protooncogene is associated with histologic subtypes in human ovarian epithelial tumors of borderline malignancy. Cancer Res 53:1489, 1993
67. Teneriello MG, Ebina M, Linnoila RI et al: p53 and Ki-ras gene mutations in epithelial ovarian neoplasms. Cancer Res 53:3103, 1993
68. Ichikawa Y, Nishida M, Suzuki H et al: Mutation of k-ras protooncogene is associated with histologic subtypes in human mucinous ovarian tumors. Cancer Res 54:33, 1994
69. Fujita M, Enomoto T, Inoue M et al: Alteration of the p53 tumor suppressor gene occurs independently of k-ras activation and more frequently in serous adenocarcinomas than in other common epithelial tumors of the human ovary. Jpn J Cancer Res 85:1247, 1994
70. Kupryjanczak J, Bell DA, Yandell DW: p53 expression in ovarian borderline tumors and stage I carcinomas. Am J Clin Pathol 102:671, 1994
71. Burchuck A, Kohler MF, Hopkins MP et al: Overexpression of p53 is not a feature of benign and early-stage borderline epithelial ovarian tumors. Gynecol Oncol 52:232, 1994
72. Kappes S, Milde-Langosch K, Kressin P et al: p53 mutations in ovarian tumors, detected by temperature-gradient gel electrophoresis, direct sequencing, and immunohistochemisty. Int J Cancer 64:52, 1995
73. Zheng J, Benedict WF, Xu HJ et al: Genetic disparity between morphologically benign cysts contiguous to ovarian carcinomas and solitary cystadenomas. J Natl Cancer Inst 87:1146, 1995
74. Kiyokawa T: Alteration of p53 in ovarian cancer: its occurence and maintenance in tumor progression. Int J Gynecol Pathol 13:311, 1994
75. Koshiyama M, Konishi I, Mandai I et al: Immunohistochemical analysis of p53 protein and 72kDa heat shock protein (HSP72) expression in ovarian carcinomas. Correlation with clinicopathology and sex steroid receptor status. Virchows Arch A Pathol Anat Histopathol 425:603, 1995
76. Klemi PJ, Takahashi S, Joensuu H et al: Immunohistochemical detection of p53 protein in borderline and malignant serous ovarian tumors. Int J Gynecol Pathol 13:228, 1994
77. Eccles DM, Russell SEH, Haites HE et al: Early loss of heterozygosity on 17q in ovarian cancer. Oncogene 7:2069, 1992

78. Dodson MK, Hartman LC, Cliby W et al: Comparison of loss of heterozygosity patterns in invasive low-grade and high-grade epithelial ovarian carcinomas. Cancer Res 53:4456, 1993

79. Rodabaugh KJ, Blanchard G, Welch WR et al: Detailed deletion mapping of chromosome 6q in borderline epithelial ovarian tumors. Cancer Res 55:2169, 1995

80. Taylor RR, Linnoila RI, Gerardts J et al: Abnormal expression of the retinoblastoma gene in ovarian neoplasms and correlation to p53 and K-ras mutations. Gynecol Oncol 58:307, 1995

81. Andersen ES, Nielsen K, Nielsen RH: Borderline epithelial tumours of the ovary. Abstract IGCS, International Gynecologic Cancer Society, Third Biennial Meeting Cairns, Australia, 1991

82. Kühn W, Kaufmann M, Feichter GE et al: DNA flow cytometry, clinical and morphological parameters as prognostic factors for advanced malignant and borderline ovarian tumors. Gynecol Oncol 33:360, 1989

83. Baak JPA, Chan KK, Stolk JG, Kenemans P: Prognostic factors in borderline and invasive ovarian tumors of the common epithelial type. Pathol Res Pract 182:755, 1987

84. Komitowski D, Janson C, Szamaborsky J, Czernobilsky B: Quantitative nuclear morphology in the diagnosis of ovarian tumors of low malignant potential (borderline). Cancer 64:905, 1989

85. Makar APh, Kaern J, Kristensen GB et al: Evaluation of serum CA 125 level as a tumor marker in borderline tumors of the ovary. Int J Gynecol Cancer 3:299, 1993

86. Henriksen R: Ovarian carcinogenesis. A study of markers for growth mechanisms in epithelial ovarian tumors. Acta Universitatis Upsaliensis. Uppsala 1994

87. Marcelli AR, Demopoulos RI, Goswami S, Mittal KR: Comparison of p53 and MIB1 expression in benign and borderline areas of ovarian serous tumors. Int J Gynecol Pathol 15:39 1996

88. Dodson MK, Hartmann LC, Cliby WA et al: Comparison of loss of heterozygosity patterns in invasive low-grade and high-grade epithelial ovarian carcinomas. Cancer Res 53:4456, 1993

89. Kim TM, Benedict WF, Xu H-J et al: Loss of heterozygosity on chromosome 13 is common only in the biologically more aggressive subtypes of ovarian epithelial tumors and is associated with normal retinoblastoma gene expression. Cancer Res 54:605, 1994

90. Hanigan MH, Frierson HF, Brown JE et al: Human ovarian tumor express gamma-glutamyl transpeptidase. Cancer Res 54:286, 1994

91. Link CJ, Kohn E, Reed E: The relationship between borderline ovarian tumors and epithelial ovarian carcinoma: epidemiologic, pathologic, and molecular aspects. Gynecol Oncol 60:347, 1996

92. Schildkraut JM, Thompson WD: Familial ovarian cancer; a population-based case control study. Am J Epidemiol 128:45, 1988

93. Russell P: Borderline epithelial tumors of the ovary: a conceptual dilemma. Clin Obstet Gynecol 11:259, 1984

94. Harris R, Whittemore A, Itnyre J et al: Characteristics treating to ovarian cancer risk: collaborative analysis of 12 US case-control studies. III. Epithelial ovarian tumors of low malignant potential in white women. Am J Epidemiol 136, 1204, 1992

95. Rossing MA, Daling JR, Weiss NS et al: Ovarian tumors in a cohort of infertile women. N Engl J Med 331:771, 1994

CHAPTER 11

THE ROLE OF RADIATION THERAPY IN THE MANAGEMENT OF OVARIAN CANCER

Marcus E. Randall
Gillian M. Thomas
Daniel S. Kapp

EDITORS' INTRODUCTION

Despite several decades of treatment of ovarian cancer patients with radiation therapy, its proper role in the management of this disease is not clearly established. In the mid-1970s, the use of external beam radiation therapy began to wane significantly. Several forces converged at that time to account for this phenomenon: (1) disappointment and frustration with the results of primary postoperative whole abdominal radiation therapy; (2) the finding of a superior therapeutic ratio with the drug melphalan compared with that with radiation therapy in a prospective randomized clinical trial at M.D. Anderson Cancer Center; (3) the introduction of new chemotherapeutic agents—such as doxorubicin, cisplatin, and hexamethylmelamine—coupled with the hope for better patient outcomes; and (4) the proliferation of medical oncologists, including strong leadership from the cohort at the National Cancer Institute.

Unfortunately, the body of literature on the treatment of ovarian cancer amassed up to and including this period suffered from the same types of problems that plagued many early studies on ovarian cancer: retrospective nature, poor study design, inadequate surgical staging, lack of uniform pathologic diagnosis, and suboptimal statistical methods. As interest in the use of this modality was seriously declining, however, radiation oncologists at the Princess Margaret Hospital in Toronto, most notably, Alon

Dembo, were extolling the virtues of radiation therapy for ovarian cancer through reports of a series of clinical trials that demonstrated continued promise for this treatment strategy. These investigators also made several important observations and contributions in this area, such as the finding that the open-field technique was less morbid than the moving-strip technique. Nevertheless, such claims were unable to stop the momentum of the pendulum swinging toward chemotherapy as standard primary postoperative treatment. Although radiation therapy as the primary postoperative treatment for ovarian cancer has never regained a foothold since the 1970s, investigators at a few institutions, such as the Princess Margaret Hospital and Stanford, represented by our contributors on this subject, continued to employ this modality. A major theme of subsequent publications on this topic was careful patient selection based on stage and residual tumor diameter. Like chemotherapy, radiation therapy appeared to be most appropriate for patients with small residual disease. Then, in the 1980s, with the first wave of disappointment generated by reports of clinical trials investigating platinum-based combination chemotherapy, there was a resurgence of interest in radiation as salvage therapy for patients with small-volume persistent disease at second-look surgery. Along the way, a few phase II studies on combined radiation therapy and chemotherapy have also been conducted, most notably by the Gynecologic Oncology Group. (GOG).

In addition, during the 1980s, standard treatment for ovarian dysgerminoma dramatically changed. Until that time, radiation therapy had been the standard postoperative treatment for all patients with this rare tumor except those with stage I disease (some experts even advocated radiation therapy for larger stage I dysgerminomas because of the clinical impression that they were more likely to recur). In fact, ovarian dysgerminomas are exquisitely sensitive to radiation, and the results with this modality were indeed excellent. In the mid-1980s, however, reports began to emerge demonstrating equally excellent outcomes with platinum-based chemotherapy. Of course, the major advantage of chemotherapy over radiation therapy is potential preservation of fertility—an attribute of extreme importance in a young population. Thus, over the past decade or so, chemotherapy has almost supplanted radiation therapy as standard postoperative treatment for patients with metastatic dysgerminoma.

Against this background, we asked our contributors, all of whom are world leaders in the study of radiation therapy for ovarian cancer, to comment on the current clinical applications for this modality and their recommendations for future clinical trials in this area.

QUESTIONS

1. What is the evidence supporting the use of radiation therapy as primary postoperative treatment for epithelial ovarian cancer?
2. What is the role, if any, of radiation therapy in the salvage setting?
3. What is the role, if any, of combined modality chemotherapy/radiation therapy for ovarian cancer?
4. Is there currently any role for radiation therapy in the treatment of (1) ovarian dysgerminoma, or (2) sex cord-stromal tumors?
5. What are your recommendations for future directions and clinical trials in this area?

QUESTION 1

What is the evidence supporting the use of radiation therapy as primary postoperative treatment for epithelial ovarian cancer?

MARCUS E. RANDALL
GILLIAN THOMAS

Primary radiation therapy in abdomen-confined ovarian carcinoma

Management of ovarian carcinoma is significantly affected by extent of disease. Because well-staged patients with ovarian carcinoma limited to the abdomen (stage I to III) have quite variable prognoses, firm data regarding management options and treatment results in patient subsets are limited. However, patients with stage I, grade 3, and stage II to III tumors as a group have relapse rates high enough to warrant therapy in addition to surgery. Historically, both intraperitoneal radiocolloids and external whole abdominal irradiation (WAI) have been used.

^{32}P as Primary Treatment

The use of intraperitoneal radiocolloids theoretically offers the possibility of delivering high doses of radiation to peritoneal surfaces, which is appropriate given the recognized transperitoneal route of dissemination of ovarian cancer. ^{32}P was the most attractive isotope because it is a pure β emitter (with short-penetrating electrons) and lacks the hazards of γ radiation that accompanied the use of ^{198}Au. Unfortunately, despite the intuitive appeal of the use of intraperitoneal radioisotopes, a therapeutic value has not been clearly established for this treatment. Given the short penetrating power of ^{32}P (to a few cell layers only), the dose to the retroperitoneal nodes is negligible and the radiation dose distribution over the peritoneum is often variable and unpredictable, often because of the presence of adhesions. There are data from randomized trials supporting the continued use of ^{32}P in early-stage patients. One study in the United States (GOG protocol 95) randomized patients with high-risk early disease between ^{32}P intraperitoneally and three cycles of cisplatin/cyclophosphamide. This study took 7 years to complete accrual and is awaiting data maturation prior to analysis. No randomized trials of radioisotopes against a control receiving no treatment have been performed. A retrospective multivariate analysis of the Norwegian Radium Hospital data showed a nonsignificant excess of relapses in patients who received ^{32}P or ^{198}Au, compared to pelvic radiation therapy or no treatment in stages I and II.[1] In a randomized study conducted by the National Cancer Institute of Canada (NCIC) in which ^{32}P was given in addition to pelvic radiation therapy, unacceptable bowel toxicity was encountered and this treatment arm was abandoned.[2] A randomized prospective study on ^{32}P versus cisplatin in high-risk patients (mostly stage I and II) revealed 5-year disease-free survivals of 81% and 75% with ^{32}P and cisplatin, respectively[3] (Table 11–1). The authors favored cisplatin because it was associated with less bowel toxicity, although patients receiving cisplatin had slightly inferior median survival, median time to recurrence, and percentage of patients relapsing. These differences were not statistically significant.

A recently published large, randomized Italian study compared cisplatin 50 mg/m^2 every 28 days for six cycles to ^{32}P in patients with stage IA, II, IIB, and IC disease. In this study with a median observation time of 76 months, there was no difference in overall survival, but the use of cisplatin reduced the recurrence risk to 16% as compared to 32% for those treated with ^{32}P. The difference between the results for survival compared to those for relapse are related to a subsequent risk of dying after relapse which was significantly increased in the patients originally randomized to the cisplatin arm. Despite the lack of survival benefit for adjuvant cisplatin, it was favored over ^{32}P because it decreased the relapse rate.[4]

TABLE 11-1
Stage I to II Ovarian Cancer Randomized Trials Using Intraperitoneal Phosphorus-32

STUDY	PATIENTS INCLUDED	TREATMENT	OUTCOME
Young et al[1a]	IG3, stage II	IP ^{32}P (n = 73)	80% 5-yr DFS
		Melphalan (n = 68)	80% 5-yr DFS
GOG 95	High-risk stage I–II	IP ^{32}P	Pending
		Cisplatinum	Pending
Vergote et al[3]	Stage I–II (92%)	IP ^{32}P (n = 141)	80% 5-yr DFS
	Stage IIIA (8%)	Cisplatinum × 6 (n = 171)	75% 5-yr DFS
	No residuum	WAI (n = 28)	86% 5-yr DFS
Bolis et al[4]	Stage IC (n = 176)	Cisplatinum × 6	81% DFS
		IP ^{32}P	56% DFS

Abbreviation: DFS, Disease-free survival.

The conclusion from the available data is that there is no clear evidence for a therapeutic benefit associated with the use of ^{32}P. Given the problems with bowel toxicity in some series, uneven distribution of radiocolloid, and lack of dose to the retroperitoneal nodes, WAR seems more appropriate if radiation is selected as the treatment of choice.

External Radiation Therapy as Primary Treatment

Long considered an effective therapy for ovarian carcinoma, WAI was largely displaced by cytotoxic chemotherapy following publication of a randomized trial showing the equivalency (not superiority) of radiation therapy and melphalan.[5] Some investigators, however, have questioned whether this change was premature, particularly in view of the substantial improvements in radiation therapy equipment and technique since that time.[6,7]

Although acute and possibly late toxicities with WAI are of concern, this modality offers theoretical and practical advantages over ^{32}P such as coverage of abdominal lymph nodes, more homogeneous dose distribution, and ability to cover all peritoneal surfaces irrespective of postoperative adhesions. These features make WAI a management option for selected patients with early and more advanced abdomen-confined disease. Published data from randomized prospective trials and retrospective studies suggest that WAI is curative in a substantial percentage of patients with stage I to III disease who have been optimally debulked.

Table 11–2 shows the results for randomized trials comparing treatment with WAI to treatment that included chemotherapy. These studies largely entered stage I and II patients, although many were not thoroughly staged by current standards and considerably more stage III patients were included than acknowledged. Three of the four trials did not compare WAI to chemotherapy alone but rather to pelvic radiation therapy plus chemotherapy with a single alkylating agent. It is unclear whether the pelvic radiation therapy impacted outcomes negatively, favorably, or not at all.

The results for several retrospective series utilizing WAI as primary therapy are shown in Table 11–3. Consistently demonstrated are 5- and 10-year survival rates and median survivals at least equivalent to those obtained with modern systemic agents. Difficulties encountered in applying the results of these randomized and nonrandomized trials to current clinical practice include, in some or all studies, use of chemotherapy, with a single alkylating agent lack of stratification prior to randomization leading to imbalances in treatment arms, limited statistical analysis, short follow-up, and inadequate radiation therapy. Given these shortcomings, the lack of consensus regarding

TABLE 11-2
Randomized Trials Using Whole Abdominal Irradiation in Stage I to III Ovarian Carcinoma

STUDY	STAGE	TREATMENT	OUTCOME
Klaassen et al[2]	I–IIIB (n = 257)	WAI (n = 107)	62% 5-yr DFS
		Pelvis RT plus melphalan (n = 106)	61% 5-yr DFS
Smith et al[5]	I (n = 42)	WAI	85% 2-yr DFS
		Melphalan	90% 2-yr DFS
	II (n = 66)	WAI	55% 2-yr DFS
		Melphalan	58% 2-yr DFS
	III (n = 40)	WAI	53% 2-yr DFS
		Melphalan	35% 2-yr DFS
Dembo et al[8]	I–III (n = 101)	WAI	81% 5-yr survival
	Completed BSOH	Pelvic RT plus chlorambucil	51% 5-yr survival
Sell et al[9]	I–II (n = 118)	WAI	63% 4-yr survival
		Pelvic RT plus cyclophosphamide	55% 4-yr survival

Abbreviations: RT, Radiation therapy; DFS, disease-free survival; BSOH, bilateral salpingo-oophorectomy and hysterectomy; WAI, whole abdominal irradiation.

the role of WAI is understandable. However, outcomes from these trials and series suggest strongly that WAI remains an important modality in the treatment of patients with stage I and II and selected stage III ovarian carcinoma felt to be at significant risk of relapse who have minimal residual disease following initial surgery.

Patient Selection

The detailed analysis of prognostic factors among patients treated with WAI stands as a major contribution from Dembo.[14] Considering pathologic type, stage, histologic grade, amount of residual disease following initial surgery, and patient age as independent and interdependent variables, Dembo placed patients into low, intermediate, and high-risk subgroups using a combination of stage, residual disease, and histology (Table 11–4).

Radiation Therapy Technique, Doses, and Fields

External beam radiation therapy techniques for ovarian carcinoma have evolved considerably over the past two decades. Limited treatment volumes such as pelvic radiation therapy have been recognized as inadequate based on prospective surgical staging information.[21] The appropriate treatment volume must include all peritoneal surfaces, accounting for beam divergence, patient movement, and setup variations.[22] The propensity of ovarian carcinoma to spread to the undersurface of the diaphragm requires that liver shielding be limited or absent. The ability to achieve large field sizes without patient movement has led to the replacement of moving strip techniques with open field opposed anterior and posterior fields and to a lower daily dose (typically 100 to 150 cGy/day). These refinements appear to have reduced the late morbidity from WAI.[23]

Care should be taken to include the entire peritoneal cavity in the radiation fields. Appropriate kidney localization and blocking should be undertaken to make sure that tolerance is not exceeded. Whole abdominal doses should be limited to 25 to 30 Gy. The use of routine pelvic boosts should be avoided, although boosts to sites of gross disease following initial surgery are recommended.

An important prognostic factor is adequacy of the radiation therapy. Lanciano and Randall[24] published a compiled list of series in

TABLE 11-3
Nonrandomized Trials Using WAI in Stage I to III Ovarian Carcinoma

STUDY	STAGE	RESIDUUM	OUTCOME	MEDIAN SURVIVAL (YR)
Martinez et al[10]	I–III (n = 152)	≤2 cm	66% 5-yr FFR	>4
Leers and Kock[11]	III	None or small		>6
Weiser et al[12]	II–III (n = 102)	None ≤2 cm	59% 10-yr survival 42% 10-yr survival	>10 6
Goldberg and Peschel[13]	II–III (n = 74)	Favorable group	79% 10-yr survival	>10
Dembo[14]	II (n = 36) III (n = 101)	≤2 cm ≤2 cm	58% 5-yr survival 45% 5-yr survival	>5
Fuller et al[15]	I–III (n = 106)	≤2 cm	71% 10-yr DFS	>10
Van Bunningen et al[16]	High-risk I–II (n = 85)	None	Stage I–IIA: 91% 5-yr DFS Stage IIB–C: 56% 5-yr DFS	>6 >6
Lindner et al[17]	I–III (n = 84)	Usually <2 cm	Stage I: 80% 5-yr survival Stage II: 64% 5-yr survival Stage III: 35% 5-yr survival	>5 >5 3
Hart et al[18]	I–II (n = 31)	Unknown	Stage I: 81% 5-yr survival Stage II: 36% 5-yr survival	>5
Hammond et al[19]	I–III (n = 59)	≤2 cm		5.5
Macbeth et al[20]	I–III (n = 57)	≤2 cm	57% 5-yr survival 49% 5-yr DFS	>5

Abbreviations: FFR, Freedom from relapse; DFS, disease-free survival.

TABLE 11-4
Prognostic Groupings for Stage I, II, III Ovarian Carcinoma[a]

STAGE	RESIDUUM	SER + CLR, WD	MUC + END	SER + CLR, PD, UND
I PD	0	—	Intermediate risk	Intermediate risk
II	0	Intermediate risk	Intermediate risk	Intermediate risk
II	Small	Intermediate risk	Intermediate risk	High risk
III	0	Intermediate risk	Intermediate risk	High risk
III	Small	Intermediate risk	High risk	High risk

Abbreviations: PD, Poorly or moderately differentiated or grades 2 and 3; WD, well-differentiated; MUC, mucinous carcinoma, END, endometrioid carcinoma; CLR, clear cell carcinoma; UND, undifferentiated carcinoma.

[a] *Definition of two patient subgroups according to stage, residuum, and histologic features in stages I, II, and III with BSOH performed (i.e., small or no macroscopic residuum). Patients with stage I, grade 1, tumors are excluded. In 36% of patients classified as having small residuum, the lesions were 2 cm or larger. (From Dembo[14])*

which radiation therapy (not always WAI) was administered to patients with stage I to III ovarian carcinoma. The superiority of outcomes in series administering WAR using current concepts and techniques was clearly evident. In the randomized series from the NCIC there was a clear correlation between violations of WAR protocol and outcome.[2]

DANIEL S. KAPP

The role of radiation therapy as primary postoperative treatment for epithelial ovarian cancer

Over the past 30 years strong evidence has accumulated supporting the role of postoperative whole abdominopelvic radiation therapy (WAR) in the treatment of selected patients with epithelial ovarian cancer. The patient selection criteria for postoperative WAR is based on the amount of residual disease prior to radiation and the limitations of normal tissue tolerance. Patients satisfying vigorous selection criteria have achieved long-term survival rates comparable to those obtained with postoperative chemotherapy in similarly selected patient groups. To ensure optimum results with WAR careful attention must be directed to appropriate field size, dose, and amount and location of residual disease.

Field Size

Evidence of a need for the use of radiation fields including the whole abdominal pelvic volume rather than more limited pelvic field treatment comes from four sources: (1) results of staging studies on patterns of spread of epithelial ovarian cancer, (2) analysis of patterns of failure in nonrandomized studies comparing WAR with pelvic radiation, (3) results of randomized trials comparing WAR versus pelvic radiation, and (4) quality assurance analysis of WAR fields.

STAGING STUDIES Through roentgenologic and surgical staging evaluation including biopsies of the para-aortic lymph nodes and the diaphragmatic surfaces has revealed occult disease in these areas in patients who were otherwise felt to have stage I or II disease.[25–28] For example, Knapp and Friedman,[25] reported a 13% (3 of 24 patients) incidence of positive para-aortic lymph node biopsies in patients with otherwise stage I disease. Similarly, Knipscheer[26] reported a 25% incidence (5 of 20) of para-aortic nodal involvement in patients with otherwise stage I epithelial ovarian cancer. In the latter study para-aortic lymph node involvement was noted in 4 of 17 patients with otherwise stage IA or IB disease and 1 of 3 patients with otherwise stage IC disease.

Results of systematic restaging were reported in 100 patients with a diagnosis of stage IA to IIB epithelial ovarian cancer, 92 of whom were believed to be free of disease.[27] Thirty-one of these patients were upstaged. Repeat laparotomies in 68 patients revealed para-aortic involvement in 12%, omental involvement in 11%, other intra-abdominal disease in 9%, and diaphragmatic involvement in 3%.[27]

PATTERNS OF FAILURE IN NONRANDOMIZED STUDIES Several series have demonstrated a high rate of failure in the untreated upper abdomen when patients with epithelial ovarian cancer received lower abdominal or pelvic radiation following initial surgery. Schray et al[29] reported their results for lower abdominal radiotherapy as primary postoperative treatment in 82 patients with stage I to III cancer. Thirty-seven percent of all relapses occurred in the untreated upper abdomen. For 36 patients with no gross residual disease, 4 of 7 relapses occurred in the upper abdomen; for 26 patients with minimal residual disease of less than 2 cm, 5 of 13 relapses were in the upper abdomen. In patients with stage I and II disease 10 of 19 failures were in the upper abdomen.

Fuller et al[15] retrospectively compared the results for WAR (42 patients) with those for various subtotal abdominopelvic techniques (64 patients) in women who received primary postoperative radiation therapy. In a favorable subgroup of 32 patients with stage I to IIIA disease, no postoperative residual, less than

2 cm pelvic residum and/or less than 0.5 cm abdominal residum, a 71% 10-year actuarial relapse-free survival was reported following WAR compared with 40% for patients (46) who were treated by subtotal abdominopelvic techniques ($P \leq 0.02$). When adjustments were made for differences in stage, grade, and postoperative residual disease volumes by the method of Cox, the survival improvement associated with the use of WAR in favorable patients became even more significant ($P \leq 0.003$).

RANDOMIZED TRIALS The results of the above retrospective studies which strongly suggested the value of WAR in comparison to smaller-field postoperative treatments were confirmed in randomized trials conducted at the Princess Margaret Hospital.[8] Patients with stage IB and II disease were randomized to receive pelvic radiation, pelvic radiation plus chlorambucil for 2 years, or WAR. Patients with asymptomatic stage III disease were randomized between the latter two treatments. For the 132 patients in this study in whom the bilateral salpingo-oophorectomy and hysterectomy was completed, the 5-year actuarial relapse-free survival rate was approximately 30% higher in patients treated with WAR (78%), compared with those treated with pelvic radiation therapy alone (47%) or pelvic radiation plus chlorambucil (45%). Similarly there was an approximately 25% improvement in long-term control of the upper abdomen (plus or minus distant metastases) (0 of 50 failures) in those receiving WAR compared to pelvic radiation alone (27% failures) or pelvic radiation plus chlorambucil (25% failures). Pelvic failures (plus or minus abdominal) were similar for all three groups (20 to 27%).[8]

QUALITY ASSURANCE STUDY Further support for the curative potential of WAR is provided from the quality assurance analysis of the radiation fields used in the treatment of patients in the NCIC clinical trial in early-stage ovarian cancer.[2] This study included patients with stage I or IIA high-risk epithelial ovarian carcinoma (rupture of malignant ovarian cyst, grade 3 cancer, extracystic excrescences, or positive peritoneal cytology) or stage IIB or III with disease confined to the pelvis. Following surgical staging, patients were randomized to WAR, melphalan, or intraperitoneal chromic phosphate. All patients also initially received pelvic radiation. A detailed review of the coverage of the WAR portals was undertaken with scores given for inadequacy of coverage of the diaphragms, lateral borders of the abdomen, and pelvis. Although no significant differences in survival rates were observed among the three treatment arms, patients with higher violation scores on quality assurance for coverage of the whole abdominal target volume had significantly poorer survival ($P = 0.01$) and disease-free survival ($P = 0.02$) than those with lower violation scores. Patients without violations in coverage of the whole abdominal target volume had a 5-year survival rate of 76% compared with 32% for those with a high score (≥ 6) for field violations. These results support the hypothesis that properly administered whole abdominal pelvic radiation with relatively low doses as used in this study (2250 cGy) can result in high survival rates for selected patients with epithelial ovarian cancer.

The value of computerized tomography (CT) scan treatment planning studies to ensure adequate coverage of the entire peritoneal surface in WAR for ovarian neoplasm has subsequently been investigated.[30] Twenty-one consecutive patients were prospectively studied comparing fields based on routine simulation films, with those drawn following CT scans demonstrating the peritoneal target volumes. Dose-volume histograms were calculated for the amount of target volume missed by the routine simulation film-generated fields. For all patients, treatment plans with simulation films missed the peritoneal volumes compared with CT scans with a medium of 137.9 cm^3 volume missed (range 1 to 837.3 cm^3). The use of CT planning and three dimensional dosimetry to ensure optimal peritoneal coverage warrants further study.

Radiation Dose

NORMAL TISSUE LIMITATIONS The dose that can be safely given to the whole abdominal pelvic field is limited by the normal tissue tolerance of critical organs included within this volume. The dose associated with a 5% rate of renal complications occurring within 5 years of treatment ($TD_{5/5}$) is approximately 20 Gy, while the dose associated with a 50% risk for kidney complication over the same time span ($TD_{50/5}$) is approximately 25 Gy.[31] This severely limits the dose that can be given in the areas in front of and behind the kidneys using our standard anterior-posterior and posterior-anterior opposed fields. The $TD_{5/5}$ (25 Gy) and the $TD_{50/5}$ (40 Gy) of the liver set upper limits for doses to the entire liver.[31] Somewhat higher doses are tolerated for smaller cone-down boosts (e.g., to the diaphragmatic surfaces of the liver). Spinal cord tolerance doses ($TD_{5/5}$ = 45 Gy) limit the doses to the para-aortic lymph nodes if only anterior-posterior opposed fields are utilized. Oblique field off-cord boosts can be given to areas of more bulky disease. Intestinal tolerance ($TD_{5/5}$ = 45 to 50 Gy) also limits overall upper abdominal peritoneal surface doses. The higher tolerances of the rectum ($TD_{5/5}$ = 60 Gy) and urinary bladder ($TD_{5/5}$ = 60 Gy) permit higher pelvic doses to be given and safely allow boost doses to limited cone-down pelvic fields that may encompass parts of these organs. The use of intraoperative radiation therapy permits the dose to surrounding normal tissues to be minimized and facilitates even higher doses to be safely given to limited regions containing bulk residual disease.

RADIATION DOSES FOR TUMOR CONTROL Extrapolating from previous experience in the treatment of adenocarcinoma of the breast and squamous cell carcinoma of the head and neck, Wharton and Fletcher[32] have suggested that the dose needed for a 50% chance of tumor control (TCD_{50}) of subclinical disease is approximately 30 Gy and that 90% control (TCD_{90}) would be obtained with 50 Gy. For 2-cm residual masses the TCD_{50} was 50 Gy, while the TCD_{90} was 60 Gy. For masses between 2 and 4 cm the TCD_{50} was approximately 60 Gy, with a TCD_{90} of 70 Gy. More recent attempts to update these estimates have yielded similar results. A composite from 62 dose-response curves for control of macroscopic residual tumors revealed a mean TCD_{50} of 50 Gy and a median TCD_{50} of 51.9 Gy.[33] From an analysis of 28 studies on elective therapy for possible microscopic residual cancer after surgical removal, the mean TCD_{50} was 39.3 Gy and the median TCD_{50} was 37.9 Gy.[33] Similarly, dose-response data for control of subclinical disease were compiled by Withers et al[34] and indicated that high control rates for subclinical metastases could be obtained for doses of 50 Gy in 2-Gy fractions. They also noted that worthwhile benefits could be achieved with lower doses. Their tumor control probability curves shared a shallow shoulder and an intercept near zero, suggesting that even low doses on the order of 30 Gy had approximately a 50% chance of eliminating recurrences. Since there may be great variability in the number of clonogens remaining in sites of occult residual disease or after gross surgical debulking (1.0 to 10^8 cells) relatively low doses of radiation may be useful, particularly when the clonogenic number is at the low end of this range.[35]

The results of several studies, including those by Schray et al, which used lower abdominal radiation therapy for the treatment of stage I to III epithelial cancers, support these dose-response concepts.[29] Employing postsurgical radiation therapy with doses between 50 Gy and 55 Gy, control within the treated lower abdomen was 97% in patients with no residual disease, 84% in patients with residual disease less than 2 cm and 55% in patients with residual disease greater than 2 cm.[29]

Sites of Residual Disease

Because of the normal tissue limitations on radiation dose as described above, the sites of residual disease also influence the outcome of postoperative radiation therapy in epithelial ovarian cancers.[36] Patients with residual disease sites that can be treated with higher total doses (e.g., para-aortic lymph nodes, pelvic residuum) have a better prognosis than those with residuum in other sites (e.g., upper abdomen). Fuks[37] reported on a series of 10 patients who had para-aortic node involvement as their only site of stage III disease. These women were treated with pelvic radiation plus para-aortic nodal radiation (doses of 50 to 55 Gy) and achieved a 5-year survival rate of 53%. This was similar to the survival obtained in patients with stage II disease treated with postoperative radiation therapy, and considerably higher than that for other stage III patients with peritoneal metastases.

Schray and colleagues[29] analyzed their results for postoperative radiation therapy in patients with disease limited to the lower abdomen and pelvis as defined at the time of surgical staging. These women received full-dose lower abdominal radiation therapy (mostly in the range of 50 to 54 Gy). Eighty-two had stage I to III disease and had an overall freedom from relapse survival of 57% at 10 years. The freedom from relapse was a function of residual disease and ranged from 79% in patients with no residual disease to 49% for those with less than 2 cm residuum, to 24% with those with greater than 2 cm residuum. Martinez et al reported similar results in an updated analysis.[10] For patients with stage II disease (by definition, disease limited to the pelvis only), those with no residual disease at the time of radiation had a 5-year relapse-free survival of 83% compared to those with minimal residual disease (< 2 cm) who had a 5-year survival of 64%. In stage III patients with no residual disease, a 68% 5-year survival was obtained, but with minimal residual disease they had only a 54% 5-year survival. In patients with more bulky disease (>2 cm) poor 5-year survival rates (20%) were reported. Additional studies have also shown that patients with residual disease limited to the pelvis or minimal residual disease in the abdomen have improved survivals following WAR, compared with patients treated with various subtotal abdominopelvic techniques.[15]

Results of Radiation Therapy in Various Subgroups

Over the past 16 years numerous trials from around the world have demonstrated high long-term survivals achieved with postoperative WAR in subsets of favorable patients with optimally debulked disease (usually taken as residual disease <2 cm or <2 cm in the pelvis and/or <0.5 cm in the upper abdomen). Patient selection criteria for the use of WAR were somewhat more variable in terms of stage, grade, and histologic subtype. These factors, as well as the thoroughness of surgical staging and the quality of the radiation therapy, contribute to the variation in the results obtained. Many authors have attempted to define an intermediate-risk subgroup of patients treated with WAR similar to that originally defined by Dembo.[14] This intermediate-risk group represents approximately one-third of the total population of patients with ovarian cancer[14] and has a 5-year survival rate following WAR of approximately 60 to 80%. Considerably poorer results are noted for a high-risk group of patients who had bulky (>2 cm) postsurgical residual disease. Table 11–5 summarizes the results of postoperative treatment of epithelial ovarian cancer with WAR for selected subgroups of patients.

Complications of WAR

In general, the use of WAR as primary postoperative treatment is well tolerated with modest acute complications and less than a 10% risk of serious late complications. A review of 598 patients treated at the Princess Margaret Hospital with WAR for ovarian cancer revealed acute nausea and vomiting in 61%, which was severe in only 6% of the entire group.[23] Diarrhea was noted in 68% of patients but was severe in only 6%. Only 10% of patients did not complete the planned WAR treatment, most frequently because of myelosuppression (16 patients). Late complications included diarrhea (14%) and symptomatic pneumonitis (4%). Bowel obstruction developed in 4.2%, and 2.7% of patients required surgery for their bowel problems. Multivariate analysis failed to identify any significant prognostic factors for bowel obstruction. Moving-strip technique (versus open-field radiation technique) was associated with a higher incidence of chronic diarrhea and pneumonitis.[23] No pa-

TABLE 11-5
Long-Term Survival in Selected Epithelial Ovarian Cancer Patients Treated with WAI

STUDY/YEAR	SELECTION CRITERIA		NO. OF PATIENTS	SURVIVAL RATE	COMMENTS
	STAGE	OTHER			
Haas et al[38] (1980)	I		29	96% 5 yr	81% >2-yr SR for stage III patients with no palpable residual tumor
	II		13	60% 5 yr	
	III		37	60% 5 yr	
Dembo[14] (1985)	I–III	Intermediate-risk group	224	75% 5 yr	5-yr SR for stage III patients with no or uncertain residuum, <2 cm or ≥2 cm residuum were 48%, 43%, and 18% respectively
	II–III	High-risk group	117	19% 5 yr	
Leers and Kock[11] (1987)	I–III	No or only small residuum	127	71% 5 yr	5-yr SR for completely staged patients was 78% compared with 61% for those incompletely staged
Fuller et al[15] (1987)	I–IIIA	No residuum	20	77% 10 yr	Overall 71% 5-yr SR
	I–IIIA	<2 cm pelvic and/or <0.5 cm abdominal residuum	12	62% 10 yr	
Weiser et al[12] (1988)	II–III	No gross residuum	24	69% 5 yr (59% 10 yr)	
	II–III	<2 cm residuum	24	48% 5 yr (42% 10 yr)	Stage III patients with ≤2 cm residuum had 10-yr SR of 40%
	II–III	>2 cm residuum	20	15% 5 yr (10% 10 yr)	
Macbeth et al[20] (1988)	I–III	No gross residuum (stage III had limited disease outside pelvis)	57	57% 5 yr	
van Bunningen et al[16] (1988)	I, IIA	Moderately or poorly differentiated	85	75% 5 yr (NED)	IA, IB, IIA: 91% 5-yr NED SR; IC, IIB, IIC: 50% 5-yr NED SR
	IIB, IIC	All grades; no gross residuum			

(*Continues*)

TABLE 11-5
(Continued)

STUDY/YEAR	SELECTION CRITERIA: STAGE	SELECTION CRITERIA: OTHER	NO. OF PATIENTS	SURVIVAL RATE	COMMENTS
Klaassen et al[2] (1988)	I or IIA	With rupture, excrescences, grade 3, or positive cytology	107	62% 5 yr	Patients with no whole abdominal target volume violations: 76% 5-yr SR
	IIB or III	With disease confined to pelvis			
Goldberg and Peschel[13] (1988)	I–III	Intermediate-risk group[a]	60	77% 10 yr	Results comparable to Princess Margaret Hospital risk grouping
	I–III	High-risk group[a]	14	7% 10 yr	
Lindner et al[17] (1990)	I–III	Intermediate-risk group[a]	59	75% 5 yr	Overall 64% 5-yr SR
	I–III	High-risk group[a]	16	20% 5 yr	
Sell et al[8] (1990)	IB, IC, II		60	63% 4 yr	Intermediate risk group[a]: 62% 4-yr SR
Hammond et al[19] (1992)	I–III	≤2 cm residuum	59	45% 5 yr (serous tumors)	Patients with no or minimal residuum: 60% 5-yr SR
Thomas et al[39] (1994)	T_1–T_3	No residuum (54); microscopic (4); ≤2 cm (4)	62	67% 5 yr	5-yr SR for T_1, T_2, T_3 were 87%, 63%, 50%, respectively

Abbreviations: SR, Survival rate; NED, no evidence of disease.
[a] *As per classification of Dembo.*[14]

tients died of radiation-induced second malignancies. This is in contrast to patients with epithelial ovarian cancers treated with chemotherapy (especially melphalan) in whom a high incidence of second cancers has been reported.[40] Similar rates of acute toxicity and late complications were reported in the other series cited in Table 11–5.

QUESTION 2

What is the role, if any, of radiation therapy in the salvage setting?

MARCUS E. RANDALL
GILLIAN M. THOMAS

Sequential chemotherapy and radiation therapy in advanced disease

There is a strong theoretical basis supporting the use of combined multimodality therapy for the treatment of advanced ovarian cancer. That theory suggests that if there is no cross-resistance of the tumor to various modalities, one can obtain maximal cell kill and therapeutic index by exploiting the cytoreductive capacity of all three modalities, namely, surgery, chemotherapy, and radiation, in ovarian cancer, providing they could be combined in a form having acceptable toxicity and without diminishing their individual efficacy. The rationale for the use of consolidation therapy after initial surgery and chemotherapy has been the observation by many groups that approximately 50% of patients without pathologically documented residual disease at second-look laparotomy following primary chemotherapy subsequently relapse and die of disease.[41–45] Overall cure rates in advanced disease using the standard accepted therapy of surgery followed by chemotherapy are still only 20 to 30%.[46] That radiation therapy should be considered a modality for exploring for consolidation treatment of patients with no overt residual disease or microscopic residual disease is reasonable, given that it has been shown to be of curative value as the sole postoperative therapy in certain subsets of patients.[14] It was, therefore, natural to consider that combinations of surgery, chemotherapy, and radiation can offer a possible treatment advantage and are therefore worthy of exploration in advanced disease.

The other setting in which there was a theoretical basis for the use of sequential multimodality therapy is as salvage treatment for patients with residual disease of varying amounts after initial surgery, chemotherapy, and possible further cytoreduction at second-look laparotomy.

Efficacy

The literature is replete with reports of single-arm observational studies on groups of patients treated initially with debulking surgery followed by chemotherapy usually consisting of platinum or platinum analog-containing combinations, subsequent surgery to assess response with planned maximal cytoreduction, and WAI with or without boosts to the pelvis or sites of bulk residuum. Most of these studies have small patient numbers, lack satisfactory controls, and have short follow-up durations. A recent review[47] documented that patient numbers were often small in these series, between 8 and 44.[48–75] The selection of patients was by no means uniform, with some series including patients with no residuum and others including patients with microscopic or macroscopic residual disease in sites throughout the abdomen and pelvis, or even patients with recurrent disease after surgery and multiple courses of chemotherapy.[64–66,75] Others excluded patients with greater than 5 mm residuum.[50,53,72] Many patients received prolonged chemotherapy initially, with up to 22 courses of cyclophosphamide and platinum,[74] and most series reported 6 to 12 courses of second-line chemotherapy after first-line failure.[55] Patients with induction chemotherapy-resistant tumors were included in some series.

The volume most commonly irradiated was the whole abdomen and pelvis, but techniques varied from open-field irradiation most commonly to moving-strip or sequential split-field therapy.[56,62,67,71] WAI doses varied between 20 Gy and 30 Gy.[56,66,67,69,74] Most studies planned a routine boost to the pelvis regardless of the site of residual disease. Several series also employed a boost to the para-aortic nodes.[48,59,60] The results of these studies have been variously interpreted as positive, negative, or equivocal by the individual investigators. Thus, it is disappointing that although a large number of patients have been treated in many series with multimodality therapy including salvage consolidation therapy, it is impossible from these uncontrolled data to reach any definite conclusions about the value of such a strategy or to precisely define the patients who might benefit from it. Overall, the balance of evidence in these studies is against a significant curative benefit for radiation therapy as salvage or consolidation therapy, at least in the situations where it has been used. However, because of the diversity of criteria for patient selection, the variability of the chemotherapy, surgery, and radiation employed, sweeping negative generalizations about results of trials should be interpreted with caution.

The literature contains only four randomized trials that have as their stated purpose a randomized comparison of WAI with further chemotherapy in patients with small volumes of residual disease after second-look laparotomy, sometimes with cytoreduction.[49–52] The study by Bruzzoni et al randomized 20 patients to radiation therapy and 21 to three further courses of platinum-based chemotherapy if there was no or minimal residual disease at second-look laparotomy. Unfortunately, the two arms were not well balanced for the amount of residual disease after second-look operation, with more patients in the chemotherapy arm without residual disease. The median follow-up was only 22 months, and although the authors have concluded that there is a survival advantage for the chemotherapy, the numbers are too small to draw meaningful conclusions. An Italian study[51] reported in abstract form only compared twice daily fractionated WAI to cisplatin/cyclophosphamide/epirubicin as consolidation therapy after first-line cisplatin-based chemotherapy. Only 64 of 79 patients are evaluable, numbers too small to allow for meaningful conclusions to be drawn. In a similar study conducted by the North Thames Group,[50] 117 patients with less than 2 cm disease after five cycles of carboplatin were randomized between consolidative WAI and a further five cycles of carboplatin. The authors concluded that there was no significant advantage for consolidation with radiation compared to that of continuing with the same chemotherapy. This study is significantly flawed since nearly 20% of patients eligible for randomization were not randomized to the appropriate treatment. Furthermore, the inclusion of a significant number of patients with macroscopic, although less than 2-cm, residual disease in the upper abdomen, precludes the possibility of a survival advantage when radiation therapy is used. A discussion of the possible selection factors predicting benefits from consolidation therapy follows.

In summary, the balance of evidence to date from nonrandomized and randomized trials suggests that there is unlikely to be a large survival benefit for WAI following platinum-based chemotherapy and surgery. Similar data exist for the use of intraperitoneal chromic phosphate when used in the salvage or consolidation setting. The data from Varia et al[76] suggest a possible survival benefit but multiple other studies[77–79] do not provide evidence of benefit.

Before completely discarding sequential multimodality therapy, it is important to examine alternate explanations for failure to show improvement in survival other than the ineffectiveness of the therapy or the strategy employed. It is also important to try to characterize patients who might benefit from sequential treatment. Most series had insufficient patients to perform meaningful analyses of possible prognostic factors determining the observed outcome, but the analysis by Schray et al[60] was useful. A multivariate analysis of factors significant for disease-free survival established significance for tumor grade, initial amount of residuum prior to chemotherapy, patient age and, most importantly, amount of residual disease at the time of radiation therapy. While the numbers were small, it appeared that the percentage surviving and survival time were related to the presence or absence of or one or more of these significant factors. If no favorable factors were present, 0% (0 of 17) remain disease-free, with one factor present 29% (n = 14), with two factors present 53% (8 of 15), and with three factors present 67% (4 of 6). Rosen et al,[66] in a small series, suggested that tumor grade might correlate with survival. Data extracted from 28 literature series of sequential therapy, based on 473 patients and with sufficient information to estimate the volume of residual disease, suggested that survival was predicted by the amount of tumor residuum prior to radiation therapy: no residuum 76%, microscopic or less than 5 mm 49%, and macroscopic only 17%.[47] Thus, in order to critically examine whether sequential therapy has therapeutic value, patient selection should be confined to those most likely to benefit from curative-intent WAI given as the sole postoperative therapy. Multifactorial classification of patients developed, refined, and validated in Toronto delineates patients most likely to benefit from primary postoperative chemotherapy.[14,80–82] Radiation therapy is appropriate only as the sole postoperative therapy for patients with no macroscopic disease in the upper abdomen and with small (less than 1 cm) or no macroscopic residual disease in the pelvis. If radiation therapy is not beneficial as initial therapy because of biological factors that may be operative, it would be even less beneficial in similar patients who have already received extensive surgery, including secondary debulking and chemotherapy, to which resistance may have already been demonstrated.

Thus, it is probable that treatment strategies employing sequential multimodality therapy including WAI will benefit only a small, select group of patients. Patient selection should be based on identification of those most likely to fail after negative second-look laparotomy combined with an assessment of the likelihood of benefit from radiation therapy.

It would be appropriate to study the role of radiation therapy patients who have a negative second-look laparotomy after chemotherapy but who are at high risk for late relapse, such as patients with large residual stage III presentations before chemotherapy, those over 50 years of age, and those with grade 3 tumors.[83] Other patients who might benefit are those with microscopic positive second-look laparotomies where the tumor is well differentiated.

The constituent modalities of sequential therapy to be investigated must be chosen to minimize acute and late toxicities.

Radiation Therapy Technique and Accompanying Toxicity

The choice of radiation therapy technique and the dose for sequential therapy are critical to provide the maximum therapeutic ratio. The high degree of toxicity from WAI encountered in some studies has resulted in delayed or incomplete treatment and might be another explanation for the observed treatment failure in some studies.

Reports on the use of WAI after chemotherapy have suggested higher bowel complication rates than when radiation therapy is used alone. Surgical detail is lacking, but many patients in the published series have undergone three or four laparotomies, often with maximal attempts at cytoreduction prior to radiation therapy.[56] In one series, one-third of patients had undergone pelvic exenteration as part of their sequential therapy.[64] While primary cytoreductive surgery is important in the initial treatment of patients with advanced ovarian cancer, it is unlikely that second, third, and fourth attempts to surgically debulk will contribute to survival although they will likely contribute to increased bowel toxicity. Similarly, protracted courses of multiagent chemotherapy lead to a decreased probability that adequate-dose radiation therapy can be completed in a timely fashion, if at all.[66] There is now general agreement that extending chemotherapy past six cycles is unlikely to provide additional benefit but will likely contribute to further suppression of bone marrow function. Last, inappropriately high radiation doses both to the upper abdomen and pelvis may lead to an increasing risk of complications if multimodality therapy is used. The use of WAI doses in excess of 22 to 25 Gy in 22 to 25 fractions may result in unacceptable long-term morbidity for surviving patients. A study from Toronto suggested that higher radiation doses given to patients following multiple previous abdominal explorations or second-look laparotomies correlated with an increasing risk of complications.[84] If sequential multimodality therapy is to be tested, it is important to minimize the risk of complications and maximize the probability of completing radiation therapy by restricting the radiation dose in patients who have had second-look surgery and by limiting the chemotherapy to six courses of the best available agents. Complication rates are acceptable when these guidelines are followed, and serious complications occur in 10 to 13% of patients. It is unclear that the routine addition of a pelvic boost to consolidation or salvage radiation therapy is useful. If this is the only known site of residual disease, it may be a reasonable strategy, but if there is no gross residual disease, the value of boosting the pelvis is unclear. When macroscopic disease is present in the upper abdomen, we do not believe that salvage radiation therapy should be employed. However, if the site of macroscopic residuum prior to chemotherapy is in a site other than the pelvis, it may not be unreasonable to boost this site with some additional treatment.

Strategies for Investigating Sequential Multimodality Treatment

Research strategies that require investigation are the result of a better knowledge of tumor biology and the identification of Taxol as an effective agent in treating ovarian carcinoma. To date, there have been no reported studies on patients treated with WAI following Taxol chemotherapy; therefore, short- and long-term complications with this strategy are unknown. However, since Taxol is becoming first-line chemotherapy for most patients, it seems appropriate to initiate phase I studies to investigate the tolerance of such sequential treatment before looking at its role in randomized studies.

Unfavorable biological phenomena might limit the curative potential of radiation therapy given on a daily basis for salvage or consolidation. While it is hoped that subsequent radiation therapy may provide cytotoxicity independent of that from cisplatin chemotherapy, tumor cellular cross-resistance may exist between the two.[85] Thus, tumor persisting after cisplatin chemotherapy may be relatively radioresistant also. Prolonged cytoreductive therapy may be associated with accelerated proliferation of clonogenic tumor cells.[86] This means that protraction of planned radiation therapy may result in diminished local control rates. This may be a particularly important factor when this modality is used in a salvage setting where the large radiation volume and tolerance of the bowel limit the radiation dose that can be given daily or cumulatively. Therefore there is a rationale for attempting to overcome the theoretical problem of accelerated proliferation and the resultant increase in residual clonogenic cells by the use of multiple daily fractions of radiation. Limited data are available pertinent to the use of hyperfractionated WAI as salvage treatment.[74] It appears that a tolerable regimen has been established—3,040 cGy at 80 cGy per fraction twice daily—but the utility of such an approach remains to be demonstrated.[87] Unfortunately, the design and conduct of trials for establishing the utility of sequential surgery, chemotherapy, and radiotherapy are not trivial. Such studies could be performed only under the auspices of a large cooperative group.

Palliative radiation therapy in ovarian cancer

Recurrent or persistent ovarian carcinoma following curative-intent chemotherapy is, unfortunately, common. Although median survivals are typically short among patients with widespread disease refractory to further chemotherapy, patients with more localized recurrences, particularly those limited to the pelvis, are likely to have appreciably longer survivals.[88,89] Davidson et al[90] reported their experience with limited-field radiation therapy in patients with localized persistent or recurrent disease, finding it to be well tolerated with limited acute or late morbidity, even in patients heavily pretreated with systemic and intraperitoneal chemotherapy. Furthermore, median actuarial survival and progression-free survival of 40 and 14 months, respectively, were observed. Although the ultimate in-field recurrence rates were high, the authors concluded that limited-field radiation therapy is an appropriate management option in patients with recurrent or persistent pelvic or retroperitoneal disease.

Other authors have evaluated the potential of radiation therapy for palliative symptoms related to recurrent ovarian cancer. May et al[89] studied 38 patients with chemotherapy-refractory disease who were treated palliatively with 55 courses of T.[89] Vaginal bleeding, dyspnea, symptomatic brain metastases, bowel obstruction of a localized nature, and pain were effectively palliated in most cases. Responses were not seen in patients with lower-extremity edema. Corn et al[91] analyzed 33 patients irradiated with palliative intent to 47 sites, also evaluating potential prognostic factors relating to radiation therapy response. An overall palliative response of 79% was reported, complete in 51%. Pulmonary symptoms, vaginal and rectal bleeding, and pain showed palliative response rates of at least 75%. Higher performance status and radiation dose (biologically effective dose ≥44, $\alpha/\beta = 10$) were significantly associated with complete symptomatic response. Both these series emphasized the importance and effectiveness of short overall treatment times in patients with limited life expectancies; Corn et al suggested a regimen of 35 Gy in 14 fractions.

The frequency and management of cerebral metastasis from ovarian cancer have become subjects of debate. With increasingly effective systemic therapy, the ability of the central nervous system (CNS) to act as a sanctuary site limiting penetration of chemotherapy could account for the greater incidence of CNS relapse reported by a number of authors.[92–97] Hardy and Harvey have even postulated a role of prophylactic cranial radiation therapy in patients achieving a complete remission with chemotherapy.[98] Other series have reported the continued rarity of CNS relapse in ovarian cancer.[99–100] Although the preponderance of the evidence suggests a somewhat higher incidence than previously appreciated, CNS relapse remains sufficiently uncommon to make a role for prophylactic cranial radiation therapy unlikely.

Whole-brain radiation therapy has been considered standard management in patients with documented cerebral metastases. Recently, the relative efficacy of radiation therapy and chemotherapy has been questioned based on a series of three patients without extracranial disease treated with carboplatin chemotherapy, one of whom achieved a complete initial response.[101] However, Corn et al reported on a series of 32 patients who received radiation therapy for symptomatic brain metastases, finding symptomatic responses in 23 patients which were maintained until death in 71%. Morbidity from radiation therapy was limited to short-term side effects, and survival was significantly greater in patients with a Karnofsky performance status of 70 or greater.[102] Rodriguez et al[103] performed a meta-analysis combining patient data from their institution with that of other published series for a total of 67 patients. While recognizing the limitations of the methodology, they concluded that the addition of chemotherapy and/or surgical resection to whole-brain radiation therapy provides significantly longer survivals than radiation therapy alone. Based on these larger well-analyzed series, it seems premature to abandon this modality for treatment of ovarian cancer metastatic to the brain.

DANIEL S. KAPP

Role of radiation therapy in the salvage setting

Tumor Bulk

The potential for a long-term survival and cure using WAR following chemotherapy failures has best been demonstrated in patients with microscopic disease following repeat surgery (see Mychalczak and Fuks[104] and Thomas[47] for reviews). It may be the treatment of choice for such patients who are platinum refractory[105] or who have residual disease limited to only the pelvis.[61,106,107]

Similar prognostic factors influence the outcome of WAR for recurrent disease as noted for its use following initial surgery. These include the initial stage (especially stages I, II, III versus stage IV disease),[67,105] patient age,[39] amount of residual disease following initial debulking surgery,[60] tumor grade,[60,105,108] and perhaps most important, the amount of residual disease immediately prior to WAR. Table 11–6 summarizes the results of 28 series in which WAR was employed as salvage therapy in patients who had failed initial chemotherapy. An attempt has been made to delete patients that were included in earlier reports from the same institution and to reclassify (when necessary) patients into groupings based on the amount of residual disease noted prior to the onset of salvage WAR. Care was also taken to exclude patients from this table in whom repeat staging failed to reveal persistent disease and in whom WAR was used as consolidation rather than salvage

TABLE 11-6
Survival after WAR for Persistent or Recurrent Epithelial Cancers Following Chemotherapy Failure

STUDY/YEAR	SURVIVAL[a] MICROSCOPIC RESIDUUM	<0.5–1.0 CM RESIDUUM	>1 CM RESIDUUM	FOLLOW-UP TIME
Hainsworth et al[59] (1983)	3/11	0/5	0/1	9–20 mo
Greiner et al[57] (1984)	—	5/9	1/4	7–64 mo
Hacker et al[53] (1985)	4/16	2/6	0/8	18–48 mo
Steiner et al[109] (1985)	4/6	—	—	10–40 mo
Hoskins et al[56] (1985)	0/6	0/1	0/1	8–20 mo
Peters et al[55] (1986)	2/9	0/7	0/6	34–52 mo
Rustin et al[72] (1987)	1/4	—	—	14–59 mo
Kuten et al[62] (1988)	12/18	—	—	2-yr actual SR
Fuks et al[48] (1988)	2/11	—	—	Median 66 mo
Solomon et al[64] (1988)	2/7	4/7	0/4	4–53 mo
Green et al[110] (1988)	—	—	0/3	Median >2 yr
Schray et al[60] (1988)	8/21	—	8/31 (≤2 cm)	30–79 mo
Kersh et al[70] (1988)	3/3	7/10	1/4	Median 58 mo
Cain et al[69] (1988)	5/9	0/1	—	2–47 mo
Cheung et al[111] (1988)	5/9	—	—	12–34 mo
Shelley et al[112] (1988)	6/15	—	—	13–25 mo
Reddy et al[61] (1989)	9/16	5/14	—	5–55 mo
Hoffman et al[113] (1989)	0/6	1/5	—	4–30 mo
Stephenson and Buchler[114] (1989)	—	3/10	0/5	Median 43 mo
Chauvet et al[115] (1989)	6/12	—	2/5 (2 mm–2 cm)	—
Kucera et al[116] (1989)	1/10	0/4	1/2	3–45 mo
Bolis et al[88] (1989)	6/18	0/8	—	10–105 mo
Linstadt et al[63] (1990)	2/6	—	0/6	13–42 mo
Eifel et al[108] (1990)	5/25	—	0/12 (gross residuum)	Up to 49 mo
Chiara et al[54] (1991)	5/11	—	3/10 (<2 cm)	4–58 mo
Rothenberg et al[67] (1992)	—	2/9	—	Up to 72 mo
Thomas et al[39] (1994)	15/43	—	—	Median 67 mo
Fein et al[117] (1994)	4/11	—	2/17 (<2 cm)	Up to 9 yr
Total	110/303	29/96	18/119	
Percent	36.3	30.2	15.1	

[a] *Number of patients surviving (without progression if data available)/number at risk.*

therapy (see Question 3). Patients were divided into three separate groups: microscopic residual, minimum macroscopic residual (usually < 0.5 or 0.1 cm), and macroscopic residual (> 1 cm or up to 2 cm where indicated). The impact of the extent of residual disease on outcome is clearly seen: patients treated for microscopic residual had a recurrence-free survival of approximately 36%, which fell to approximately 15% for those with macroscopic residuals up to 2 cm. The wide variations noted between trials reflect in part the small number of patients within each trial, varying treatment techniques and doses (e.g., single fraction per day versus multifraction per day treatment, use of boost doses to the pelvis and other sites of bulk residual disease, coverage of entire peritoneal cavity with WAR fields, and percentage of patients failing to complete WAR), and patient selection factors in terms of initial stage, grade, and amount and site of residual disease at the time of their *initial* staging laparotomy. Thoroughness of restaging and tumor debulking may also impact on the results of salvage WAR. Two situations require specific mention: patients with predominant pelvic mass after chemotherapy and patients who are platinum refractory.

PREDOMINANT PELVIC MASS Analogous to the potential for improved survival noted with initial WAR treatment in patients with post-surgical residual confined to the pelvis, significantly higher salvage rates have also been noted with salvage WAR for patients with solely pelvic failures following initial surgery and chemotherapy. The pelvic location of such recurrences permits through debulking to be attempted, and the tolerance of pelvic structures for radiation (compared to the limitations imposed by small bowel, kidney, and liver with upper abdominal recurrences) allow higher boost doses to be delivered. This issue has been explored in sequential updated analyses of the influence of site of recurrence in patients treated with WAR as a salvage modality at the Rush-Presbyterian-St. Luke's Medical Center.[61,106,107] In their initial series, 30 patients with either residual ovarian cancer after second- or third-look laparotomy or recurrence after a negative second-look were treated with WAR (25 Gy to the upper abdomen with a boost to the involved gross disease to 40 Gy total and/or a boost to the para-aortic nodes to 45 Gy).[61] Pelvic boosts up to 60 to 70 Gy total were given with implants, external beam irradiation, or intraoperative irradiation. Following debulking procedures prior to radiation, 16 patients had microscopic residuum while 14 had macroscopic residuum. In 12 patients the pelvis was the only site of residuum while 14 patients had upper abdominal disease and pelvic disease and 4 patients had upper only abdominal residuum. Actuarial 2-year survival rates were significantly improved when the residual was in the pelvis alone (92%) compared with patients with upper abdominal involvement (31%, $P < 0.05$). Similarly, the recurrence-free survival for patients with pelvic disease only was 75% compared with 15% for those with upper abdominal involvement ($P < 0.05$). Patients who received a pelvic boost had only a 45% failure rate, compared to 83% for patients who did not receive a pelvic boost.[61]

The second update of this experience included a total of 40 patients with recurrent epithelial cancer of the ovary and 4 with recurrent primary adenocarcinoma of the peritoneal cavity.[107] The pelvis was the only site of residual disease in 14 patients, while 30 had abdominal involvement with or without pelvic residuum. Site of residual disease again strongly correlated with outcome following salvage WAR. The 4-year survival rate for patients with pelvic-only residuum was 48%, compared to 7% when the upper abdomen was involved ($P < 0.025$). The 4-year recurrence-free survival was 56% for patients with pelvic disease only, while none of the patients with upper abdominal disease were recurrence-free at 4 years ($P < 0.005$).

The most recent update of this series included 51 patients (47 with epithelial ovarian carcinoma, 4 with primary carcinoma of the peritoneal cavity) with a median follow-up of 53 months for the surviving patients.[106] Twenty patients had disease limited to the pelvis, and 31 had disease involving the upper abdomen. Statistically significant differences were again noted in the 4-year actuarial and recurrence-free survival in patients with pelvic involvement only (60% and 54%, respectively), compared with upper abdominal involvement (16% and 4%; $P = 0.0019$ and 0.0002, respectively). These series strongly support the role of salvage WAR with a pelvic boost in patients with pelvic recurrences following chemotherapy.

PLATINUM-REFRACTORY TUMORS The potential influence of persistence or recurrence within 6 months after treatment with platinum-based chemotherapy regimens on subsequent salvage treatment with WAR has recently been reported by Cmelak et al.[105] Of 41 women with persistent or recurrent epithelial ovarian cancers after initial treatment with surgical debulking and chemotherapy, 22 failed platinum-based regimens within 6 months after completion of chemotherapy or failed to have a complete response with such regimens (platinum-refractory group). Disease-specific survival was found to be statistically significantly related to initial stage and residual tumor size at the time of WAR but not to prior platinum failure. The 5-year disease-specific survival for platinum-refractory patients was 50%, compared with 41% for the entire patient group. At least for this study group, the previously postulated cross-resistance to radiation therapy following failure of platinum regimens did not appear to exist and/or to have clinical relevance.[118,119]

QUESTION 3

What is the role, if any, of combined modality chemotherapy/radiation therapy for ovarian cancer?

MARCUS E. RANDALL
GILLIAN M. THOMAS

There are theoretical mechanisms by which concurrent chemotherapy and radiation therapy can achieve enhancement of tumor cell kill. They have been enunciated by Steele and Peckham[120] and include, (1) modification of initial radiation damage, (2) inhibition of repair of radiation damage in tumor cells, (3) exploitation of induced cell synchrony, (4) reoxygenation following drug treatment and before irradiation, (5) improved drug access following irradiation, and (6) decrease in tumor volumes caused by radiation, leading to more rapid proliferation and greater chemosensitivity of tumor cells.[121] Other mechanisms that may also be operational are radiation modifications of chemotherapy cell kill, indirect cytotoxicity through possible tumor vascular toxic effects from the chemotherapy, and radiation and chemotherapeutic reduction of tumor repopulation. Concurrent use of chemotherapy and radiation exploits the possible additivity of the two different therapies. Agents such as 5-fluorouracil (5-FU) appear to be toxic to tissue such as epithelium and tumor which respond acutely to radiation, but not to late-reacting tissues which are the source of late radiation injury. Thus, if combinations are acutely tolerable, they could lead to therapeutic improvements. Concurrent administration may also possibly facilitate interaction or synergy in the case of independent cytotoxic drugs and radiation, or sensitization in the case of sensitizing agents. Multiple drugs are of interest with respect to their ability to act in concert with radiation. There are suggestions that hydroxyurea, an S-phase cell cycle-specific inhibitor of DNA synthesis, acts as a radiation potentiator by three possible mechanisms: (1) destroying cells in the relatively resistant S-phase of the cell cycle, (2) causing an accumulation of surviving cells at the G_1-S interface, a relatively radiosensitive portion of the cell cycle, and (3) by inhibiting the repair of tumor cells sublethally damaged by radiation. A study by the GOG suggested that combinations of hydroxyurea and radiation in the treatment of stage IIIB squamous cell carcinoma of the cervix have resulted in a 6-month improvement in the median progression-free interval and some long-term survival advantage.[122] Cisplatinum is another potentially useful agent for concomitant therapy with postulated mechanisms for cisplatin potentiation of radiation, including inhibition of repair of sublethal radiation damage, inhibition of the passage of cells through the radioresistant G_1-S phase of the cell cycle with the rest of cells in the radiosensitive phase and possibly independent hypoxic cell cytotoxicity. A third drug that has been explored extensively in trials of concurrent radiation and chemotherapy is 5-FU. Both in vivo and in vitro data demonstrate increased cytotoxicity of radiation in the presence of 5-FU, particularly with adenocarcinoma cells.[123] The cellular mechanisms of 5-FU-radiation interaction have not been clearly identified, and indeed some investigators have found only additive activity of these two agents resulting from independent cell kill by each one.[123–126] Mitomycin C has also been used concurrently with radiation therapy in other tumor sites, including carcinoma of the esophagus and anal canal. Definitive data from a phase III randomized trial indicates that the addition of mitomycin C to 5-FU and radiation therapy in the management of advanced anal canal cancer improves outcome. While there is no evidence for direct interaction between mitomycin C and radiation, a combination of the two agents may result in additive cytotoxicity as demonstrated by Rockwell.[127] The activity of mitomycin C as an adjunct to radiation therapy might not be correlated with its overall effectiveness as a single agent but rather with its selective activity against the hypoxic cell subset. Finally, extensive evidence[128–130] suggests that Taxol potentiates the cell kill produced by radiation therapy in addition to its role as a highly effective independent cytotoxic for epithelial ovarian cancer.

Despite all this theoretical information and information from multiple other tumor sites exploring the role of concurrent irradiation and chemotherapy, there are no studies on epithelial ovarian cancer examining their combined role with WAI. It seems appropriate to explore concurrent combinations of cisplatin with radiation therapy and Taxol with radiation therapy in view of the potential for enhancement as well as their independent cytotoxic activity. These studies should explore both intravenous and intraperitoneal drug administration, the latter to exploit the possible pharmacologic advantage of higher locally achievable drug doses. Important concepts in combining concurrent radiation therapy and chemotherapy include the principle of avoiding interruption in radiation therapy schedules or reduction in total doses in radiation when drugs are added, since both of these are likely to result in a declining therapeutic ratio for the combination.

The ability of cisplatin to enhance the cytotoxicity of low-dose continuous irradiation using ^{32}P has been demonstrated in vitro. This finding led Patillo et al[130] to combine fractionated ^{32}P (5 mCi) with monthly platinum chemotherapy in 30 patients with advanced disease. Complete and partial response rates were 47% and 40%, respectively. Therapy was well tolerated and produced a 3-year survival rate of 63%. This work suggests another avenue for investigation in selected patients with ovarian carcinoma.[131]

DANIEL S. KAPP

Combined modality chemotherapy/radiation therapy for epithelial ovarian cancer

CONSOLIDATION WITH RADIATION IN PATHOLOGICAL COMPLETE RESPONDERS Second-look laparotomy studies have shown that despite the finding of a pathologic complete response to chemotherapy, subsequent relapse rates of between 30% and 63% are noted with prolonged follow-up.[45,132–134] Therefore it is logical to treat patients with pathologic complete response with consolidation WAR. Table 11–7 summarizes the results of 17 trials in which chemotherapy was followed by WAR in patients with negative second-look laparotomies. The overall average crude survival rate was 70.4%, indicating the potential value of this combined modality approach.

RETROSPECTIVE COMPARATIVE STUDIES Several retrospective analyses have also suggested a significant clinical benefit of a planned combined chemotherapy/WAR approach compared with either chemotherapy or WAR alone. Goldhirsch et al[71] reported their results in 195 patients with stage IIB, IIC, III, and IV epithelial ovarian cancers

TABLE 11-7
Survival after Consolidative WAR in Patients with Negative Second-Look Laparotomy Following Chemotherapy for Epithelial Ovarian Cancer

STUDY/YEAR	NO. OF PATIENTS	NO. OF PATIENTS SURVIVING	FOLLOW-UP
Greiner et al[57] (1984)	15	14	7–64 mo
Rosen et al[66] (1986)	4	4	3–71 mo
Menczer et al[73] (1986)	10	9	Median >56 mo
Coltart et al[75] (1986)	3	2	19–37 mo
Rustin et al[72] (1987)	7	5	14–59 mo
Kuten et al[62] (1988)	5	5	2-yr actuarial SR 100%
Fuks et al[48] (1988)	14	6	Median 66 mo
Green et al[110] (1988)	10	10	Median 33 mo
Kersh et al[70] (1988)	4	1	Median 58 mo
Shelley et al[112] (1988)	12	8	13–25 mo
Goldhirsch et al[71] (1988)	24	19	24–73 mo
Haie et al[68] (1989)	23	14[a]	32–129 mo
Chauvet et al[115] (1989)	8	3	—
Bruzzone et al[49] (1990)	9	6	1–46 mo
Franchin et al[136] (1990)	11	7[b]	33–80 mo
Chiara et al[54] (1990)	9	6	4–58 mo
Thomas et al[39] (1994)	38	26	Median 67 mo
Total	206	145 (70.4%)	

Abbreviations: SR, Survival rate; NED, no evidence of disease.
[a] *Based on 63% 6-year NED SR.*
[b] *Based on 67% 5-year SR.*

treated with surgery and chemotherapy.[71] Forty-five patients achieved pathologically confirmed complete responses. Consolidation with WAR was then given based on the choice of each institution involved in the study: 24 patients received WAR (25 to 30 Gy), and 21 received no further treatment. The 3-year progression-free survival was 83% for women who received WAR, compared with 49% for those who received no additional radiation treatment ($P = 0.03$). When the two groups were adjusted for stage, histologic grade, and residuum at first operation, a statistically significant reduction in relapses for the group receiving consolidation WAR was still noted ($P = 0.03$).

The role of consolidation WAR following radical tumor debulking and cisplatin-based chemotherapy in stage III ovarian cancer was also analyzed for patients who were clinically free of disease (based on physical examination, CT scanning, and tumor marker levels) but who did not undergo second-look laparotomy.[135] At the completion of chemotherapy, women who were clinically free of disease were informed of the possible risks and benefits of WAR, and those who were willing to receive this therapy were treated to 30 Gy to the upper abdomen and 51.6 Gy to the pelvis. The outcome for 10 stage III patients who received chemotherapy/radiation therapy was compared with that for 11 stage III patients (matched for age, histology, grade, lymph node involvement, and residual disease after initial surgery) who received chemotherapy only. At 3 years, the relapse-free survival for patients receiving chemotherapy/radiation therapy was superior to that for those who received chemotherapy only (78% vs 28%), although the differences were not statistically significant ($P = 0.11$).

An additional study compared the outcome of 44 patients with high-risk optimally cytoreduced stage II and III epithelial ovarian cancer who were treated with six cycles of cisplatin-based chemotherapy followed by WAR (in 33 patients) to 48 historical control patients who were treated with WAR alone.[137] The median survival rate for women treated with combined therapy was 5.7 years, compared to 2.4 years for those treated with WAR alone ($P = 0.13$). The median time to relapse was increased more than twofold in the combined treatment group (3.0 years), compared with that for WAR-treated patients (1.4 years). At 5 years, 43% of the combined treatment group remained relapse-free, compared to 22% of those treated with WAR alone.

RANDOMIZED TRIALS Five prospective randomized trials have investigated the potential value of consolidative WAR following chemotherapy. The results of three have appeared only in meeting abstracts,[50,51,138] while the other two had a relatively limited number of patients.[49,52] Bruzzone et al[49] randomized 41 patients with stage III and IV disease who had no or minimal residual disease at second-look laparotomy following three cycles of chemotherapy to either three additional courses of the same chemotherapy (21 patients) or to WAR (20 patients). After second-look surgery 25 women had no residual disease, 12 had microscopic residual disease, and 4 had macroscopic disease less than 2 cm. Disease progression was observed in 55% of patients treated with consolidative WAR and in 29% of patients treated with chemotherapy, but these differences were not statistically significant ($P = 0.08$). Disease-related deaths occurred in 45% of women in the WAR arm and in 14% in the chemotherapy arm ($P = 0.02$). Unfortunately, a separate subset analysis was not done comparing the consolidative treatments in patients with pathologic complete responses or microscopic disease only, the patients most likely to benefit from consolidative WAR.

Mangioni et al[51] demonstrated a possible advantage of consolidation with cisplatin-based chemotherapy regimens (37 evaluable patients) versus consolidation treatment with relatively low-dose WAR (27 evaluable patients) in patients with stage III ovarian cancer who had minimum residual disease (≤ 3 positive sites either in the pelvis or in the abdomen). The relapse rates were 55% for the patients treated with WAR, compared with 38% for those treated with chemotherapy. Here too, statistical analyses based on the amount of residual disease at the time of the consolidative treatment were not provided, and so the results of this study remain difficult to interpret.

In contrast to these results, Lawton et al[52] reported no difference in survival in patients randomized after five courses of cisplatinum to receive second-look laparotomy and then either WAR (56 patients) or 1-year treatment with chlorambucil chemotherapy (53 patients). Overall survival at 2 years was 35%, with no differences in the two treatment arms noted. Only 5 women in the WAR group compared to 12 in the chlorambucil treatment arm had negative second-look laparotomies. The potential benefit of WAR in the negative second-look patients was not evaluated separately. Similarly, Lambert and co-workers[50] reportedly demonstrated no significant differences between consolidation therapy with carboplatinum or WAR.

Compared to these studies with insufficient patient numbers to permit meaningful subset analysis based on the amount of residual disease after initial chemotherapy, Sorbe et al[138] have reported their initial results in 742 patients with stage III epithelial ovarian carcinoma. All patients received four cycles of cisplatin-based chemotherapy. The subgroup of patients with pathologic complete responses at second-look laparotomy (98 patients) were randomized to receive WAR (20

Gy to the whole abdomen and 40 Gy to the lower abdominal pelvic fields), six cycles of chemotherapy similar to the induction therapy, or no further treatment. The overall 3-year survival rates were 83% after WAR, 76% after chemotherapy, and 73% after no further treatment ($P = 0.12$). Progression-free survival was significantly better in the WAR group compared to that in the control group ($P = 0.04$) but not statistically different from that in the chemotherapy group ($P = 0.17$). Also, the number of recurrences was lowest among the WAR-treated patients. Patients with microscopic residuum at second look (74 patients) were randomized to WAR or chemotherapy. The 3–year survival rate was 46% after WAR, which was not statistically significantly different from that obtained after additional chemotherapy (56%, $P = 0.57$). The final long-term results of this trial should provide useful information on the value of combined chemotherapy/radiation therapy in the treatment of patients with pathologic complete responses or microscopic residual disease.

QUESTION 4

Is there currently any role for radiation therapy in the treatment of (1) ovarian dysgerminoma or (2) sex cord-stromal tumors?

MARCUS E. RANDALL
GILLIAN THOMAS

Dysgerminoma

Dysgerminomas comprise approximately 50% of ovarian germ cell tumors, with 70% diagnosed while confined to one ovary (stage IA). Adequate work-up requires, at a minimum, CT of the abdomen and pelvis, chest x-ray, serum marker assays, and routine lab work. Lymphangiography, if available, can add important information and should be obtained in patients with apparent stage I disease. Using lymphangiography, De Palo and coworkers demonstrated a 35% rate of upstaging among stage I and II patients.[140]

Exquisitely radiosensitive, dysgerminomas often spread in an orderly fashion to the retroperitoneal and pelvic lymph nodes. In years past, these features resulted in the frequent administration of para-aortic and hemipelvic radiation therapy in early-stage disease.[141] However, in patients felt to require adjuvant treatment (typically completely resected stages greater than IA), systemic therapy has essentially replaced radiation therapy, largely to preserve fertility in this young patient population. It remains to be seen whether this advantage will persist in view of advances in fertility including embryo transfer. Other theoretical advantages of chemotherapy over radiation therapy include its ability to treat subclinical hematogenous and/or transperitoneal disease and its efficacy in potentially present but unrecognized nondysgerminomatous elements. Possible disadvantages of chemotherapy are the emergence of tumor radioresistance during chemotherapy exposure[118] and compromised hematologic tolerance should radiation therapy become necessary.

Although consistent efficacy in large numbers of patients with long follow-ups remains to be demonstrated, patients with extensive abdomen-confined disease are also candidates for initial treatment with chemotherapy.[142,143] However, since many women with advanced disease will be surgically rendered infertile, large-field radiation therapy remains a valid and effective treatment strategy. Long-term relapse-free survivals of at least 60% have been reported, even in stage III disease.[141,144,145] There is evidence that even better results are obtained using modern megavoltage equipment with treatment delivered to more generous volumes.[144,145] Furthermore, overall survival figures are substantially higher because of the effectiveness of chemotherapy or radiation therapy salvage.

Generally, patients with stage IB to III dysgerminoma treated with radiation therapy primarily or in a salvage setting should receive WAI since there is a high incidence of intraperitoneal disease and treatment morbidity with modest doses is increased minimally compared to pelvic and para-aortic radiation therapy.[14] Typically, 20 to 30 Gy in 100 to 150-cGy fractions is given, followed in some cases by 15 to 20-Gy boosts to the pelvis and known sites of gross disease. Using doses in this range delivered with a variety of techniques and fields including moving strip, Mitchell et al[146] retrospectively reviewed the M. D. Anderson Cancer Center experience with dysgerminomas to determine the effects of radiation therapy. Compared to unirradiated controls, patients experienced long-term gastrointestinal effects limited to an increase in frequency of bowel movements. No bowel obstructions were observed among 43 irradiated patients at a median follow-up of over 12 years. Of 19 patients with uteri and contralateral ovaries intact, intact menstrual function was noted in 14, although none had conceived. No significant urinary dysfunction or cases of second malignancies were reported.

The authors favor 25 Gy delivered over 5 weeks to the entire abdomen using 1 Gy/day with appropriate shielding of the kidneys and boosts of 10 to 15 Gy for sites of residual disease over 5 cm in maximum diameter. The routine use of pelvic boosts should be discontinued.

The up-front use of chemotherapy in dysgerminoma is a relatively recent development, and the role of subsequent radiation therapy is unclear. Whether consolidation radiation therapy should be used for previous sites of bulky disease completely responding to chemotherapy is controversial, and data are nonexistent. The authors favor its use only for single sites of disease greater than 10 cm prior to chemotherapy or when an elevated β-human chorionic gonadotropin in a pure dysgerminoma fails to return to normal. Even more difficult is the management of a stage II to III patient with bulky residual disease showing no or limited responsiveness to chemotherapy. Salvage surgery has been used with some success in selected patients.[147] For others, large-field radiation therapy, preferably initiated after no more than three or four cycles of chemotherapy, might be more appropriate, but again adequate data are unavailable at this time. Documentation of active disease with fine needle aspiration biopsy is appropriate in this setting.

Granulosa cell tumor

Pure granulosa cell tumor follows an indolent course in many cases. However, Fox et al[149] performed a detailed review of 92 cases, determining clinical and pathologic factors associated with an unfavorable outcome including age over 40, presentation with abdominal symptoms, a palpable mass, a solid large tumor, bilateral tumors, extraovarian spread, and a high mitotic rate.[148] Additional evidence of the adverse prognostic significance of high mitotic rate ($\geq$10 per 10 high-power fields) was presented by Malmstrom et al.[149] In Evans'[150] review of 118 patients, patients with stage II and III disease had recurrence rates of at least 35%, with a mean time to recurrence of 6 years.[150] Analysis of failure patterns revealed an overwhelming tendency for recurrence within the abdominal cavity. Unfortunately, salvage rates after recurrence are very low. Therefore, a strong case for adjuvant therapy exists, assuming effective treatment is available.

Adjuvant therapies administered in this disease have included chemotherapy and radiation therapy. The ability to evaluate the efficacy of either is limited by the rarity of the disease, the tendency for late recurrences, and the absence of prospective randomized trials. Although the use of chemotherapy continues to be studied by the GOG and others, its role in granulosa cell tumors is not well defined at present.

Clinically relevant radiosensitivity of granulosa cell tumor has been documented.[151,152] Furthermore, a number of series have supported the value of adjunctive radiation therapy in various patient groups.[153–155] However, uncertainties and inconsistencies in patient selection, prognostic factors, radiation therapy approach, and follow-up, as well as the lack of an untreated control group, make interpretation difficult.

In the absence of prospective randomized trials in well-defined patient populations, it is reasonable to base management decisions on known prognostic factors such as stage and mitotic rate. Data from Stenwig et al[159] suggest that pelvic radiation therapy alone is of no value as adjuvant treatment in stage I granulosa cell tumors. In view of the low recurrence rate in surgical stage I patients, this finding is not surprising. However, in women with tumor spillage, high mitotic rate, and advanced stage, the literature supports adjunctive radiation therapy as a valid management option, particularly in younger patients with a good performance status. WAI with the open-field technique is suggested in view of the known spread and recurrence patterns. Although no dose-response relationship is documented in granulosa cell tumor, a midplane dose of 2,550 cGy at 150 cGy/day approaches tolerance for this volume. Pelvic boosts increase complication rates and should not be used routinely.[87] However, boosts to sites of positive margins or gross disease are appropriate.

Clearly, additional work is needed to better determine the preferred approaches and respective roles of chemotherapy and radiation therapy. Controlled trials with large numbers of patients will be required to address these issues—a difficult task in view of the rarity of granulosa cell tumor.

DANIEL S. KAPP

The role of radiation in the treatment of dysgerminomas

The extreme radiosensitivity of ovarian dysgerminomas and their propensity for early lymphatic spread rather than diffuse peritoneal seeding has resulted in very high cure rates with postoperative radiation. Five- and 10-year survival rates greater than 90% have been reported for a composite of series of patients treated initially with conservative surgery alone for stage IA dysgerminomas[141,160] and a survival rate of 82% for 64 patients with stage II to IV dysgerminoma (abstracted from series reported between 1976 and 1982) has been achieved with surgery and postoperative radiation therapy.[160] Since the surgical staging of patients in these early series was probably incomplete by our current standards and serum markers for nondysgerminomatous elements (e.g., α-fetoprotein) were not always obtained, one can anticipate even better results stage for stage if modern surgical staging techniques and marker studies to exclude nondysgerminomas or mixed germ cell tumors are employed. Table 11–8 summarizes the very high cure rates reported in series from the past 10 years for patients predominately treated with surgery and postoperative radiation therapy for pure dysgerminomas. The standard postsurgical radiation treatment in earlier years was, for most patients with greater than stage IA disease, WAR (25 Gy) with possible boosts (10 Gy) to sites of bulky pelvic or para-aortic nodal disease.[141] Such treatments resulted in sterility. However, since the spread of dysgerminomas is more likely confined to the regional pelvic and para-aortic lymph nodes, in selected well-staged patients more conservative fertility-sparing radiation treatment has been used. Postoperative fields confined to the lymph nodes of the ipsilateral hemipelvis and the para-aortic nodes have been successfully employed.[140,145,161–164] With such ovary-sparing radiation techniques excellent survivals have been reported and fertility preserved, and many patients have been able to bear children.[145] It is with these more recent studies that the current chemotherapy regimens should be compared.

The late side effects of postoperative radiation treatment of dysgerminoma of the ovary have been reviewed by Mitchell et al.[146] Forty-three women treated for dysgerminomas were evaluated for late toxicity and compared to 55 matched controls in reference to bowel, bladder, thyroid, menstrual, reproductive, sexual, and growth function. These women had been treated with relatively high doses of WAR (up to 40 Gy), and many received pelvic and para-aortic boosts and mediastinal and supraclavicular treatment. No deaths secondary to the radiation therapy were noted nor were there any secondary malignancies or

TABLE 11-8
Survival of Dysgerminomas with Radiation Therapy as Primary Adjuvant Treatment: Summary of Experience Reported Since 1987

STUDY/YEAR	STAGE	NO. OF PATIENTS	SURVIVAL	FOLLOW-UP
De Palo et al[140] (1987)	I	13	100% NED	Median 77 mo
	III	12	61.4% NED 5 yr 89.5% 5 yr	Median 67 mo
Santoni et al[163] (1987)	I	21	11/12	60 mo
	II	1	0/1	60 mo
	III	7	5/6	60 mo
	All	29	90%	At 2 yr
LaPolla et al[165] (1987)	I	10	100% NED	Median 100 mo
	II–IV	11	9/11	Median 60 mo
Buskirk et al[161] (1987)	IA_1	18	100%	60 mo
	IA_1–IV	35	94.3%	60 mo
Lawson and Adler[162] (1988)	All (4 with distant metastases)	14	72%	54 mo
Gallion et al[160] (1988)	All (1 recurrent)	7	100% NED	35–240 mo
Dilhuydy et al[166] (1990)	All	10	80% 10 yr	3–129 mo
Björkholm et al[145] (1990)	All	60	83% 5 yr	Mean 228 mo
Susnerwala et al[167] (1991)	I	10	100%	4–108 mo
	II	6	100%	3–81 mo
	III	7	3	61–91 mo
	IV	1	1	81 mo
	Recurrent	3	3	53–66 mo
	All primary	24	88%	At 108 mo
Zaghloul and Khattab[168] (1992)	I	4	100% 5 yr	
	II	2	100% 5 yr	
	III	13	66% 5 yr	
	IV	3	67% 5 yr	
	All	22	76% 5 yr	Median 67 mo
About et al[169] (1993)	All	17	94% 5 yr	—
Teinturier et al[164] (1993)	I	14	100% 5 yr	13–360 mo
	II–III	18	100% 5 yr	6–192 mo
	IV	3	1/3	6–95 mo
	All	35	94.5% 5 yr	102 mo
Ayhan et al[170] (1995)	All	32	78.5%	—

Abbreviations: NED, No evidence of disease.

bowel complications requiring surgery. An increased number of patients in the radiation therapy group reported more than two bowel movements per day (58% vs 19%; $p = 0.0002$), while fewer reported constipation (40% vs 66%; $P = 0.014$). There were no statistically significant differences between the radiated patients and the controls in terms of bladder function except for a higher incidence of urinary tract infections in control patients (28% vs 61%; $P = 0.013$). No thyroid disorders were noted related to radiation therapy, and only one patient had delayed bone growth. The greatest effect of the treatment was on fertility, with no patients having conceived. However, most patients with intact uteri bled monthly on hormonal replacement so that oocyte in vitro fertilization may permit them conception if they so desire.[171] Although there is a slight increase in dyspareunia in the treated group, most patients were satisfied with their sexual functioning.

Unfortunately, comparable information on the late sequelae of chemotherapy used in the treatment of dysgerminoma of the ovary for a large series of patients (other than data on preservation of fertility) is not available. Toxicity data from 20 patients with dysgerminomas treated in GOG trials revealed significant acute toxicity.[139] All patients had alopecia, significant hematopoietic toxicity, and some degree of nausea and vomiting. An allergic reaction was noted in one patient in response to etoposide, and a severe but reversible neurotoxicity developed following a drug overdose of vincristine. In another small series of patients, one of six treated with chemotherapy for recurrent dysgerminoma died of treatment-related neutropenia.[143]

Substantial toxicity has been observed in patients treated with similar chemotherapy regimens for other germ cell tumors of the ovary.[173] Five treatment-related deaths were reported among 97 patients treated on GOG protocols. Two were from pulmonary fibrosis, two were from myelosuppression with infection, and one was sudden death from an unknown cause. Cortical blindness and seizures have also been reported in a patient with ovarian dysgerminoma, who was treated with cisplatin/vinblastine/bleomyocin.[174] Individual institutional trials have revealed similar acute toxicities in addition to sleep disturbances,[175] severe myalgias, severe bladder pain, and urinary frequency.[176] If one could extrapolate from the late toxicities following cisplatin/vinblastine/bleomyocin treatments reported in males with analogous testicular germ cell tumors, long-term neural toxicities including sensory and hearing loss,[177] Raynaud-like phenomenon and/or gastrointestinal problems should be anticipated.[178] There also appears to be a dose-response relationship between etopside exposure and the risk of secondary leukemia.[179, 180]

Currently, radiation therapy following surgery remains a viable alternative to chemotherapy in the treatment of dysgerminoma. Prospective trials, including quality-of-life determinations, will be necessary for determination of the optimum treatment. Radiation therapy may be the postoperative treatment of choice in women who are infertile (e.g., those with dysgenetic ovaries),[181] in those in whom fertility is not an issue, and in those those who can be treated with ovary-conserving radiation techniques. Radiation therapy remains an excellent treatment for palliation of painful bone metastases[182] following chemotherapy failure, in metastatic disease requiring emergency intervention (e.g., spinal cord compression), and in sites of disease not effectively reached by chemotherapy (e.g., leptomeningeal metastases). For example, Jolles et al[183] reported a patient with a leptomeningeal recurrence who had failed chemotherapy. She responded to craniospinal radiation and was free of disease for 2 years following radiation therapy.

The role of radiation in the treatment of stromal cell tumors

There are no randomized studies on adjuvant radiation therapy or chemotherapy for stromal cell tumors of the ovary. The propensity for late recurrences and death after 5 years in patients with granulosa cell tumors makes the interpretation of studies with limited follow-up difficult.[149,150,184–186] For example, Evans et al[149] report that the mean time from diagnosis to first recurrence was 6 years.[150] However, the radiosensitive nature of granulosa cell tumor has been established, and long-term responses have been noted following relatively low radiation doses.[151,155–157,187–189] Many series

TABLE 11-9
The Role of Radiation Therapy in the Treatment of Granulosa Cell Tumor of the Ovary

STUDY/YEAR	NO. OF PATIENTS	OUTCOME
Moreton and Leddy[189] (1948)	11 (8 from literature)	7 NED 1–15 yr; 1 died of liver metastases at 5 yr; 2 recurrent at 2.5, 6 yr 1 died of unknown cancer at 16 yr; long-term survival noted in 3 inoperable patients (9, 9, 16 yr)
Haines and Jackson[188] (1950)	8	4 remain alive; 1 with rapid regression of pelvic metastases
Duckett et al[187] (1953)	4	1 with initial omental metastases A&W at 4 yr; 1 A&W at 12 yr; 1 with metastases to rectum—A&W 11.5 yr; 1 with metastases to pelvic viscera and vagina expired at 2 yr with carcinomatosis
Stoll[192] (1956)	1	Multiple courses of abdominal and thoracic XRT for treatment of metastases—with tumor regression over 5-yr period
Engle[157] (1958)	12	4 long-term survivors (12–18 yr); 2 A&W at 3 yr; all 6 had extensive disease
Sjöstedt and Wahlen[186] (1961)	104	5-yr SR higher in patients treated with surgery and radiation (85.6%) compared with 52 patients treated with surgery alone (82.7%); excluding patients with metastases noted at surgery, 5-yr SR are 89.6% vs 82.7% for combined treatment vs surgery alone
Simmons and Sciarra[156] (1967)	2 (recurrent)	1 NED for 9 yr after XRT—recurred and reirradiated—well for 5+ yr; 1 NED for 6 yr after XRT
Dinnerstein and O'Leary[194] (1968)	7	Individual outcomes not given, but "liberal use of postoperative external radiation recommended"
Norris and Taylor[185] (1968)	6	Pelvic XRT given for persistent tumor; tumor shrank in 4; 5 survived >4 yr after XRT; 1 died of metastatic breast cancer
Kalavathi[151] (1971)	1	Extensive peritoneal cavity recurrence controlled for 2 yr
Goldston et al[155] (1972)	5 stage I	Radiation to pelvis (4) plus abdomen (1); 2 recurred at 5.5, 16 yr; 2 A&W at 2, 6 yr
	3 stage III	Radiation to pelvis—NED 15, 21, 26 yr
	2 stage IV	Palliative radiation; died 3, 6 yr
Fox et al[148] (1975)	11	3 alive at 0.5, 2, and 20 yr
Schwartz and Smith[153] (1976)	18	Better SR in 18 patients who received postoperative radiation than in 19 who did not

(*Continues*)

TABLE 11-9
(Continued)

STUDY/YEAR	NO. OF PATIENTS	OUTCOME
Pankratz et al[158] (1978)	48	Better SR in 48 patients who received postoperative radiation than in 13 who did not (even though XRT patients had higher stages)
Stenwig et al[159] (1979)	67	For stage I patients better results for surgery alone then surgery plus XRT; for more advanced stages, recommend adding XRT
Björkholm and Silfverswärd[190] (1981)	198	For stage I patients with unruptured tumors no benefit from XRT; for stage I patients with ruptured tumors, XRT reduced the number of deaths due to tumor recurrences (12/37 vs 4/5 for surgery alone)
Ohel et al[191] (1983)	45	Postoperative radiation had no effect on 5-yr SR; 50% in patients with XRT; 55% in 63 patients without XRT
Kumar et al[152] (1986)	1	Complete response for 2+ yr for liver metastases treated with XRT
Malström et al[149] (1994)	48	Overall 5-yr survival was 90%; since 89% of patients had received adjuvant XRT, its value cannot be estimated

Abbreviations: A&W, Alive and well; NED, no evidence of disease; XRT, radiation therapy, SR, survival rate.

support the role of radiation therapy as postoperative adjuvant treatment (Table 11–9). The benefit of postoperative radiation is most apparent in stage I patients with ruptured tumors[190] and in patients with more advanced-stage disease.[153, 158] In well-staged patients with stage IA disease, no benefit from postoperative radiation therapy has been noted.[148, 150, 159, 190, 191] Similarly, stage IA granulosa tumors of the ovary in children have been managed with unilateral salpingo-oopherectomy with good results.[192] Long-term palliation of intra-abdominal, pulmonary, and liver metastases with radiation therapy has also been reported.[152, 193] Until further information is available on long-term results of chemotherapy, postoperative radiation therapy for patients with stage IC to III granulosa cell tumor remains a worthwhile option.

Less information is available on the role of radiation in the treatment of other sex cord-stromal cell tumors. Schwartz and Smith[153] have reported successful treatment with WAR of a patient with a retroperitoneal recurrence of a Sertoli-Leydig tumor who remained without evidence of further recurrence 67 months following radiation therapy. They recommended that all patients with stage IB to III Sertoli-Leydig tumor with residual disease less than 2 cm receive WAR with a pelvic boost. Because of the rarity of sex cord-stromal tumors of the ovary, national studies will be required to gain more information on their optimum treatment.

QUESTION 5

What are your recommendations for future directions and clinical trials in this area?

MARCUS E. RANDALL
GILLIAN THOMAS

Future directions

The data reviewed in the earlier parts of this chapter clearly indicate that radiation therapy is highly effective in the management of approximately one-third of patients with ovarian cancer. Multiple studies have delineated the pretreatment prognostic factors predicting patient groups that have a significant probability of cure when WAI is used as the sole postoperative treatment.[80, 81] The most important factor that predicts the success of this therapy is the amount of residual disease after initial surgery. With current standard radiation fractionation schedules, the dose of radiation that can be applied to the abdomen and pelvis is limited by the tolerance of the normal tissues. Conventional teaching and interpretation of dose-control relationships suggested that doses of 45 to 50 Gy in 2-Gy fractions are necessary to achieve an overall 90% reduction in the incidence of metastases that were small but macroscopic.[195] Radiobiological modeling supported by data from the clinical literature on multiple tumor sites has demonstrated that the dose-response curve for control of subclinical metastases is in fact different from that for macroscopic disease. The curve for control is linear and shallow and extrapolates to a dose intercept not demonstrably different from zero. The slope of this curve is compatible with a model in which there is heterogeneity in the metastatic tumor cell burden outside the primary field, which varies from 1 to 10^8 or 10^9, where the tumor is at the border of clinical detectability. The implication is that worthwhile rates of control can still be achieved with lower than optimal doses of 45 to 50 Gy and that the degree of biologic effectiveness of elective treatment is measured directly by the percentage reduction in failure rate. Available data pertinent to the control of subclinical ovarian cancer treated with WAI indicate that doses of 2250 to 2500 cGy in 100-cGy fractions lead to a reduction in metastatic rate of 38 to 40%.[15,34,196] A model of the heterogeneity of residual tumor cell burden in ovarian cancer and the subsequent response to less than optimal doses of radiation therapy provides an understanding of the efficacy and limitations of conventional radiation in ovarian cancer. It provides an explanation of why these lower doses have led to cure in a substantial proportion of patients. The model implies that radiation therapy should be commenced as soon after surgery as possible in order to treat the tumor at the stage of lowest tumor cell burden.

To further exploit the utility of radiation in ovarian cancer, two possible conceptual approaches need to be examined. The first is to attempt modifications of radiation therapy, such that a biologically higher effective radiation dose can be delivered to the upper abdomen and pelvis, yet still be within the tolerance of the normal tissues. This could theoretically be achieved using altered fractionation schemes or with adjunctive use of chemotherapeutic agents likely to have radiation-sensitizing properties. Finally, both altered fractionation schemes and sensitizing chemotherapy could be exploited together. The second major concept worthy of discussion is the development of strategies leading to the exploitation of each of the effective modalities of treatment in order to maximize benefit. The use of radiation therapy in ovarian cancer has met with considerable resistance and has been underutilized. Furthermore, the use of effective doses of radiation or combining radiation with drugs such as Taxol, platinum, or 5-FU has also been met with resistance because of concerns about the ability to deliver "effective" doses of chemotherapy. Since chemotherapy may be no more effective in curing ovarian cancer than radiation therapy, it seems shortsighted to focus on response rates and relapse-free intervals produced by chemotherapy and discard radiation therapy from the treatment armamentarium. While radiation is a locoregional treatment and chemotherapy is a systemic treatment, the predominant pattern of intra-abdominal failure in ovarian cancer still means that effective locoregional treatments have a part to play in ovarian cancer as well as systemic therapy. In the case of no other solid tumor has a therapy that produces very high response rates (and indeed high cure rates in patients with microscopic residual disease) been discarded from the treatment armamentarium in the manner in which radiation therapy for ovarian cancer has been discarded. The remainder of this chapter will review potential strategies for exploiting the use of radiation therapy for ovarian cancer.

Altered fractionation schemes

When radiation therapy is used as the sole postoperative management in ovarian cancer, severe late gastrointestinal complications rise significantly when the abdominal dose exceeds 25 Gy and the pelvic dose exceeds 45 Gy in 100-cGy fractions. Similarly, the risk of complications increases substantially from 3 or 4% at the lower doses to 25 to 30% when multiple laparotomies are performed prior to radiation treatment. Thus, simple escalations of total radiation dose using standard fractionation schemes are unlikely to yield an improved therapeutic ratio. Radiobiological modeling however, suggests that a higher dose of radiation can be delivered with acceptable complications if multiple daily fractions of radiation are given with a lower dose at each fraction.[197]

Fein et al[117] use an altered radiation fractionation scheme to treat 28 patients with stage III epithelial ovarian carcinoma previously treated with cisplatin-based chemotherapy. They received 0.8 Gy per fraction twice daily to a total dose of 30.2 Gy to the whole abdomen and pelvis, and 20 of the 28 received additional radiation therapy to the pelvis to a mean dose of 15 Gy. Many of these patients had been extensively pretreated both surgically with two to four laparotomies and had had between 6 and 28 cycles of chemotherapy prior to radiation therapy. Despite extensive pretreatment, patients tolerated therapy well. Only two required treatment breaks, and four required surgery for small bowel obstruction. Radiobiological modeling suggests that such a regimen would offer late effects comparable to those of standard once daily dosing while offering a higher effective biological dose. Eifel et al[108] reported their experience with altered fractionation to the whole abdomen and pelvis after chemotherapy in which two fractions per day of 1 Gy were given to a total of 30 Gy with 3-week rest period after 15 Gy.[108] It is likely that most experimental altered fractionation schemes in this setting will not incorporate a planned split in the course of irradiation because of the possibility that interruptions may allow accelerated clonogenic proliferation which would decrease the biological effectiveness of any given total dose in addition to the possibility of increasing complication rates.[198]

Randall et al[87] published results of a phase II GOG study in which optimal stage III patients received three cycles of cisplatin-based chemotherapy followed by surgical reassessment and hyperfractionated WAI.[87] Interestingly, this study documented a 40% disease progression rate during chemotherapy. The WAI regimen (80 cGy twice daily to 30.4 Gy) was found to be very well tolerated acutely. Late complications were seen only in patients receiving a pelvic boost. Median and disease-free survivals were at least comparable to results achieved using chemotherapy only in earlier GOG trials.

Clearly, further phase I investigations of altered fractionation schemes are required. Those to be tested should aim at delivering biologically more effective doses to the volume without increasing late tissue effects. The ability to improve the therapeutic index with the use of daily small-fraction multiple radiation is predicated on data and modeling suggesting that small fraction sizes differentially spare late tissue damage for a given level of tumor control and acute toxicity and that shortening overall treatment time reduces the likelihood of treatment failure due to tumor proliferation occurring during a course of radiation therapy. Subsequent testing of such schemes in randomized trails either against standard radiation therapy or against the best available chemotherapy would most appropriately be performed in patient subsets in which there is already a clear indication that standard radiation provides a substantial curative benefit, namely, those with intermediate-risk epithelial ovarian cancer. If such trials showed an improvement in outcome for these patient subsets, the obvious extension would be to use the altered fractionation schemes in patients with slightly more residual disease than those in the intermediate-risk group.

DANIEL S. KAPP

Future directions in clinical trials and ovarian cancer

Technical: Further development and employment of three-dimensional treatment planning techniques and quality assurance for treatment fields are essential to verify that the entire abdominopelvic treatment volume is being adequately covered. Areas of particular concern include adequate coverage of the diaphragms and lateral coverage of the peritoneal cavity. In slender patients care must also be taken not to underdose the anterior peritoneal surface due to the buildup region of high-energy photon beams. Precise shielding of the kidneys and the liver (where indicated) could also be accomplished with three-dimensional techniques. Respiratory gated treatment may permit less normal lung to be irradiated while providing adequate diaphragmatic coverage. The use of on-line portal imaging will provide daily real-time checks for patient motion and adequacy of coverage. Future developments including modulated conformal therapy[199] may permit boosting of high-risk peritoneal surfaces while limiting kidney and liver parachymal doses. Stereotactic techniques and intraoperative radiation or brachytherapy implants may permit boosts to sites of recurrent or persistent disease without exceeding normal tissue tolerance.[200]

Radiobiologic Considerations

Additional studies on the optimization of treatment schedules using field-within field, hyperfractionation, or accelerated fractionation techniques[65,74,108] tailor-made to measured tumor kinetic parameters are warranted. Predictive assays for both tumor and normal tissue intrinsic radiosensitivity may also permit individualization of patient treatment.[201] The use of monoclonal antibodies, hypoxic cell sensitizers, and hypoxic cell toxins should be considered, especially in patients with measurable recurrent disease after second-look surgery where the outcome is almost universally poor. For example, the use of tirapazamine in combined chemotherapy and radiation treatment is particularly intriguing since this hypoxic cell toxin may be supra-additive to both radiation and cisplatin chemotherapy.[201] The potential use of regional hyperthermia in conjunction with cisplatin or carboplatin chemotherapy in recurrent ovarian is currently being explored.[202, 203] Finally the role of aggressive cytoreductive surgery for recurrent or persistent tumor should be prospectively investigated.[204]

Randomized Trials

The relatively high 5-year survival rates (73%) obtained with postsurgical WAR in intermediate-risk group patients[82] warrant confirmation in prospective trials (stratified by patient age, stage, grade, histologic type, and postsurgical residuum comparing WAR to modern chemotherapy regimens (e.g., cisplatin/Taxol combinations). WAR may indeed have particular value in the treatment of patients with minimum tumor residum limited to the pelvis or to the para-aortic lymph nodes or in optimally debulked patients with grade III clear-cell carcinomas (which are relatively poor responders to cisplatin chemotherapy).[205]

Additional prospective trials are also needed to evaluate the use of consolidative WAR in patients with pathologic complete responses to chemotherapy. Patient subgroups with a high risk of subsequent failure include those with large (>2 cm) prechemotherapy residual disease, those with grade III or clear-cell tumors, and older patients. Such women would be candidates for consolidative WAR treatments. A control group receiving no additional treatment should be included in such trials. Since the incidence of serious gastrointestinal complications has been correlated with abdominal radiation dose, pelvic dose, and employment of second-look laparotomy,[84] the value of pelvic boosts in such patients should be prospectively studied.

Similarly, additional prospective randomized trials are needed to define the potential role of combined chemotherapy/WAR in patients with microscopic residual disease at second-look laparotomy. The use of intraoperative radiation boosts to the sites of microscopic residual disease may be of particular value in this situation. The employment of hemopoietic growth factors may also facilitate timely deliverance of WAR, especially in patients failing after multiple cycles of chemotherapy with poor bone marrow reserve. Techniques should be further developed to exclude patients with macroscopic residual disease from second-look procedures and subsequent WAR consolidation. The use of serial CA 125 assays has been studied in a small series of stage III patients, and none of eight such patients achieving postchemotherapy CA 125 values of less than 35 U/ml had residual disease greater than 1 cm at second-look laparotomy.[206] However other series have demonstrated macroscopic tumors even in patients with CA 125 values measuring less than 35 U/ml.[172, 207] Therefore the development of other noninvasive techniques such as radioimmunoscintigraphy[207] in conjunction with serial tumor markers may help identify patients with minimal residual disease for trials with consolidative WAR, forgoing the additional risk of second-look laparotomy. Finally, investigational strategies need to be prospectively evaluated for patients with suboptimally debulked initial tumors or suboptimally debulked recurrences. It is for these women that multiple modality approaches including the use of radiosensitizers, hypoxic cell toxins, and hyperthermia should be explored in conjunction with sequential chemotherapy/WAR.

EDITORS' COMMENTARY

Both sets of authors provide substantial evidence supporting the use of radiation therapy as primary postoperative treatment for epithelial ovarian cancer. They make their case based on very good tolerance with acceptable morbidity coupled with promising results in patients who have been left with minimal residual disease after optimal debulking surgery. The limitations of this modality with regard to normal tissue tolerance and sites of residual tumor are well outlined. Information from the literature on this topic is nicely summarized in tabular form. In addition, both authors emphasize careful patient selection. Of course, the obvious strategy needed to resolve this ongoing debate about the role of radiation therapy as primary postoperative treatment is to conduct a prospective randomized study comparing WAR with contemporary platinum-based chemotherapy in a good-prognostic group. Such a study was initiated a few years ago by the GOG but was discontinued prematurely because of inadequate patient accrual most likely related to biases among the participating investigators.

Studies to date on the use of WAR as salvage therapy for patients with persistent small-volume disease at second-look surgery (after surgery and platinum-based chemotherapy) have also yielded disappointing results. In several reports, morbidity in the form of intestinal injury has been unacceptably high, and the salvage rate has been poor. Here, Dr. Kapp presents a somewhat more optimistic perspective than Drs. Randall and Thomas. The issue of WAR as consolidation therapy for patients who have negative second-look findings but poor prognostic factors and those with persistent well-differentiated microscopic tumor is also discussed. Both groups review the role of radiation therapy as palliative therapy for patients with a predominant pelvic mass. Drs. Randall and Thomas also discuss the need for further study of concomitant chemotherapy and radiation therapy. We agree with their recommendation for more pilot studies in this area.

With regard to the radiotherapeutic treatment of ovarian dysgerminoma, both sets of authors agree that it is a viable alternative to chemotherapy. Again, Dr. Kapp is more enthusiastic about its current role than Drs. Randall and Thomas. It appears that, for patients who receive postoperative radiation therapy, the incidence of morbidity is low, which is undoubtedly related to the relatively low dose required. Nevertheless, it is difficult for the authors to argue against the potential benefit of chemotherapy with regard to fertility preservation. Of course, for patients who have undergone bilateral salpingo-oophorectomy and hysterectomy because of bilateral ovarian involvement and older patients who have completed childbearing, the choice of postoperative therapy is based on the morbidity profile of each treatment modality. For patients with granulosa cell tumors, the authors refer to available limited information demonstrating activity for radiation therapy. Both groups agree that cooperative group studies are needed in this area to further delineate the role of radiation therapy. We agree with their conclusion on this subject. The major problem in interpreting the literature on this subject, other than the scarcity of data, is that in many cases radiation therapy is used in an adjuvant fashion to treat patients without measurable disease or is used in conjunction with chemotherapy (either sequentially or concomitantly). At M. D. Anderson Cancer Center, we are currently reviewing our experience with radiation therapy alone in patients with measurable disease.

Future research in this area, as outlined by the authors, should include further study of altered fractionation schemes, concomitant chemotherapy and radiation therapy, innovative radiotherapeutic techniques, and randomized trials comparing radiation therapy with chemotherapy in several settings, including primary postoperative treatment and consolidation of patients with compete pathologic response or persistent microscopic disease. We support these recommendations but understand that the successful conduct of some of these trials will be difficult because of lingering biases.

References

1. Dembo AJ, Davy M, Stenwig AE et al: Prognostic factors in patients with stage I epithelial ovarian cancer. Obstet Gynecol 75(2):263, 1990

1a. Young RC, Walton LA, Ellenburg SS et al: Adjuvant therapy in stage I and stage II epithelial ovarian cancer: results of two prospective randomized trials. NEJM 332:1021, 1990

2. Klaasen D, Shelley W, Starreveld A et al: Early stage ovarian cancer: A randomized clinical trial comparing whole abdominal radiotherapy, melphalan, and intraperitoneal chromic phosphate: a National Cancer Institute of Canada Clinical Trials Group report. J Clin Oncol 6:1254, 1988

3. Vergote IB, Vergote-De Vos LN, Abeler VM et al: Randomized trial comparing cisplatin with radioactive phosphorus or whole-abdomen irradiation as adjuvant treatment of ovarian cancer. Cancer 69:741, 1992

4. Bolis G, Colombo N, Pecorelli S et al: Adjuvant treatment for early epithelial ovarian cancer: results of two randomised clinical trials comparing cisplatin to no further treatment or chromic phosphate (^{32}P). Ann Oncol 6:887, 1995

5. Smith JP, Rutledge, FN, Delclos L: Postoperative treatment of early cancer of the ovary: a random trial between postoperative irradiation and chemotherapy. Natl Cancer Inst Monogr 42:149, 1975

6. Randall ME: A call to WAR. J Natl Cancer Inst 85:440, 1993

7. Thomas GM: Radiotherapy in early ovarian cancer. Gynecol Oncol 55:S73, 1994

8. Dembo AJ, Bush RS, Beale FA et al: Ovarian carcinoma: improved survival following abdominopelvic irradiation in patients with a completed pelvic op-

eration. Am J Obstet Gynecol 134: 793, 1979

9. Sell A, Bertelsen K, Andersen JE et al: Randomized study of whole-abdomen irradiation versus pelvic irradiation plus cyclophosphamide in treatment of early ovarian cancer. Gynecol Oncol 37:367, 1990
10. Martinez A, Schray MF, Howes AE et al: Postoperative radiation therapy for epithelial ovarian cancer: the curative role based on a 24-year experience. J Clin Oncol 3:901, 1985
11. Leers WH, Kock HCLV: The evaluation of postoperative irradiation in patients with early-stage ovarian cancer. Gynecol Oncol 28:41, 1987
12. Weiser, EB, Burke TW, Heller PB et al: Determinants of survival of patients with epithelial ovarian carcinoma following whole abdomen irradiation (WAR). Gynecol Oncol 30:201, 1988
13. Goldberg N, Peschel RE: Postoperative abdominopelvic radiation therapy for ovarian cancer. Int J Radiat Oncol Biol Phys 14:425, 1988
14. Dembo AJ: Abdominopelvic radiotherapy in ovarian cancer: a 10-year experience. Cancer 55:2285, 1985
15. Fuller DB, Sause WT, Plenk HP, Menlove RL: Analysis of postoperative radiation therapy in stage I through III epithelial ovarian carcinoma. J Clin Oncol 5:897, 1987
16. Van Bunningen B, Bouma J, Kooijman C et al: Total abdominal irradiation in stage I and II carcinoma of the ovary. Radiother Oncol 11:305, 1988
17. Lindner H, Willich H, Atzinger A: Primary adjuvant whole abdominal irradiation in ovarian carcinoma. Int J Radiat Oncol Biol Phys 19:1203, 1990
18. Hart S, Ben-Baruch G, Herczeg E et al: Abdominopelvic radiation for stage I–II ovarian cancer. Eur J Gynaecol Oncol 10:416, 1989
19. Hammond R, Bull C, Houghton CRS et al: Primary adjunctive whole abdominal radiotherapy in epithelial ovarian cancer: results of 10-years' experience. Aust NZ J Obstet Gynaecol 32:267, 1992
20. Macbeth FR, MacDonald H, Williams CJ: Total abdominal and pelvic radiotherapy in the management of early stage ovarian carcinoma. Int J Radiat Oncol Biol Phys 15:353, 1988
21. Buchsbaum HJ, Brady MF, Delgado G, et al: Surgical staging of carcinoma of the ovaries. Surg Gynecol Obstet 169:226, 1989
22. Fuller DB, LaRouere J, Perez-Tamayo C et al: Optimal coverage of peritoneal surface in whole abdominal radiation for ovarian neoplasms. Int J Radiat Oncol Biol Phys 17:607, 1989
23. Fyles AW, Dembo AJ, Bush RS et al: Analysis of complications in patients treated with abdominopelvic radiation therapy for ovarian carcinoma. Int J Radiat Oncol Biol Phys 22:847, 1992
24. Lanciano RM, Randall ME: Update on the role of radiotherapy in ovarian cancer. Semin Oncol 18:233, 1991
25. Knapp RC, Friedman EA: Aortic lymph node metastases in early ovarian cancer. Am J Obstet Gynecol 119: 1013, 1974
26. Knipscheer RJJL: Para-aortal lymph nodes dissection in 20 cases of primary epithelial ovary carcinoma stage I (FIGO): influence on staging. Eur J Obstet Gynecol Reprod Biol 13:303, 1982
27. Young RC, Decker DG, Wharton JT et al: Staging laparotomy in early ovarian cancer. JAMA 250:3072, 1983
28. Young RC, Fisher RI: The staging and treatment of epithelial ovarian cancer. Can Med Assoc 119:249, 1978
29. Schray MF, Cox RS, Martinez A: Lower abdominal radiotherapy for stages I, II and selected III epithelial

ovarian cancer: 20 years experience. Gynecol Oncol 15:78, 1983

30. LaRouere J, Perez-Tamayo C, Fraass B et al: Optimal coverage of peritoneal surface in whole abdominal radiation for ovarian neoplasms. Int J Radiat Oncol Biol Phys 17:607, 1989
31. Rubin P: The dose-limiting organs in radiation oncology. p.2. In: Radiation Biology and Radiation Pathology Syllabus. American College of Radiology, Chicago, 1975
32. Wharton JT, Fletcher GH: The principles of radiation therapy for malignant pelvic lesions. Surg Clin North Am 58:181, 1978
33. Okunieff P, Morgan D, Niemierko A, Suit HD: Radiation dose-response of human tumors. Int J Radiat Oncol Biol Phys 32:1227, 1995
34. Withers HR, Peters LJ, Taylor JMG: Dose-response relationship for radiation therapy of subclinical disease. Int J Radiat Oncol Biol Phys 31:353, 1995
35. Marks LB: A standard dose of radiation for "microscopic disease" is not appropriate. Cancer 66:2498, 1990
36. Kapp DS: The role of the radiation oncologist in the management of gynecologic cancer. Cancer 51:2485, 1983
37. Fuks Z: External radiotherapy of ovarian cancer: standard approaches and new frontiers. Semin Oncol 2:253, 1975
38. Haas JS, Mansfield CM, Hartman GV et al: Results of radiation therapy in the treatment of epithelial carcinoma of the ovary. Cancer 46:1950, 1980
39. Thomas L, Pigneux J, Chauvergne J et al: Evaluation of whole abdominal irradiation in ovaian carcinoma with a four orthogonal fields technique. Int J Radiat Oncol Biol Phys 30:1083, 1994
40. Einhorn N, Nilsson B, Holmberg K et al: Risk of second tumors in a cohort of patients with ovarian carcinoma. Int J Gynecol Cancer 6:313, 1996
41. Rubin SC, Hoskins WJ, Hakes TB et al: Recurrence after negative second-look laparotomy for ovarian cancer: analysis of risk factors. Am J Obstet Gynecol 159:1094, 1988
42. Gershenson DM, Copeland LJ, Wharton JT et al: Prognosis of surgically determined complete responders in advanced ovarian cancer. Cancer 55: 1129, 1985
43. Podratz KC, Malkasian GD, Wiegand HS et al: Recurrent disease after negative second-look laparotomy in stage III and IV ovarian carcinoma. Gynecol Oncol 29:274, 1988
44. Roberts WS, Hodel K, Rich WM et al: Second-look laparotomy in the management of gynecologic malignancy. Gynecol Oncol 13:345, 1982
45. Podczaski E, Manetta A, Kaminski P et al: Survival of patients with ovarian epithelial carcinomas after second-look laparotomy. Gynecol Oncol 36:43, 1990
46. Omura GA, Blessing JA, Ehrlich CE et al: A randomized trial of cyclophosphamide and doxorubicin with or without cisplatin in advanced ovarian carcinoma: a Gynecologic Oncology Group study. Cancer 57:1725, 1986
47. Thomas GM: Is there a role for consolidation or salvage radiotherapy after chemotherapy in advanced epithelial ovarian cancer? Gynecol Oncol 51: 97, 1993
48. Fuks Z, Rizel S, Biran S: Chemotherapeutic and surgical induction of pathological complete remission and whole abdominal irradiation for consolidation does not enhance the cure of stage III ovarian carcinoma. J Clin Oncol 6:509, 1988
49. Bruzzone M, Repetto L, Chiara S et al: Chemotherapy versus radiotherapy in the management of ovarian cancer patients with pathological complete response or minimal residual disease at

second look. Gynecol Oncol 38:392, 1990

50. Lambert HE, Rustin GJS, Gregory WM et al: A randomized trial comparing single agent carboplatin with carboplatin followed by radiotherapy for advanced ovarian cancer: North Thames Ovary Group study. Ann Meet Br Oncol Assoc, July 1991
51. Mangioni C, Epis A, Vassena L et al: Radiotherapy (RT) versus chemotherapy (CH) as second line treatment of minimal residual disease (MRD) in advanced epithelial ovarian cancer (EOC). Proc Int Gynecol Cancer Soc 49:1987
52. Lawton F, Luesley D, Blackledge G et al: A randomized trial comparing whole abdominal radiotherapy with chemotherapy following cisplatinum cytoreduction in epithelial ovarian cancer: West Midlands Ovarian Cancer Group Trial II. Clin Oncol 2:4, 1990
53. Hacker NF, Berek JS, Burnison CM et al: Whole abdominal radiation as salvage therapy for epithelial ovarian cancer. Obstet Gynecol 65:60, 1985
54. Chiara S, Orsatti M, Franzone P et al: Abdominopelvic radiotherapy following surgery and chemotherapy in advanced ovarian cancer. Clin Oncol 3:340, 1991
55. Peters WA III, Blasko JC, Bagley CM Jr et al: Salvage therapy with whole abdominal irradiation in patients with advanced carcinoma of the ovary previously treated by combination chemotherapy. Cancer 58:880, 1986
56. Hoskins WJ, Lichter AS, Whittington R et al: Whole abdominal and pelvic irradiation in patients with minimal disease at second-look surgical reassessment for ovarian carcinoma. Gynecol Oncol 20:271, 1985
57. Greiner R, Goldhirsch A, Davis BW et al: Whole-abdomen radiation in patients with advanced ovarian carcinoma after surgery, chemotherapy and second-look laparotomy. J Cancer Res Clin Oncol 107:94, 1984
58. Piver MS, Barlow JJ, Lee FT, Vongtama V: Sequential therapy for advanced ovarian adenocarcinoma: operation, chemotherapy, second-look laparotomy and radiation therapy. Am J Obstet Gynecol 122:355, 1975
59. Hainsworth JD, Malcolm A, Johnson DH et al: Advanced minimal residual ovarian carcinoma: abdominopelvic irradiation following combination chemotherapy. Obstet Gynecol 61:619, 1983
60. Schray MF, Martinez A, Howes AE et al: Advanced epithelial ovarian cancer: salvage whole abdominal irradiation for patients with recurrent or persistent disease after combination chemotherapy. J Clin Oncol 6:1433, 1988
61. Reddy S, Hartsell W, Graham J et al: Whole abdomen radiation therapy in ovarian carcinoma: its role as a salvage therapeutic modality. Gynecol Oncol 35:307, 1989
62. Kuten A, Stein M, Steiner M et al: Whole abdominal irradiation following chemotherapy in advanced ovarian carcinoma. Int J Radiat Oncol Biol Phys 14:273, 1988
63. Linstadt DE, Stern JL, Quivey JM et al: Salvage whole-abdominal irradiation following chemotherapy failure in epithelial ovarian carcinoma. Gynecol Oncol 36:327, 1990
64. Solomon HJ, Atkinson KH, Coppleson JVM et al: Ovarian carcinoma: abdominopelvic irradiation following reexploration. Gynecol Oncol 31:396, 1988
65. Kong JS, Peters LJ, Wharton JT et al: Hyperfractionated split-course whole abdominal radiotherapy for ovarian carcinoma: tolerance and toxicity. Int J Radiat Oncol Biol Phys 14:737, 1988
66. Rosen EM, Goldberg ID, Rose C et al: Sequential multi-agent chemotherapy and whole abdominal irradiation for

stage III ovarian carcinoma. Radiother Oncol 7:223, 1986

67. Rothenberg ML, Ozols RF, Glatstein E et al: Dose-intensive induction therapy with cyclophosphamide, cisplatin, and consolidative abdominal radiation in advanced-stage epithelial ovarian cancer. J Clin Oncol 10:727, 1992
68. Haie C, Pejovic-Lenfant MH, George M et al: Whole abdominal irradiation following chemotherapy in patients with minimal residual disease after second look surgery in ovarian carcinoma. Int J Radiat Oncol Biol Phys 17:15, 1989
69. Cain JM, Russell AH, Greer BE et al: Whole abdomen radiation for minimal residual epithelial ovarian carcinoma after surgical resection and maximal first-line chemotherapy. Gynecol Oncol 29:168, 1988
70. Kersh CR, Randall ME, Constable WC et al: Whole abdominal radiotherapy following cytoreductive surgery and chemotherapy in ovarian carcinoma. Gynecol Oncol 31:113, 1988
71. Goldhirsch A, Greiner R, Dreher E et al: Treatment of advanced ovarian cancer with surgery, chemotherapy, and consolidation of response by whole-abdominal radiotherapy. Cancer 62: 40, 1988
72. Rustin GJS, Minton M, Southcott B et al: Surgery, chemotherapy and whole abdominal radiotherapy in the management of advanced ovarian carcinoma. Clin Radiol 38:269, 1987
73. Menczer J, Modan M, Brenner J et al: Abdominopelvic irradiation for stage II–IV ovarian carcinoma patients with limited or no residual disease at second-look laparotomy after completion of cisplatinum-based combination chemotherapy. Gynecol Oncol 24:149, 1986
74. Morgan L, Chafe W, Mendenhall W, Marcus R: Hyperfractionation of whole-abdomen radiation therapy: Salvage treatment of persistent ovarian carcinoma following chemotherapy. Gynecol Oncol 31:122, 1988
75. Coltart RS, Nethersell ABW, Brown CH: A pilot study of high dose abdominopelvic radiotherapy following surgery and chemotherapy for stage III epithelial carcinoma of the ovary. Gynecol Oncol 23:105, 1986
76. Varia M, Rosenman J, Venkatrama S et al: Intraperitoneal chromic phosphate therapy after second-look laparotomy for ovarian cancer. Cancer 61:919, 1988
77. Reddy S, Sutton GP, Stehman FB et al: Ovarian carcinoma: adjuvant treatment with P-32. Radiology 165:275, 1987
78. Soper JT, Wilkinson RH, Bandy LC et al: Intraperitoneal chromic phosphate ^{32}P as salvage therapy for persistent carcinoma of the ovary after surgical restaging. Am J Obstet Gynecol 156:1153, 1987
79. Potter ME, Partridge EE, Shingleton HM et al: Intraperitoneal chromic phosphate in ovarian cancer: risks and benefits. Gynecol Oncol 32:314, 1989
80. Dembo AJ, Bush RS: Choice of postoperative therapy based on prognostic factors. Int J Radiat Oncol Biol Phys 8:893, 1982
81. Dembo AJ, Bush RS, Brown TC: Clinicopathological correlates in ovarian cancer. Bull Cancer 69:292, 1982
82. Carey M, Dembo AJ, Fyles AW, Simm J: Testing the validity of a prognostic classification in patients with surgically optimal ovarian carcinoma: a 15-year review. Int J Gynecol Cancer 3:24, 1993
83. Shelly WE, Carmichael JC, Brown LB et al: Adriamycin and cisplatin in the treatment of stage II and IV epithelial ovarian carcinoma. Gynecol Oncol 29:208, 1988
84. Whelan TJ, Dembo AJ, Bush RS et al: Complications of whole abdominal and

pelvic radiotherapy following chemotherapy for advanced ovarian cancer. Int J Radiat Oncol Biol Phys 22:853, 1992

85. Louie KG, Behrens BC, Kinsella TJ et al: Radiation survival parameters of antineoplastic drug-sensitive and resistant human ovarian cancer cell lines and their modification by buthionine sulfoximine. Cancer Res 45:2110, 1985

86. Withers HR, Taylor JMG, Maciejewski B: The hazard of accelerated tumor clonogen repopulation during radiotherapy. Acta Oncol 27:131, 1988

87. Randall ME, Barrett RJ, Spirtos NM, et al: Chemotherapy, early surgical reassessment, and hyperfractionated abdominal radiotherapy in stage III ovarian cancer: results of a Gynecologic Oncology Group study. Int J Radiat Oncol Biol Phys 34:139, 1996

88. Bolis G, Zanaboni F, Russo A et al: The impact of whole-abdomen radiotherapy on survival in advanced ovarian cancer patients with minimal residual disease after chemotherapy. Gynecol Oncol 39:150, 1990

89. May LF, Belinson JL, Roland TA. Palliative benefit of radiation therapy in advanced ovarian cancer. Gynecol Oncol 37:408, 1990

90. Davidson SA, Rubin SC, Mychalczak B et al: Limited-field radiotherapy as salvage treatment of localized persistent or recurrent epithelial ovarian cancer. Gynecol Oncol 51:349, 1993

91. Corn BW, Lanciano RM, Boente M et al: Recurrent ovarian cancer: effective radiotherapeutic palliation after chemotherapy failure. Cancer 74:2979, 1994

92. Dauplat J, Nieberg RK, Hacker NF. Central nervous system involvement in epithelial ovarian carcinoma. Cancer 60:2559, 1987

93. Stein M, Steiner M, Klein B et al: Involvement of the central nervous system by ovarian carcinoma. Cancer 58:2066, 1986

94. Ziegler J, Gliedman P, Fass D et al: Brain metastases from ovarian cancer. J Neurooncol 5:211, 1987

95. Deutsch M, Beck D, Manor D et al: Metastatic tumor following negative second look operation in ovarian carcinoma. Gynecol Oncol 27:116, 1987

96. Ross WM, Carmichael VA, Shelley WE: Advanced carcinoma of the ovary with central nervous system relapse. Gynecol Oncol 30:398, 1988

97. LeRoux PD, Berger MS, Eliot P et al: Cerebral metastases from ovarian carcinoma. Cancer 67:2194, 1991

98. Hardy JR, Harvey VJ: Central metastases in patients with ovarian cancer treated with chemotherapy. Gynecol Oncol 33:296, 1989

99. Larson D, Copeland L, Moser R et al: Central nervous system metastases in epithelial ovarian carcinoma. Obstet Gynecol 68:746, 1986

100. Bruzzone M, Campora E, Chiara S et al: Cerebral metastases secondary to ovarian cancer: still an unusual event. Gynecol Oncol 49:37, 1993

101. Cooper KG, Kitchener HC, Parkin DE: Cerebral metastases from epithelial ovarian carcinoma treated with carboplatin. Gynecol Oncol 55:318, 1994

102. Corn BW, Greven KM, Randall ME et al: The efficacy of cranial irradiation in ovarian cancer metastatic to the brain: analysis of 32 cases. Obstet Gynecol 86:955, 1995

103. Rodriguez GC, Soper JT, Berchuck A et al: Improved palliation of cerebral metastases in epithelial ovarian cancer using a combined modality approach including radiation therapy, chemotherapy, and surgery. J Clin Oncol 10:1553, 1992

104. Mychalczak BR, Fuks Z: The current role of radiotherapy in the manage-

ment of ovarian cancer. Hematol Oncol Clin North Am 6:895, 1992

105. Cmelak AJ, Cox RS, Kapp DS: Long term survival with whole abdominopelvic irradiation (WAI) in platinum-refractory ovarian cancer, abstract. Int J Radiat Oncol Biol Phys, suppl. 1. 36:176, 1996
106. Baker K, Reddy S, Lee MS et al: Salvage whole abdominal radiation therapy for ovarian cancer: a twelve year experience, abstract. Int J Radiat Oncol Biol Phys, suppl. 1. 36:176, 1996
107. Reddy S, Lee MS, Yordan E et al: Salvage whole abdomen radiation therapy: its role in ovarian cancer. Int J Radiat Oncol Biol Phys 27:879, 1993
108. Eifel PJ, Gershenson DM, Delclos L, et al: Twice-daily split-course abdominopelvic radiation therapy after chemotherapy and positive second-look laparotomy for epithelial ovarian carcinoma. Int J Radiat Oncol Biol Phys 21:1013, 1991
109. Steiner M, Rubinov R, Borovik R et al: Multimodal approach (surgery, chemotherapy, and radiotherapy) in the treatment of advanced ovarian carcinoma. Cancer 55:2748,1985
110. Green JA, Warenius HM, Errington RD et al: Sequential cisplatin/cyclophosphamide chemotherapy and abdominopelvic radiotherapy in the management of advanced ovarian cancer. Br J Cancer 58:635, 1988
111. Cheung AYC: Salvage radiotherapy for carcinoma of the ovary following chemotherapy. Gynecol Oncol 30:15, 1988
112. Shelley WE, Starreveld AA, Carmichael JA et al: Toxicity of abdominopelvic radiation in advanced ovarian carcinoma patients after cisplatin/cyclophosphamide therapy and second-look laparotomy. Obstet Gynecol 71:327, 1988
113. Hoffman MS, Greenberg H, Finan M et al: Whole-abdomen radiation as a second-line therapy for epithelial ovarian cancer. Gynecol Oncol 35:73, 1989
114. Stephenson JA, Buchler DA: Abdominopelvic irradiation for persistent advanced ovarian carcinoma. Int J Radiat Oncol Biol Phys 17:385, 1989
115. Chauvet B, Fignon A, Lansac J et al: Radiothérapie après chimiothérapie et deuxième laparotomie dans le traitement des cancers de l'ovaire é un stade avancé. Ann Radiol 32:131, 1989
116. Kucera PR, Berman ML, Treadwell P et al: Whole-abdominal radiotherapy for patients with minimal residual epithelial ovarian cancer. Gynecol Oncol 36:338, 1990
117. Fein DA, Morgan LS, Marcus RB, Jr, et al: Stage III ovarian carcinoma: An analysis of treatment results and complications following hyperfractionated abdominopelvic irradiation for salvage. Int J Radiat Biol Phys 29(1):169, 1994
118. Britten RA, Peacock J, Warenius HM. Collateral resistance to photon and neutron irradiation is associated with acquired *cis*-platinum resistance in human ovarian tumor cells. Radiother Oncol 23:170, 1992
119. Schwartz JL, Rotmensch J, Beckett MA et al: X-ray and *cis*-diammiedichloroplatinum (II) cross-resistance in human tumor cell lines. Cancer Res 48:5133, 1988
120. Steele GG, Peckham MJ: Exploitable mechanisms in combined radiotherapy-chemotherapy: the concept of additivity. Int J Radiat Oncol Biol Phys 5:85, 1979
121. Murad AM, Triginelli SA, Ribalta JCL: Phase II trial of bleomycin, ifosfamide, and carboplatin in metastatic cervical cancer. J Clin Oncol 12(1):55, 1994
122. Malfetano J, Keys H, Kredentser et al: Weekly cisplatin and radical radiation therapy for advanced, recurrent, and poor prognosis cervical carcinoma. Cancer 71(11):3703, 1993

123. Berry RJ: Effects of some metabolic inhibitors on x-ray dose-response curves for the survival of mammalian cells in vitro, and on early recovery between fractionated x-ray doses. Br J Radiol 39:348, 1966

124. Bagshaw MA: Possible role of potentiators in radiation therapy. Am J Roentgenol 85(5):822, 1961

125. Vermund H, Hodgett J, Ansfield FJ: Effects of combined roentgen irradiation and chemotherapy on transplanted tumors in mice. Am J Roentgenol 85(3):559, 1961

126. Nakajima Y, Miyamoto T, Tanabe M et al: Enhancement of mammalian cell killing by 5-fluorouracil in combination with x-rays. Cancer Res 39:3763, 1979

127. Rockwell S: Cytotoxicities of mitomycin C and x-rays to aerobic and hypoxic cells in vitro. Int J Radiat Oncol Biol Phys 8:1035, 1982

128. Steren A, Bernd-Uwe S, Perras J et al: Taxol sensitizes human ovarian cancer cells to radiation. Gynecol Oncol 48:252, 1993

129. Tishler RB, Schiff PB, Geard CR, Hall EJ: Taxol: a novel radiation sensitizer. Int J Radiat Oncol Biol Phys 22:613, 1992

130. Leibmann J, Cook JA, Fisher J et al: In vitro studies of Taxol as a radiation sensitizer in human tumor cells. Cancer Res 52:3495, 1992

131. Pattillo RA. Collier BD, Abdel-Dayem H et al: Phosphorus-32-chromic phosphate for ovarian cancer: I. fractionated low-dose intraperitoneal treatments in conjunction with platinum analog chemotherapy. J Nucl Med 36:29, 1995

132. Copeland LJ, Gershenson DM: Ovarian cancer recurrences in patients with no macroscopic tumor at second-look laparotomy. Obstet Gynecol 68:873, 1986

133. Hoskins PJ, O'Reilly SE, Swenerton KD et al: Ten-year outcome of patients with advanced epithelial ovarian carcinoma treated with cisplatin-based multimodality therapy. J Clin Oncol 10:1561, 1992

134. Sutton GP, Stehman FB, Einhorn LH et al: Ten-year follow-up of patients receiving cisplatin, doxorubicin, and cyclophosphamide chemotherapy for advanced epithlial ovarian carcinoma. J Clin Oncol 7:223, 1989

135. Pickel H, Petru E, Lahousen M et al: Consolidation radiotherapy following carboplatin-based chemotherapy in radically operated advanced ovarian cancer: a pilot study. Am J Clin Oncol 14:184, 1991

136. Franchin G, Tamolo S, Scarabelli C et al: Whole abdomen radiation therapy after a short chemotherapy course and second-look laparotomy in advanced ovarian cancer. Gynecol Oncol 41: 206, 1991

137. Ledermann JA, Dembo AJ, Sturgeon JFG et al: Outcome of patients with unfavorable optimally cytoreduced ovarian cancer treated with chemotherapy and whole abdominal radiation. Gynecol Oncol 41:30, 1991

138. Sorbe B, Tropé C, Nordal R et al: Chemotherapy versus radiotherapy as consolidation treatment of ovarian carcinoma stage III at surgical complete remission from induction chemotherapy, abstract. Proc ASCO 15:287, 1996

139. Williams SD, Blessing JA, Hatch KD, Homesley HD: Chemotherapy of advanced dysgerminoma: trials of the Gynecologic Oncology Group. J Clin Oncol 9:1950, 1991

140. De Palo G, Lattuada A, Kenda R et al: Germ cell tumors of the ovary: the experience of the National Cancer Institute of Milan. I. Dysgerminoma. Int J Radiat Oncol Biol Phys 13:853, 1987

141. Thomas GM, Dembo AJ, Hacker NF, DePetrillo AD: Current therapy for

dysgerminoma of the ovary. Obstet Gynecol 70:268, 1987

142. Gershenson DM: Management of early ovarian cancer: germ cell and sex cord-stromal tumors. Gynecol Oncol 55:S62, 1994
143. Culine S, Lhomme C, Kattan J et al: Cisplatin-based chemotherapy in dysgerminoma of the ovary: thirteen-year experience at the Institut Gustave Roussy. Gynecol Oncol 58:344, 1995
144. Rogo KO, Persson H, Stendahl U: Dysgerminoma of the ovary: treatment results in northern Sweden. Eur J Gynaecol Oncol 11:43, 1990
145. Bjorkholm E, Lundell M, Gyftodimos A, Silfversward C: Dysgerminoma: the Radiumhemmet series 1927–1984. Cancer 65:38, 1990
146. Mitchell MF, Gershenson DM, Soeters RP et al: The long-term effects of radiation therapy on patients with ovarian dysgerminoma. Cancer 67:1084, 1991
147. Munkarah A, Gershenson DM, Levenback C et al: Salvage surgery for chemorefractory ovarian germ cell tumors. Gynecol Oncol 55:217, 1994
148. Fox H, Agrawal K, Langley FA: A clinicopathologic study of 92 cases of granulosa cell tumor of the ovary with special reference to factors influencing prognosis. Cancer 35:231, 1975
149. Malmström H, Hogberg T, Risberg B, Simonsen E: Granulosa cell tumors of the ovary: prognostic factors and outcome. Gynecol Oncol 52:50, 1994
150. Evans AT III, Gaffey TA, Malkasian GD, Annegers JF: Clinicopathologic review of 118 granulosa and 82 theca cell tumors. Obstet Gynecol 55:231, 1980
151. Kalawathi N: Granulosa cell tumour—hormonal aspects and radiosensitivity. Clin Radiol 22:524, 1971
152. Kumar P, Good R, Linder J: Complete response of granulosa cell tumor metastatic to the liver after hepatic irradiation: a case report. Obstet Gynecol 67:95S, 1986
153. Schwartz PE, Smith JP: Treatment of ovarian stromal tumors. Am J Obstet Gynecol 125:402, 1976
154. Malkasian GD, Webb MJ, Jorgenson EO: Observations on chemotherapy of granulosa cell carcinomas and malignant ovarian teratomas. Obstet Gynecol 44:885, 1974
155. Goldstone WR, Johnston WW, Fetter BF: Clinicopathologic studies in feminizing tumors of the ovary. I. Some aspects of the pathology and therapy of granulosa cell tumors. Am J Obstet Gynecol 112:422, 1972
156. Simmons RL, Sciarra JJ: Treatment of late recurrent granulosa cell tumors of the ovary. Surg Gynecol Obstet 124:65, 1967
157. Engle RB: Roentgen treatment of granulosa cell carcinoma of the ovary. Am J Roentgenol 80:793, 1958
158. Pankratz E, Boyes DA, White GW et al: Granulosa cell tumors: a clinical review of 61 cases. Obstet Gynecol 52:718, 1978
159. Stenwig JT, Hazekemp JT, Beecham JT: Granulosa cell tumors of the ovary: a clinicopathologic study of 118 cases with long-term follow-up. Gynecol Oncol 7:136, 1979
160. Gallion HH, van Nagell JR, Jr, Donaldson ES, Powell DE: Ovarian dysgerminoma: report of seven cases and review of the literature. Am J Obstet Gynecol 158:591, 1988
161. Buskirk SJ, Schray MF, Podratz KC et al: Ovarian dysgerminoma: a retrospective analysis of results of treatment, sites of treatment failure, and radiosensitivity. Mayo Clin Proc 62:1149, 1987
162. Lawson AP, Adler GF: Radiotherapy in the treatment of ovarian dysgerminomas. Int J Radiat Oncol Biol Phys 14:431, 1988

163. Santoni R, Cionini L, D'Elia F et al: Dysgerminoma of the ovary: a report on 29 patients. Clin Radiol 38:203, 1987

164. Teinturier C, Gelez J, Flamant F et al: Pure dysgerminoma of the ovary in childhood; treatment results and sequelae. Med Pediatr Oncol 23:1, 1994

165. LaPolla JP, Benda J, Vigliotti AP, Anderson B: Dysgerminoma of the ovary. Obstet Gynecol 69:859, 1987

166. Dilhuydy JM, Lagarde P, Chauvergne J et al: Le dysgerminome ovarien pur. Bilan d'une expérience et définition d'une stratégie thérapeutique. Bull Cancer 77:213–224, 1990

167. Susnerwala SS, Pande SC, Shrivastava SK, Dinshaw KA: Dysgerminoma of the ovary: review of 27 cases. J Surg Oncol 46:43, 1991

168. Zaghloul MS, Khattab TY: Dysgerminoma of the ovary: good prognosis even in advanced stages. Int J Radiat Oncol Biol Phys 24:161, 1992

169. About I, Bugat R, Naja A et al: Dysgerminomes purs de l'ovaire: analyse rétrospective de dix-sept cas traités au Centre Claudius Regaud de 1974 à 1989. Ann Chir 47:631, 1993

170. Ayhan A, Tuncer ZS, Yanik F et al: Malignant germ cell tumors of the ovary: Hacettepe hospital experience. Acta Obstet Gynecol Scand 74:384, 1995

171. Navot D, Laufer N, Kopolovic J et al: Artificially induced endometrial cycles and establishment of pregnancies in the absence of ovaries. N Engl J Med 314:806, 1986

172. van der Burg MEL, Lammes FB, Verweij J: The role of CA 125 in the early diagnosis of progressive disease in ovarian cancer. Ann Oncol 1:301, 1990

173. Williams SD, Blessing JA, Moore DH et al: Cisplatin, vinblastine, and bleomycin in advanced and recurrent ovarian germ-cell tumors: a trial of the Gynecologic Oncology Group. Ann Intern Med 111:22, 1989

174. Young DC, Mitchell A, Kessler J, Christman JE: Cortical blindness and seizures possibly related to cisplatin, vinblastine, and bleomycin treatment of ovarian dysgerminoma. J Am Osteopath Assoc 93:502, 1993

175. Gershenson DM, Morris M, Cangir A et al: Treatment of malignant germ cell tumors of the ovary with bleomycin, etoposide, and cisplatin. J Clin Oncol 8:715, 1990

176. Schwartz PE, Chambers SK, Chambers JT et al: Ovarian germ cell malignancies: the Yale University experience. Gynecol Oncol 45:26, 1992

177. Hansen SW, Helweg-Larsen S, Trojaborg W: Long-term neurotoxicity in patients treated with cisplatin, vinblastine, and bleomycin for metastatic germ cell cancer. J Clin Oncol 7:1457, 1989

178. Fosså SD, Aass N, Kaalhus O et al: Long-term survival and morbidity in patients with metastatic malignant germ cell tumors treated with cisplatin-based combination chemotherapy. Cancer 58:2600, 1986

179. Nichols CR, Breeden ES, Loehrer PJ et al: Secondary leukemia associated with a conventional dose of etoposide: review of serial germ cell tumor protocols. J Natl Cancer Inst 85:36, 1993

180. Pedersen-Bjergaard J, Daugaard G, Hansen SW et al: Increased risk of myelodysplasia and leukaemia after etoposide, cisplatin, and bleomycin for germ-cell tumours. Lancet 338:359, 1991

181. Troche V, Hernandez E: Neoplasia arising in dysgenetic gonads. Obstet Gynecol Surv 41:74, 1986

182. Watanabe T, Makiyama Y, Nishimoto H et al: Metachronous ovarian dysgerminoma after a suprasellar germ-cell tumor treated by radiation therapy. J Neurosurg 83:149, 1995

183. Jolles CJ, Karayianis S, Smotkin D, Delia JE: Advanced ovarian dysgerminoma with cure of tumor persistent in meninges. Gynecol Oncol 33:389, 1989

184. Diddle, AW: Granulosa- and theca-cell ovarian tumors: prognosis. Cancer 5:215, 1952

185. Norris HJ, Taylor HB: Prognosis of granulosa-theca tumors of the ovary. Cancer 21:255, 1968

186. Sjöstedt S, Wahlén T: Prognosis of granulosa cell tumours. Acta Obstet Gynecol Scand, suppl. 6. 40:3, 1961

187. Duckett HC, Davis CD, Fetter BF: Granulosa cell carcinoma of the ovary: clinical and pathological review of seventeen patients. Obstet Gynecol 2: 611, 1953

188. Haines M, Jackson I: Granulosa-cell tumour of the ovary: an analysis of 40 cases. J Obstet Gynecol Br Emp 57:737, 1950

189. Moreton RD, Leddy ET: Granulosa-cell tumor of the ovary with special reference to radiosensitivity. Am J Roentgenol 59:717–726, 1948

190. Björkholm E, Silfverswärd C: Prognostic factors in granulosa-cell tumors. Gynecol Oncol 11:261, 1981

191. Ohel G, Kaneti H, Schenker JG: Granulosa cell tumors in Israel: a study of 172 cases. Gynecol Oncol 15:278, 1983

192. Zaloudek C, Norris HJ: Granulosa tumors of the ovary in children: a clinical and pathologic study of 32 cases. Am J Surg Pathol 6:513, 1982

193. Stoll BA: The radiosensitivity of granulosa-cell tumour of the ovary. Med J Austr 1:1004, 1956

194. Dinnerstein AJ, O'Leary JA: Granulosa-theca cell tumors: a clinical review of 102 patients. Obstet Gynecol 31:654, 1968

195. Fletcher GH: Textbook of radiotherapy. p. 195. 3rd Ed Lea and Febiger, Philadelphia, 1980

196. Dembo AJ: Radiotherapeutic management of ovarian cancer. Semin Oncol 11:238, 1984

197. Thames HD, Peters LJ, Withers HR, Fletcher GH: Accelerated fractionation vs hyperfractionation: rationales for several treatments per day. Int J Radiat Biol Phys 9:127, 1983

198. Sigmon WR, Randall ME, Olds WW et al: Increased chronic bowel complications with split-course pelvic irradiation. Int J Radiat Oncol Biol Phys 28:395, 1994

199. Bortfeld T, Boyer AL, Schlegel W et al: Realization and verification of three-dimensional conformal radiotherapy with modulated fields. Int J Radiat Oncol Biol Phys 30:899, 1994

200. Konski AA, Neisler J, Phibbs G et al: A pilot study investigating intraoperative electron beam irradiation in the treatment of ovarian malignancies. Gynecol Oncol 38:121, 1990

201. Kapp DS, Giaccia AJ: New directions for radiation biology research in cancer of the uterine cervix. Monogr Natl Cancer Inst 21:131, 1996

202. Formenti SC, Shrivastava PN, Sapozink M et al: Abdomino-pelvic hyperthermia and intraperitoneal carboplatin in epithelial ovarian cancer: feasibility, tolerance and pharmacology. Int J Radiat Oncol Biol Phys 35:993, 1996

203. Leopold KA, Oleson JR, Clarke-Pearson et al: Intraperitoneal cisplatin and regional hyperthermia for ovarian carcinoma. Int J Radiat Oncol Biol Phys 27:1245, 1993

204. Bristow RE, Lagasse LD, Karlan BY: Secondary surgical cytoreduction for advanced epithelial ovarian cancer: patient selection and review of the literature. Cancer 78:2049, 1996

205. Recio FO, Piver MS, Hempling RE, Driscoll DL: Lack of improved survival plus increase in thromboembolic

complications in patients with clear cell carcinoma of the ovary treated with platinum versus nonplatinum-based chemotherapy. Cancer 78:2157, 1996

206. Pirtoli L, Risso G, Inaudi P et al: A role for tumor markers in therapeutic decisions after chemotherapy induction of objective remission in stage III epithelial ovarian neoplasms. Int J Biol Markers 6:107, 1991

207. Method MW, Serafini AN, Averette HE et al: The role of radioimmunoscintigraphy and computed tomography scan prior to reassessment laparotomy of patients with ovarian carcinoma: a preliminary report. Cancer 77:2286, 1996

CHAPTER 12

THE ROLE OF RADIOISOTOPE THERAPY IN THE MANAGEMENT OF OVARIAN CANCER

John T. Soper
William J. Spanos, Jr.

EDITORS' INTRODUCTION

Since ovarian cancer remains confined to the peritoneal cavity during most of its natural history, various approaches to regional therapy have been evaluated over the past two to three decades. One of these is the use of intraperitoneal radiotherapy. Studies initially used ^{198}Au but found this γ emitter to be excessively toxic. Subsequent to this most studies with radioisotopes have utilized ^{32}P which is a β emitter with a depth of penetration of 2 to 3 mm. Thus, it is agreed that regional radiotherapy should be reserved for patients with very low-volume macroscopic disease or microscopic disease, or as an adjunct in patients with a pathologic complete response following primary therapy. Additionally, patients undergoing regional radiotherapy must have a peritoneal cavity without significant adhesive peritonitis to prevent loculation of radioactivity leading to excessive toxicity. The number of patients meeting the above criteria is so small that most studies have inadequate statistical power, lack adequate control groups, and cannot be stratified for other known prognostic factors such as stage and grade.

We have asked our reviewers to comment on the use of intraperitoneal radioisotopes in three groups of patients: (1) patients undergoing primary treatment of stage I and II disease, (2) patients with microscopically positive second-look findings following primary therapy, and (3) patients with negative second-look findings. The largest number of patients fall in the first group, allowing some basic recommendations. In the latter two groups of patients continued controversy is anticipated because of the small amount of data currently available.

QUESTIONS

1. What is the role, if any, of radioisotopes in treating patients with early-stage epithelial ovarian cancer?
2. What is the role, if any, of radioisotopes in treating patients with (1) microscopically positive second-look findings or (2) negative second-look findings?
3. Are there any other major issues in this area? What are the future directions?

QUESTION 1

What is the role, if any, of radioisotopes in treating patients with early-stage epithelial ovarian cancer?

JOHN T. SOPER

It has long been recognized that epithelial ovarian carcinoma often spreads to involve peritoneal surfaces via intraperitoneal fluid. The entire peritoneal cavity is at risk for metastatic spread, recognized on gross examination in patients with advanced epithelial ovarian carcinoma and in cytologic assessment of washings or blind biopsies of the peritoneum in a substantial proportion of women with disease clinically confined to the ovary or pelvis. Intraperitoneal therapy of epithelial ovarian carcinoma is appealing because distribution of materials throughout the intraperitoneal cavity follows the same mechanics of dissemination as intraperitoneal metastases. Both chemotherapy and radioisotopes have been used for this purpose.

Since the 1950s, when radioactive chromic phosphate (^{32}P) became available, it has become the preferred radiopharmaceutical for intraperitoneal treatment. A pure β emitter, ^{32}P is a suspension rather than a true colloid. It has average β energy of 0.69 MeV and average tissue penetration of approximately 1.4 to 3.0 mm, with a half-life of 14.3 days.[1] Studies using phantoms, dogs, and patients have established that ^{32}P is adsorbed by peritoneal surfaces within a few hours of administration.[2] Optimal distribution is obtained when it is premixed and administered in more than 1 liter of fluid[1,2]

Toxicity from ^{32}P has been largely related to a combination of low-grade peritonitis and probable radiation effects on the serosa of the small intestine. In patients who receive intraperitoneal ^{32}P as their only treatment modality, 6 to 14% develop moderately severe abdominal pain requiring narcotic or nonsteroidal analgesics, and less than 5 to 6% develop bowel obstruction requiring surgical intervention.[1,3–7] The risk of bowel obstruction increases when patients have extensive adhesiolysis before administration of ^{32}P and when ^{32}P is given in conjunction with pelvic radiotherapy.[1,3] The development of leukemia has not been reported in patients who receive only ^{32}P. In a single small study using fractionated dosing of ^{32}P in combination with single-agent cisplatin, no unusual toxicity from this combined treatment was reported.[8]

Both intraperitoneal ^{32}P and whole abdominopelvic radiotherapy (WAR) are used in the treatment of patients with epithelial ovarian carcinoma. Advantages of ^{32}P over WAR include case of administration, cost, and relative absence of bone marrow toxicity (Table 12-1).[1] In contrast, WAR administers a more homogeneous dose to the peritoneal cavity and retroperitoneal structures, at the expense of myelotoxicity and bowel toxicity.[1] Intraperitoneal ^{32}P is often used in situations where WAR is being considered, when treating patients with minimal intraperitoneal tumor burden.

Despite a long history of use in the treatment of patients with epithelial ovarian carcinoma, too few randomized studies have been

TABLE 12-1
Comparison of ^{32}P and War as Therapy of Ovarian Carcinoma

Advantages of ^{32}P
Cost
Ease of administration
Absence of myelosuppression
Lower incidence of bowel complications
Advantages of WAR
Homogeneous radiation doses to peritoneal cavity and lymph nodes

Abbreviations: ^{32}P, radioactive chronic phosphate; WAR, whole abdominopelvic radiotherapy.

completed to allow firm conclusions regarding the efficacy of intraperitoneal ^{32}P. It should be emphasized that no randomized study has compared the efficacy of ^{32}P to a nontreatment arm in any subset of patients with epithelial ovarian carcinoma. This chapter will briefly review the various situations in which intraperitoneal ^{32}P can be considered for the treatment of patients with ovarian carcinoma, including its use in initial adjuvant treatment of early disease, consolidation therapy in patients with negative second-look laparotomy, and as secondary treatment of patients with persistent ovarian carcinoma at the time of reassessment laparotomy.

Initial adjuvant therapy of early ovarian carcinoma

Optimal primary management of epithelial ovarian carcinoma begins with a comprehensive staging laparotomy that includes removal of all visible tumor, total abdominal hysterectomy with bilateral salpingo-oophorectomy, omentectomy, complete peritoneal exploration with washings for cytology and peritoneal biopsies; and selective pelvic and periaortic lymph node sampling. In the absence of comprehensive staging, approximately 15 to 20% of patients with presumed stage I and up to 43% of patients with presumed stage II epithelial ovarian carcinoma have occult advanced-stage disease.[9,10] Unfortunately, most series of patients treated with adjuvant ^{32}P for early disease had consisted of patients with suboptimal staging procedures treated in a nonrandom fashion.

Initial reports from small series of patients with putative stage I lesions treated with intraperitoneal ^{32}P indicated survival of approximately 90% and appeared to provide circumstantial evidence for efficacy of this treatment when compared to previous reports of patients treated with surgery alone.[1] Many of the early studies were hampered by relatively short-term follow-up. Series described by Soper et al[5] and Piver et al[11] with longer-term follow-up reported life table progression-free survival of 75% and 79%, respectively, beyond 5 years. Two randomized series (Table 12-2) compared intraperitoneal ^{32}P to other treatment modalities in patients with early epithelial ovarian carcinoma who had not undergone comprehensive staging laparotomies.[3,6]

In the study reported by Klaassen et al,[3] patients with putative stage I and II and microscopic residual stage III ovarian carcinomas had equivalent survival whether randomized to intraperitoneal ^{32}P, WAR, or a single alkylator combined with pelvic radiotherapy. They initially treated 44 patients in the ^{32}P arm with pelvic radiotherapy but closed this arm to patient accrual after 5 women (11%) developed either small bowel obstruction or bowel fistulas that required surgical correction.[3]

Vergote et al[6] randomized patients with putative stage I and II and completely debulked stage III lesions to receive intraperitoneal ^{32}P or six cycles of single-agent cisplatin.[6] Patients with borderline malignant potential lesions comprised approximately 10% of both treatment arms. Patients with adhesions precluding diffuse intraperitoneal distribution of ^{32}P received WAR. Bowel obstruction requiring surgical correction occurred in 4% of patients receiving ^{32}P compared to 10% and 1% for those receiving WAR and cisplatin, respectively. Survival was equivalent in both arms.[6]

TABLE 12-2
Randomized Trials of ^{32}P Adjuvant Therapy in Early Ovarian Carcinoma

STUDY	STAGE	TREATMENT ARMS[a]	SURVIVAL (%)	P
Klaassen et al[3]	I–III[b]	WAR (107)	62	
		PEL + MEL (106)	61	NS
		^{32}P + PEL (44)	66	
Vergote et al[6]	I–III[b]	Cisplatin (171)	83	
		^{32}P (169)[c]	81	NS
Young et al[4]	I, II[d]	MEL (68)	81	
	(high risk)	^{32}P (73)	79	NS

Abbreviations: WAR, Whole abdominopelvic radiotherapy; NS, No significant difference.
[a] *Number of patients is shown in parentheses.*
[b] *Incomplete surgical staging; includes patients with stage IIIA disease.*
[c] *28 patients received WAR and 5 received cisplatin because ^{32}P was not given.*
[d] *Comprehensive surgical staging; includes stage I, grade 3, and stages I and II, all grades.*

In our series of patients with putative stage I and II epithelial ovarian carcinoma treated with intraperitoneal ^{32}P as the only adjuvant therapy after primary surgery, seven (58%) of 12 patients who relapsed had lymph node metastasis as the first sign of recurrence, including 2 of 3 patients who developed late recurrences.[5] Our results emphasize the inadequate distribution of ^{32}P to the retroperitoneal lymph nodes. Intraperitoneal ^{32}P is not appropriate therapy for women with apparent early-stage epithelial ovarian cancer who have not received comprehensive surgical staging.

Only one mature study reported to date has randomized patients undergoing comprehensive staging laparotomy to intraperitoneal ^{32}P and chemotherapy. The Gynecologic Oncology Group/Ovarian Cancer Study Group (GOG/OCSG) study randomized patients with high-risk disease (stage I, grade 3, and all stage IC and II) to receive either intraperitoneal ^{32}P or 18 months of melphalan (Table 12-2). Disease-free and overall survivals were the same in both treatment arms.[4]

Preliminary results of an Italian cooperative study indicate no difference in the survival of patients who had undergone comprehensive staging laparotomy and were treated with either ^{32}P or cisplatin for high-risk stage I epithelial ovarian carcinomas. These results, presented in abstract form only, indicate a significant improvement in disease-free survival among patients receiving cisplatin. Overall survival was equivalent in both arms, however, because patients who relapsed after intraperitoneal ^{32}P were often successfully treated with platin regimens. Finally, a GOG study that randomized patients with high-risk stage I or II epithelial ovarian carcinoma after comprehensive surgical staging to receive intraperitoneal ^{32}P versus three cycles of cisplatin cyclophosphamide combination chemotherapy has completed patient accrual. Results of this study have not been presented because follow-up is not mature.

In summary, the use of intraperitoneal ^{32}P in initial adjuvant treatment of early ovarian carcinoma should be reserved for patients who have undergone comprehensive staging laparotomy with negative retroperitoneal biopsies. Although the majority of patients in this situation are usually offered cytotoxic chemotherapy, available data indicate that survival is very similar in patients receiving intraperitoneal ^{32}P. We currently use intraperitoneal ^{32}P for patients with high-risk stage I and II epithelial ovarian carcinomas who do not qualify for chemotherapy protocols and/or who refuse cytotoxic chemotherapy.

WILLIAM J. SPANOS, JR.

The role of radioisotopes in patients with epithelial ovarian cancer

The spread pattern of ovarian cancer, particularly in the early stages, is dominantly peritoneal. This makes it ideal for treatment by any cytotoxic agent that can be concentrated at the peritoneal surface. This concept of concentrating treatment at the peritoneal surface began with the use of colloidal ^{198}Au but now includes intraperitoneal chemotherapy as well as other radioisotopes. Early reports on the use of colloidal ^{198}Au for intraperitoneal treatment of ovarian cancer indicated palliation and improved survival in early-stage patients.[12–14] However, because of the high-energy γ component of the gold isotope, there was a significant incidence of moderate to severe complications usually involving the gastrointestinal tract. A second isotope of phosphorus (^{32}P) has become the preferred radioisotope in the intraperitoneal treatment of ovarian cancer. ^{32}P has been the basis of literature reports on intraperitoneal radioisotopes in patient management for the last two decades. The attractiveness of ^{32}P as a intraperitoneal radioisotope is the low-energy β (electron) radiation with a limited effective depth of penetration of less than 5 mm. Phosphorus is an element normally present in the body and is readily fixed to tissues within a short time after exposure. Various studies have been done in the past to determine the dose that ^{32}P delivers to the abdominal cavity. Probably the most detailed study on peritoneal distribution has been done by Currie et al.[2] His results indicated that doses in the range of 3,000 to 4,000 cGy are achievable with ^{32}P. The distribution pattern of ^{32}P is not uniform, however, it does follow the usual fluid circulation pattern within the abdominal cavity and therefore tends to be concentrated in places that are most at risk for peritoneal spread of ovarian cancer.

Early-Stage Epithelial Ovarian Cancer

Early ovarian cancer includes stages IA through II. In addition to variation and prognosis by stage, other important prognostic variables influencing the outcome of early-stage ovarian cancer include grade, histology, and completeness of surgical staging. The number of permutations available for prognostic subgrouping makes it unlikely that any single institution with a limited number of patients can convincingly demonstrate advantages for any single modality of treatment whether it be chemotherapy or ^{32}P.

Table 12-3 is a listing of recent single-institution reports[5,11,16,17] of the use of ^{32}P as intraperitoneal treatment for patients with early-stage ovarian cancer. The number of patients in each of these studies is small, and they have a varying mix of distribution of patients between various subsets of stages I and II. The follow-up times are quite variable. The projected 5-year survival results show a fairly consistent 85 to 95% for stage I. Stage II results are much more variable, ranging from 50 to 100% with very small numbers in each group. It is important to note the number of patients included in these studies that would now be classified as low risk for relapse (stage IA or IB, grades 1 and 2, and low malignant potential). Duke University and Roswell Park provided sufficient information to allow estimation of the patient population at low risk for relapse. The other three series included patients with a low grade or low malignant potential, but the investigators did not subdivide them by stage and therefore the percentage of patients could not be accurately estimated. For the series that did provide information, 14 to 30% of the patients treated fell into this very favorable subgroup. If the use of ^{32}P were confined to patients at higher risk, the 5-year survivals might differ from the overall values. The toxicity from ^{32}P seen in these series is uniformly low (<5%).

Three different randomized trials compared ^{32}P to another form of treatment, usually single-agent chemotherapy: (1) National Cancer Institute of Canada (NCIC),[3] (2) GOG of

TABLE 12-3
^{32}P Treatment for Early-Stage Epithelial Ovarian Cancer

REFERENCE	NO. OF PATIENTS	LOW RISK[a]	STAGE[b]	FOLLOW-UP	RESULTS	^{32}P DOSE (mCi)	COMP
University of Alabama[15]	23	7 (30%)	I (18) II (6)	8 mo–8 yr	17/18[c] NED 4/4[d] NED	10–15	Not stated
Indiana University[16]	15	Not stated	I (10) II (2) III (3)[e]	9–77 mo (26½ mo median)	15/15 NED	15	3.5%
St. Joseph Hospital Atlanta[17]	16	Not stated	I (8) II (8)	16–78 mo (38 mo median)	I (87.5%) II (50%)	15	None
Duke University[5]	49	7 (14%)	I (42) II (7)	3 yr minimum (9 yr median)	I (84%) II (86%)	15	2%
Roswell Park[11]	25	Not stated	I (25)	5 yr minimum	84% 5 yr 75% 10 yr	15	
University of Oregon[12]	50	Not stated	IB (12) IC (18) II (18)[f]	5 yr minimum	I (73% 5 yr) II (73% 5 yr)	15	2%

Abbreviations: NED, No evidence of disease; LMP, Low malignant potential; Comp, Complications.
[a] *Low risk defined as stage IA gastrointestinal or stage I LMP.*
[b] *Number of patients is shown in parentheses.*
[c] *Salvaged with platinum-based chemotherapy.*
[d] *Two patients lost to follow-up.*
[e] *Completely resected.*
[f] *Nine also received pelvic radiation therapy.*

the United States,[4,18] and (3) the Norwegian Radium Hospital (NRH).[6]

The trial from the NCIC will be discussed separately since there was no arm with ^{32}P alone. This lack of a ^{32}P-only arm restricts any conclusions about the effectiveness of ^{32}P on survival. However, the study is of value with regard to the toxicity of ^{32}P combined with pelvic radiation. In the NCIC study, the arm with ^{32}P and pelvic radiation was prematurely discontinued because of excessive toxicity (12% late bowel toxicity requiring surgery) and concluded that whole pelvic radiation should not be given in addition to ^{32}P.

The two other randomized trials that included ^{32}P in the treatment of early-stage ovarian carcinoma are listed in Table 12-4. Of the two studies, only the GOG study limited the patients to stages I and II. In the Norwegian study, 27 patients with stage III disease were included (^{32}P 9; cisplatinum 18). The other significant difference in the Norwegian study is the low dose of ^{32}P which ranged from 7 mCi to 10 mCi. This is a significantly lower dose than the standard of 15 mCi commonly used in the United States.

Both randomized trials compared ^{32}P with single-agent chemotherapy. The GOG used melphalan and the NRH used cisplatinum as single-agent chemotherapy. Both studies concluded that ^{32}P was equally effective as single-agent chemotherapy. However, the recommendations of the two studies were significantly different. The GOG concluded that the cost of the procedure, ease of delivery, and single-treatment format favored ^{32}P as the

TABLE 12-4
^{32}P Treatment for Early Epithelial Ovarian Cancer Randomized Trials

REFERENCE	NO. OF PATIENTS	MODALITY	STAGE[a]	FOLLOW-UP	5-YR RESULTS (%)	^{32}P DOSE (mCi)	^{32}P COMP (%)
GOG 1[4]	73 68	^{32}P Melphalan	I (52) II (89)	3 yr minimum (6 yr median)	80 (DFS)	15	6
GOG 2[18]	48 45	^{32}P Melphalan	II (93)	5 yr minimum	75	15	6
Vergote[6]	169 171	^{32}P Cisplatin	I (265) II (48) III (27)	24–90 mo (62 mo median)	82	7–10	6[b]

Abbreviations: Comp, Complications.
[a] *Number patients is shown in parentheses.*
[b] *The 9% of patients successfully treated by medical management are included.*

adjunctive treatment of choice for early-stage ovarian cancer. The NRH concluded that single-agent cisplatinum was the treatment of choice because of the late toxicity associated, with ^{32}P, however, this conclusion regarding late toxicity requires additional comment. Not only was a higher incidence of toxicity reported with ^{32}P but the increase in toxicity occurred at doses of ^{32}P lower than those used by the GOG. The GOG trial reports a late toxicity rate of 6% small bowel obstruction requiring surgery, and the Norwegian trial reports 9% bowel obstruction. However, only 4.5% of patients required surgery, and the rest were successfully managed by nonsurgical means. Therefore, the bowel complication incidence is probably no greater than that reported by GOG and may be less. It has been repeatedly shown that the toxicity of ^{32}P is significantly dependent upon technique of delivery and care of the patient during the time period immediately following ^{32}P treatment.[19–21]

Determination of intra-abdominal flow patterns has long been recommended as a baseline standard for assessment of the ability to deliver ^{32}P safely. The Norwegian trial did not assess peritoneal distribution prior to delivery of ^{32}P, which could have affected the toxicity since loculation of fluid is known to occur as a result of reformation of adhesions or catheter migration.

Subsequent to the report on the overall group with high-risk stage I and II ovarian adenocarcinoma, the GOG reported separately on the subset of stage II patients (Table 12-3). These results are based on a minimum 5-year follow-up and show a 75% 5-year survival with no difference between ^{32}P and melphalan.

On the basis of nonrandomized studies using historic controls, ^{32}P provides improved 5-year survival. ^{32}P clearly is as effective as single-agent nonplatinum chemotherapy for high-risk stage I and II patients based on randomized trials from the GOG and from Norway. Using proper management techniques and protocols for the delivery of ^{32}P results in minimal toxicity and a low incidence of complications. A 15-mCi dose of ^{32}P is well tolerated and should be the minimum dose recommended, not withstanding the Norwegian trial. Future trials considering multiagent chemotherapy in this group of patients should also include a ^{32}P arm as a control.

QUESTION 2

What is the role, if any, of radioisotopes in treating patients with (1) microscopically positive second-look findings or (2) negative second-look findings?

JOHN T. SOPER

Intraperitoneal ^{32}P as salvage therapy for persistent disease after second-look laparotomy

Effective second-line treatment for patients with persistent disease identified at second-look laparotomy (SLL) is currently undefined. Proposed strategies for treatment include administration of systemic or intraperitoneal chemotherapy, WAR, and intraperitoneal ^{32}P administration for selected patients. Several small series of patients with persistent disease identified at SLL have been reported, comprised of mixed populations of patients with microscopic and macroscopic residual disease.[22,23–25] In the series reported by Soper et al[25] and Potter et al,[15] median disease-free survivals of 2 to 2½ years were observed in patients with either microscopic persistent disease or macroscopic disease that was completely resected at SLL. In these two series combined, 0 of 9 patients with small macroscopic residual disease survived beyond 3 years. Likewise, Varia et al[20] noted relapses in 7 of 17 patients receiving intraperitoneal ^{32}P for "minimal" residual disease at SLL.[22] Both Potter et al and Varia et al reported very poor survival for patients with grade 3 lesions who received salvage ^{32}P, in contrast to excellent survival among patients with grade 1 or 2 lesions and those with early original stage.[22,25] In all small series reported to date, several patients received radiotherapy or chemotherapy in addition to "salvage" ^{32}P. However, patients with microscopic residual disease at SLL tend to have favorable survival rates, particularly those with well-differentiated lesions.[16] Although intraperitoneal ^{32}P is a reasonable option to offer patients with no gross disease residual at SLL who refuse additional treatment, it appears that the survival after salvage intraperitoneal ^{32}P in this setting probably reflects the biology of the disease rather than the therapeutic efficacy of the intraperitoneal ^{32}P.

Intraperitoneal ^{32}P as consolidation therapy after negative second-look laparotomy

During the 1970s and 1980s, SLL was popularized as a means of identifying patient response to induction chemotherapy. Initial reports indicated favorable survival in patients with negative SLL, however, later reports describing advanced-stage patients with longer follow-up indicated relapse rates approaching 50 to 60% in those with negative SLL after chemotherapy for advanced-stage disease.[11] Some retrospective studies appear to demonstrate improved survival in patients who received intraperitoneal ^{32}P after negative second-look laparotomy, compared to historic or contemporary controls.[22,26] For example, Varia et al reported that 4-year survival for patients with negative SLL was 89% for 43 patients receiving ^{32}P versus 67% for 14 who did not receive further therapy.[22] The difference in survival was significant only for patients treated after 1979. Their population included women with stage I and II lesions. In contrast, a recent report by Peters et al,[24] found no improvement in disease-free survival when intraperitoneal ^{32}P was used after negative SLL in patients with advanced-stage ovarian carcinoma, compared to historic controls. Although the theory behind using intraperitoneal ^{32}P consolidation therapy to treat undetected intraperitoneal microscopic deposits of disease following induction chemotherapy is attractive, data supporting or refuting this practice await maturation of a recently completed GOG randomized trial.

WILLIAM J. SPANOS, JR.

The role of radioisotopes in patients undergoing second-look laparotomy or with stage III epithelial carcinoma of the ovary

Approximately 60 to 75% of patients presenting with epithelial ovarian carcinoma present as stage III. Multiagent chemotherapy converts 30 to 40% (optimal debulking) of patients with stage III ovarian carcinoma of the ovary to no residual disease on re-exploration after 6 to 12 courses.[28] Unfortunately, in spite of this success, patients with negative findings at SLL have a subsequent failure rate of 40 to 60%. Since the residual peritoneal disease in these women is low volume, it follows that ^{32}P may be an effective addition to the standard management plan for patients with stage III ovarian cancer. Table 12-5 is a summary of reports from the literature on the use of ^{32}P following SLL. In all but one of these reports there is a mixture of patients with stages I through IV. An explanation of the reason for second-look surgery in lower-stage patients was not given. Because of the unusual mix of patients in these series, a comparison of the overall results of ^{32}P following second-look surgery between series is not valid. The University of Louisville series[31] was a prospective nonrandomized trial evaluating the results of ^{32}P after SLL. This trial was confined to patients with stage III disease, with routine use of ^{32}P in all individuals undergoing a second-look procedure where the residual disease was reducible to 0.5 cm or less, and it involved a relatively uniform patient population. However, there was no untreated patient group in this series for comparison.

Distillation of the stage III subset of patients receiving ^{32}P after SLL from these series provides a more uniform basis for comparison of results. Since residual disease is one of the most significant prognostic factors at SLL, these results will be discussed below based on residual disease status.

Microscopic positive second-look laparotomy

The presence of residual microscopic disease at SLL following chemotherapy carries a negative prognosis. The discovery of microscopic disease on random biopsies may represent a sampling difference when compared with negative findings. Since microscopic disease at SLL represents persistent tumor, additional therapy is indicated. Whether it is given in an adjuvant setting or withheld until clinical relapse is subject to debate. ^{32}P has been employed by several centers as additional treatment for microscopic residual findings at SLL.

Indiana University[32] used ^{32}P in treating 15 patients with microscopic disease at SLL. Eight of 15 patients remained with no evidence of disease (NED) after 16 to 56 months' follow-up. The Duke University experience[25] using ^{32}P as salvage therapy in 10 patients with microscopic residual disease at SLL resulted in a 4-year disease-free survival of 50%. The University of Alabama[15] trial used ^{32}P as salvage therapy for 28 patients with microscopic residual disease at SLL and included a mixture of recurrent stage I and II (7 patients) and stage III (21 patients). The 4-year disease-free survival was 42%. The University of Louisville series[31] had 15 stage III patients with microscopic residual disease at SLL treated with ^{32}P and the 4-year survival was 46%. The University of North Carolina[30] reports on 34 stage III patients with minimal residual disease at SLL in this series that included 14 patients who did not receive ^{32}P for comparison. For the 20 patients treated with ^{32}P, disease-free survival at 5 years was 31%. At 5 years there were no disease-free patients who had not received ^{32}P ($P = 0.05$).

The potential advantage of ^{32}P as salvage therapy in patients with microscopic residual disease at SLL over second-line chemotherapy cannot be established by the above data. In the above series survivals range from 31 to 50% following ^{32}P and may not differ significantly from those in the MD Anderson series reported by Copeland et al.[33] (In a personal communication, Dr. Copeland stated that many of these patients had benign disease.) In that series, the 5-year disease-free survival was 70% for 50 patients with microscopic findings at SLL, and a similar survival curve was obtained for those with negative findings at SLL. All but four patients received additional treatment at varying times following SLL. In addition, Copeland demonstrated a highly sig-

TABLE 12-5
^{32}*P Following Second-Look Laparotomy*

REFERENCE	NO. OF PATIENTS	STAGE[a]	RESIDUAL[a]	FOLLOW-UP	SURVIVAL
Duke University[5]	23[b]	IB, 2C (2) 3 (19) 4 (2)	Micro (10) Macro (13)	24 mo median	57% (4 yr)
Medical University of South Carolina[29]	14	I,II (8) III (4) Unknown (2)	Negative	24 mo minimum (4 yr median)	100% (4 yr)
University of North Carolina[30]	30	I,II (10) III (20)	Minimum	58 mo mean	31% (DFS) for stage III
University of North Carolina[20]	51	I,II (39) III (12)	Negative (51)	18 mo minimum (58 mo median)	82% (5 yr)
Pudget Sound Oncology Consortium[24]	34	I,II (8) III (26)	Negative	19 mo minimum (31 mo median)	62% (4 yr)
University of Louisville[31]	56	III (56)	Negative (27) Micro (15) Gross (14)	24 mo minimum (48 mo median)	Negative 75% (4 yr) Micro 46% (4 yr) Macro 30% (4 yr)
Indiana University[16]	14	I (1) III (12) IV (1)	Micro (14)	12 mo minimum (24 mo median)	53% (2 yr)
University of Oregon[12]	9	III (9)	Not stated	5 yr minimum	50% (5 yr)

Abbreviations: DFS, Disease-free survival
[a] *Number of patients is shown in parentheses.*
[b] *Salvage therapy.*

nificant effect of grade on disease-free survival for patients with microscopic findings at SLL. Therefore, grade should be a consideration in comparing results, but this is not possible with the small series reported above.

In spite of the difficulty in establishing efficacy on the basis of the above series, there are two appealing aspects of ^{32}P in this setting: (1) ^{32}P can be given as a single treatment at the time of SLL and has low toxicity when administered properly. (2) ^{32}P does not affect bone marrow reserve and thus does not preclude later consideration of additional chemotherapy. Since its effectiveness is very dependent on bulk of disease, the decision to use ^{32}P cannot be delayed until the patients show clinical signs of progression.

Periaortic nodes

Recommended initial staging for stage III epithelial ovarian cancer includes sampling of periaortic nodes. Based on lymphangiogram studies, approximately 30% of stage III patients have positive periaortic nodes.[34] Does the presence of positive periaortic nodes at initial staging exclude consideration of ^{32}P at SLL? The answer is not clear. Certainly, ^{32}P has no effect on periaortic nodes. Can additional external beam radiation be given to periaortic nodes after ^{32}P therapy? In the series described by Spanos et al,[31] select group of patients with stage III disease and positive periaortic nodes on initial staging received external beam radiation to 45 Gy following ^{32}P and no additional late toxicity was noted. The effect on survival or the pattern of relapse is unclear.

Overview of use of ^{32}P following second-look laparotomy

The use of SLL following chemotherapy for stage III epithelial ovarian cancer is in itself controversial. The added morbidity of this procedure has to be balanced by demonstrated improvement in disease-free survival. The theoretical potential for ^{32}P to increase the cure rate for patients with negative or microscopic residual disease or decrease the abdominal relapse rate for patients with reducible gross disease continues to be tantalizing, particularly since ^{32}P does not interfere with later salvage chemotherapy. The above-mentioned series are suggestive of a benefit to disease-free survival or survival. However, because of multiple prognostic factors and small patient numbers, ^{32}P cannot be shown to improve patient outcome sufficiently to justify SLL for the purpose of using ^{32}P alone. Blind administration of ^{32}P without knowledge of the status of intra-abdominal disease or the status of adhesions is not recommended. If in the judgment of a gynecologic oncologist SLL is justified for reasons other than using ^{32}P, the ^{32}P should be considered additional adjunctive therapy or salvage therapy. Otherwise, standard use of ^{32}P following SLL should occur in the context of prospective single institution or multi-institution trials where treatment protocols can be standardized and prognostic factors controlled.

Negative SLL

Patients with microscopically negative findings at SLL following chemotherapy have a 40 to 60% abdominal failure rate. ^{32}P can be considered a continuation of adjuvant management in this setting. The following reports from the literature discuss the use of ^{32}P in negative SLL. All but one trial includes a mixture of stages I through III. In some of the reports, the results for stage III patients can be separated from those for other patients.

The Medical University of South Carolina[29] trial included four stage III patients treated by ^{32}P following negative SLL. There were no recurrences after a mean follow-up of 4 years. The Puget Sound Oncology Consortium[24] reported on 26 patients with stage III disease treated with ^{32}P following negative SLL. The relapse rate was 58% with a median follow-up of 31 months. However, five relapses occurred outside the peritoneal cavity and would not have been influenced by ^{32}P. Of these five relapses, the number of extraperitoneal relapses in the stage III subset of patients was not given. The University of North Carolina[24] reported on patients treated with ^{32}P following negative SLL. In that series there were 12 stage III patients, however, the results for these patients were not reported separately from those for the stage I and II patients. The series from the University of Louisville[28] included 23 patients with negative SLL. The 5-year survival was 75% with a median follow-up of 48 months.

The impact of ^{32}P on relapse rates following negative SLL cannot be determined from the above scattered data and the small patient numbers. An accurate estimate of the effect of ^{32}P in this setting awaits completion of a randomized trial conducted by the GOG comparing ^{32}P with observation for patients with negative findings at SLL.

QUESTION 3

Are there any other major issues in this area? What are the future directions?

WILLIAM J. SPANOS, Jr.

Future directions for intra-abdominal radioisotopes

The current limitation on the use of intra-abdominal radioisotopes is the ability to deliver sufficient dose uniformly to the tumor without additional damage to normal structures.

Radioisotope Dose

The current dose recommendation for ^{32}P is somewhat arbitrary, the most commonly used dose in the United States being 15 mCi. There have been institutional variations in this dose to adjust for patient size. The GOG trial used 15 mCi of ^{32}P. The Norwegian trial used 7 to 10 mCi which varied by patient size. Both series report similar bowel toxicity rates (6 and 4.5%, respectively). The single-institution series listed in Table 12-5 also reports similar low late toxicity rates ranging from 0 to 13%. All but one trial[25] reported toxicity rates less than 6%. The toxicity of ^{32}P does not appear to depend on dose within the 7- to 15-mCi range. It can be significantly, reduced by procedures that account for intra-abdominal fluid volume, verification of intra-abdominal flow pattern, and a strict patient positioning protocol. Additional gains in minimizing toxicity have been suggested by the administration of ^{32}P during the immediate postoperative period before adhesions can form.[19-20] Since the toxicity of ^{32}P within the 7- to 15-mCi dose range appears to depend more on procedure than on dose, higher doses may be possible without a significant increase in toxicity. A dose-seeking protocol with a gradual increase in ^{32}P should be considered.

Chemosensitization

Since ^{32}P and all other nonspecific radioisotopes deliver similar doses to the tumor and to adjacent normal tissue, additional methods of improving the therapeutic gain to the tumor need to be considered. One potential method of increasing therapeutic gain for ^{32}P is the systemic or intraperitoneal addition of a chemotherapeutic agent known to have radiation-sensitizing properties during the effective biologic half-life of ^{32}P. This concept is in early stages of investigation with one preliminary report[35] on effectiveness in animal models with cisplatin and ^{32}P available.

Radioisotope-Tagged Monoclonal Antibodies

One of the most appealing concepts of increasing the therapeutic ratio for radioisotopes is marriage of the radioisotope to a monoclonal antibody specific for epithelial ovarian cancer. If the sensitivity and specificity of the monoclonal antibody are high and the monoclonal antibody-radioisotope combination is biologically stable, the potential improvement in therapeutic ratio could be substantial. This has been a very active area of investigation. The biologic basis was laid with the use of radioisotope-tagged monoclonal antibodies employed in a diagnostic setting. Sensitivity and specificity results have ranged from 65% to 98%.[36-41] A large variety of monoclonal antibodies to epithelial ovarian cancer are available for investigation. The most commonly used radioisotopes have been ^{111}In, ^{131}-I, and ^{125}-I.

Animal studies using murine ovarian cancer models have produced results varying from no therapeutic advantage[42] to significant tumor regression and prolonged survival.[43,44] Specific tumor uptake of radioisotope compared to that in normal tissue was widely variable in one study.[45]

Phase I and II human studies using radioisotope-tagged monoclonal antibodies have been reported from several centers. Patient numbers have ranged from 7- to 52,[46-54] and a marked variation in tumor uptake was seen in series[50,51] where multiple biopsies were taken. Dose-limiting toxicity of myelosuppression was reported in some series,[46,53] and others described minor gastrointestinal, thyroid, and musculoskeletal symptoms.[47,49,54] Tumor response has varied significantly from encouraging responses[49,51] to minimal or no evidence of response.[48,49]

The appeal of radioisotope-tagged monoclonal antibodies remains high, however, the optimal combination of isotope and antibody is far from established. The toxicity profile of this approach is not clear and will need careful documentation in ongoing trials. Despite the expectation of targeted uptake predicted by theory, actual tumor uptake levels are quite variable in both animal and human series. Despite the variability of radioisotope uptake, tumor uptake is still higher than for non-tagged isotopes.

EDITORS' COMMENTARY

As noted in chapter 3 on early-stage ovarian cancer, studies of the role of ^{32}P have been hampered by the low number of eligible patients, making studies of extremely low statistical power. Furthermore, in the decade required for accrual, if new, active therapies have become available, investigators may not enter patients to what they consider suboptimal therapy. One additional problem is lack of proper staging in studies performed more than 15 years ago. Probably 20% of stage I patients and up to 50% of stage II patients actually have cryptic stage III disease, making end results appear worse than they really are. Conversely, many of these studies include patients with borderline tumors, making end results appear better than they would if the patients had had invasive carcinoma.

In discussing the use of ^{32}P as an adjunct to the treatment of high-risk, early-stage disease, Dr. Soper underlines the need for rigorous staging in terms of having a homogeneous population for trials but additionally to avoid placement of patients with tumor implants and retroperitoneal nodes in such trials. These patients are the ones most likely to relapse since there are few data supporting significant radiation to tumor deposits located in this area. Dr. Spanos feels that ^{32}P provides an improved 5-year survival but admits that this conclusion is based on nonrandomized studies. He believes that intraperitoneal ^{32}P is well-tolerated and thus appropriate for use in patients with early-stage disease. Dr. Soper, on the other hand, utilizes this treatment only in patients who are not candidates for protocol or who refuse chemotherapeutic management. We note the Norwegian trial in which outcomes with platinum and ^{32}P were similar, but toxicities were somewhat higher in the patients treated with ^{32}P. Additionally, data from the Italian trial suggest that cisplatin has a better therapeutic index than ^{32}P based on both improved progression-free survival and reduced toxicity in the ^{32}P arm. The Italian study is the first to suggest an outcome advantage for patients treated with any form of therapy over simple observation.

^{32}P has also been used as consolidation therapy after negative SLL. Both authors agree, and we concur, that there are not enough data on the use of ^{32}P in a negative second-look setting to make any conclusions or recommendations. A recently completed GOG study evaluated observation versus ^{32}P after negative SLL. Several more years of data maturity are necessary before any of the results of this trial will be forthcoming. At this point in time there does not seem to be a role for consolidation with ^{32}P outside a clinical trial.

In commenting on the use of ^{32}P in patients with microscopically positive second-look operations, both authors agree that not enough data are available to make firm conclusions. Dr. Spanos feels this is a reasonable approach in such patients based on the need for a single treatment and the lack of hematologic toxicity from the therapy, making future chemotherapy possible. Dr. Soper believes, and we concur, that the variable outcome for patients with microscopically positive second-look surgery depends more on the biology of the disease than on the therapeutic efficacy of the ^{32}P.

Thus, a well-defined role for intraperitoneal ^{32}P in the treatment of ovarian cancer remains to be defined. Additionally, such therapy is suitable only for a small subset of patients, those with low-volume disease and a peritoneal cavity that allows adequate distribution of the radiocolloid.

References

1. Rosenshein NB, Leichner PK, Vogelsgang G: Radiocolloids in the treatment of ovarian cancer. Obstet Gynecol Surv 34:708, 1979
2. Currie JL, Bayne F, Harris C et al: Radioactive chromic phosphate suspension: studies on distribution, close absorption, and effective therapeutic

radiation in phantoms, dogs, and patients. Gynecol Oncol 12:193, 1981

3. Klaassen D, Shelley W, Starreverd A et al: Early stage ovarian cancer: randomized clinical trial comparing whole abdominal radiotherapy, melphalan, and intraperitoneal chromic phosphate. A National Cancer Institute of Canada Clinical Trials Group report. J Clin Oncol 6:1254, 1988
4. Young RE, Walton LA, Ellenberg SS et al: Adjuvant therapy in stage I and stage II epithelial ovarian cancer: results of two prospective randomized trails. N Engl J Med 322:1021, 1990
5. Soper JT, Berchuck A, Clarke-Pearson DL: Adjuvant intraperitoneal chromic phosphate therapy for women with apparent early ovarian carcinoma who have not undergone comprehensive surgical staging. Cancer 68:725, 1991
6. Vergote IB, Vergote-De Vos LN, Abeler VM et al: Randomized trial comparing cisplatin with radioactive phosphorus or whole abdomen irradiation as adjuvant treatment of ovarian cancer. Cancer 69:741, 1992
7. Soper JT, Berchuck A, Dodge R et al: Adjuvant therapy with intraperitoneal chromic phosphate (^{32}P) in women with early ovarian carcinoma after comprehensive surgical staging. Obstet Gynecol 79:993, 1992
8. Patillo RA, Collier BD, Abdel-Dayem H et al: Phosphorus-32 chromic phosphate for ovarian cancer: I. Fractionate low-dose intraperitoneal treatments in conjunction with platinum analog chemotherapy. J Nucl Med 36:29, 1995
9. Young RE, Decker DG, Wharton JT et al: Staging laparotomy in early ovarian cancer. JAMA 250:3072, 1983
10. Buchsbaum MS, Brady MF, Delgado G et al: Surgical staging of carcinoma of the ovaries. Surg Gynecol Obstet 169:226, 1989
11. Piver MS, Lele SB, Bakshi S et al: Five and ten year estimated survival and disease-free rates after intraperitoneal chromic phosphate; stage I ovarian adenocarcinoma. Am J Clin Oncol 11:515, 1988
12. Aure JC, Hoeg K, Kolstad P: Radioactive colloidal gold in the treatment of ovarian carcinoma. Northwest Med 66:1040, 1967
13. Decker DG, Webb MJ, Holbrook MA: Radiocolloid treatment of epithelial cancer of the ovary: late results. Am J Obstet Gynecol 115:751, 1973
14. Perez CA, Walz BJ, Jacobson PL: Radiation therapy in the management of carcinoma of the ovary. Natl Cancer Inst Monogr 42:119, 1975
15. Potter ME, Partridge EE, Shingleton HM et al: Intraperitoneal chromic phosphate in ovarian cancer: risks and benefits. Gynecol Oncol 32:314, 1989
16. Reddy S, Sutton GP, Stehman FB et al: Ovarian carcinoma: adjuvant treatment with ^{32}P. Radiology 165:275, 1987
17. Powell JL, Burrell MO, Kirchner AB: Intraperitoneal radioactive chromic phosphate ^{32}P in the treatment of ovarian cancer. South Med J 80:1513, 1987
18. Walton LA, Yadusky A, Rubinstein L et al: Stage II carcinoma of the ovary: an analysis of survival after comprehensive surgical staging and adjuvant therapy. Gynecol Oncol 44:55, 1992
19. Spanos WJ Jr, Day T, Abner A et al: Complications in the use of intra-abdominal ^{32}P for ovarian carcinoma. Gynecol Oncol 45:243, 1992
20. Varia M, Rosenman J, Venkatraman S et al: Intraperitoneal chromic phosphate therapy after second-look laparotomy for ovarian cancer. Cancer 61:919, 1988
21. Bakri YN, Given FT, Peeples WJ et al: Complications from intraperitoneal radioactive phosphorus in ovarian malignancies. Gynecol Oncol 21:294, 1985
22. Bolis G, Beni S, Fevali G et al: Multicentric controlled trial in patients with epi-

thelial ovarian cancer stage I, abstract 157. Proc Int Gynecol Cancer Soc, 1989

23. Spencer TR, Marks RD, Fenn JO et al: Intraperitoneal ^{32}P after negative second-look laparotomy in ovarian carcinoma. Cancer 63:243, 1989
24. Peters WA, Smith MR, Cain JM et al: Intraperitoneal ^{32}P is not effective consolidation therapy after a negative second-look laparotomy for epithelial carcinoma of the ovary. Gynecol Oncol 47:146, 1992
25. Soper JT, Wilkinson RH, Bendy LC et al: Intraperitoneal chromic phosphate ^{32}P as salvage therapy for persistent carcinoma of the ovary after surgical restaging. Am J Obstet Gynecol 156:1153, 1987
26. Clarke-Pearson DL, Kohler MF, Hurteau JA et al: Surgery for advanced ovarian cancer. Clin Obstet Gynecol 37:439, 1994
27. Rogers L, Varia M, Halle J et al: ^{32}P following negative second-look laparotomy for epithelial ovarian cancer. Gynecol Oncol 50:141, 1993
28. Potter ME, Hatch KD, Soong SJ et al: Second-look laparotomy and salvage therapy: a research modality only? Gynecol Oncol 44:3, 1992
29. Spencer TR Jr, Marks RD Jr, Fenn JO et al: Intraperitoneal ^{32}P after negative second-look laparotomy in ovarian carcinoma. Cancer 63:2434, 1989
30. Rogers L, Varia M, Halle J et al: ^{32}P following second-look laparotomy for epithelial ovarian cancer. Int J Radiat Oncol Biol Phys 19(1):167, 1990
31. Spanos WJ Jr, Day T Jr, Jose B et al: Use of ^{32}P in stage III epithelial carcinoma of the ovary. Gynecol Oncol 54:35, 1994
32. Smirz LR, Stehman FB, Ulbright TM et al: Second-look laparotomy after chemotherapy in the management of ovarian malignancy. Am J Obstet Gynecol 152:661, 1985
33. Copeland LJ, Gershenson DM, Wharton JT et al: Microscopic disease at second-look laparotomy in advanced ovarian cancer. Cancer 55:472, 1985
34. Musumeci R, DePalo G, Kenda R et al: Retroperitoneal metastases from ovarian carcinoma: reassessment of 365 patients studied with lymphography. Am J Radiol 134:449, 1980
35. Pattillo R, Collier BD, Ruckert A et al: Ovarian cancer. ^{32}P and its new role in adjuvant chemotherapy. Proc Am Assoc Cancer Res 36:243, 1995
36. Hunter RE, Doherty P, Griffin TW: Use of indium-111 labeled OC-125 monoclonal antibody in the detection of ovarian cancer. Gynecol Oncol 27(3): 325, 1987
37. Rubin SC, Kostakoglu L, Divgi C et al: Biodistribution and intraoperative evaluation of radiolabeled monoclonal antibody MX35 in patients with epithelial ovarian cancer. Gynecol Oncol 51(1): 61, 1993
38. Maguire RT, Pascucci VL, Maroli AN et al: Clinical assessment of ^{111}In-CYT-103 immunoscintigraphy in ovarian cancer. Gynecol Oncol 48(3):285, 1993
39. Qian H, Feng J, Cui H et al: Clinical evaluation of radioimmunoimaging with ^{131}I-COC183B2 monoclonal antibody against ovarian carcinoma by intraperitoneal injection. Gynecol Oncol 47(2): 216, 1992
40. Hempling RE, Piver MS, Baker TR: Immunoscintigraphy using ^{111}InCyt103 prior to second look laparotomy in ovarian cancer: a pilot study. Am J Clin Oncol 17(4):331, 1994
41. Chaudhuri TR, Zinn KR, Morris JS et al: Detection of ovarian cancer by ^{198}Au-labeled human monoclonal antibody. Cancer, suppl 3.73:878, 1994
42. Manetta A, Satyaswaroop PG, Hamilton T et al: Therapeutic effect of a radiolabeled monoclonal antibody on human

ovarian cancer xenograft in nude mice. Gynecol Oncol 32(3):368, 1989

43. Molthoff CF, Pinedo HM, Schluper HM et al: Influence of dose and schedule on the therapeutic efficacy of ^{131}I-labeled monoclonal antibody 139H2 in a human ovarian cancer xenograft model. Int J Cancer 50(3):474, 1992
44. Kairemo K, Ljunggren K, Strand SE et al: Radioimmunotherapy with ^{90}Y-labeled monoclonal antibodies in a nude mouse ovarian cancer model. Acta Oncol 32(7–8):801, 1993
45. Breitz HB, Durham JS, Fisher DR: Radiation-absorbed dose estimates to normal organs following intraperitoneal ^{186}Re-labeled monoclonal antibody: methods and results. Cancer Res 55 suppl 23:5817s, 1995
46. Kavanagh JJ, Rosenblum MG, Kudelka AP et al: Yttrium-labeled antibodies in the treatment of epithelial ovarian cancer, abstract. pp. 16–17, Fourth Annual Symposium: Current Status and Future Directions of Immunoconjugates. Diagnostic and Therapeutic Applications in Benign and Malignant Disorders. January 23–26, 1992, Key Biscayne, FL, 1992
47. Partridge E, Meredith R, Alvarez R et al: Phase I study of intraperitoneal lutetium-177 (LU-177) monoclonal CC49 for ovarian cancer. Proc Ann Meet Am Assoc Cancer Res 35:A3008, 1994
48. Ward B, Mather S, Shepherd J et al: The treatment of intraperitoneal malignant disease with monoclonal antibody guided ^{131}I radiotherapy. Brit J Cancer 58(5):658, 1988
49. Finkler NJ, Muto MG, Kassis AI et al: Intraperitoneal radiolabeled OC 125 in patients with advanced ovarian cancer. Gynecol Oncol 34(3)339, 1989
50. Rosenblum MG, Kavanagh JJ, Burke TW et al: Clinical pharmacology, metabolism, and tissue distribution of ^{90}Y-labeled monoclonal antibody B72.3 after intraperitoneal administration. J Nat Cancer Inst 83(22):1629, 1991
51. Buckman R, DeAngelis C, Shaw P et al: Intraperitoneal therapy of malignant ascites associated with carcinoma of ovary and breast using radioiodinated monoclonal antibody 2G3. Gynecol Oncol 47(1):102, 1992
52. Hird V, Maraveyas A, Snook D et al: Adjuvant therapy of ovarian cancer with radioactive monoclonal antibody. Brit J Cancer 68(2):403, 1993
53. Muto MG, Finkler NJ, Kassis AI et al: Intraperitoneal radioimmunotherapy of refractory ovarian carcinoma utilizing iodine-131-labeled monoclonal antibody OC125. Gynecol Oncol 45(3): 265, 1992
54. Crippa F, Bolis G, Seregni E et al: Single-dose intraperitoneal radioimmunotherapy with the murine monoclonal antibody I-131 MOv18: clinical results in patients with minimal residual disease of ovarian cancer. Eur J Cancer 31A(5):686, 1995

CHAPTER 13

PALLIATIVE CARE AND QUALITY OF LIFE CONSIDERATIONS IN THE MANAGEMENT OF OVARIAN CANCER

Joanna Mary Cain
Lari B. Wenzel
Bradley J. Monk
David Cella

EDITORS' INTRODUCTION

As treatments have become more complex and aggressive, patients, regulatory agencies, and funding agencies have begun to ask important questions about quality of life (QOL) in patients on various treatment protocols. For example, certain drugs that do not lead to an increased length of life have been approved on the basis of their association with a perceived improvement in QOL so long as they do not have any significant toxicity. On the other hand, funding and regulatory agencies have refused to support new therapies that are excessively toxic or lead to large decrements in QOL even in the face of modest apparent survival advantage.

QOL issues also are important in the palliative mode. Certain therapies that have *no* chance of improving survival end points may have an acceptable therapeutic index based on a reasonable balance between the toxicity of the intervention and the resolution of symptoms secondary to that intervention. With this in mind we have asked our experts to comment on how candid physicians should be in discussing the prognosis for patients with a newly diagnosed illness. At the other end of this disease spectrum we have asked for a discussion about when it is appropriate to discontinue therapy and when one should initiate hospice care. Included with this topic is the issue of deciding when palliative chemotherapy is appropriate. We have also asked our authors to discuss what current options are available for assessment of QOL in patients with ovarian cancer. Finally, two major issues that deserve special mention because of their frequent occurrence in patients with terminal ovarian cancer involve the management of recurrent ascites and the use of palliative surgery in the treatment of bowel obstruction.

It is clear that in the next decade QOL measures will be as important as the more classic end points of response rate and survival. Significant work still appears to be needed to adequately measure QOL. Nonetheless, such measurements are currently mandated when two potential therapies are perceived to have a divergent impact on QOL.

QUESTIONS

1. How candid should we be in discussing prognoses for patients with newly diagnosed advanced-stage epithelial ovarian cancer?
2. Please discuss when it is appropriate to discontinue therapy for a patient with progressive ovarian cancer. When should the hospice alternative be considered?
3. What are the current options for assessment of quality of life in ovarian cancer patients?
4. Please discuss options for management of recurrent ascites.
5. How do we best select patients for palliative surgery?

QUESTION 1

How candid should we be in discussing prognoses for patients with newly diagnosed advanced-stage epithelial ovarian cancer?

JOANNA MARY CAIN

The initial diagnosis: a crisis point

She is 44 years old and the mother of an 11-year-old boy and a 13-year-old girl. A prominent attorney, she is used to being in charge of her career and the functioning of her family. Her illness has been diagnosed as high-grade serous cystadenocarcinoma with liver and lung parenchymal metastases. She is angry with everyone involved in her care but "wouldn't go anywhere else" and wants "everything" done. You need to discuss treatment and prognosis with her. What will you say?

The purpose of discussing diagnosis, treatment, and prognosis with patients is to inform and educate them in a manner that restores and fosters their ability to make decisions regarding their care. Proscriptions against using the word *cancer* or couching the discussion in euphemisms that fail to reveal the gravity of the situation are not appropriate. Is it true not only that patients who are not told of a cancer diagnosis already know their diagnosis,[1] but also that their ability to cope and make decisions is improved by the use of direct, unambiguous language in disclosing information.[2] Truthfulness and accurate presentations from the beginning of the patient-physician relationship establish a trust relationship that will be essential when making the numerous decisions to come during the course of care.

The parameters of this initial discussion need attention. Clearly, patients still heavily sedated following surgery may only be able to comprehend "Yes, it was the cancer we discussed. When you are more awake, we'll talk about the next steps to take." A patient who is awake and alert clearly deserves a broader discussion not only explaining risks and benefits of the proposed course of treatment but also exploring the types of risks and side effects they are willing to trade for a diminution in quality of life or an increase in length of survival. Mazer's[3] work suggests that in making decisions patients are very capable of weighing risk versus benefit and mortality against their own short and long-term QOL. Restoring the ability to make choices about their care through carefully timed informative discussions not only respects autonomy but also rebuilds a sense of control that is lost when a diagnosis of cancer is given.

The need to open the door to conversations that explore the patient's perception of her own QOL cannot be overstated. How individual patients judge their own experience of living (QOL) varies widely. One may choose a novel therapy with high potential risks and unknown benefits because of a desire to contribute knowledge or benefit to others. Another may reject surgery with a high curative value and few side effects because of an unwillingness to face even small perceived changes in her experience of living. As Cassell[4] points out, people have family ties, a past, a cultural background, a future, relationships, and roles that all play a part in their experience of illness and suffering. "People suffer from what they have lost of themselves in relation to the world of objects, events, and relationships," he observes. In as much as the diagnosis and the therapy change each of these connections, they are a potential source of suffering and diminished QOL for patients. Lack of acknowledgment of and attention to this experience in the context of living reduces the effectiveness and trustworthiness of physicians as caregivers. Failure to begin to assess this aspect of patient health at the time of the initial diagnosis not only is a failure to offer medical benefit but also adds to the burden of suffering a woman experiences.

That these initial conversations should take place in a setting that restores patient dignity and control and establishes a respectful relationship between patient and physician should go without saying. However, the fact that diagnosis and prognosis are still delivered during "rounds" or in a fashion that discourages further communication suggests that guidelines need to be stated. These include the "who, what, where, and when"[5] that physicians are ethically obligated to explain in all discussions from disclosure of the initial diagnosis to conversations dealing with end-of-life issues.

The who, what, where, and when of patient care discussions

Who should be included? This should be completely up to the patient unless she is not capable of making decisions regarding her own care. However, the desire to spare family and friends who are the caregivers from bad news is as misplaced as the desire to spare patients from the same bad news. Unless friends and family members are children or have extremely diminished health or mental functioning, the ambiguity, uncertainty, and anxiety that accompanies a lack of information may not be what the patient intends. It is worthwhile pointing this out if family members are being excluded on this basis, particularly if they are to be involved in subsequent caregiving in the home setting.

What to say has already mentioned—the truth. The depth of information and the timing of its delivery vary depending on physician assessment of the patient's ability to comprehend, consider, correlate, and communicate (the elements of decision-making competence). Deciding when further information cannot be understood or considered during such conversations is a fine art requiring skill, experience, and an ability to understand the meaning of the patient's words and gestures.

Honesty and hope

Concerns about the need to preserve hope can lead to the use of euphemisms or less than full disclosure over time, and as already stated, this approach leads to less successful coping. The focus of such discussions should not be achieving a balance between honesty and hope fullness but rather how hope can be a vehicle for transcending the suffering brought about by a diagnosis or prognosis. Therefore it is more important to consider how physicians can lend strength to overcome suffering rather than increase suffering by lying or by deceit fulness in failing to disclose important information.

Lending strength requires *not* that a physician be less than honest but that the truth be disclosed over a period of time in a setting where the patient has the support required and with repetition as information is assimilated in the small amounts that can be understood. Representing a threat to one's personhood. Patients are then able to develop their own coping strategies to overcome this threat. If their strategy is hope against all odds—"Doctor, I know I'm dying but there still can be a miracle," the answer is, "Yes, there can be." The medical information is clearly understood, but lending support to overcome suffering is an appropriate medical role at this point. These strategies for dealing with the suffering a terminal diagnosis brings in and of itself will be as varied as the individuals treated. Some patients may be dysfunctional in making decisions—denial being the best example—and these women require gentle encouragement to consider an alternative approach. Denying patients an opportunity to choose another strategy only inflicts harm. Forcing a patient to adopt your own view of the odds does not take into consideration the tangential harms and the personal framework patients must deal with and corrodes a relationship that must endure through the palliative therapy or care to come. For a patient who denies the diagnosis and the disease, battering at the doors of denial only makes it less likely that they will ever return to hear the information when they are ready. So maintaining hope is thus better understood as lending strength to overcome suffering—the complex suffering of individuals that has to do with the relationship between the whole person and the illness and nothing to do with the medical information itself.[6]

Timing, determining when information should be disclosed, deserves further comment. The preceding discussion suggests that timing is critical, and judging what portion of the information should be disclosed is an art. To adequately address these issues it is reasonable to expect multiple meetings over time with varying amounts of information. An open-ended meeting with adequate time allocated confirms the patient's belief that the physician will be "there for me." This support alone can be part of restoring wholeness when there is no longer a possibility that health can be restored.

LARI B. WENZEL
BRADLEY J. MONK
DAVID CELLA

QOL issues

QOL considerations should not be isolated from treatment planning and implementation. The controversies inherent in ovarian cancer treatment suggest that understanding and measuring QOL are particularly important and deserve serious consideration when determining the cost/benefit ratio associated with treatment options.[7]

There are important QOL considerations in the management of ovarian cancer at many levels. In high-risk women, testing for gene mutations related to ovarian cancer (e.g., BRCA1) is associated with many ethical and psychosocial issues. Screening for ovarian cancer has not proven to be of value, even for women at high risk. In early-stage disease, the value of adjuvant therapy must be weighed against the drawbacks associated with acute toxicity and, more importantly, delayed and late effects of treatment. In advanced disease, which is the condition of most patients, there are considerable concerns related to the competing positive and negative effects of surgical and chemotherapeutic treatments, and it is often necessary to address palliative care issues as well. Most women with ovarian cancer present with advanced disease and require a multimodal treatment approach. Consequently, psychosocial and physical concerns directly affecting QOL are usually present throughout the course of treatment. Just after diagnosis, a significant proportion of women experience psychological distress often accompanied by impaired physical functioning. Women with persistent disease rate their QOL lower than that of those who respond to treatment.[8] Indeed, persistent and recurrent disease are more difficult to cope with than the initial diagnosis.[8,9]

This discussion focuses on four key QOL issues in ovarian cancer: (1) discussing poor prognosis and disease management, (2) deciding when to discontinue cytotoxic or cytoreductive treatment and shift to a palliative or hospice approach, (3) use of palliative surgery, and (4) QOL measurement.

Discussing poor prognosis and disease management

Key times at which patient emotional vulnerability is greatest include initial diagnosis, diagnosis of recurrent disease, and discovery of disease progression, all times at which symptoms of depression and anxiety typically rise.[10] Deleterious QOL effects often persist and worsen throughout the course of advanced ovarian cancer, particularly as physical functioning declines, further increasing vulnerability. A diagnosis of recurrence heightens psychological vulnerability and dashes hope, further negatively affecting QOL. These are important considerations, particularly when acknowledging that most patients with advanced disease will ultimately have a recurrence and that 5-year survival rates are roughly 25 to 30%.[11]

Discussing disease management with patients at diagnosis and again upon recurrence or discovery of disease progression is challenging. On the one hand, there is an impulse to protect them from the distress and emotional upheaval that attend these events, but on the other hand, there is a desire to be honest with them and prepare them for what lies ahead. Achieving a balance between honesty and maintaining hope can seem impossible at times, often because physicians tend to project their own concerns onto the patient and assume she will give up hope. In reality, hope is a very robust emotional stance that is rarely dashed by open, compassionate discussion of prognosis and treatment options. When there are no remaining viable cytotoxic treatment options, there are still many palliative options that can achieve meaningful therapeutic ends. It is helpful for patients to hear such optimism in the face of a generally poor prognosis.

As the patient's illness advances, feelings of helplessness due to loss of control and fear of dying may resurface. At this point the physician can openly recognize the patient's fear and grief and internally acknowledge his or her own attitude toward her impending death.[10] Ironically, doctors and other staff tend to spend less time with patients as their disease progresses and they deteriorate into a terminal condition. This is presumably because they feel helpless (and perhaps even threatened) when confronted with the imminence of death. Many fail to realize the effectiveness of compassion and active palliative care. Actively participating in symptom management and compassionate listening help ease the patient's mind and allow her to ask questions that help plan realistically for the future and maintain a sense of control. Although most patients know when they are dying and can verbalize this realization, they also retain hope. The physician is uniquely poised to encourage and reinforce a patient's hope without giving false or insincere reassurance.

A recent study[12] focusing on end-of-life preferences of gynecologic cancer patients reported that only 5% of 108 patients would stop fighting after receiving a poor prognosis with no medically recommended treatment options left. Most (78%) of these patients expressed a resolve to continue fighting against their disease even under the poorest prognostic circumstances. Perhaps management involves rallying resources to assist with this fight and in the care of the dying patient. Appropriate use of colleagues familiar with care for the dying can relieve the physician of some of the responsibility of being the sole provider of hope, care, and sensitive attention to incurable problems.

QUESTION 2

Please discuss when it is appropriate to discontinue therapy for a patient with progressive ovarian cancer.

When should the hospice alternative be considered?

JOANNA MARY CAIN

Discontinuing curative therapy: refocusing goals toward palliative care

There is a point in most patient's care at which further chemotherapy would have side effects that would overwhelm any benefit. At this point it is fallacious to refer to a difference between curative and palliative intent for such chemotherapy, as few people ultimately achieve cure for this disease. There is, rather, a point at which interventions such as certain chemotherapies or extensive surgery have little chance of success and must be weighed against ever-increasing side effects such as pain. In the ethics literature this is often the point at which medical futility is first encountered, and that literature regarding ethics of aggressive intervention in hopeless situations will be used to expand our discussion. That ethic does not, however, condemn the use of palliative chemotherapeutic drugs or less extensive surgery (e.g., colostomy) in circumstances where other goals of medicine such as symptom management or prolongation of life to achieve a certain objective (e.g., a daughter's graduation) can be achieved.

Futility

Treatments that offer no benefit to patients are clearly not obligatory. However, in these discussions we find ourselves perched on the line between how much benefit is obtained—even if only little—and at what cost in terms of risk and QOL. Given the previous discussion regarding hope—we need to distinguish hopelessness from futility. "Futility refers to an objective quality of an action; hopelessness describes a subjective attitude. Hope and hopelessness bear more relation to desire, faith, denial, and other psychological responses than to the objective possibility or probability that the actions being contemplated will be successful."[13] Futile medical interventions are those that have a remote possibility of a good outcome but which experience or reasoning suggests are "highly improbable and cannot be systematically produced."

Considering interventions such as chemotherapy, then, leaves us with additional guidelines for choosing to forgo further chemotherapy or more aggressive surgery. First, there is no obligation to offer treatment that is of no benefit. Second, the patient's goals and perception of quality of life dictate the levels of risk versus benefit they find acceptable. Third, there also are therapies that may offer a rare chance of success, although success is highly improbable and in the experience of the physician is not likely. If these are the circumstance surrounding further chemotherapy or more aggressive surgery, the discussion should center around changing the goals of management to those consistent with the best of palliative care—not with a potential cure. When the medical goal of curing the disease or even containing its progress cannot substantially be met, the goals of comfort, alleviation of pain, and relief of suffering are still left to be aggressively addressed.

Based on this argument, there is *no* single point for all patients at which they have completed a certain number of therapeutic interventions sum that further control of the disease is impossible. While the cancer is increasingly less likely to respond to second-, third-, or fourth-line agents, this is not necessarily an indication of their potential efficacy in the individual patient. Previous responses to a similar agent, the development of an entirely new therapy, or the presence of only a localized recurrence might sway the discussion toward an additional trial of therapy to control the disease process. Ovarian cancer is a disease entity that requires treatment to be individualized to the needs and presentation of each patient in ways that other disease processes do not.

Additionally, a clearly defined trial of therapy with parameters and goals thoroughly discussed by physician and patient may aid in the transition from a curative or controlling therapy to a purely palliative strategy. This approach may also be helpful in evaluating the palliative benefit of therapies otherwise considered aggressive in this setting. The parameters to be set are (1) the medical goal being addressed (control, pain relief, return to normal function); (2) the patient goal being addressed (time to see children, desire to eat even if minimally); (3) the length of the trial that will determine whether or not the strategy is successful (one cycle of chemotherapy, 2 weeks of total parenteral nutrition [TPN]); and (4) the acceptable outcome and the measurement system to be used (slow disease process, stable CA 125 level, better control of nausea). Even interventions such as paracentesis, antibiotics, and total parenteral nutrition can be viewed as short term trials that can be considered both patient and physician set GOALS in terms of their success in improving symptoms. These therapeutic trials are especially helpful in dealing with patients with whom the physician has had a relationship or has highly valued short-term goals that might be met if the trial is successful.

Do-Not-Resuscitate Policies: Withholding and Withdrawing Therapy

Withholding or withdrawing therapy after the failure of a clearly defined and agreed upon trial is often more palatable to patients and their families as they must agree that the goals have not been achieved. Not offering medically futile therapies (withholding) is ultimately the same as terminating medically futile therapy (withdrawing) and is therefore regarded as ethically the same. The basic idea is that this intervention does not meet a goal of medicine or a goal articulated by the patient.

The use of do-not-resuscitate (DNR) consent forms and procedures is based on the same reasoning. In the case of metastatic, progressive cancers, the rate of survival following cardiopulmonary resuscitation is virtually zero. Therefore, offering a coordinated series of medical maneuvers to address cardiopulmonary failure is not only *not* obligatory but also may subject the patient to additional pain and suffering.

It is important to note, however, that this discussion refes solely to cardiopulmonary resuscitation. The list of interventions that often appears in DNR documentation often confuses the issue, as the medical futility of these interventions may not be apparent. For example, the list may have items regarding the administration of vasoactive substances, blood products, antibiotics, and so on, and as stated above, these procedures may be entirely appropriate even in terminal palliative care if they clearly address a goal. Packed red blood cells given as a trial to a patient to allow her to be more alert and able to complete conversations with family members is an example. Additionally, items on the list may be the focus of trials of therapies with clearly demarcated limits.

An additional concern of particular importance in designing DNR orders for patients with ovarian cancer is the institutional policy for DNR as part of an anesthetic induction.[14–16] The patient may have a well-documented DNR order based on medical futility and patient and family preferences. She may be undergoing an indwelling subclavian line placement or a colostomy, to directly address terminal symptoms such as pain and may have clearly requested that no resuscitation should be done in the case of sudden, unexpected cardiopulmonary arrest. On the other hand, the anesthesiologist may take the position that the administration of all anesthesia is inherently resuscitative in nature and that to not resuscitate the patient would be a failure to adhere to the standards of the discipline. This is an area of active debate at many institutions because there is no clear national policy. How to balance, on the one hand, the ethical obligations of all physicians while honoring the patient's choices regarding her care (e.g., DNR in the operating room) can be a vexing issue. The additional difficulty of having to weigh unwanted resuscitation against palliative surgery may be an overwhelming burden for an already ill woman. It is important to consider these ramifications and individual institutional policies when palliative surgeries are considered.

LARI B. WENZEL
BRADLEY J. MONK
DAVID CELLA

Gynecologic oncology training should include more guidance on managing the transition from cytotoxic or cytoreductive treatment to palliative ovarian cancer treatment. In fact, most experts in palliative care agree that there is not, and should never be, a clear demarcation between therapies with curative versus life-extending versus palliative intent. Ideally, patients in curative or life-extending treatment settings are also given active supportive care. Similarly, patients in palliative care settings should be given therapy that is as active in orientation as front-line curative treatment. It is best to consider *every* patient a person who requires palliation, or improvement in QOL, all along the treatment trajectory. The relative prominence of a palliative mind-set of course naturally increases in those unfortunate patients who do in fact deteriorate and die, but it should always be present. Keeping this palliative mind-set throughout the illness enables the physician to be more emotionally available and responsive to patient queries regarding personal values and treatment preferences for second and third-line treatments as well as end-of-life issues.

Cure, or even long-term remission, is unlikely in the majority of ovarian cancer patients. Therefore, any benefit of debulking or cytotoxic therapy must be assessed by balancing the following parameters: extension of survival time, extension of progression-free survival time, toxicity of treatment, symptom relief, and overall impact upon QOL. For the early-stage patient, virtually any aggressive therapy is acceptable if it can significantly improve the cure rate. For patients with widely metastatic disease, palliation of symptoms is the primary concern. Patients between these two groups (i.e., most women with ovarian cancer) pose the greatest challenge to the clinician attempting to integrate QOL considerations into treatment plans. This requires the combining of time, toxicity, and QOL impact into a clinical summary that can be used to evaluate the overall benefit of therapy.

Although some women failing initial therapy have meaningful responses to second-line therapy, rarely do such women achieve long-term survival. In fact, despite high initial response rates to platinum-based chemotherapy, most patients with advanced ovarian carcinoma die of drug-resistant disease. One experimental approach used in treating drug-resistant disease involves administration of high-dose chemotherapy with autologous bone marrow transplantation or peripheral blood stem cell support.[11] A new high-dose regimen was evaluated in patients with relapsed or refractory ovarian cancer in order to define toxicities and responses.[17] Patients received mitoxantrone, carboplatin, and cyclophosphamide followed by autologous bone marrow transplantation. Overall, 89% responded, with complete responses seen in 88% versus 47% of platinum-sensitive versus platinum-resistant disease. The median survival for all 30 patients was 29 months, and after 3 years 23% were still alive without disease.[17] The regimen appeared to be safe and superior to other therapy for platinum-sensitive disease. Toxicities included mild to moderate nausea, alopecia, prolonged anorexia, ototoxicity, diarrhea, mucositis, herpetic conditions, bacteremia, and sepsis. Although use of this regimen is advocated for exploration earlier in the management of advanced ovarian cancer, no QOL assessment was provided to compare short-term toxicity to long-term QOL changes.

If high-dose chemotherapy followed by autologous stem cell transplant extends survival time by a small amount compared to standard therapy but is also associated with increased toxicity and impairment of QOL, its overall value to the patient becomes questionable. If, on the other hand, survival time is not improved by autologous stem cell transplantation but there is an increase in progression-free survival, it is important to determine whether that improvement is associated with (an assumed) improvement in QOL

There are other possible outcomes with regard to the primary end points (survival and progression-free survival), some of which would render QOL data less useful. For example, if there is no difference in overall survival or in progression-free survival, it is unlikely that the added cost and toxicity of autologous stem cell transplantation would be acceptable to patients, providers, or health care payers unless the unlikely event of dramatic improvement in QOL were to occur. As Thigpen[18] noted, until a randomized study demonstrates the efficacy of high-dose chemotherapy, the cost, the toxicity and the available evidence pointing to a lack of improved results with dose escalation beyond conventional treatment levels suggest that this approach should not be used outside a clinical trial. Such a trial has recently been activated by the GOG (Protocol 164). Salvage therapy has ultimate value only if it can generate a cure, improve survival with acceptable toxicity, and/or improve QOL.[19] In this trial QOL will be assessed using the Functional Assessment of Cancer Therapy (FACT) measurement system, including the ovarian cancer and bone marrow transplantation subscales (see Question 3 a for description).

QUESTION 3

What are the current options for assessment of quality of life in ovarian cancer patients?

LARI B. WENZEL
BRADLEY J. MONK
DAVID CELLA

Chemotherapy studies that have examined QOL

A 1978 QOL assessment of 57 patients with stage III or IV disease examined a now resolved controversy regarding the risks and benefits of 5-fluorouracil (5-FU)/melphalan (FUME), actinomycin D/ 5-FU/melphalan (ACFUME), and actinomycin D 5-FU/cyclophosphamide (ACFUCY). This clinical trial revealed that patients on FUME had a longer median duration of survival with an attendant improvement in lifestyle and activity, and less toxicity (mouth ulcers, diarrhea, vomiting, hematologic toxicity, hospitalization).[20] These results provided justification to omit actinomycin D from future use, resulting in a significant decrease in gastrointestinal side effects.

A later study stratified patients by residual tumor (≤ 1 cm vs > 1 cm) and stage (III vs IV) to receive cisplatin (C) with either epirubicin (E) or doxorubicin (D) every 4 weeks for eight courses. QOL was monitored by visual analog scales and did not differ significantly between the two groups. Thus, CE patients compared to CD patients had nearly identical survival, no significant differences in clinical response rate or negative second-look laparotomy rate, and equivalent QOL but experienced less cardiotoxicity and thrombocytopenia. The CD regimen therefore had the more favorable therapeutic index.[21]

Impact of treatment on QOL was also examined relative to short, intensive cisplatin-based chemotherapy administered to an unselected group of 68 patients with stage III to IV ovarian cancer.[22] Treatment impact was assessed by the *T*ime *W*ithout *S*ymptoms or *T*oxicity (TWiST) Index in relation to the individual length of progression-free survival. Although the median was 18 months and the median overall survival 22 months, the median duration of TWiST was 10 months, indicating that about 8 months were lost to symptoms related to treatment or hospital admissions for chemotherapy or laparotomy. The authors conclude that 28% of the cumulative period of progression-free survival is consumed by the treatment and its side effects. Specific platinum-related side effects included general malaise, loss of appetite, and change in taste. Neurotoxicity, which occurred in most patients, profoundly affected well-being.

McGuire et al[19] compared cisplatin/cyclophosphamide to cisplatin/paclitaxel, and progression-free survival and overall survival were significantly longer in the cisplatin/paclitaxel group. This observation has led to adoption of a combination of paclitaxel and a platinum compound as the standard therapy for ovarian cancer patients. The study also reported more frequent alopecia, neutropenia, fever, and allergic reactions in the cisplatin/paclitaxel group. Peripheral neurotoxicity was also more common in the paclitaxel group. This research presents clear evidence of a long-term survival benefit weighted against greater short-term discomfort secondary to toxicities hampering aspects of QOL during treatment. These side effects were considered tolerable because of the significant survival benefit afforded women who received the cisplatin/Taxol regimen. It appears that patients are willing to endure substantial disruption in QOL in exchange for an increase in likelihood of survival or even progression-free survival.

One of the most important concerns related to QOL in ovarian cancer is the current controversy involving the potential QOL benefits of carboplatin versus those of cisplatin as the platinum compound of choice in treating advanced ovarian cancer. Until recently, standard care for patients with advanced ovarian cancer was cyclophosphamide and a platinum compound. In addition to the fact that no significant difference was found in survival between patients receiving carboplatin and those receiving cisplatin, patients on carboplatin have less nausea and vomiting, less neurotoxicity, and less anorexia. Consequently, it is necessary to test the efficacy of carboplatin/Taxol versus cisplatin/Taxol because of QOL variables associated with significant treatment toxicities. These comparison data can help evaluate whether survival is lengthened with Taxol and a more easily tolerated platinum agent, enhancing QOL while not reducing survival.

It is increasingly being recognized that the convenience, timing, administration, and dose intensity of chemotherapy can greatly affect different QOL parameters. For example, treatments with Taxol requiring hematologic support and/or prolonged infusion are more expensive and can have a negative impact on the QOL of patients undergoing therapy.[11] With the goal of assessing convenience and comfort, a 6-month prospective study on 53 patients with advanced breast or ovarian cancer determined whether the site (either hospital or home) and method of chemotherapy administration influenced their QOL. Hospital-administered chemotherapy was more disruptive to QOL.[23]

Illustrating the importance of dose intensity to QOL, a substudy of a phase III randomized trial comparing intensive and nonintensive dosing schedules of cyclophosphamide and cisplatin was conducted in patients with advanced epithelial ovarian cancer. The purpose of the study was to determine if differences existed in patients' perceptions of QOL between the four-course intensive arm and the eight-course nonintensive arm. Two hundred patients completed the Functional Living Index—Cancer (FLIC) prior to randomization, during each course of therapy, and 6 weeks after therapy or at the time of second-look laparotomy, whichever came first.[24] Most (64%) patients reported improved QOL after the first course, but fewer patients reported improvement on the intensive regimen and the magnitude of improvement was smaller. Patients in the intensive group reported significantly more frequent severe nausea. Results indicated that the intensive regimen had a greater negative impact on perceived QOL than the nonintensive regimen.[24] Such results may temper enthusiasm for an intensive regimen if it is only marginally better than a nonintensive regimen in terms of response and survival.

QOL measurement

There are many ways to assess QOL in women with advanced cancer. A detailed review of available methods, most of which rely upon patient self-report, is beyond the scope of this discussion and can be found elsewhere.[27] Much has been learned about the QOL of women with ovarian cancer, some of which has already been highlighted. Compared to other cancer patients, patients receiving chemotherapy for ovarian cancer have significantly greater impairment in physical, role, and social functioning and more fatigue and pain than patients with breast or lung cancer.[28] Ovarian cancer is a disease that frequently carries uncomfortable and disabling abdominal symptoms. This, of course, has an adverse effect upon QOL, especially when these symptoms are reflective of incurable disease. There is therefore need for a brief, yet comprehensive questionnaire to measure QOL in women with ovarian cancer.

One example of a multidimensional, combined generic and disease-specific QOL questionnaire for use with these patients is the Functional Assessment of Cancer Therapy (FACT) measurement system. The FACT-G (FACT-General) questionnaire is a 34-item self-report measure developed specifically for cancer patients and designed to be used in a variety of settings, including clinical trials. It is comprised of five subscales (physical well-being, social well-being, emotional well-being, functional well-being, and relationship with doctor) which can be analyzed separately or summed to produce a total QOL score. It has demonstrated reliability, validity, and responsiveness to change over time.[27,29,30] Two additional subscales have been designed to measure aspects of QOL particular to ovarian cancer and to bone marrow transplantation. The FACT-O (FACT-G plus 12 items specific to ovarian cancer) is currently being used in many clinical trials of ovarian cancer (e.g., GOG 152 and 164). The FACT-BMT (FACT-G plus 20 items specific to bone marrow transplantation) detects problems associated with the transplant experience and has been successfully tested with a group of mixed-diagnosis patients upon hospital admission for bone marrow transplantation, most of whom received an autologous transplant.[28] The FACT-O questionnaire can be found in the appendix to this chapter. Data from the first 163 patients entered into GOG 152 (described earlier) are summarized in Table 13–1. It is noteworthy that the QOL of the ovarian cancer sample is quite comparable to the average QOL of the initial FACT-G standardization sample. While statistical comparisons would be inappropriate because of sample and sampling differences, a casual comparison of sample means and variances suggests no difference between groups. Also of interest is that this is the first reporting of the ovarian cancer subscale, which is summed as the total of 11 out of the 12 items in the subscale. This decision was made because removal of the one item relating to treatment side effects (hair loss) resulted in an improvement in the internal consistency of the subscale (see Table 13–1).

A trial outcome index has been created by combining the FACT-O and/or FACT-BMT subscale scores with two of the FACT-G subscales (physical well-being and functional well-being). A similar trial outcome index was recently created using the FACT lung cancer subscale, and it was found to be highly reliable and sensitive to change in performance status rating.[30] The trial outcome index is appealing for medical trial outcome evaluation because it focuses on physical symptoms and abilities which, when compared to emotional and social well-being, are no more important to people but are more dramatically changed by cancer and its treatment. A subset of patients also completed the FACT-BMT at hospital discharge and again approximately 100 days after initial assessment. Preliminary results indicate that the FACT-BMT demonstrates validity and reliability as well as sensitivity to clinically significant change in performance status.[28]

Summary

Many of the current controversies in ovarian cancer risk assessment, screening, diagnosis, and treatment have QOL considerations at their core. Genetic testing and screening pose their own unique and unchartered risks and benefits. Critics suggest that the psychological costs are harmful, with little opportunity for concrete benefits. Proponents argue that many women express a desire for genetic testing as well as screening and could obtain great relief with definitive knowledge of their status. However, programs have not been perfected and professionals have not been sufficiently educated to provide comprehensive genetic counseling.

More familiar areas of controversy persist regarding optimal treatments for ovarian cancer patients. Traditionally, end points in cancer research have included response rate, progression-free survival, survival, and toxicity.

TABLE 13-1
Baseline FACT-O Scores of Patients Entered on GOG 152[a]

SCALE/SUBSCALE	NO. OF ITEMS	MEAN SCORE	STANDARD DEVIATION	STANDARDIZATION SAMPLE[c] MEAN SCORE	STANDARDIZATION SAMPLE[c] STANDARD DEVIATION
Physical well-being	7	20.4	5.7	20.5	5.5
Social/family well-being	7	23.8	3.7	21.9	4.8
Relationship with doctor	2	7.6	1.0	6.9	1.5
Emotional well-being	5	15.0	3.7	14.8	3.9
Functional well-being	7	17.6	6.1	18.0	6.1
FACT-G total score	28	84.4	14.7	82.1	15.9
Ovarian cancer subscale	11[b]	32.6	5.2	Not available	

[a] *After 3 weeks of paclitaxel/cisplatin therapy;* n = *163; median age = 58 years.*

[b] *The ovarian cancer subscale contains 12 items, one of which is not added into the total (I am bothered by hair loss). For the 11 item subscale, Chronbach's* $\alpha = 0.62$.

[c] *Data from Cella et al.*[28]

An additional critical variable of evaluation now also includes QOL, defined as the subjective evaluation of one's physical, social, and emotional well-being.

Many advances have been made in the surgical and chemotherapeutic approaches to ovarian cancer, extending survival for a predominantly incurable disease. QOL assessments can help determine optimal first-line therapy by examining general and specific QOL issues in ovarian cancer.

Generally, QOL data suggest that as physical functioning declines so too does psychological functioning. Frequent clinical and QOL assessment of ovarian cancer patients ensures that the clinician will continues to keep QOL considerations at the forefront of decision making. These clinical considerations should be interwoven with our appreciation of the advantages and disadvantages of state-of-the art treatments, including second-look surgeries, new chemotherapy agents and combinations, scheduling and dosing of chemotherapy, debulking surgery, and symptom management. In short, our knowledge of the disease and its optimal treatment to date provides us with sufficient information to initiate multidisciplinary treatment plans that actively attend to QOL. Subsequent treatment goals can than be discussed and realistically set to enhance QOL for women with cancer.

Guthrie's (1985)[31] comment still applies today: "It is essential that we remember at all times that we are treating patients who happen to have cancer and not cancers that happen to have patients attached. A method of analysis which combines length of survival with quality of life should be used in [future] trials, to enable clinicians to evaluate our treatments more carefully with regard to the requirements of patients."

QUESTION 4

Please discuss options for the management of recurrent ascites.

JOANNA MARY CAIN

Management of recurrent ascites

Certain symptoms are more common in patients dying of ovarian cancer and are worthy of further comment here. One particularly difficult problem is balancing the removal of ascites for relief of pressure-related pain and gastric compression and the consequent intravascular volume depletion and tissue edema that occur with continual removal of protein. Studies dealing with repeated paracenteses have not shown a decrease in serum proteins, but these studies involved patients in a relatively good nutritional state.[32] In the terminal phase, replacement of lost protein with total parenteral nutrition or intravenous albumin is unlikely to resolve the difficulty of accumulation of peripheral tissue fluids from intravascular protein loss. Furthermore, the use of parenteral nutrition must be evaluated in the entire context of patient goals. The length of time the patient is likely to survive and the intervals of removal of fluid may warrant consideration of an indwelling port or other options for control of ascites.

Unfortunately, the other options for control of ascites may carry side effects that may be unwelcome at this point in the patient's course. For example, various chemotherapeutic and immunotherapeutic agents have been used to control ascites in the intraperitoneal space.[33,34] Some success has occurred with mitoxantrone, although the length of control is unclear. LeVeen shunts and their more contemporary counterparts have been employed primarily for ascites associated with liver disease.[35,36] Unfortunately, in that setting there was no advantage over conservative measures using paracentesis and diuretics. An additional problem with these shunts is short-lived patency.

Symptoms of thirst related to dehydration are often of concern in the terminal phase of ovarian cancer where obstruction and nausea limit the ability to take oral fluids. Quite often, the response to these symptoms is to increase the amount intravenous fluids with a consequent increase in extracellular fluid and pain from limb swelling. Burge[37] attempted to correlate symptoms of thirst and other correlates of dehydration (such as actual intake, fluid status, and electrolytes) in the terminal course of illness and found very poor correlation among symptoms, laboratory findings, and replacement by the intravenous route. In addition, it should be pointed out that use of fluid replacement to normalize an electrolyte imbalance—if there are no direct symptoms—does not meet the goal of end-of-life care, which is to improve the quality of the remaining time. Trials involving fluid replacement for specific symptoms should be undertaken, as noted previously, with clearly defined end points and time intervals.

The restlessness and anxiety that are often the hallmarks of the last 24 hours of life are symptoms that are distressing to both family and patient, and therapy with oral or intravenous anxiolytics or subcutaneous drugs such as midaxolam[38,39] may be of great benefit to patients and their caregivers. Concern that the use of these drugs will shorten life is misplaced when they are used appropriately and are clearly intended for the relief of particular symptoms.[40]

Where death will occur

The choice of where they would like death to occur depends on the patient's family structure (or lack of it), on their financial status, and on multiple other socioeconomic factors. For the most part, patients prefer to die at home.[41] However, the impact of changes in health care financing is seen in the location of where patients die, just as it is seen in the shortened length of hospital stays and the decreased number of admissions on the day before surgery. When Medicare's prospective payment system was enacted, patients were shifted from the acute care setting to nursing home settings to die, the assumption being that this is more cost-effective.[42,43] As we move forward with managed health care systems, we must address the misapprehension that greater savings are obtained when all deaths occur at home or in nonhospital settings.[44] In fact, the invisible but easily identified costs of time taken off work by other family members or friends to care for the patient, out-of-pocket expenses for everything from additional laundry to partially covered medication, medical equipment, or respite care suggest that the figures that guide policy save only insurers money and fail to address the economic impact on families or on the overall economy. Physicians must advocate for adequate analysis of coverage and full costs of care, as well as evaluation of care in all settings.

During the weeks and days before death patients and their families have to deal with multiple losses. Patients must contend with the loss of their traditional family role and their sense of self as they become increasingly more dependent on others to care for them and with the loss of a future with those dear to them.[45] The care required goes far beyond the traditional parameters encompassed by an oncology practice. For some physicians, this phase, in which the goal of therapy is not potential cure and prevention of death and where the role is not medical and science advisor but often equally provider of psychological support and symptom management, is simply not what they envisioned or desired when they entered the discipline.[46] Physicians must, regardless of their feelings in this regard, advocate access to adequate support systems in the terminal phase of an illness.

If the physicians are not the appropriate caregivers in the terminal phase, the appropriate caregiver must be identified.

Suicide and terminal cancer

There is an increasing cultural trend toward support of patient suicide and physician-assisted suicide based on the assumption that taking one's life can be a rational choice.[47] Regardless of the beliefs of an individual physician in this regard, their major obligation is to ensure that patients make decisions with the fullest ability to consider the choices and subsequent consequences and is of particular importance in this setting.[48–50] In particular, the high incidence of depression in patients having a desire to die is significant. A trial of antidepressant therapy is a reasonable consideration given this concern. As Chochinov et al[48] note, this "does not necessarily imply that a desire for death is implicitly 'irrational' but the reasoning processes of depressed patients are characteristically biased by negative mental sets that may affect their capacity to make well-considered life and death decisions."

Summary

The essential points of this discussion are the following. First, the road to palliative care begins at the point of diagnosis, not at the point at which no further controlling or curative care can be delivered. Second, however, we mark the steps along this road in terms of QOL—these sign posts are different, for individual patients and we are responsible for providing interpretation and guidance. Excellence of palliative care is judged not by how well each individual symptom is managed but by how directly the suffering of individual patients is addressed. It is judged by whether or not we can restore wholeness to the terminal course of ovarian cancer.

LARI B. WENZEL
BRADLEY J. MONK
DAVID CELLA

Although epithelial ovarian cancer is a surface-spreading disease that rarely invades vital organs, partial or complete bowel obstruction is often seen at the time of initial diagnosis or, more frequently, in association with recurrent disease. Obstruction may be secondary to extrinsic compression of the small bowel or hypoperistalsis due to mesenteric and bowel surface implants. The symptoms, which are almost always present, are intestinal colic, continuous abdominal pain, nausea, and vomiting. In most cases, nausea and vomiting can be relieved by conservative measures, and intestinal symptoms usually resolve after primary cytoreductive surgery and multiagent cisplatin-based cytotoxic chemotherapy.

Despite the high objective response rate of primary untreated ovarian cancer to several platinum-based combination chemotherapeutic regimens, most patients with advanced disease ultimately develop intraperitoneal recurrence and require a salvage regimen for palliation of symptoms. A number of therapeutic strategies have been used in such patients, some of including retreatment with cisplatin or carboplatin, or the use of paclitaxel, ifosfamide, hexamethylmelamine, oral etoposide, 5-FU/leucovorin, or tamoxifen.[51] Multiple clinical factors must be considered when selecting the most appropriate salvage therapy. Unfortunately, in patients previously treated with cisplatin, other chemotherapeutic agents are not likely to be effective in relieving symptoms of bowel obstruction or ascites.

For most patients who present with bowel obstruction secondary to recurrent intraperitoneal cancer, initial management should include proper radiographic documentation of the obstruction, hydration, correction of any electrolyte abnormalities, parenteral alimentation, and intestinal intubation. In some patients the obstruction may be relieved with this conservative approach. However, palliative surgery is usually considered in almost every patient at some time before disease progression and death. When surgery is indicated, the type of surgery depends on the extent of disease as well as on the number and location of obstructions. If the obstruction is principally contained in one area, this area can be either resected (if secondary cytoreduction is indicated) or bypassed. Since the success of secondary cytoreduction depends on the chemosensitivity of the residual disease present after debulking surgery, intestinal bypass is generally preferable to resection because most patients present after multiple failed attempts at cytotoxic therapy resulting in chemoresistant cancer. In addition, intestinal bypass surgery such as an enterocolostomy is usually associated with reduced morbidity when compared to a radical resection.[52–54] At the time of operation, the bulb of the long tube can frequently be palpated and used to identify the small bowel proximal to the obstruction. This small bowel can then be anastomosed in a side-to-side fashion to the most appropriate area of colon, bypassing the site of obstruction. Obviously, it is paramount to obtain a preoperative barium enema to ensure that there is no obstruction of the lower colon distal to the bypass site. In rare cases, the colon may be incased in tumor, necessitating a colostomy with or without bypass surgery.

Sadly, multiple sites of obstruction are common in patients with recurrent epithelial ovarian cancer. More than one-half have small bowel obstruction, one-third have colon obstructions, and one-sixth have both.[52–54] If multiple sites of obstruction are present, resection of several segments of intestine is usually not indicated. In such cases, an ileostomy or even a proximal jejunostomy may be necessary to provide adequate intestinal diversion. On the contrary, if the extent of disease is so great that the morbidity of intestinal surgery seems excessive, stomach decompression with a gastrostomy may be effective in palliating symptoms of obstruction and ascites such as pressure, nausea, vomiting, and pain. When the stomach and/or anterior abdominal wall are not involved with tumor, drainage tubes can frequently be placed percutaneously, avoiding the morbidity of a laparotomy.[55]

Since malignant ascites is almost always the result of intraperitoneal cancer, treatment of these effusions generally involves therapy directed against the associated malignant neoplasm. However, treatments are occasionally directed specifically toward the palliation of symptoms related to malignant ascites, particularly when the intraperitoneal cancer is refractory to all known treatments. The traditional treatment with diuretics, salt, and fluid restriction is rarely effective. Therefore, patients usually undergo repeated paracentesis, resulting in an imbalance of protein and electrolytes. For this reason novel therapies such as intraperitoneal immunotherapy[58] and drainage using a double-valve Denver peritoneal venous shunt[25] have been proposed to palliate the symptoms associated with malignant ascites. In a selected series involving 42 patients treated with a peritoneal venous shunt over a 5-year period, shunting the peritoneal fluid into the vascular space relieved symptoms with neither new hematogenous metastases nor evidence of disseminated intravascular coagulation. Interestingly, the median survival of patients with breast and gynecologic cancer after surgery was significantly longer than that of patients with primary gastrointestinal neoplasms, resulting in an improvement in QOL.[27,28]

A hope for cure is no longer possible once a woman develops recurrent disease associated with symptomatic bowel obstruction and ascites. However, a sense of optimism and hope are still common, not for a cure, but toward a goal of symptom relief and palliation with chemotherapy, surgery, tube drainage, or supportive care. Only through careful patient selection and insight into the toxicity associated with these therapies can this hope be realized and QOL optimized.

QUESTION 5

How do we best select patients for palliative surgery?

JOANNA MARY CAIN

Surgery as a palliative intervention

The preceding discussions have set the stage for considering surgery a potential palliative intervention. Cunningham et al[59] pointed out that relieving bowel or gastric obstruction with a percutaneous gastrostomy can be effective in alleviating pain in the terminal phase of ovarian cancer. Placement of an implanted port for paracentesis can also decrease the need for additional painful procedures. However, the advantages and disadvantages need to be continually weighed.[60,61] Additional postoperative pain and obtundation from anesthetics and the additional pain medicines prescribed for that period may not be the outcomes a patient desires if the benefit is short-lived. Surgery for simple debulking as a means of pain or disease control when it is clear that secondary optimal reduction or effective local therapy cannot be achieved meets neither the goal of reducing pain nor the goal of disease control and should not be part of a palliative care program.

Pain control

The area of foremost concern and one of the greatest contemporary failings of medicine is pain management. Even when specific interventions were designed to improve end-of-life care, adequate pain management was absent in up to a third of dying patients.[62] Relief of pain is one of the most fundamental goals of medicine and may be the only goal that can be met in the end-of-life care of patients. Developing an adequate information base and a network of knowledgeable colleagues to provide maximal pain control is therefore obligatory for any physician participating in end-of-life care.[63,64] It is up to every physician to help overcome the public perception that physicians' efforts in addressing pain relief are less relentless and less effective than their pursuit of a cure for the disease.[65]

The first step in management of pain requires identification of the source and type of pain. Is it diaphragmatic pressure from ascites? Paracentesis may help. Is it a local neural invasion from an extraperitoneal tumor? Is it neuropathic pain or pain related to direct tissue damage? A simplified identification scheme appears in Table 13-2.

There are four important aspects of pain control in the terminal phase. First, if possible, the type of pain involved should be identified and addressed specifically. Second, continous adjustment will be required—the type of pain medication, the amount of medication, and the patient's tolerance are all continually changing variables.[67] Continuous adjustment of pain relief requires repeated comprehensive assessment of pain control—not only baseline pain but also breakthrough pain.[68] The use of rescue doses for interval increases in pain above the baseline is an important component of planned analgesic therapy. Third, rapid use of the next potency level on the analgesic scale for inadequate pain relief is required. Finally, doses must be adequate to achieve reliable

TABLE 13-2
Identification of Pain

TYPE OF PAIN	COMMON SYMPTOMS	PAIN THERAPY STRATEGY
Neuropathic pain	Burning, cramping, sharp, stabbing pain	Include antidepression or anticonvulsant If regional (e.g., pelvic only) consider continual epidural If all fails, segmented neurocotomy
Bony pain	Severe continuous bony pain often increasing with movement or pressure	Local radiation Use of antiinflammatory agents, NSAIDS, or corticosteroids Consider palmidonate[66]
General pressure	Tight feeling in abdomen or chest Poorly localized pain	Treat source of pressure locally (e.g., paracentesis, thoracentesis, or relief of bowel or gastric obstruction) Standard pain management scale
Tissue damage: organs	Pain from metabolic dysfunction of organ-capsular involvement	Assess organ system for overall benefit or harm of interventions and patient goals Examples: bile duct stints, ureteral stints, pleurodesis, radiation of sidewall lesion

pain-free state. Brescia, et al[67] documented a wide range of doses required for adequate pain control in advanced cancer patients as well as the lack of predictability of cancer pain, underscoring both the need for flexible management and wider dose ranges than in acute pain settings (such as postoperative pain relief).

Terminal care

The closer a patient come toward death, the greater the demands on her family and on her' physicians. "Keeping the patient clean, caring for the skin, preventing the formation of bed sores, treating neuropsychiatric symptoms, controlling peripheral and pulmonary edema, aggressively reducing nausea and vomiting, using intravenous medications, fighting the psychosocial forces that can lead to family fragmentation—all can tax the ingenuity and equanimity of the most skilled health professionals. [They] are still called on to use intensive measures—extreme responsibility, extraordinary sensitivity, and heroic compassion."[63]

LARI B. WENZEL
BRADLEY J. MONK
DAVID CELLA

Selecting patients for palliative surgery

Although combined surgery and chemotherapy produces a 70 to 85% response rate in patients with advanced disease, most ultimately have recurrences and 5-year survival rates are 25 to 30%.[11] Therefore, palliative care continues to be a priority in managing ovarian cancer.

Primary cytoreductive surgery

Although 50 to 60% of patients with advanced disease can undergo effective cytoreduction, there is controversy regarding the impact of cytoreductive surgery on overall survival, the optimal surgical approach, and the impact on QOL. Recently, this controversy has been extended to risks versus benefits of systemic pelvic and para-aortic lymphadenectomy, where the possibility of postoperative morbidity increases, perhaps limiting longer-term aspects of functioning.[69,70] In general, women who undergo successful cytoreduction appear to have improved QOL with decreased symptoms from large masses and respond more favorably to postoperative chemotherapy.[11] However, few studies have addressed QOL related to surgical approaches to ovarian cancer.

Debulking Surgery for Tumors Larger than 2 cm

Comparing 19 debulked and 17 nondebulked ovarian cancer patients, Blythe and Wahl[71] evaluated patient acceptance of ostomy, activity level, employment, confinement, enjoyment of life, and consumption of a regular diet. QOL was estimated independently by the oncologist, oncology nurse, and enterostomal therapist. Objective criteria included frequency of thoracentesis, paracentesis, surgical procedures, nonchemotherapy-related hospital admissions, and bowel obstructions per patient survival months. The authors concluded that extensive surgery in carefully selected patients is worthwhile and that QOL was acceptable regardless of quantity. The weaknesses of the study include its lack of random assignment, small sample size, and sole use of provider ratings of QOL. Nevertheless, it represents an early (1982) attempt to consider patient QOL explicitly in evaluating treatment outcome.

Interval Cytoreductive Surgery

The debate regarding benefits of cytoreduction following a short course of induction chemotherapy persists. Many investigators claim that benefits include improved survival and potential improvement in QOL.[72–74] To address the continuing debate, the GOG is conducting a multicenter, two-arm trial comparing interval cytoreductive surgery following three of six cycles of paclitaxel/cisplatin to six cycles of paclitaxel/cisplatin alone (GOG 152). QOL data collected on 163 patients with stage IIIC suboptimally debulked epithelial ovarian carcinoma were analyzed to determine the QOL concerns of this population after receiving three courses of paclitaxel/cisplatin. These data serve as baseline scores to allow comparison of women who receive interval surgery versus those who simply receive three more courses of paclitaxel/cisplatin. As the study is ongoing, it is premature to make any comparisons at this time, but preliminary baseline data are helpful in determining the reliability of these data in this population of patients and in planning for study analyses. These preliminary FACT-O data are presented later. Additional surgery, particularly that with limited efficacy, can be burdensome to the patient with recurrent ovarian cancer. Janicke et al[76] conclude that combined surgery and chemotherapy can improve the course of the disease, even in recurrent ovarian cancer. While this would logically translate into improved QOL, this has never been empirically demonstrated, and indeed may never be. Based upon the literature and on experience,[51] investigators at M. D. Anderson Cancer Center conclude that patients who fail primary treatment are not good candidates for secondary resection.[77] This conclusion is based largely on the unavailability of effective second-line chemotherapy, and it is not clear if or how the addition of paclitaxel to current platinum-based regimens might affect this position.

Secondary Debulking for Recurrent Ovarian Cancer

Unfortunately, recurrent ovarian cancer occurs even after negative findings at second-look laparotomy. Recently, however, factors associated with a survival advantage are being identified for women with a documented previously complete surgical response[75] or optimal secondary cytoreduction. In addition, radical surgical procedures also appear to prolong survival time in some patients with recurrent ovarian cancer.[76] Patients who had a complete resection of cancer tissue in the primary operation and those who experienced a disease-free interval of more than 12 months after the primary operation (18 months in another study[51]) are a most likely to benefit from a second operation. Radical surgery in these patients may enhance the usually limited efficacy of second-line chemotherapy.

The study cited above was sensitive to QOL issues, recognizing that additional surgery could prove burdensome to patients with recurrent ovarian cancer. Performance status, using the Eastern Cooperative Oncology Group (ECOG) scale at 6-month intervals after the operation, suggested that 48% of patients were assigned an ECOG score of 0 to 2 (i.e., ambulatory and active at least half the waking day), and this continued through 12 months after surgery. After 1 year, 38% of surviving patients had ECOG scores of 0 to 2. Unfortunately, no QOL data were collected on those with recurrences receiving only second-line chemotherapy without the operation. The authors conclude that the combined therapeutic efforts of an extended surgical procedure and chemotherapy can improve the course of the disease even in recurrent ovarian cancer. While this would logically translate into improved QOL, this has never been empirically demonstrated.

As an alternative to chemotherapy, correction of an intestinal blockage can occasionally be achieved by re-exploration and bowel bypass or enterostomy. Patients must be carefully selected, and surgery should be as conservative as possible. Unfortunately, it is difficult to determine which individuals might benefit from palliative surgery and thereby experience an improvement in QOL. Indeed, intestinal obstruction due to recurrent ovarian cancer remains a very refractory problem in gynecologic oncology and is the most common cause of death in women with ovarian cancer. The median survival after intestinal surgery for an intestinal obstruction secondary to ovarian cancer ranges from 2.5 to 7 months. Thus, palliative surgery is usually hazardous at best and frequently associated with substantial morbidity, with approximately 15% and 35% of patients experiencing major and minor complications, respectively.[77]

In an attempt to identify women with recurrent ovarian cancer most likely to achieve a substanial improvement in QOL after palliative intestinal surgery, Jong and colleagues[80] studied 53 patients with advanced ovarian cancer and bowel obstruction treated between 1982 and 1992. Successful palliation was achieved in 27 (51%) patients and was associated with the absence of four prognostic factors: palpable abdominal and pelvic masses, ascites exceeding 3 L, multiple obstructive sites, and preoperative weight loss greater than 9 g. Age, time interval between diagnosis of ovarian cancer and bowel obstruction, state of disease at initial diagnosis, tumor type and grade, site and degree of obstruction, presence of gross residual tumor after initial operation, and preoperative use of chemotherapy or radiotherapy did not indicate the success or failure of palliative surgery in this particular series.[80] Other reports have shown that patients whose life expectancy is very short (e.g., less than 2 months) are also poor candidates for surgical relief of bowel obstruction.[79] Good nutritional status, young age, and the absence of rapidly accumulating ascites are other features that may be suggestive of a favorable postoperative outcome.[80]

EDITORS' COMMENTARY

All contributors agreed that the patient and her family need to be made aware of the diagnosis and its potential implications. Dr. Cella and colleagues point out the robustness of hope and suggests that complete information and hope can triumph over deception and futility. Dr. Cain agrees that full disclosure is mandatory but suggests that this disclosure should occur at intervals and in a setting where the patient has adequate family support.

The contributors point out that movement from curative to palliative intent occurs biologically when the patient has persistent or recurrent disease. Nevertheless, the point at which the physician should discourage rather than encourage palliative approaches may differ significantly from patient to patient. For example, an older patient with confirmed drug-resistant disease may be encouraged to discontinue toxic drug therapy and enter hospice care early in the course of her recurrence, while a younger patient with prior response to therapy and family goals to be met may be encouraged to receive even third and fourth-line chemotherapy. All of this discussion should take place in the context of patient needs and expectations.

Dr. Cella and colleagues give an extensive discussion of published studies that examined QOL and then review some of the current instruments available for assessment of this end point. They explain the need for QOL measures, particularly in patients undergoing salvage and probably noncurative therapy or very aggressive primary therapy.

All contributors point out the difficulty in treating patients with chronic ascites and bowel obstruction secondary to recurrent disease. Treatment in these individuals needs to be individualized. Some guidelines for exclusion of patients for surgical intervention are presented, and we basically agree that drug resistance, multiple areas of obstruction, and poor nutritional status strongly argue against surgical intervention in a palliative mode. Treatment of chronic ascites is also problematic. Chronic protein malnutrition supervenes with repeated paracentesis. Salvage chemotherapy has been relatively ineffective either systemically or intraperitoneally in the management of this problem. Chronic indwelling peritoneoatrial shunts are associated with an unacceptably high incidence of disseminated intravascular coagulation. Paracentesis may be the best option until intervals between them become short, at which point more appropriate management may be directed at control of the discomfort from the abdominal distention.

It should be clear to the reader that the area of QOL has been poorly described in most previous clinical studies but will become more important as therapeutic options increase in both number and aggressiveness. Certainly QOL issues should be strongly considered in any randomized study that attempts to improve outcomes. Improvement in QOL is just as important as improved response rate and disease-free survival.

APPENDIX 13–1

FUNCTIONAL ASSESSMENT OF CANCER THERAPY—OVARY

FACT-O (Version 3)

Below is a list of statements that other people with your illness have said are important.
By circling one number per line, please indicate how true each statement has been for you during the past 7 days.

PHYSICAL WELL-BEING	not at all	a little bit	some-what	quite a bit	very much
1. I have a lack of energy	0	1	2	3	4
2. I have nausea	0	1	2	3	4
3. Because of my physical condition, I have trouble meeting the needs of my family	0	1	2	3	4
4. I have pain	0	1	2	3	4
5. I am bothered by side effects of treatment	0	1	2	3	4
6. I feel ill	0	1	2	3	4
7. I am forced to spend time in bed	0	1	2	3	4

8. Looking at the above 7 questions, how much would you say your **PHYSICAL WELL-BEING** affects your quality of life? (circle one number)

0 1 2 3 4 5 6 7 8 9 10

Not at all **Very much so**

SOCIAL/FAMILY WELL-BEING	not at all	a little bit	some-what	quite a bit	very much
9. I feel distant from my friends	0	1	2	3	4
10. I get emotional support from my family	0	1	2	3	4
11. I get support from my friends and neighbors	0	1	2	3	4
12. My family has accepted my illness	0	1	2	3	4
13. Family communication about my illness is poor	0	1	2	3	4
14. I feel close to my partner (or the person who is my main support)	0	1	2	3	4
15. Have you been sexually active during the past year? No ___ Yes ___ If yes: I am satisfied with my sex life	0	1	2	3	4

16. Looking at the above 7 questions, how much would you say your **SOCIAL/FAMILY WELL-BEING** affects your quality of life? (circle one number)

0 1 2 3 4 5 6 7 8 9 10

Not at all **Very much so**

Note: Items 1 to 34 comprise the FACT-G; items 35 to 47 comprise the Ovarian Cancer Subscale. Items 8, 16, 19, 26, 34, and 47 are experimental in nature and therefore not scored.
(From Rush-Presbyterian-St. Luke's Medical Center, with permission.)

FACT-O (Version 3)

Please indicate how true each statement has been for you <u>during the past 7 days</u>.

<u>RELATIONSHIP WITH DOCTOR</u>	not at all	a little bit	some-what	quite a bit	very much
17. I have confidence in my doctor(s)	0	1	2	3	4
18. My doctor is available to answer my questions	0	1	2	3	4

19. Looking at the above 2 questions, how much would you say your **RELATIONSHIP WITH THE DOCTOR** affects your quality of life? (circle one number)

0 1 2 3 4 5 6 7 8 9 10

Not at all **Very much so**

<u>EMOTIONAL WELL-BEING</u>	not at all	a little bit	some-what	quite a bit	very much
20. I feel sad	0	1	2	3	4
21. I am proud of how I'm coping with my illness	0	1	2	3	4
22. I am losing hope in the fight against my illness	0	1	2	3	4
23. I feel nervous	0	1	2	3	4
24. I worry about dying	0	1	2	3	4
25. I worry that my condition will get worse	0	1	2	3	4

26. Looking at the above 6 questions, how much would you say your **EMOTIONAL WELL-BEING** affects your quality of life? (circle one number)

0 1 2 3 4 5 6 7 8 9 10

Not at all **Very much so**

<u>FUNCTIONAL WELL-BEING</u>	not at all	a little bit	some-what	quite a bit	very much
27. I am able to work (include work in home)	0	1	2	3	4
28. My work (include work in home) is fulfilling	0	1	2	3	4
29. I am able to enjoy life	0	1	2	3	4
30. I have accepted my illness	0	1	2	3	4
31. I am sleeping well	0	1	2	3	4
32. I am enjoying the things I usually do for fun	0	1	2	3	4
33. I am content with the quality of my life right now	0	1	2	3	4

34. Looking at the above 7 questions, how much would you say your **FUNCTIONAL WELL-BEING** affects your quality of life? (circle one number)

0 1 2 3 4 5 6 7 8 9 10

Not at all **Very much so**

FACT - O (Version 3)

Please indicate how true each statement has been for you during the past 7 days.

	ADDITIONAL CONCERNS	not at all	a little bit	some-what	quite a bit	very much
35.	I have swelling in my stomach area	0	1	2	3	4
36.	I am losing weight	0	1	2	3	4
37.	I have control of my bowels	0	1	2	3	4
38.	I have been vomiting	0	1	2	3	4
39.	I am bothered by hair loss	0	1	2	3	4
40.	I have a good appetite	0	1	2	3	4
41.	I like the appearance of my body	0	1	2	3	4
42.	I am able to get around by myself	0	1	2	3	4
43.	I am able to feel like a woman	0	1	2	3	4
44.	I have cramps in my stomach area	0	1	2	3	4
45.	I am interested in sex	0	1	2	3	4
46.	I have concerns about my ability to have children	0	1	2	3	4

47. Looking at the above 12 questions, how much would you say these **ADDITIONAL CONCERNS** affect your quality of life? (circle one number)

0 1 2 3 4 5 6 7 8 9 10

Not at all **Very much so**

FACT-O scoring guidelines

Instructions:
1. Record answers in "item response" column.
2. Perform reversals as indicated to obtain "item scores."
3. Multiply the sum of the item scores by the number of items in the subscale, then divide by the number of items answered. This produces the subscale score.
4. Add FACT-G score from FACT-G scoring guide to obtain **TOTAL.**

Additional Subscale	**Item Number**	**Item Reverse?**		**Item Response**	**Item Score**
FACT-O (Ovarian)	35	4	-	_______	=_______
	36	4	-	_______	=_______
	37	0	+	_______	=_______
	38	4	-	_______	=_______
	39	4	-	_______	=_______
	40	0	+	_______	=_______
	41	0	+	_______	=_______
	42	0	+	_______	=_______
	43	0	+	_______	=_______
	44	4	-	_______	=_______
	45	0	+	_______	=_______
	46	4	-	_______	=_______

Sum ITEM SCORES ==> [_____] x 12 ÷ [_____] = [_____]
Enter number of items answered _______↑

Enter FACT-G score =================> [_____]

Add to get **TOTAL FACT-O SCORE** =========> [_____]

References

1. Cassilith BR, Zupkis RV, Sutton-Smith K et al: Information and participation sequences among cancer patients. Ann Intern Med 92:832–836, 1980
2. Dunn SM, Patterson PU, Butow PN et al: Cancer by another name: a randomized trial of euthansia and uncertainty in communicating with cancer patients. J Clin Oncol 11:989–996, 1993
3. Mazur D, Hickam D: Patient preferences: survival as quality of life considerations. J Gen Intern Med:8:374–377, 1993
4. Cassell E: The nature of suffering and the goals of medicine. N Engl J Med 306:639–645, 1982
5. Cain J, Stacy L, Jusenius K, Figge D: The quality of dying: financial, psychological, and ethical dilemmas. Obstet Gynecol 76:149–152, 1990
6. Clark PG: Quality of life, values and teamwork in geriatric care: do we communicate what we mean? Gerontology 35:402–411, 1995
7. Cella DF: Quality of life: the concept. J Palliative Care 8(3):8–13, 1992
8. Guidozzi F: Living with ovarian cancer. Gynecol Oncol 50:202, 1993
9. Cella DF, Mahon SM, Donovan MI: Cancer recurrence as a traumatic event. Behavioral Med 16:15–22, 1990
10. Small ES, Anderson B, Watring WG et al: Ovarian carcinoma: management of stress in patients and physicians. Gynecol Oncol 15:160, 1983
11. Ozols RF: Outcome issues in ovarian cancer. Oncology, 9 (suppl). 9:135, 1995
12. Brown D, Roberts JA, Elkins TE et al: Hard choices: the gynecologic cancer patient's end-of-life preferences, Gynecol Oncol 55:355–362, 1994
13. Schneiderman LJ, Jecker NS, Jonsen AR: Medical futility: its meanings and ethical implication. Ann Intern Med 112:949–954, 1990
14. Walker RM: DNR in the OR: resuscitation as an operative risk. JAMA 266: 2407–2412, 1991
15. Cohen CB, Cohen PJ: Do-not-resuscitate orders in the operating room. N Engl J Med 325:1879–1882, 1991 carcinoma. Obstet Gynecol 61:327–330, 1983
16. Puay ME, Llewellyn-Thomas H: Assessing preferences about the DNR order: does it depend how you ask? Med Decis Making 15:209–216, 1995
17. Stiff P, Bayer R, Camarda M et al: A phase II trial of high-dose mitoxantrone, carboplatin, and cyclophosphamide with autologous bone marrow rescue for recurrent epithelial ovarian carcinoma: analysis of risk factors for clinical outcomes. Gynecol Oncol 57:278, 1995
18. Thigpen JT: High-dose chemotherapy with autologous bone marrow support in ovarian carcinoma: the bottom line, more or less. Gynecol Oncol 57:275, 1995
19. McGuire WP, Hoskins WJ, Brady MF et al: Cyclophosphamide and cisplatin compared with paclitaxel and cisplatin in patients with stage III and stage IV ovarian cancer. N Eng J Med 334:1, 1996
20. Lele SB, Piver S, Barlow J: Chemotherapy in ovarian carcinoma recurrent after radiation therapy. Obstet Gynecol 51:101–104, 1978
21. Homesley H, Harry D, O'Toole R et al: Randomized comparison of cisplatin (C) plus epirubicin (E) or doxorubicin (D) for advanced ovarian cancer: a multicenter trial. Proc ASCO 9:627, 1990
22. Willemse PH, Van Lith J, Mulder NH et al: Risks and benefits of cisplatin in ovarian cancer: a quality-adjusted survival analysis. Eur J Cancer 26:345, 1990
23. Payne SA: A study of quality of life in cancer patients receiving palliative chemotherapy. Soc Sci Med 35:1505, 1992
24. Waiczak JR, Brady M: Comparison of quality of life in ovarian cancer patients

participating in a national cooperative group phase III randomized trial. Proc ASCO 10:A1185, 1991

25. Li KW, Wong WS: Double valve Denver peritoneal venous shunt used in ovarian malignant ascites: a case report. Chinese Med J 102:300–302, 1989
26. Campioni N, Pasquali Lasagni R, Vituccl C et al: Peritoneovenous shunt and neoplastic ascites: a 5-year experience report. J Surg Oncol 33:31–35, 1986
27. Cella DF, Bonomi AE: Measuring quality of life: 1995 updete. Oncology 9 (Suppl): 47–60, 1995
28. McQuellon RP, Russell GB, Cella DF et al: Quality of life measurement in bone marrow transplantation: Development of the Functional Assessment of Cancer Therapy Bone Marrow Transplant (FACT-BMT) scale. Bone Marrow Transplantation 19:357–368, 1997
29. Cella DF, Tulsky DS, Gray G et al: The Functional Assessment of Cancer Therapy scale: development and validation of the general measure. J Clin Oncol 11(3):570–579, 1993
30. Celia DF, Bonomi AE, Lloyd SR et al: Reliability and validity of the Functional Assessment of Cancer Therapy—Lung (FACT-L) quality of life instrument. Lung Cancer 12:199–220, 1995
31. Guthrie E. Ovarian cancer. In Bleehen NM (ed): Chemotherapy in Multicentre Studies. Springer-Verlag, Berlin, 1985
32. Lifshitz S, Buchsbaum, HJ: The effect of paracentesis on proteins. Gyn Oncol 4:347–353, 1976
33. Lorusso V, Catino A, Gargano G et al: Mitoxantrone in the treatment of recurrent ascites of pretreated ovarian cancer. Eur J Gynecol Oncol 15:75–80, 1994
34. Stuart GC, Nation JG, Snider DD, Thunberg P: Intraperitoneal interferon in the management of malignant ascites. Cancer 71:2027–2030, 1993
35. LeVeen HH, Wapnick S, Grosbert S, Kinney MJ: Further experience with the peritoneovenuous stent for ascites. Ann Surg 184:574–581, 1976
36. Stanley MM, Odie S, Lee KK et al: Peritoneovenuous stenting as compared with alveoli cirrhosis and massive ascites. N Engl Med 321:1632–1638, 1989
37. Burge F: Dehydration symptoms of palliative care patients. J Pain Manage 8:454–464, 1993
38. Enck R: The last few days. Am J Hospice Palliative Care July/August: 11–13, 1992
39. Amesburg BDW, Dunphy KP: The use of sub Q midalolaman in the home care setting. Palliative Med 3:299–301, 1989
40. Truog RD, Verde CB, Mitchell C, Grier H: Barbituates in the care of the terminally ill. N Engl J Med 327:1678–1681, 1992
41. Townsend J, Frank AO, Fermont D et al: Terminal cancer care and patients preferral for place of death: a prospective study. Br Med J 301:415–417, 1990
42. McCusker J: Where cancer patients die: an epidemiologic study. Public Health Rep 96:170–176, 1983
43. Sager MA, Easterling DV, Kindiz DA, Anderson OW: Changes in the location of death after passage of Medicare's prospective payment system. N Engl J Med 320:433–439, 1989
44. Emanuel EJ, Emanuel LL: The economics of dying: the illusion of cost savings at the end of life. N Engl J Med 330:540–544, 1994
45. Aldridge D: Families, cancer, and dying. Fam Pract 4:212–218, 1987
46. Mount B: Dealing with our losses. J Clin Oncol 4:1127–1134, 1986
47. Siegel K, Tuckel P: Rational suicide and the terminally ill cancer patient. Omega 15:263–269, 1984
48. Chochinov HM, Wilson KG, Enns M et al: Desire for death in the terminally ill. Am J Psychia 152:1185–1191, 1995
49. Hietanen P, Lonnquist J: Cancer and suicide. Ann Oncol 2:19–23, 1991

50. Hendin H, Kiermau G: Physician-assisted suicide: the dangers of legalization. Am J Psychiatr 150:143–145, 1993
51. Morris M, Gershenson DM, Wharton JT et al: Secondary cytoreductive surgery for recurrent epithelial ovarian cancer. Gynecol Oncol 34(3): 334–338, 1989
52. Castaldo TW, Petrilli ES, Ballon SC et al: Intestinal operation in patients with ovarian carcinoma. Obstet Gynecol 139:80–84, 1981
53. Krebs HB, Goplerud DR: Surgical management of bowel obstruction in advanced ovarian carcinoma. Obstet Gynecol 61:327–330, 1983
54. Clarke-Pearson DL, Chin NO, DeLong ER et al: Surgical management of intestinal obstruction in ovarian cancer. I. clinical features, postoperative complications, and survival. Gynecol Oncol 26:11–18, 1987
55. Rubin SC, Benjamin I, Hoskins WI et al: Intestinal surgery in gynecologic oncology. Gynecol Oncol 34:30–33, 1989
56. Ripamonti C: Management of bowel obstruction in advanced cancer. Current Opin Oncol 6:351–357, 1994
57. Campagnutta E, Cannizzaro R, Gallo A et al: Palliative treatment of upper intestinel obstruction by gynecological malignancy: the usefulness of percutaneous endoscopic gastrostomy. Gyn Oncol 62:103–105, 1996
58. Stuart GC, Nation JG, Snider DD, Thunberg P: Intraperitoneal interferon in the management of malignant ascites. Cancer 71:2027–2030, 1993
59. Cunningham MJ, Bromberg C, Kredentser DC et al: Percutaneous gastrostomy for decompression in patients with advanced gynecological malignancies. Gynecol Oncol 59:273–276, 1995
60. Markman, M: Surgery for support and palliation in patients with malignant disease. Sci Oncol 22:91–94, 1995
61. Chan A, Woodruff R: Intestinal obstruction in patients with widespread intraabdominal malignancy. J Pain Symptom Manage 7:339–342, 1992
62. Hammes B, Cain J: Ethics and pain management: clinical applications. J Pain Symptom Manage 8:7–12, 1993
63. Wanzer SH, Federman DD, Adelstein SJ et al: N Engl Med 320:844–849, 1989
64. Cain JM, Hammes B: Ethics and pain management: respecting patient wishes. J Pain Symptom Manage 8:1–6, 1993
65. Payne R, Foley KM: Cancer pain. Med Clin North Am 71:153–352, 1987
66. Purohit OP, Anthony C, Radstone CR et al: High dose intravenous pamidronate for metastatic bone pain. Br J Cancer, 70:3:554–558, 1994
67. Brescia FJ, Portenoy RK, Ryan M et al: Pain, opiod use, and survival in hospitalized patients with advanced cancer. J Clin Oncol 10:149–155, 1992
68. Portenoy RK, Hagen NA: Breakthrough pain: definition, prevalence and characteristics. Pain 41:273–281, 1990
69. Hacker NF: Systemic pelvic and para-aortic lymphadenectomy for advanced ovarian cancer—therapeutic advance or surgical folly? Gynecol Oncol 56:325, 1995
70. Scarabelli C, Gallo A, Zarrelli A et al: Systematic pelvic and paraaortic lymphadenectomy during cytoreductive surgery in advanced ovarian cancer: potential benefit on survival. Gyecol Oncol 56:328, 1995
71. Blythe JG, Wahl TP: Debulking surgery: does it increase the quality of survival? Gynecol Oncol 14:396, 1982
72. Carson LF, Rubin SC: Secondary cytoreduction—thoughts on the "pro" side. Gynecol Oncol 51: 127, 1993
73. van der Burg MEL, van Lent M, Kobierska A et al: Intervention debulking surgery (IDS) does improve survival in advanced epithelial ovarian cancer (EOC): An EORTC gynecologic cancer cooperative group (GCCG) study. Proc ASCO 12:258, 1993

74. Pecorelli S: Proc 24th Ann Meeting Felix Rutledge Soc, abstract 23, 1993
75. Vaccarello L, Rubin SD, Viamis V et al: Cytoreductive surgery in ovarian carcinoma patients with a documented previously complete surgical response. Gynecol Oncol 57:61, 1995
76. Janicke F et al: Radical surgical procedure improves survival time in patients with ovarian cancer. Cancer 70:2129, 1992
77. Burke TW, Morris M: Secondary cytoreductive surgery for ovarian cancer. Obstet Gynecol Clin North Am 21(1):167–178, 1994
78. Markman M: The use of chemotherapy as palliative treatment for patients with advance ovarian cancer. Semin Oncol, suppl 3 22:325–29, 1995
79. Farias-Eisner R, Kim YB, Berek JS: Surgical management of ovarian cancer. Semin Surg Oncol, 10:268–275, 1994
80. Jong P, Sturgeon J, Jamieson CG: Benefit of palliative surgery for bowel obstruction in advanced ovarian cancer. Can J Surg 38:454–457, 1995

CHAPTER 14

POST-THERAPY SURVEILLANCE IN PATIENTS WITH EPITHELIAL OVARIAN CANCER

Victoria L. Seewaldt
Barbara A. Goff
Benjamin E. Greer
Jonathan M. Niloff

EDITORS' INTRODUCTION

Follow-up after primary therapy in ovarian cancer is poorly defined. It is comprised of history and physical examination including bimanual pelvic examination, serial assessment of serum CA 125 level or other tumor marker, reassessment or second-look laparotomy, and occasionally one or more imaging studies; and has no clear impact on outcome parameters including quality and quantity of life.

The CA 125 tumor marker has been the most extensively studied and has both positive and negative effects on the treatment of patients with ovarian cancer. In terms of prognosis it appears clear that rapid decay of a tumor marker indicates a good prognosis, while slow decay into the normal range or lack of normalization connotes a poor prognosis. Virtually all patients with elevated marker levels at completion of primary therapy have persistent disease even if it is not clinically detectable. Unfortunately, upward of 50% of patients with normal marker levels at completion of therapy would be found to have persistent disease if submitted to reassessment laparotomy. Finally, in the vast majority of patients, sequential elevations of this tumor marker following clinical and/or pathologic complete remission presage clinical recurrence with an average lead time of 3 to 5 months, with some patients not developing clinical recurrence for up to 2 years. There has been no clinical study, however, clearly documenting that institution of salvage therapy at the time of initial marker elevation improves either quality or quantity of life, compared to institution of therapy at the time the patient develops radiographic evidence or symptomatic evidence of recurrence. Further, it is unlikely that such a clinical study will ever be performed since most patients with sequential elevations of CA 125 tumor marker strongly desire salvage therapy even without any assurance that it can improve their survival.

Second-look or reassessment laparotomy allows the earliest possible identification of persistent disease following primary therapy. Nevertheless, proving that therapies directed at patients with small-volume persistent disease have an influence on survival has been problematic. The natural history of small-volume persistent disease is quite variable, with some patients receiving no therapy at the time of a positive second look not developing clinical recurrence for up to 3 years. The only potential value of second-look laparotomy appears to be in the selection of patients who are the best candidates for intraperitoneal therapy. Even this approach has not clearly been shown to have an impact on survival and is probably valid only for patients who have microscopic persistent disease.

The questions posed to our experts asked them to recommend specific procedures and specific frequencies of follow-up studies. Additionally we have asked them to specify how to treat patients with serial elevations of tumor marker following primary therapy with and without clinical findings or symptoms of recurrence.

QUESTIONS

1. What are the options and what is your recommendation for patients with epithelial ovarian cancer who have completed primary therapy?
2. What, in your opinion, should be the treatment of a patient with an elevated serum CA 125 level (1) at a level of 100 units/ml and (2) with serial values showing a rise from 25 to 500 units/ml? Should any patients with an isolated abnormal serum CA 125 level (without any other clinical findings) be treated with chemotherapy? Should such patients be candidates for clinical trials?
3. Are there any other major issues pertinent to this subject? If so, what are they?

QUESTION 1

What are the options and what is your recommendation for patients with epithelial ovarian cancer who have completed primary therapy?

VICTORIA L. SEEWALDT
BARBARA A. GOFF
BENJAMIN E. GREER

The dilemma of detecting peritoneal disease

In evaluating surveillance strategies for the detection of recurrent ovarian cancer, it is important to consider the anatomic sites where disease is most likely to recur. The most common sites for ovarian cancer recurrence are the abdominal cavity (>90%)[1] and the vaginal apex (>50%).[2] Unlike patients with breast cancer, women with ovarian cancer rarely have pulmonary or intrahepatic recurrences.[3] One of the most difficult aspects of detecting relapsed ovarian cancer is its diffuse distribution throughout the peritoneal cavity. Although the total number of malignant cells present in the peritoneum may be quite large, the area over which they are distributed is also large. Therefore, the number of malignant cells per unit area in the peritoneal cavity may be low, even in the face of significant tumor burden. Screening modalities such as computer tomography (CT) and magnetic resonance (MR) imaging currently play an important role in detecting the recurrence of many cancers such as breast cancer, lymphomas, and sarcomas. Unfortunately, these imaging techniques are less effective in detecting recurrent ovarian cancer because they are best suited to imaging discrete tumor nodules and have difficulty imaging the diffusely distributed disease typical of recurrent ovarian cancer.

Screening modalities

Second-Look Surgery

Second-look laparotomy is a surgical procedure performed to evaluate the disease status of patients who are clinically free of disease following primary therapy. The advantage of this technique is that the peritoneal cavity can be examined directly for the presence of diffuse recurrent disease. Its disadvantages are that it is an invasive surgical procedure and is able to document disease status only at a single point in time.

In the past, second-look laparotomy has been commonly performed either to document a complete response to cytotoxic chemotherapy or to demonstrate chemotherapy-resistant disease. Barter and Barnes[4] present an extensive review of the second-look laparotomy procedure, summarizing results from 71 published reports describing 5,190 patients with a history of ovarian cancer who underwent second-look surgery from 1980 to 1990. Their data demonstrate that more than 50% of patients had residual disease at second-look laparotomy and that 75% of all residual disease was macroscopic. The percentage of patients found to have persistent disease at second-look surgery increased with the stage of disease: 16% of patients with FIGO stage I disease compared to 67% of patients with FIGO stage IV disease had persistent disease. The risk of subsequent recurrence following second-look laparotomy also increased with disease stage. Nine percent of patients with FIGO stage I and II disease compared to 32% of patients with FIGO stage III and IV disease had recurrent disease following second-look surgery. The majority of recurrences occurred within 2 years following negative second-look laparotomy, although later relapses were documented. Median survival ranged from 11 months to 32 months following recurrence.

Indications for routine second-look laparotomy have decreased in recent years because of the availability of a reliable tumor marker, CA 125. Second-look surgery in the management of epithelial ovarian cancer, however, remains a controversial topic. Clearly, findings at the time of second-look laparotomy can indicate prognosis and ultimate survival. However, there is little evidence in the literature that this procedure improves survival.[5] Unfortunately, studies that do not find a benefit for second-look laparotomy were not designed to specifically evaluate the impact of second-look surgery on overall survival. After primary therapy, 50% of patients with advanced ovarian cancer and CA 125 levels less than 35 units/ml have detectable disease. Although recurrent disease develops in 30 to 50% of patients with negative second-look surgery, the value of this procedure may be to identify patients with negative or microscopic residual disease, drug-responsive tumors, and possibly more favorable tumor biology.[6] These are the patients who are ideal candidates for additional chemotherapy or dose-intensive therapy, and they may present an opportunity to improve overall survival rates. In a study by Copeland et al,[7] patients with microscopic residual ovarian cancer at second-look laparotomy who went on to receive additional chemotherapy had 2- and 5-year survival rates of 96% and 71%, respectively. At our institution, the decision to recommend second-look laparotomy is individualized for each patient. In general, we believe that second look surgery should be performed in patients with advanced ovarian cancer who are good candidates for consolidation therapy, especially when opportunities to participate in prospective clinical trials are available.

Pelvic Examination

Bimanual pelvic examination is the least expensive and least invasive method for detecting recurrent ovarian cancer. While pelvic examination is of questionable value as a routine screening procedure for the initial detection of ovarian cancer, we feel that it plays an important role in surveillance for recurrent disease. Bimanual examination is limited as a screening tool because of the low incidence of ovarian cancer in healthy women and the relatively high prevalence (1.5%) of benign adnexal abnormalities.[8] This situation, however, is reversed for women who have been diagnosed with advanced ovarian cancer, as 60 to 80% relapse within 5 years, and therefore the incidence of malignant disease is far greater than the prevalence of benign abnormalities.

Pelvic examination has generally been found to be comparable or superior to ultrasound and CT for the detection of suspected or recurrent ovarian cancer. In one prospective multicenter study, the differential diagnostic potential of pelvic examination was compared to that of ultrasound and serum CA 125 assay in postmenopausal women with suspected ovarian cancer.[9] A total of 228 patients were evaluated preoperatively, and the individual accuracy of pelvic examination, ultrasound, and serum CA 125 assay in discriminating between benign and malignant pelvic masses was approximately the same (76%, 74% and 77%, respectively). Based on logistic regression analysis, the power of pelvic examination appeared to be the most relevant factor (adjusted odds ratio 9.2), followed by serum CA 125 assay (odds ratio 5.6) and ultrasound (odds ratio 4.6).

At our institution we also evaluated the relative abilities of pelvic examination and CT to detect the presence of recurrent ovarian cancer in women receiving paclitaxel for platinum-resistant ovarian cancer (NCI-TRC 9103).[10] We found that pelvic examination was superior to CT for detecting vaginal apex recurrence and comparable or superior for detecting pelvic recurrence. Pelvic examination detected a vaginal apex mass in 33 of 100 patients, whereas CT scanning was able to detect none of 21 vaginal apex masses 5 cm or less and was able to detect only 7 of 12 vaginal apex masses greater than 5 cm.

We feel that pelvic examination is an important component of ovarian cancer surveillance, but surprisingly, this procedure is not performed routinely, despite its proven benefit. Nodularity or small vaginal apex masses that can be missed by CT or ultrasound are easily detected by physicians with experience in performing pelvic examination. The major limitation of this procedure is that it is unable to detect diffuse peritoneal disease. For this reason we feel that pelvic examination should not be utilized as the sole criterion for detecting recurrent disease and is best used in combination with a serologic marker such as CA 125.

CA 125

CA 125 is a glycoprotein expressed on the surface of epithelial ovarian cancer cells and has been clinically useful in monitoring response to chemotherapy.[11,12] It has been less effective in detecting small-volume disease. The advantages of CA 125 determination as a surveillance test for recurrent ovarian cancer are its low cost, availability, and minimal discomfort and invasiveness, whereas the disadvantage is its low sensitivity. Serum CA 125 level is determined primarily by two factors: amount of antigen shed by an individual tumor and volume of disease present. As a result, while nearly 90% of patients with advanced epithelial ovarian cancer have elevated circulating levels of CA 125, less than 50% of patients with stage IA and IB disease have elevated CA 125 levels.

There is currently no consensus regarding the routine use of CA 125 assay in the follow-up of patients with ovarian cancer. Virtually all patients with an elevated serum CA 125 level (≥35 units/ml) prior to second-look laparotomy have residual tumor, however, approximately 50% of patients with normal CA 125 levels (<35 units/ml) also have disease present.[13–15] Overall, CA 125 (serum level ≥35 units/ml) has a 44% sensitivity, 96% specificity, and 65% accuracy in detecting residual disease prior to second-look laparotomy.[4] In order to increase the sensitivity of CA 125 in detecting recurrent disease, a multicenter trial evaluated the prognostic implications of high normal serum CA 125 levels (20 to 35 units/ml) before second-look laparotomy for patients with stage III and IV epithelial ovarian cancer.[16] Recurrent disease was documented in 55 of 95 patients with serum CA 125 levels less than or equal to 35 units/ml. Forty-nine percent of the 82 patients with serum CA 125 levels less than 20 units/ml had recurrent disease, whereas 12 of 13 patients (92%) with serum CA 125 levels of 20 to 35 units/ml had recurrent disease. These data suggest that slight elevations following primary therapy might be predictive of recurrent or persistent disease.[17]

Ultrasound

Ultrasound is a relatively inexpensive imaging modality which has been utilized to confirm the presence of recurrent ovarian cancer. It is limited by an inability to detect small-volume disease and is somewhat operator dependent. The sensitivity of ultrasound has been reported to range from 20% to 89% with a specificity of 75 to 100%, verified by findings at second-look laparotomy.[4] Ultrasound has limited sensitivity for peritoneal disease and is unable to reliably detect prevertebral lymph nodes less than 3 cm in greatest diameter, peritoneal masses less than 2 cm in diameter, and mesenteric masses less than 5 cm in diameter.[18]

High-frequency transvaginal ultrasound provides increased resolution relative to conventional transabdominal ultrasound.[18,19] In preliminary studies, the sensitivity and specificity of this technique appear to be superior to that of transabdominal ultrasound. However, this modality has not yet been evaluated for its ability to detect recurrent ovarian cancer, and therefore no conclusive recommendations can be made in regard to its use as a surveillance technique.

CT Scanning and MR Imaging

CT is generally unable to detect disease less than 1 to 2 cm and for this reason is not a sensitive tool for posttherapy surveillance in patients with a history of epithelial ovarian cancer. As previously mentioned, CT scanning is particularly ineffective in detecting vaginal apex recurrences and at our center failed to detect vaginal apex masses 5 cm or less. In comparison with findings at second-look laparotomy CT scans have a sensitivity of 44%, a specificity of 86%, and an overall diagnostic accuracy of 63%.[4]

Why is CT so insensitive in detecting recurrent ovarian cancer? This procedure has optimal resolution when detecting the presence of tumor in an organ of uniform density (e.g., liver) or in an organ where the density of the organ is significantly different from that of the tumor (e.g., lung). However, the peritoneal cavity is the most likely site for recurrent disease and, unlike the situation in breast cancer, lung and intraparenchymal liver metastases are rare. Unfortunately, the abdominal cavity is not of uniform density and the density of recurrent tumor is not significantly different from that of the surrounding bowel. This makes CT scanning a particularly poor imaging choice for the detection of recurrent ovarian cancer. The exception to this is the case where a patient has a tumor nodule that cannot be evaluated by any other modality and the nodule dimensions are being evaluated to assess tumor response to a specific therapy.

MR imaging has the ability to detect masses greater than 1 to 2 cm and has relatively better soft tissue resolution relative to CT.[18] However, MR imaging is significantly more expensive than either CT or ultrasound and there are few data evaluating its ability to detect recurrent epithelial ovarian cancer. Therefore, recommendations regarding the use of MR imaging must be deferred at the present time.

New Imaging Methods

Positron emission tomography (PET) is a new imaging method that detects metabolic and biochemical activity. Preliminary data suggest that PET imaging may provide data complementary to that obtained with anatomic methods such as CT, however, information on this technique at this point in time are limited at best. In one study PET and CT scans were performed on 51 patients with suspected ovarian cancer.[20] In these individuals, PET imaging had an 83% sensitivity, 80% specificity, and 82% accuracy. In comparison CT had an 82% sensitivity, 53% specificity, and 72% accuracy. The positive predictive value for patients in whom both CT and PET scans were positive was 95%, and the negative predictive value was 100%. In a second study, PET scans detected disease not revealed by CA 125 assay, or ultrasound.[21] However, the small number of patients evaluated in this study limits its ability to predict the utility of this procedure in general. Further prospective evaluation of the efficacy and cost-effectiveness of PET imaging will be necessary to determine its utility in detecting recurrent epithelial ovarian cancer.

Immunoscintigraphy is a second new imaging technique currently being tested for its ability to detect recurrent ovarian cancer. It utilizes radionuclide-conjugated monoclonal antibodies that specifically recognize adenocarcinoma cells. Limited data suggest that immunoscintigraphy may have predictive value comparable to that of CT scanning, but too few data are available at this time to make specific recommendations.

New Serologic Testing

One area of active research that holds promise for the surveillance of recurrent epithelial cancer is the development of new serologic markers of the disease. For example, a recent study has shown that patients with both breast and ovarian cancer have elevated serum levels of the HER-2/*neu* oncogene product.[22] Other researchers report[23] that tumor necrosis factor and its receptor were found to be elevated in the serum of patients with ovarian cancer. The presence of elevated serum tumor necrosis soluble receptor was shown to have a higher sensitivity, specificity, and positive predictive value for detecting disease than the presence of CA 125 in patients with epithelial ovarian cancer.[24]

BRCA1

It is estimated that 5 to 10% of all ovarian cancers result from hereditary predisposition, with the germline inheritance of a mutation conferring autosomal dominant susceptibility.[25–28] Recently it has been demonstrated that some hereditary breast and ovarian cancers are linked to the BRCA1 locus on chromosome 17q21.[27–31] Mutation analysis of the BRCA1 gene in ovarian cancers supports the hypothesis that BRCA1 mutations are frequently involved in the etiology of hereditary ovarian carcinomas but occur rarely in sporadic tumors.[32] These data, however, do not exclude the possibility that downstream targets of the BRCA1 gene or genes modulating BRCA1 expression may be involved in sporadic ovarian cancer.

The linkage of hereditary ovarian cancer to a specific mutation presents an exciting opportunity to better understand the molecular biology of ovarian cancer carcinogenesis. It is likely that knowledge gained in the future will to lead to novel therapeutic strategies and new marker for detecting the presence of recurrent disease. For this reason, methods utilized in posttherapy surveillance of epithelial ovarian cancer may be radically different in the future.

Summary

At the present time there is no definitive test for detecting the presence of microscopic recurrent epithelial ovarian cancer. For this reason there remains significant controversy as to what constitutes optimal posttherapy surveillance. It is likely that in the future, as new surveillance tests are developed, recommendations for the detection of recurrent epithelial ovarian cancer will change. Our suggestions for posttherapy surveillance in patients with a history of epithelial ovarian cancer are summarized in Table 14-1.

TABLE 14-1
Surveillance Recommendations for Patients with Epithelial Ovarian Cancer

MODALITY	1–2 YEARS (MO)	3–5 YEARS (MO)	AFTER 5 YEARS (MO)
Physical and pelvic examination	3	4–6	6–12
CA 125 assay	3	4–6	6–12

Following initial surgery and chemotherapy, the decision to perform second-look laparotomy should be individualized for each patient. We feel that investigators who design research protocols involving high-dose chemotherapy or autologous bone marrow transplantation should strongly consider the inclusion of second-look laparotomy in order to accurately risk-stratify patients.

During the first 2 years following initial therapy we recommend that patients be evaluated every 3 months because most patients with a history of epithelial ovarian cancer have recurrences within the first 2 years. At each visit patients should have a complete history and physical, pelvic, and rectovaginal examinations. In addition, those with elevated pretreatment CA 125 levels should undergo CA 125 testing at each visit. From 2 to 5 years following initial therapy we recommend that patients be evaluated every 4 to 6 months, and 5 years we evaluate patients every 6 to 12 months. In addition, we recommend yearly mammograms, stool guaiac at each visit, and screening for colorectal carcinoma as advised by the American Cancer Society. Patients with a strong family history of ovarian cancer and/or breast and ovarian cancer should be referred to a geneticist for evaluation of BRCA1 mutations and family counseling.

JONATHAN M. NILOFF

The question posed is not answerable. There is no standard or generally accepted post-therapy surveillance regimen for patients with epithelial ovarian cancer. Furthermore, there are no meaningful data that directly address this issue. Certainly, no prospective studies have been conducted. Follow-up regimens have been prescribed in investigational protocols evaluating new therapies, however, it must be remembered that these protocols are designed to determine the outcome of the study treatment modality and do not have optimization of patient outcome as their primary goal. Because of the lack of available data, firm recommendations for post-therapy surveillance cannot be made. I will discuss the options, drawing indirect inferences from the available data.

In selecting a post-therapy surveillance regimen, one must first define the goal. We will assume that the primary objective is to achieve for the patient the best quantity and quality of life possible, given the currently available therapeutic modalities. Data are not being collected for investigational purposes. The limitations of second-line therapy need to be recognized. The psychological impact of repeated testing—good and bad—must be considered because each encounter reminds the patient of her disease. Although some women ultimately find negative follow-up reassuring, for many it produces anxiety. This anxiety is certainly magnified when recurrent the tumor is detected but no effective therapy is available. Finally, we all work in an increasingly cost-conscious health care environment. Our expenditure of money and resources on post-therapy surveillance needs to be matched with a commensurate improvement in survival or quality of life. The latter is difficult to quantitate, and good data addressing this issue are currently not available.

Surveillance modalities

Surveillance techniques include history and clinical examination, serum tumor marker assays, and imaging studies. potential imaging modalities are sonography, CT scanning,immunoscintigraphy, and MR imaging. A selection from among these options at defined time intervals constitutes a post-therapy surveillance regimen. One might consider modifications to the regimen depending on the disease stage, grade of tumor, or comorbid phenomena.

History and Physical Examination

Symptoms of recurrent ovarian cancer, as in the primary disease, are usually subtle and more commonly absent. Vague gastrointestinal dysfunction, pain, and pressure phenomena are the most common, when present. However, they are often difficult to distinguish from the late effects of prior therapy.

In the vast majority of cases epithelial ovarian cancer recurs in the peritoneal cavity. Therefore, procedures for detecting recurrence should focus on abdominal and pelvic examinations.

Imaging Modalities

Imaging modalities include sonography, CT scanning, MR imaging, and immunoscintigraphy. Ultrasound has inadequate sensitivity for post-therapy surveillance and therefore is not indicated for use in routine follow-up.[33]

The potential usefulness of CT scanning can be indirectly derived from data evaluating its use prior to second-look laparotomy. De Rosa et al[34] reported sensitivity of 47% and specificity of 87%, and Silverman et al[35] reported a similar sensitivity and specificity of 40% and 99%, respectively.

CT scanning was limited in detecting small-volume tumors. The data suggest that the modest sensitivity of this together with its high cost precludes its use as a routine serial test in post-therapy surveillance.[36] It is, however, a valid modality for evaluating patients with physical findings or CA 125 levels suggestive of recurrence.

Several studies have evaluated MR imaging for use in assessing intra-abdominal tumor status. However, none have determined the efficacy of serial MR scanning during post-therapy surveillance. In a study by Fuerstner et al[37] on MR imaging identified tumor in 20 of 29 patients with surgically documented disease. Sensitivity for lesions smaller than 2 cm was only 35%. Overall, the accuracy of CT and MR scanning seems to be similar,[33,38,39] as neither detects small-volume tumors. At present, because of its limitations in sensitivity, its cost, and its time requirement MR imaging should be reserved for the evaluation of problematic cases with elevated CA 125 levels and indeterminate CT scans. In time it may replace CT as the primary imaging modality.[40]

There has been increased interest in immunoscintigraphy over the last several years, but currently there is no role for this imaging modality in the serial evaluation of post-therapy asymptomatic patients. Performance of this test using mouse antibody may induce a human anti-mouse antibody response, precluding future use of CA 125 assay in these patients.[41]

Tumor markers

The best-studied tumor marker is CA 125. Serum CA 125 levels are elevated in more than 80% of women with epithelial ovarian cancer.[6] Serial levels reflect changing tumor burden, rising or falling with progression or regression of disease, respectively, in more than 90% of cases.[6,12,43]

CA 125 levels obtained during post-therapy surveillance often identify patients destined to manifest a clinical recurrence.[44–47] In one study, CA 125 levels became elevated prior to clinical recurrence in 94% of patients with a median lead time of 3 months,[44] and more than one-third of patients had lead times in excess of 6 months. This has been confirmed by other investigators.

It is important to recognize that a CA 125 level in the normal range does not guarantee the absence of tumor.[13,14] The sensitivity and specificity of the assay depend on the reference value selected, which is of course arbitrary. About one-half of patients with CA 125 levels in the normal range at the completion of primary chemotherapy have small-volume persistent tumor, usually 1 cm or less in maximum diameter.[13] In considering use of this assay for post-therapy surveillance, the important question is not whether occult tumor is present or absent but whether and when the patient is likely to suffer a clinical or symptomatic recurrence and how this event may influence survival. These are probably the more important parameters for women with incurable tumors for whom palliation and short-term survival are the goals.

CA 125 values obtained at specific times are useful in predicting recurrence and survival. As indicated above, these levels become elevated in 93% of women prior to clinical recurrence.[44] The rate of fall of serial CA 125 levels or serum half-life values reflects chemosensitivity and is a strong predictor of survival.

Two-year actuarial survivals with CA 125 half-lives of less than 20 days, 20 to 40 days, and more than 40 days obtained during primary chemotherapy were 76, 48, and 7 months, respectively,[48] and similar relationships have been reported by other investigators.[45,49–53] CA 125 levels obtained at completion of primary therapy are also predictive of the risk of recurrence and survival. In one study patients with elevated CA 125 levels at this time had a 60% chance of clinical recurrence within the next 4 months.[44] In contrast, patients with CA 125 levels in the normal range had only a 5% risk of manifesting clinical recurrence over the same 4-month period.

Several studies have evaluated the use of multiple markers simultaneously in addition to CA 125. Some have demonstrated a modest improvement in following patients with ovarian cancer, but others have no observed benefit at all.[54] Given the increased cost and lack of clear efficacy, the use of complementary serum markers should be reserved for patients whose tumors have been demonstrated to not manifest CA 125.

A posttherapy surveillance regimen

The goal of post-therapy surveillance is the timely detection of recurrence. It is useful if it facilitates earlier institution of therapy and translates into improved quality of life through palliation of potential symptoms or prolongation of survival. The success of this strategy depends on the efficacy of second-line therapy. Although, as discussed elsewhere in this book, second-line therapies are available, cures are the exception.[55–57] An informal survey has indicated a wide variation in follow-up regimens. Typically, surveillance is more intensive initially and then becomes less frequent as the tumor-free interval increases. This is based on the expected natural history of the disease and the consequent risk of recurrence, however, therapeutically it may be paradoxical. Patients with early recurrence, within the first 6 to 12 months, commonly manifest platinum resistance and do not exhibit a survival advantage from secondary cytoreductive surgery. In contrast, patients with later recurrences are more commonly chemotherapy responsive. Some reports suggest an improvement in survival when such patients have had secondary cytoreductive operations.[58–60] Therefore, although the risk of recurrence and consequently the yield of surveillance diminishes with time, the potential for meaningful therapy may be greater. Early detection of late recurrences may permit earlier intervention when cytoreductive surgery is technically easier and the tumor burden for subsequent chemotherapy is less.

The selection of an actual posttherapy surveillance regimen is arbitrary and is not encumbered by any prospective cost-effectiveness data. Initially, tumor-free patients are evaluated clinically every 2 to 3 months for the first year and at 3 to 4-month intervals for 3 to 4 years thereafter. The schedule can be further liberalized after 5 years, and some clinicians decrease surveillance intensity earlier than 5 years. I favor a simple approach of examining patients with frank ovarian carcinoma at 3-month intervals for the first 2 to 3 years, depending on the stage, and then every 4 months until 5 years have elapsed. The surveillance interval then becomes 6 months (Table 14-2). Each visit includes a clinical examination and a serum CA 125 assay. Additional markers are of no value unless the patient's tumor has been demonstrated previously to be CA 125-negative and another marker to be positive. An example is carcinoembryonic antigen (CEA) in some mucinous tumors. Tests showing elevated CA 125 levels should always be repeated, as transient unexplained elevations are often observed. Some are related to intercurrent illnesses. A sustained and rising CA 125 level is a strong predictor of recurrence. Imaging studies are not obtained unless symptoms, physical findings, or an elevated CA 125 level suggests recurrence. The imaging study of choice is probably a CT scan. It is often useful to obtain a baseline scan initially in order to differentiate postsurgical changes from recurrent tumor. MR imaging may find a role as an alternate imaging modal-

TABLE 14-2
Suggested Surveillance Regimen for Patients with Epithelial Ovarian Cancer

SCREENING MODALITY	2–3 YEARS (MO)	3–5 YEARS (MO)	AFTER 5 YEARS
Clinical examination	3	4	6
CA 125 assay	3	4	6
CT	When examination or CA 125 level suggests recurrence		

ity in the future for women considered likely to have a recurrence.

Modification of the suggested regimen may be appropriate in two specific circumstances. The first is in the case of early-stage patients treated with unilateral salpingo-oophorectomy who still have the contralateral ovary in situ. Because of the additional risk of bilaterality, sonographic imaging of this ovary at 6- to 12-month intervals may be considered. The second special case involves borderline tumors. They have a lower absolute risk of recurrence but a greater risk of late recurrence than invasive epithelial tumors. Therefore, it is reasonable to evaluate them less frequently, but follow-up must continue indefinitely. CA 125 assay may be less efficacious with borderline tumors, but a greater role for imaging studies has not been demonstrated.

QUESTION 2

What, in your opinion, should be the treatment of a patient with an elevated serum CA 125 level (1) at a level of 100 units/ml and (2) with serial values showing a rise from 25 to 500 units/ml? Should any patients with an isolated abnormal serum CA 125 level (without any other clinical findings) be treated with chemotherapy? Should such patients be candidates for clinical trials?

VICTORIA L. SEEWALDT
BARBARA A. GOFF
BENJAMIN E. GREER

We feel that CA 125 is a sensitive marker of recurrent disease in patients with epithelial ovarian cancer whose CA 125 level has been elevated prior to therapy. Serial measurement of CA 125 is particularly valuable because it can detect disease before it is evidenced by symptoms, physical findings, or radiographic abnormalities.[17] In the group of patients who have a CA 125 level of 100 units/ml following primary therapy or a rise in CA 125 level from 25 units/ml to 500 units/ml, we are likely to assume that an individual has persistent or recurrent disease. At this point we recommend performing a thorough history and physical and pelvic examinations, as well as excluding any other cause of CA 125 elevation, such as liver disease, infection, or renal disease. If the patient has had a previous site of disease detected specifically by a radiographic study, for example a chest nodule detected by chest x-ray, we repeat that study. Otherwise, we feel that there is no clear benefit in performing additional radiographic studies unless they are indicated by new findings on physical examination. Once the patient has been restaged, we then recommend the institution of further therapy.

For patients with an elevated CA 125 level in the absence of physical or radiographic evidence of disease, the decision to reinstitute chemotherapy must be made cautiously. CA 125 measurement should be repeated in several weeks to exclude the possibility of laboratory error. In patients who have elevated serum CA 125 levels at diagnosis and subsequently develop post-therapy elevations, we favor reinstitution of chemotherapy even in the absence of physical or radiographic findings. We generally reinitiate therapy if serum CA 125 rises serially from normal to above 100 units/ml. Special consideration must be given to patients who are candidates for chemotherapy protocols with appreciable mortality rates such as bone marrow transplantation and high-dose chemotherapy. In these patients we consider the possibility of second-look surgery to confirm the existence of recurrent disease. We are less hesitant to enter a patient into a clinical trial for which there is a low incidence of morbidity and mortality.

JONATHAN M. NILOFF

Management of an elevated CA 125 level in an asymptomatic patient with no palpable tumor is very problematic. First, the assay should be repeated for confirmation and to determine the rate of rise, which may give an indication of the rate of progression. A confirmed elevated CA 125 level should be further evaluated with a CT scan. Patients with radiologically confirmed large-volume recurrences are candidates for second-line therapy as discussed elsewhere in this book.

The optimal management of a patient with a confirmed elevated CA 125 level but no palpable or radiologic evidence of tumor has not been defined. I generally recommend careful follow-up with serial examinations, CA 125 determinations, and CT scans. I do not recommend chemotherapy with an elevated serum CA 125 level as the only indication of recurrence. This is a situation in which the clinician must balance the potential survival benefit of chemotherapy, with or without surgery, against the morbidity and side effects of such treatment. As suggested earlier, the therapeutic index of intervention may be greater in patients with later recurrences. However, with the currently available treatment modalities, cure is not a realistic expectation.[56]

Because of the limitations of second-line therapy, it could be argued that CA 125 levels should not be obtained at all because this information creates anxiety for the physician and the patient.[57] Some women cannot emotionally tolerate receiving no therapy once they become aware of an elevated CA 125 level. This knowledge may compromise their subsequent quality of life. In such patients with progressively rising CA 125 levels but no other manifestation of tumor who "need" to be treated, I favor an option with minimal side effects such as tamoxifen. I withhold cytotoxic chemotherapy until there is clinical evidence of tumor progression.

I do not feel that patients with elevated CA 125 levels as the only evidence of recurrence should be candidates for chemotherapy. A randomized trial comparing therapy at time of CA 125 elevation or clinical recurrence would be interesting. Survival should be the end point. It is to be hoped that this type of protocol would determine the best time to initiate second-line therapy.

QUESTION 3

Are there any other major issues pertinent to this subject? If so, what are they?

VICTORIA L. SEEWALDT
BARBARA A. GOFF
BENJAMIN E. GREER

We strongly feel that there is a need for the further development of serologic markers to detect recurrent epithelial ovarian cancer and for innovative strategies to detect microscopic recurrent disease. In addition we believe that there is a need for prospective trials for evaluating the efficacy and cost-effectiveness of various treatment strategies. More money spent on increasingly complex technology does not necessarily translate into improved patient care. A priority should be placed on training internists and medical oncologists to perform pelvic and rectovaginal exam inations in order to promote the use of this inexpensive and effective screening test.

At present we lack an effective cure for women with recurrent epithelial ovarian cancer, and for this reason there may not be an immediate need for intensive surveillance for this disease. However, as new chemotherapeutic agents are discovered and more effective treatment modalities are developed, we hope there will be an increasing need for innovative strategies for detecting microscopic recurrent disease.

JONATHAN M. NILOFF

A simple post-therapy surveillance regimen using clinical examination and serum CA 125 levels can effectively detect recurrence in most patients with epithelial ovarian cancer before clinical manifestation, and this advance warning may cause great anxiety among patients. The optimal treatment of patients with early recurrence, especially those with isolated elevated CA 125 levels remains undefined. Our diagnostic abilities have exceeded the weapons in our therapeutic armamentarium. Determination of the optimal surveillance regimen and management strategy awaits the development of new treatments and will require careful prospective study.

EDITORS' COMMENTARY

We agree with the contributors that no well-defined routine post-therapy surveillance can be recommended. Nevertheless, our experts recommend the use of physical examination and serial assessment of the CA 125 tumor marker at decreasing intervals as the patient becomes more distant from primary therapy. We also agree with the recommendation that imaging procedures have a sensitivity that is too low for incorporation into post-therapy surveillance.

We agree with our contributors that the routine use of cytotoxic chemotherapy based on serial elevation of a tumor marker without clinical or radiographic evidence of recurrent disease should be approached cautiously. Dr. Niloff is the more cautious, recommending either no therapy with tumor marker elevation or a therapy with very low toxicity such as tamoxifen. Dr. Seewaldt and colleagues recommend routine therapy with cytotoxics as soon as the CA 125 level rises to a level of 100 units/ml but verify persistent disease by a second-look surgical procedure before instituting an aggressive form of therapy such as bone marrow transplantation. Although we agree that therapy eventually needs to be instituted in a patient with an elevated marker level, we feel that deferral of this therapy until she has a symptomatic recurrence may be in her best interest. Nevertheless, from an emotional point of view immediate institution of therapy is often easier for the patient.

It is clear that the impact of salvage therapy in recurrent and persistent ovarian cancer has value in terms of tumor reduction and often in resolution of symptoms. Its impact on overall survival, however, remains questionable. Clinical trials designed to determine whether early institution versus later institution of salvage therapy has an impact on survival are needed. Only if salvage therapies can be shown to be more efficacious during early relapse can routine surveillance with current methodologies be strongly recommended. Further research in this area is urgently needed.

References

1. Ghatage P, Krepart G, Lotocki R: Factor analysis of false-negative second-look laparotomy. Gynecol Oncol 37: 172, 1990
2. Podczacki E, Manetta A, Kaminski P et al: Survival of patients with ovarian epithelial carcinomas after second-look laparotomy. Gynecol Oncol 36:43, 1990
3. Dauplat J, Hacker NF, Nieberg RK et al: Distant metastasis in epithelial ovarian carcinoma. Cancer 60:1561, 1987
4. Barter JF, Barnes WA: Second-look laparotomy. pp. 269–300. In Rubin SC, Sutton GP (eds). Ovarian Cancer. 1st Ed. McGraw-Hill, New York, 1993

5. Creasman WT: Second look laparotomy in ovarian cancer. Gynecol Oncol 55: 122, 1994
6. Podratz KC, Cliby WA: Second look surgery in the management of epithelial ovarian cancer. Gynecol Oncol 55:472, 1994
7. Copeland LJ, Gershenson DM, Wharton JT et al: Microscopic disease at second look laparotomy in advanced ovarian cancer. Cancer 55:472, 1985
8. Grover SR, Quinn MA: Is there any value in bimanual pelvic examination as a screening test? Med J Aust 162:408, 1995
9. Schutter EM, Kenemans P, Sohn C et al: Diagnostic value of pelvic examination, ultrasound, and serum CA 125 in postmenopausal women with a pelvic mass: an international multicenter study. Cancer 74:1398, 1994
10. Seewaldt VL, Cain JM, Greer BE et al: Reviving the pelvic examination for evaluating the status of ovarian carcinoma. J Clin Oncol 13:799, 1995
11. Bast RC, Feeney M, Lazarus H et al: Reactivity of a monoclonal antibody with human ovarian cancer. J Clin Invest 68:1331, 1981
12. Bast RC, Klug TL, St John E et al: A radioimmunoassay using a monoclonal antibody to monitor the course of epithelial ovarian cancer. N Engl J Med 309:883, 1993
13. Niloff JM, Bast RC, Schaetzl EM, Knapp RC: Predictive value of CA-125 antigen levels in second-look procedures for ovarian cancer. Am J Obstet Gynecol 151:981, 1985
14. Berek JS, Knapp RC, Malkasian GD et al: CA-125 serum levels correlated with second-look operations among ovarian cancer patients. Obstet Gynecol 67: 685, 1986
15. Patsner B, Orr JW, Mann WJ et al: Does serum CA-125 level prior to second-look laparotomy for invasive ovarian adenocarcinoma predict size of residual disease? Gynecol Oncol 37:319, 1990
16. Gallion HH, Hunter JE, van Nagell JR et al: The prognostic implications of low serum CA 125 levels prior to the second-look operation for stage III and IV epithelial ovarian cancer. Gynecol Oncol 46:29, 1992
17. Markman M: Follow-up of the asymptomatic patient with ovarian cancer. Gynecol Oncol 55:134, 1994
18. Cohen CJ, Jennings TS: Screening for ovarian cancer: the role of noninvasive imaging techniques. Am J Obstet Gynecol 170:1088, 1994
19. Bourne T, Campbell S, Steer C, Whitehead MI et al: Transvaginal colour flow imaging: a possible new screening technique for ovarian cancer. Br Med J 299:1367, 1989
20. Hubner KF, McDonald TW, Niethammer JG et al: Assessment of primary and metastatic ovarian cancer by positron emission tomography (PET) using 2[^{18}F]-deoxyglucose (2-[^{18}F]FDG). Gynecol Oncol 51:197, 1993
21. Casey MJ, Gupta NC, Muths CK: Experience with positron emission tomography (PET) scans in patients with ovarian cancer. Gynecol Oncol 53:331, 1994
22. McKenzie SJ, De Sombre KA, Bast BS et al: Serum levels of HER-2/*neu* (c-erb-2) correlate with overexpression of p185 neu in human ovarian cancer. Cancer 71:3942, 1993
23. Grosen EA, Granger GA, Gatanaga M et al: Measurement of soluble membrane receptors for tumor necrosis factor and lymphotoxin in the sera of patients with gynecologic malignancies. Gynecol Oncol 50:68, 1993
24. Kutteh WH, Kutteh CC: Quantitation of tumor necrosis factor-alpha, interleukin 1-beta, and interleukin-6 in the effusions of ovarian epithelial neoplasms. Am J Obstet Gynecol 167:1864, 1992

25. Schildkraout JM, Rich N, Thompson WD: Evaluating genetic association among ovarian, breast, and endometrial cancer: evidence for a breast/ovarian cancer relationship. Am J Hum Genet 45:521, 1989

26. Houlston RS, Collins A, Slack J et al: Genetic epidemiology of ovarian cancer: segregation analysis. Ann Hum Genet 55:291, 1991

27. Bewtra C, Watson P, Conway T, Read-Hippee C et al: Hereditary ovarian cancer: a clinicopathological study. Int J Gynecol Pathol 11:180, 1992

28. Narod SA, Madlensky L, Bradley L et al: Heredity and familial ovarian cancer in southern Ontario. Cancer, 74:2341, 1994

29. Narod SA, Feunteun J, Lynch HT et al: Familial breast-ovarian cancer locus on chromosome 17q21–q23. Lancet 338:82, 1991

30. Easton DF, Bishop DT, Ford D, Crockford GP: Genetic linkage analysis in familial breast and ovarian cancer: results from 214 families. The Breast Cancer Linkage Consortium. Am J Hum Genet 52:678, 1993

31. Steichen-Gersdorf E, Gallion HH, Ford D et al: Familial site-specific ovarian cancer is linked to BRAC1 on 17q12-21. Am J Hum Genet 55:870, 1994

32. Takahashi H, Behbakht K, McGovern PE et al: Mutation analysis of the BRAC1 gene in ovarian cancers. Cancer Res 55:2998, 1995

33. Kainz C, Prayer L, Gitsch G et al: The diagnostic value of magnetic resonance imaging for the detection of tumor recurrence in patients with carcinoma of the ovaries. J Am Coll Surg 178:238, 1994

34. De Rosa V, Mangoni di Stefano MF, Brunetti A et al: Computed tomography and second-look surgery in ovarian cancer patients: correlation, actual role and limitations of CT scan. Eur J Gynaecol Oncol 16:123, 1995

35. Silverman PM, Osborne M, Dunnick NR, Bandy LC: CT prior to second-look operation in ovarian cancer. Am J Roentgenol 150:829, 1988

36. Aravantinos D, Michalas S, Papazefkos V et al: Predictive values of CA 125 antigen levels and CT scan in second-look procedures for ovarian cancer. Eur J Obstet Gynecol Reprod Biol 37:265, 1990

37. Forstner R, Hricak H, Powell CB et al: Ovarian cancer recurrence: value of MR imaging. Radiology 196:715, 1995

38. Prayer L, Kainz C, Kramer J et al: CT and MR accuracy in the detection of tumor recurrence in patients treated for ovarian cancer. J Comput Assist Tomogr 17:626, 1993

39. Low RN, Carter WD, Saleh F, Sigeti JS: Ovarian cancer: comparison of findings with perfluorocarbon-enhanced MR imaging, In-lll-CYT-103 immunoscintigraphy, and CT. Radiology 195:391, 1995

40. Forstner R, Hricak H, White S: CT and MRI of ovarian cancer. Abdom Imaging, 20:2, 1995

41. Cannistra SA: ^{111}In-CYT-103 immunoscintigraphy in ovarian cancer, letter. Gynecol Oncol 51:292, 1993

42. Podczaski E, Whitney C, Manetta A et al: Use of CA 125 to monitor patients with ovarian epithelial carcinomas. Gynecol Oncol 33:193, 1989

43. Krebs H, Goplerud ER, Kilpatrick SJ et al: Role of CA 125 as tumor marker in ovarian carcinoma. Obstet Gynecol 67:473, 1986

44. Niloff JM, Knapp RC, Lavin PT et al: The CA 125 assay as a predictor of clinical recurrence in epithelial ovarian cancer. Am J Obstet Gynecol 155:56, 1986

45. Vergote IB, Bormer OP, Abeler VM: Evaluation of serum CA 125 levels in the monitoring of ovarian cancer. Gynecol Oncol 157:88, 1987

46. Cruickshank DJ, Terry PB, Fullertor WT: The potential value of CA 125 as a tumour marker in small volume, non-evaluable epithelial ovarian cancer. Int J Biol Markers 6:247, 1991

47. Gallagher CJ, Ostler P, Bowles J et al: CA 125 surrogate marker of response and indication for a trial of the early treatment of relapse, abstract. Proc Ann Meet Am Soc Clin Oncol 13:A871, 1994

48. Hawkins RE, Roberts K, Wiltshaw E et al: The prognostic significance of the half-life of serum CA 125 in patients responding to chemotherapy for epithelial ovarian carcinoma. Brit J Obstet Gynecol 96:1395, 1989

49. Lavin PT, Knapp RC, Malkasian G et al: CA 125 for the monitoring of ovarian carcinoma during primary therapy. Obstet Gynecol 69:223, 1987

50. Van Der Burg MEL, Lammes FB, Van Putten WLJ, Stoter G: Ovarian cancer: the prognostic value of the serum half-life of CA 125 during induction chemotherapy. Gynecol Oncol 30:307, 1988

51. Hunter VJ, Daly L, Helms M et al: The prognostic significance of CA 125 half-life in patients with ovarian cancer who have received primary chemotherapy after surgical cytoreduction. Am J Obstet Gynecol 163:1164, 1990

52. Rustin GJS, Genning JN, Nelstrop AE et al: Use of CA 125 to predict survival of patients with ovarian carcinoma. J Clin Oncol 7:1667, 1989

53. Sevelda P, Schemper M, Spona J: CA 125 as an independent prognostic factor for survival in patients with epithelial ovarian cancer. Am J Obstet Gynecol 161:1213, 1989

54. Bast RC Jr, Klug TL, Schaetzl E et al: Monitoring human ovarian carcinoma with a combination of CA 125, CA 19–9 and carcinoembryonic antigen. Am J Obstet Gynecol 149:553, 1984

55. Ozols RF, Rubin SC, Dembo AJ, Robboy S: Epithelial ovarian cancer. p. 769. In Hoskins WJ, Perez CA, Young RC (eds): Principles and Practice of Gynecologic Oncology. JB Lippincott, Philadelphia, 1992

56. Ozols RF: Outcome issues in ovarian cancer. Oncology Suppl. 9:135, 1995

57. Markman M: Resetting the CA 125 range for a complete response to chemotherapy: Why? Gynecol Oncol 53:281, 1994

58. Morris M, Gershenson DM, Wharton JT: Secondary cytoreductive surgery in epithelial ovarian cancer: nonresponders to first-line therapy. Gynecol Oncol 33:1, 1989

59. Berek JS, Hacker NF, Legasse LD et al: Survival of patients following secondary cytoreductive surgery in ovarian cancer. Obstet Gynecol 61:189, 1983

60. Segna RA, Dottino PR, Mandeli JP et al: Secondary cytoredution for ovarian cancer following cisplatin therapy. J Clin Oncol 11:434, 1993

CHAPTER 15

THE ROLE OF HORMONAL THERAPY IN THE MANAGEMENT OF OVARIAN CANCER

Peter E. Schwartz
John Kavanagh
Andrzej P. Kudelka
Claire F. Verschraegen

EDITORS' INTRODUCTION

Over the past two decades multiple forms of hormonal therapy have been utilized in treating patients with ovarian cancer, including estrogens, progestins, antiestrogens, androgens, antiandrogens, and gonadotropins. The value of any of these therapies remains unproven, but because of their low toxicity they are often utilized particularly in patients with poor performance status or comorbid illness. We have asked our experts to discuss the role of hormonal therapy in the treatment of patients with refractory or recurrent ovarian cancer and to comment on whether the steroid receptor status of the ovarian tumor is useful in selecting patients or predicting therapeutic outcome.

Hormones have also been used in the rare sex cord stromal tumors of the ovary. These tumors are extraordinarily unusual, and thus the numbers of patients available for study are small. Nevertheless, we have asked for a discussion of this topic.

Finally, since virtually all patients with ovarian cancer undergo a bilateral oophorectomy as part of their initial surgical procedure, surgical menopause is common and estrogen replacement therapy is often requested by patients. We have asked the authors to comment on the potential negative effects of estrogen replacement therapy in terms of causing recurrence of the cancer.

QUESTIONS

1. What is the role of hormonal therapy in the treatment of patients with refractory epithelial ovarian cancer?
2. How should steroid receptor status of ovarian cancer be used to guide therapy?
3. What is the role, if any, of hormonal therapy in the treatment of sex cord-stromal tumors of the ovary?
4. How should we counsel patients about estrogen replacement therapy after a diagnosis of epithelial ovarian cancer?
5. What should be the future directions in this area?

QUESTION 1

What is the role of hormonal therapy in the treatment of patients with refractory epithelial ovarian cancer?

PETER E. SCHWARTZ

Progestin therapy

Over the past 33 years numerous reports have appeared indicating a potential role for progestins in the management of refractory epithelial ovarian cancer. These progestins include Delalutin (17-hydroxyprogesterone in oil), oral Provera (medroxyprogesterone acetate [MPA], intramuscular Provera, and Megace (megestrol acetate).[1–15] In reviewing earlier series it is difficult to determine objective response rates based on current conventions for patients treated with these agents. Overall, 390 women have been included, 30 (8%) of whom have responded (Table 15-1). The series with the largest percentage of responders was described by Geisler[11] in 1985 using Megace.[11] Thirty-one patients responded to this therapy. However, in four subsequent series, composed of a total of 115 patients, only five objective responses to Megace were documented.[12–15] At present, progestin therapy for refractory ovarian cancer is not particularly effective in management of this disease.

Estrogen Therapy

Only one series has been reported involving the use of an estrogen-like preparation in the treatment of women with refractory ovarian cancer. In 1963 Long and Evans[16] described their experience with diethylstilbestrol (DES) in 14 patients with refractory advanced ovarian cancer, five of whom were subsequently lost to follow-up.[16] Two of the nine with follow-up demonstrated objective responses lasting more than 1 year. One patient had a papillary adenocarcinoma associated with generalized metastases, and the second patient had pseudomyxoma peritonei. Three additional patients reported an increased sense of well-being, despite a lack of objective response to the therapy. The authors speculated that perhaps DES inhibited gonadotropin release and that it was through this mechanism that it had a favorable impact in the two patients who objectively responded to this treatment.

Estrogen/Progestin

Combined estrogen and progestin therapy has been used in the management of women with advanced epithelial ovarian cancers. Jolles et al[3] reported on 65 women treated with estrogen and progestins as second-line therapy. Ethinyl estradiol 0.1 mg p.o. daily was orally given for 25 days of a 30-day cycle, and Provera 10 mg daily was given on days 8 to 25 of

TABLE 15-1
Progestin Therapy for Advanced and Recurrent Ovarian Cancer

PROGESTIN	STUDY/YEAR	NO. OF PATIENTS TREATED	NO. OF PATIENTS RESPONDING	RESPONSE (%)
Delalutin (IM)	Varga and Henriksen[1] (1964)	6	1	16
	Ward[2] (1972)	23	3	13
	Jolles et al[3] (1983)	10	1	10
Provera (PO)	Kaufman[4] (1966)	11	1	9
	Malkasian et al[5] (1977)	19	1	5
	Mangioni et al[6] (1981)	30	0	0
	Aabo et al[7] (1982)	27	1	4
	Hamerlynck et al[10] (1985)	41	1	2
Provera (IM)	Slayton et al[8] (1981)	19	0	0
	Mangioni et al[6] (1981)	33	5	15
	Tropé et al[9] (1981)	25	1	4
Megace (PO)	Geisler[11] (1985)	31	10	32
	Ahlgren et al[12] (1985)	26	1	4
	Sikic et al[13] (1986)	47	4	9
	Schwartz et al[14] (1987)	12	0	0
	Ahlgren et al[15] (1993)	30	0	0
Total		390	30	8

Abbreviations: Delalutin, 17α-hydroxyprogesterone caproate; Provera, medroxyprogesterone acetate; Megace, megestrol acetate.

the ethinyl estradiol cycle. Women received no therapy on days 26 through 30. Nine (14%) objective responses were noted. One patient who had a partial response had to discontinue therapy because of severe nausea and vomiting, and one complication involving a cerebral vascular accident was documented in a patient receiving her first course of treatment. From et al[17] used similar therapy consisting of ethinyl estradiol (0.5 mg days 1 through 7) and Provera 400 mg days 8 through 25) on a 25-day schedule and observed 4 (17%) partial responses among 23 patients. The combined estrogen and progestin therapy does not appear to be more efficacious in the management of refractory ovarian cancer than the use of progestin alone.

Antiestrogen Therapy

In 1978 a series of women began treatment with an estrogen agonist-antagonist, tamoxifen, for refractory advanced epithelial ovarian cancer at Yale-New Haven Medical Center.[18] Prior to receiving tamoxifen, all patients had received chemotherapy and many had received radiotherapy as well. The treatment plan was to give 10 mg of tamoxifen twice a day with a doubling of the dose every 4 weeks until an objective response was observed. The maximum dose administered was 320 mg daily. One partial response lasting 2 months was observed in this series, four women had stable disease lasting 11 to 30 weeks, and eight women failed to respond. Five of the eight who failed to respond had partial small bowel obstruction at the initiation of tamoxifen therapy and died within 9 weeks of beginning the protocol. The three remaining women died within 24 weeks of starting tamoxifen treatment. The first death in a tamoxifen-treated patient with stabilized disease occurred 25 weeks after initiating treatment. All women who had stabilized disease or a clinical partial response had estrogen receptor–rich tumors (23 to 169 fmol/mg of cytosol protein). However, estrogen receptor was also detected in women who had progressive disease while on tamoxifen therapy.

Ten subsequent reports have confirmed a very limited role for tamoxifen in the management of refractory advanced epithelial ovarian cancer.[15,19–27] The largest series was reported by Hatch et al[26] and represented 105 women treated on a Gynecologic Oncology Group (GOG) protocol, all of whom had refractory ovarian cancer. Ten women had complete responses, 8 had partial responses, and 40 had stable disease. Combining all series currently available (Table 15-2) reveals that 351 women have been treated with tamoxifen. A complete response rate of 4.6%, a partial response rate of 7.4%, and stabilization of disease for 30.5% was reported. These data suggest that tamoxifen may have a modest role in controlling refractory advanced ovarian cancer.

Maenpaa et al[28] have presented data suggesting that toremifene, a triphenylethylene antiestrogen that is active against breast cancer, may have a chemopotentiating effect in vitro on drug-resistant ovarian cancers. However, in a clinical study of five women with refractory epithelial ovarian cancer, toremifene given prior to cytotoxic chemotherapy produced no change in disease status in two patients (3 months, 12+ months) and progressive disease in two women. The final patient was unevaluable for response.

Androgen therapy

Kaufman[4] was the first to report the use of androgen therapy in the management of refractory epithelial ovarian cancer. This series treated women with extremely advanced recurrent disease, and no objective response was observed. Kavanagh et al[29] subsequently reported on 16 women treated with fluoxymesterone (Halotestin) and was unable to demonstrate any objective response using androgen therapy.

Gonadotropin releasing hormone analog therapy

Five series have been reported in which women with refractory epithelial ovarian cancers received gonadotropin releasing hor-

TABLE 15-2
Tamoxifen Therapy for Refractory Ovarian Cancer

STUDY/YEAR	NO. OF PATIENTS	RESPONSE COMPLETE	PARTIAL	STABLE	CR PLUS PR (%)
Schwartz et al[18] (1982)	13	0	1	4	7.7
Pagel et al[19] (1983)	29	1	7	12	27.6
Hamerlynck et al[20] (1985)	18	0	1	2	5.6
Shirley et al[21] (1985)	23	0	0	19	0
Campbell et al[22] (1985)	22	2	3		22.7
Slevin et al[23] (1986)	22	0	0	1	0
Weiner et al[24] (1987)	37	1	2	6	8.1
Osborne et al[25] (1988)	53	0	1	5	1.9
Hatch et al[26] (1991)	105	10	8	40	17.1
Ahlgren et al[15] (1993)	29	2	3	18	17.2
Van Der Velden[27] (1995)	30	2	0	10	6.7
Total	381	18	26	117	11.5

Abbreviations: CR, Complete response; PR, partial response.

mone (GnRH) analog therapy. Lind et al[30] described two partial responses in 30 women with advanced ovarian cancer lasting 40 and 105 weeks and five patients with disease stabilization lasting 25, 35, 40, 66, and 70 weeks, respectively, using Goserelin (Table 15-3). The series reported by Palmer et al[31] employed D-Trp-6 luteinizing hormone (Decapeptyl) in 39 women. Six patients (15%) demonstrated a partial response, and 5 patients (12.8%) showed stabilization of disease. Three series used Leuprolide in the treatment of women with refractory ovarian cancer.[32–34] One of 53 (1.9%) demonstrated a complete response, 7 of 53 (13.2%) demonstrated a partial response, and 19 of 53 (35.8%) demonstrated stabilization of disease. In total, 122 patients reportedly received GnRH analog therapy: one (0.8%) complete response, 15 (12.3%) partial responses, and 29 (23.8%) stabilizations of disease were observed for an objective response rate of 13.1%. There appears to be a minimal role for GnRH analog therapy in the management of refractory ovarian cancer, and that role may be limited to use in women with well-differentiated or moderately differentiated cancers, as no responses have been observed in patients with poorly differentiated carcinomas.

Aromatase inhibitors

The conversion of androgens to estrogens occurs in a variety of extragonadal tissue such as adipose tissue and brain.[35] Estrogens produced in peripheral tissue are believed to be important in the etiology of breast and endometrial cancer. The biosynthesis of estrogens is catalyzed by aromatase, an enzyme localized to the endoplasmic reticulum. Aminoglutethimide and testolactone represent first-generation aromatase inhibitors.[36] Ahlgren et al[15] treated 15 patients with aminoglutethimide 250 mg orally 4 times a day plus hydrocortisone initially 100 mg daily and then tapered to 20 mg daily as tolerated. This trial was discontinued when no objective responses were observed.

JOHN KAVANAGH
ANDRZEJ P. KUDELKA
CLAIRE F. VERSCHRAEGEN

The reproductive nature of the organ involved, epidemiologic data suggesting a hormonal causation, and the presence of steroid receptors imply that ovarian cancer may be amenable to treatment with hormone manipulation. However, the clinical data are far from clear. There is a paucity of information on the primary treatment of ovarian cancer with endocrine therapy. Rendina et al[37] used MPA in 33 chemotherapy-naive patients, many of whom had lower-grade or endometrioid tumors, and reported 18 (55%) responses. Since the advent of combination chemotherapy, primary hormonal treatment of ovarian cancer has rarely been used.

The use of progestins in refractory disease has been practiced for many years, employing

TABLE 15-3
GnRH Analog Therapy for Refractory Ovarian Cancer

STUDY	GnRH ANALOG	CLINICAL RESPONSE				TOTAL NO. OF PATIENTS
		COMPLETE	PARTIAL	STABLE	PROGRESSION	
Palmer et al[31]	Decapeptyl	0	6	5	28	39
Kavanagh et al[29]	Leuprolide	0	4	2	17	23
Bruckner et al[33]	Leuprolide	1	2	2	0	5
Miller et al[34]	Leuprolide	0	1	15	9	25
Lind et al[30]	Goserelin	0	2	5	23	30
Total (%)		1 (0.8)	15 (12.3)	29 (23.8)	77 (63.1)	122

TABLE 15-4
Progestational Agents in the Treatment of Refractory Ovarian Cancer

STUDY/YEAR	RESPONSE RATE
Aabo[7] (1982)	1/27 (4%)
Hamerlynck[10] (1985)	1/41 (2%)
Landoni[38] (1985)	9/67 (7%)
Mangioni[6] (1981)	5/63 (8%)
Sikic[13] (1986)	4/47 (9%)
Tropé[9] (1982)	1/25 (4%)
Total	21/270 (8%)

various agents in various doses. A review of trials with at least 25 patients showed response rates of 0 to 15% (Table 15-4). Although palliative effects of increased appetite and well-being occur, objective response rates are low. The addition of progestational agents to chemotherapy has not proven superior to chemotherapy alone.

The use of antiestrogens, such as tamoxifen, was logical, especially with the discovery of estrogen receptors in ovarian cancer. However, the drug has failed to show activity in heavily pretreated patients. In larger trials the response rates were 0 to 10% (Table 15-5). It is unclear from these studies whether a subset of patients benefit from the drug. Also, the definition and clinical importance of stability of disease are difficult to assess in these trials. The addition of tamoxifen to cisplatin and doxorubicin has not resulted in improved chemotherapy response.[39]

Androgen receptors are commonly present in ovarian cancer, however, a trial of fluoxymesterone in 16 patients produced no response.[40] Furthermore, the antiandrogen flutamide yielded a response rate of less than 10% in 20 patients. The combination of leuprolide acetate and flutamide also yielded a response rate of 12% in 25 patients (J. J. Kavanagh, unpublished data). This combination did not appear superior to other single-agent hormone therapy. It has been hypothesized that gonadotropins are a risk factor for the development of ovarian cancer.[41] However, recent data suggest that low serum gonadotropin levels or high androgen levels are a risk factor for the disease.[42] GnRH analogs have been evaluated in refractory epithelial ovarian cancer (Table 15-6), and the response rates in studies with more than 10 patients were between 15% and 18%. In one provocative trial, nine patients achieved stability of disease for at least 3 months with a slower increase in CA 125 levels compared to those in a control group.[43] Gonadotropin analogs thus have a level of activity similar to that of other hormonal agents.[44–46] The combination of leuprolide acetate and tamoxifen in the treatment of refractory ovarian cancer produced a 12% response rate in 17 evaluable patients. However, 29% had stabilization of disease and median duration of survival from the start of therapy was a surprising 14.4 months. The number of patients studied was too small for a subset analysis.[47]

Curiously, estrogens have only rarely been used as single-agent therapy in ovarian cancer.

TABLE 15-5
Tamoxifen in the Treatment of Refractory Ovarian Cancer

STUDY/YEAR	RESPONSE RATE
Shirley[21] (1985)	0/22 (0%)
Landoni[38] (1985)	0/55 (0%)
Slevin[23] (1986)	0/22 (0%)
Weiner[24] (1987)	3/31 (10%)
Total	3/130 (2%)

TABLE 15-6
Gonadotropin Releasing Hormone Analogs in the Treatment of Refractory Ovarian Cancer

STUDY/YEAR	RESPONSE RATE
Jager[43] (1989)	0/11 (0%) (9 stable)
Kavanagh[44] (1989)	4/23 (17%)
Kullander[45] (1986)	2/10 (20%)
Parmar[46] (1988)	6/39 (15%)
Total	12/83 (14%)

Fourteen patients received oral DES after failing radiation therapy or alkylating agent therapy, and two responded. There was a trend for patients with better differentiated tumors to react more favorably to the compound.[47a]

Addition of estrogen to another hormonal agent has been utilized in several studies. Adding a progestational agent or tamoxifen did not appear to improve response rates (Table 15-7). However, prolonged stability of disease is usually reported for a few patients in these studies.

In summary, the activity of single-agent hormonal therapy in epithelial ovarian cancer is usually 10 to 15%, and another 10 to 15% of patients demonstrate stabilization of their disease. These agents are usually used in refractory settings for palliation, and there is limited experience in the primary setting. Combination hormonal therapy using either other hormones or chemotherapy does not seem to offer an obvious advantage over the use of single agents.

QUESTION 2

How should steroid receptor status of ovarian cancer be used to guide therapy?

PETER E. SCHWARTZ

The presence of steroid receptor proteins is well established in epithelial ovarian cancer specimens. Thus, estrogen, progestin, androgen, and corticosteroid receptor proteins are observed in a high percentage of women whose epithelial ovarian cancer specimens have been analyzed for these macromolecules.[50-60] Progestin receptors are found in approximately 50% of epithelial ovarian cancer specimens studied, androgen receptors in as many as 80% of specimens studied, and corticosteroid receptors in 90% of specimens studied.[50-60]

The presence of steroid receptor protein in a tumor specimen does not guarantee that the malignancy is hormonally sensitive. There is heterogeneity between the receptor content of the primary site and its metastases.[51] Many cancer specimens studied for estrogen or progestin receptors are obtained at initial surgery. Most patients receiving progestin therapies have had advanced refractory disease before being treated with hormones. The original tamoxifen protocol for refractory ovarian cancer at Yale-New Haven Medical Center did not demonstrate that estrogen receptor positivity in the initial specimen guaranteed sensitivity to tamoxifen when the cancer became refractory to chemotherapy.[14] In 1989 the first prospective randomized trial combining cytotoxic chemotherapy (Adriamycin and cisplatin) with or without tamoxifen in the treatment of previously untreated advanced epithelial ovarian cancers was reported.[39] No survival advantage for women with estrogen and/or progestin receptor-rich tumors receiving tamoxifen was demonstrated in that prospective randomized trial.

There is limited information on the response of women to progestin therapy when they have had previously untreated epithelial ovarian cancers and progestin receptors have been detected in their cancer specimens. There are no series involving women with previously untreated epithelial ovarian cancers who have received androgen or corticosteroid therapy and correlated response with the tumor androgen or corticosteroid receptor content.

There are three series in which progestins were given as part of the initial treatment.[37,61,62] Burqvist et al[61] and Timothy[62] demonstrated that previously untreated women with epithe-

TABLE 15-7
Progestin Combinations in the Treatment of Refractory Ovarian Cancer

STUDY/YEAR	ADDITIONAL AGENT	RESPONSE RATE
Freedman[48] (1986)	Estrogen	9/65 (14%)
Jakobsen[49] (1987)	Tamoxifen	0/17 (0%)
Ward[1] (1972)	Estrogen	0/8 (0%)
Total		9/90 (10%)

lial ovarian cancer can respond to progestin therapy.[61,62] The series by Rendina et al[37] included 31 women with advanced endometrioid ovarian cancers, 30 with stage III disease, and 1 with stage IV disease. Estrogen receptors were present in 81.3% of the primary tumors, and progestin receptors were determined to be present in 72.1%. Only 14% of the tumors lacked receptors. Of the 30 women in whom objective responses could be measured, 17 responded; three had complete responses, and 14 had partial responses. In addition, eight patients showed stabilization of disease and six had progressive disease. Throughout the entire series, complete and partial responses were observed only in women whose tumors were estrogen receptor-positive or both estrogen and progestin receptor-positive. Among the eight women in whom there was no detectable level of estrogen or progestin receptor, six had progressive disease on progestin therapy and two had stable disease. Estrogen receptor level determinations may be of value in the treatment of women with endometrioid carcinoma in order to determine hormonal sensitivity. It is highly likely that receptor-positive tumors are limited to women with well-differentiated endometrioid carcinomas. Data are available suggesting that progestins have activity in first-line therapy for the management of epithelial ovarian cancers.[37,61–63] There are almost no data on estrogen and progestin receptors in non endometrioid epithelial ovarian carcinomas and the response of these cancers to progestin therapy. There is no documentation suggesting that estrogen receptor levels are useful in determining tamoxifen response. Indeed, this compound may work through mechanisms other than the estrogen receptor mechanism.[63,64] It is possible that, in the case of refractory disease, patients most likely to respond to tamoxifen are estrogen receptor–positive, as their tumors may be biologically less virulent than receptor-negative tumors. Other than in endometrioid epithelial ovarian cancer, there is no demonstrated role for determining tumor steroid receptor protein status in guiding therapy.

JOHN KAVANAGH ET AL

There is extensive literature on the presence of steroid receptors in epithelial ovarian cancer. Receptors for estrogen and progesterone are found in 50% of cases, however, the presence of these receptors does not correlate well with histologic grade of tumor or stage of disease.[65] In fact, one investigator has reported that poorly differentiated tumors have a greater likelihood of having estrogen receptors. Lymphocyte infiltration of tumors is found in the presence of progesterone receptors.[66] Endometrioid tumors have been reported to contain higher levels of progesterone and estrogen receptors.[37,67] The issue is somewhat confusing in that normal ovarian tissue and benign ovarian tumors have receptors for progesterone, estrogen, and even androgens. The level at which the tissue is considered positive varies in different studies. There is also a definite heterogeneity in the amount of receptor in primary ovarian cancer and metastases.[49,66,67] The utility of hormonal receptors in guiding therapy is compromised by the issues mentioned above and the paucity of prospective studies.

Gonadotropin receptors have been identified in epithelial ovarian cancers, usually at a relatively low level. Granulosa cell tumors have been reported to have high levels of receptors for gonadotropins,[68,69] and GnRH also have receptor sites identifiable in ovarian tumors.[70,71]

There are no available data on the correlation between presence of androgen receptors, stage, or clinical course. The use of receptor data to predict response to hormonal agents has generally been disappointing. No correlation has been shown between presence of estrogen and progesterone receptors and response to tamoxifen therapy.[21,24,39] The occurrence of these receptors in endometrioid ovarian carcinoma did predict response to progestational compounds in minimally treated patients. Receptor analysis, although of scientific interest, is not highly predictive of response to hormones or clinical evolution of disease.

QUESTION 3

What is the role, if any, of hormonal therapy in the treatment of sex cord-stromal tumors of the ovary?

PETER E. SCHWARTZ

Data are limited regarding hormonal therapy in the management of sex cord-stromal tumors of the ovary. A rationale for its use might be based on the presence of estrogen or progestin receptors in sex cord-stromal tumor specimens. A series from the Yale-New Haven Medical Center demonstrated the presence of progestin receptors in two of three granulosa cell tumors of the ovary.[72] While these tumors frequently produce estrogen, there is no evidence that they are hormonally dependent. One patient treated with progestins in the series showed prolonged stable disease in the presence of refractory advanced granulosa cell tumor. It was uncertain whether the response to progestins was a true inhibition of growth or simply a reflection of the natural history of granulosa cell tumor as a biologically indolent tumor. Malik et al.[73] demonstrated a partial response to MPA in one patient using 100 mg three times a day that lasted more than 2 years, and stabilization of disease in a second patient who required escalating doses of MPA to achieve this effect over an 8-month period. Isaacs et al.[74] described one woman with refractory granulosa cell tumor who had a complete response to MPA 200 mg three times a day lasting 42 months and a second patient whose refractory granulosa cell tumor showed a marked response to megestrol acetate 160 mg daily 5 months after initiating hormone therapy. One of three women with granulosa cell tumors treated by Maenpaa[28] with toremifene as a cytotoxic chemotherapy sensitizer demonstrated a partial response lasting 6 months. The two other toremifene-treated patients were unevaluable for response.

Granulosa cell tumors often do quite well in younger women but appear to be biologically more virulent after age 40. In a series from the MD Anderson Hospital, Schwartz and Smith[75] noted that patients treated with radiotherapy for early-stage ovarian cancers often developed recurrences more than 10 years after the original treatment. All the women who had recurrences were over age 40. One possible explanation is that sex cord-stromal tumors may be stimulated to grow under the influence of the elevated levels of gonadotropins found in postmenopausal women.[16] However, granulosa cell tumors have been shown to produce inhibin, a peptide hormone that inhibits follicle stimulating hormone (FSH) release.[76,77] Serum inhibin levels may be considerably elevated in women with active granulosa cell tumors.[77] Serum inhibin should theoretically inhibit FSH release and limit the growth of granulosa cell tumors.

Kauppila et al.[78] treated five women with granulosa cell tumors refractory to cytotoxic chemotherapy using GnRH agonist analogs. One partial response and one stabilization of disease were documented, and three patients developed progressive disease. Serum inhibin levels were elevated in three of four patients and remained relatively constant or declined during the first 3 months of therapy. Inhibin levels subsequently increased as the disease progressed.

JOHN KAVANAGH
ANDRZEJ P. KUDELKA
CLAIRE F. VERSCHRAEGEN

Granulosa cell tumors of the ovary are rare and are generally treated by surgical resection. These tumors produce estradiol and inhibin, which may be useful as tumor markers.[69] As mentioned previously, gonadotropin hormone receptors are found in these tumors.[68] Tamoxifen has induced responses in three of seven patients refractory to chemotherapy.[21]

Leuprolide acetate, a GnRH agonist, induced partial responses in two of four evaluable patients. Two women had stable disease for 3 and 16 months. Treatment was well tolerated.[71a] There is no information on the treatment of Sertoli-Leydig cell tumors with hormonal agents. The information available suggests that hormonal therapy may have a role in sex cord-stromal tumors and is worthy of further study.

QUESTION 4

How should we counsel patients about estrogen replacement therapy after a diagnosis of epithelial ovarian cancer?

PETER E. SCHWARTZ

The usual reasons for employing hormone replacement therapy in women who are postmenopausal, either spontaneously or by surgical intervention, is to provide symptomatic relief for menopausal symptoms such as hot flashes, vaginal dryness, nervous irritability, and urinary incontinence; to avoid the onset of osteoporosis; and to reduce the risk of cardiovascular disease.[79] The risk in initiating hormone replacement therapy in women with epithelial ovarian cancers is potential reactivation of the disease. The basis for this possibility is the obvious presence of estrogen receptor proteins in at least half of the ovarian cancer specimens studied. However, there are no convincing laboratory data supporting the contention that estrogens might reactivate quiescent epithelial ovarian cancers.

An English language medical literature search revealed only one series involving women in whom hormone replacement therapy was used following a diagnosis of epithelial ovarian cancer. A retrospective study by Eeles et al[80] compared a group of 78 women who received a variety of hormone replacement therapies to one consisting of 295 women with epithelial ovarian cancers who did not receive hormone replacement therapy. All four FIGO stages were present in this series, and the authors reported no significant difference in the stage distribution of the two groups of patients. More patients with well-differentiated tumors, that is, 20 of 78 (25.6%), received hormone replacement therapy compared to 42 of 295 (14.2%) women who did not receive hormone replacement therapy. Overall the group given hormone replacement therapy had histologically better differentiated tumors than those who did not ($P = 0.009$). The group who received hormone replacement therapy was statistically younger than the group who did not. Thirty-eight of 78 (48.7%) women who received hormone replacement therapy were under the age of 40, whereas 76 of 295 (25.8%) who did not receive hormone replacement therapy were under the age of 40 ($P = 0.001$). A selection bias in this series favored hormone replacement therapy in young women with well-differentiated tumors compared to those who were older and had poorly differentiated carcinomas. The median time from diagnosis to start of hormone replacement therapy was 11.25 months (range 0 to 404 months). Those receiving hormone replacement therapy had a median time of treatment of 28 months (range <1 to >200 months). The median follow-up was 42 months (range <1 to 216 months). Seventy of the 78 women received Premarin alone (32) or Premarin plus norgestrel (38). Six patients in this series received only progestin, and two received testosterone. Selecting women who were alive a minimum of 1 year after initial presentation and looking at the percentage of those who survived, it appears that hormone replacement therapy did not hurt the patients. Indeed, patients receiving hormone replacement therapy had a statistically better survival rate out to 11 years than that estimated for those who did not receive hormone replacement therapy. The *P* value for the survival difference was 0.07.

Currently available data do not suggest that hormone replacement therapy is deleterious to the health of a women who has been treated for epithelial ovarian cancer. Women under the age of 40 years with stage I disease who have retained an ovary may not experience an increase in recurrences.[81] Furthermore, epidemiologic evidence suggests that pregnancy and prolonged oral contraceptive use statistically reduce the risk of a woman developing ovarian cancer, indirect evidence suggesting that estrogens and progestins are not etiologically associated with epithelial ovarian cancer.[82] Indeed, estrogens and progestins have been used in the treatment of epithelial ovarian cancers. In terms of the safety of hormone replacement therapy following treatment of epithelial ovarian cancer, a possible exception is women with well-differentiated endometrioid carcinomas as these tumors may be hormone-sensitive.[37]

JOHN KAVANAGH
ANDRZEJ P. KUDELKA
CLAIRE F. VERSCHRAEGEN

The use of estrogens as hormonal supplementation in patients with a diagnosis of epithelial ovarian cancer has not been well studied. In a retrospective review, 78 women with ovarian cancer given hormone replacement therapy had no difference in survival compared to 295 not given replacement therapy.[80] Generally, it is thought that estrogen replacement in a typical patient with advanced ovarian cancer is not associated with adverse effects, however, this conclusion is based on clinical impressions rather than on large prospective studies. The effect of hormone replacement on patients with a history of endometrioid, borderline, or well-differentiated ovarian carcinoma remains a matter of speculation.

QUESTION 5

What should be the future directions in this area?

PETER E. SCHWARTZ

Data from studies on progestin therapy suggest that the efficacy of hormonal therapy is no different from that of chemotherapy or radiotherapy; that is, it is best when used as initial treatment.[37,61,62] Thus, one future direction in this area should be to consider progestin therapy as first-line treatment in prospective trials.

Strategies for prospective trials comparing progestin therapy to standard chemotherapy may be (1) as palliative therapy in previously untreated women who have had epithelial ovarian carcinoma and either have large residual cancers as a result of unsuccessful cytoreductive surgery or have stage IV disease, or (2) as treatment for women who are medically unable to tolerate standard chemotherapy.[83] The fact that progestin therapy is relatively free of side effects makes these women appropriate for first-line studies.

There is a need to objectively evaluate newer forms of hormonal therapy, including antiprogestins, second- and third-generation aromatase inhibitors, and antiandrogens, in the treatment of women with advanced ovarian cancer. Mefepristone (RU 486), an antiprogestin, is currently being evaluated in one unpublished series in the United States for women who have failed platinum-based chemotherapy. Anecdotal experience suggests that this drug may be active in platinum-refractory disease.

Aromatase activity has been identified in epithelial ovarian cancers as well as in breast cancers.[35,36,84] First-generation aromatase inhibitors are quite toxic,[36] however, new aromatase inhibitors (e.g. rogletimide, fadrozole, and triazole derivatives) are being evaluated in women with breast cancer.[35] In general, we have hesitated to use aromatase inhibitors in the management of ovarian cancer because of their significant side effects. As new aromatase inhibitors that are better tolerated are developed for clinical use, studies will be necessary to determine whether they can play a role in controlling advanced epithelial ovarian cancers.

There has been no documented effort to evaluate androgen antagonists in the treatment of women with refractory ovarian cancer. An English language computer search failed to reveal any trials of this nature. The presence of androgen receptors in epithelial ovarian cancer suggests that clinical trials may be appropriate.

Cytotoxic agents linked to steroid hormones have been minimally evaluated in patients with epithelial ovarian cancer. Intravenous radiolabeled, γ-emitting, 16α-iodoestradiol did not appear to be effective in the treatment of women with ovarian cancer in an earlier series[85] because of the rapid breakdown of radiolabeled iodine from the hormone. A subsequent attempt (R. Hochberg, P. C. Schwartz, unpublished observations) using radiolabeled 11-methoxy-16a-iodoestradiol administered intravenously did not reveal selective uptake of this agent by the cancer. Chemotherapeutic agents have now been chemically bound to estrogens. In vitro studies on estramustine phosphate suggest that it has activity in epithelial ovarian cancer cells in vitro.[86] It is time to study similar compounds in vivo to determine their place in hormonal therapy for the management of epithelial ovarian cancers.

JOHN KAVANAGH ET AL

Areas of future investigation may be divided into two categories. The first is increased molecular understanding of the various steroid receptors in ovarian cancer. Are they different from those in breast cancer? What are the hormone-responsive elements of the genome and what is their role as enhancers of transcription? Are there important posttranscriptional events that offer potential targets for therapeutic intervention? What is the relationship of steroid receptors to various growthlike factors, particularly epidermal growth factor and its receptor, and transforming growth factor (TGF)-α and -β? Do steroid receptors interact with yet undefined tumor suppressor genes? Additional knowledge of this nature would allow us to go beyond the simple analysis of steroid receptor quantity and the empirical testing of hormonal agents.

The second area of investigation is refinement of our present limited clinical information to allow more precise application of hormonal therapies. Are granulosa cell tumors responsive to gonadotropin analogs and antiestrogens? Do borderline and well-differentiated ovarian carcinomas respond to hormonal therapy? Are carcinomas influenced by progestational or other hormonal compounds? Can we define stability of refractory disease under hormonal treatment utilizing sequential dynamic measurements of CA 125 or other surrogate markers? The literature suggests that these questions are worthy of clinical trials in patients of good performance status who have had minimal prior chemotherapy.

EDITORS' COMMENTARY

Both authors nicely reviewed the literature on the use of various hormonal agents in the treatment of ovarian cancer. They conclude that only for antiestrogens and gonadotropins is there perhaps adequate evidence supporting their use. Dr. Schwartz feels that this therapy should be reserved only for patients with well-differentiated or moderately differentiated tumors since responses are rarely seen in individuals with poorly differentiated tumors. We agree with this conclusion and would probably limit such therapy to very frail patients or those who wish some form of therapy without the possibility of toxicity. Even with this proviso, however, there are other agents that offer a therapeutic index as good as or better than hormones based on more evidence of activity and low toxicity. These agents include gemcitabine and oral vepesid.

Neither author feels that evaluation of steroid receptors in tumor tissue is useful in guiding therapy. They both point out that steroid receptor-negative tumors may respond, while tumors most rich in steroid receptors often progress during therapy. There are also data suggesting that more poorly differentiated tumors (those that are least likely to respond) are often steroid rich.

Both authors feel that there are too few data to strongly recommend the use of hormones in the treatment of stromal cell tumors. Granulosa cell tumors often have an indolent course, and it is very difficult to determine whether patients with stable disease are benefiting from hormonal therapy or just displaying the natural history of the disease. It is our feeling that such tumors are best left untreated if the patient is asymptomatic, reserving more classic cytotoxic chemotherapy for women with more rapid disease velocity and/or symptoms.

Both authors agree that there are no data justifying the withholding of estrogen replacement therapy in a patient with ovarian cancer. Dr. Schwartz points out that the use of oral contraceptives is protective in terms of the development of ovarian cancer. He correctly opines that it is younger patients who may have an early carcinoma, undergo a fertility-sparing surgical procedure, and actually derive anticarcinogenic potential from replacement therapy. Dr. Schwartz also, however, cautions against the use of replacement therapy in women with well-differentiated endometrioid carcinomas which may be hormone-sensitive.

Both authors feel a need for understanding at a more biologic level the interaction between various hormones and receptors on tumor tissue. Additionally, they support future trials for evaluating new agents such as antiprogestins and new aromatase inhibitors.

References

1. Varga A, Henriksen E: Effect of 17-alpha-hydroxyprogesterone 17-*n*-caproate on various pelvic malignancies. Obstet Gynecol 23:51, 1964
2. Ward HWC: Progestagen therapy for ovarian carcinoma. J Obstet Gynecol Br Commonw 79:555, 1972
3. Jolles CJ, Freedman RS, Jones LA: Estrogen and progestogen therapy in advanced ovarian cancer: preliminary report. Gynecol Oncol 16:352, 1983
4. Kaufman RJ: Management of advanced ovarian carcinoma. Med Clin North Am 50:845, 1966
5. Malkasian GD, Decker DG, Jorgensen EO, Edmonson H: Medroxyprogesterone acetate for the treatment of metastatic and recurrent ovarian carcinoma. Cancer Treat Rep 61:913, 1977
6. Mangioni C, Franceschi S, LaVecchia C, D'Incalci M: High-dose medroxyprogesterone acetate (MPA) in advanced epithelial ovarian cancer resistant to first- or second-line chemotherapy. Gynecol Oncol 12:314, 1981
7. Aabo K, Pederson AG, Hald I, Dombernowsky P: High-dose medroxyprogesterone acetate (MPA) in advanced chemotherapy-resistant ovarian carcinoma: a phase II study. Cancer Treat Rep 66:407, 1982
8. Slayton RE, Pagano M, Creech RH: Progestin therapy for advanced ovarian cancer: a phase II Eastern Cooperative Oncology Group trial. Cancer Treat Rep 65:895, 1981
9. Tropé C, Johnson JE, Sigurdsson K, Simonsen E: High-dose medroxyprogesterone acetate for the treatment of advanced ovarian carcinoma. Cancer Treat Rep 66:1441, 1982
10. Hamerlynck JVTH, Maskens AP, Manioni C et al: Phase II trial of medroxyprogesterone acetate in advanced ovarian cancer: an EORTC Gynecologic Cancer Cooperative Group study. Gynecol Oncol 22:313, 1985
11. Geisler HE: The use of high-dose megestrol acetate in the treatment of ovarian adenocarcinoma. Semin Oncol 12:20, 1985
12. Ahlgren JD, Thomas D, Ellison N et al: Phase II evaluation of high dose megestrol acetate in advanced refractory ovarian cancer. Proc ASCO 4:124, 1985
13. Sikic BI, Schudder SA, Ballon SC et al: High-dose megestrol acetate therapy of ovarian carcinoma: a phase II study by the Northern California Oncology Group. Semin Oncol 13:26, 1986
14. Schwartz PE, Naftolin F: Hormone therapy. p. 613. In Berek JS and Hacker NC (eds): Practical Gynecologic Oncology. 2nd Ed. Williams & Wilkens, Baltimore, 1994
15. Ahlgren JD, Ellison NM, Gottlieb RJ et al: Hormonal palliation of chemoresis-

tant ovarian cancer: three consecutive phase II trials of the Mid-Atlantic Oncology Program. J Clin Oncol 11:1957, 1993

16. Long RTL, Evans AM: Diethylstilbestrol as a chemotherapeutic agent for ovarian carcinoma. Mo Med 60:1125, 1963
17. Fromm GL, Freedman RS, Fritsche HA et al: Sequentially administered ethinyl estradiol and medroxyprogesterone acetate in the treatment of refractory epithelial ovarian carcinoma in patients with positive estrogen receptors. Cancer 68:1885, 1991
18. Schwartz PE, Keating F, MacLusky N et al: Tamoxifen therapy for advanced ovarian cancer. Obstet Gynecol 59: 583, 1982
19. Pagel J, Rose C, Thorpe S et al: Treatment of advanced ovarian carcinoma with tamoxifen: a phase II trial, abstract. Proc 2nd Eur Conf Clin Oncol, 1983
20. Hamerlynck JVTH, Vermorken JB, van der Burg MEL et al: Tamoxifen therapy in advanced ovarian cancer: a phase II study, abstract. Proc ASCO 4:115, 1985
21. Shirey DR, Kavanagh JJ Jr, Gershenson DM et al: Tamoxifen therapy of epithelial ovarian cancer. Obstet Gynecol 66:575, 1985
22. Campbell JJ, Rome RM, Quinn MA et al: Tamoxifen for recurrent progressive epithelial ovarian tumors. Med Pediatr Oncol 13:150, 1985
23. Slevin ML, Harvey VJ, Osborne RJ et al: A phase II study of tamoxifen in ovarian cancer. Eur J Cancer Clin Oncol 22:309, 1986
24. Weiner SA, Alberts DS, Surwit EA et al: Tamoxifen therapy in recurrent epithelial ovarian carcinoma. Gynecol Oncol 27:208, 1987
25. Osborne RJ, Malik S, Slevin ML et al: Tamoxifen in refractory ovarian cancer: the use of a loading dose. Br J Cancer 57:115, 1988
26. Hatch KD, Beecham JB, Blessing JA et al: Responsiveness of patients with advanced ovarian cancer to tamoxifen: a Gynecologic Oncology Group study of second-line therapy in 105 patients. Cancer 68:269, 1991
27. Van der Velden J, Gitsch G, Wain GV et al: Tamoxifen in patients with advanced epithelial ovarian cancer. Int J Gynecol Cancer 5:301, 1995
28. Maenpaa J, Sipila P, Kangas L et al: Chemosensitizing effect on an antiestrogen, toremifene, on ovarian cancer. Gynecol Oncol 46:292, 1992
29. Kavanagh JJ, Wharaton JT, Roberts WS: Androgen therapy in the treatment of refractory epithelial ovarian cancer. Cancer Treat Rep 71:537, 1987
30. Lind MJ, Cantwell BM, Millward MJ et al: A phase II trial of goserelin (zoladex) in relapsed epithelial ovarian cancer. Br J Cancer 65:621, 1992
31. Palmer H, Rustin G, Lightman SL: Response to D-Trp-6-luteinizing hormone releasing hormone (Decapeptyl) microcapsules in advanced ovarian cancer. Br Med J 296:1229, 1988
32. Kavanagh JJ, Roberts W, Townsend P et al: Leuprolide acetate in the treatment of refractory or persistent epithelial ovarian cancer. J Clin Oncol 7:115, 1989
33. Bruckner HW, Motwani BT: Treatment of advanced refractory ovarian carcinoma with gonadotropin-releasing hormone analogue. Am J Obstet Gynecol 161:1216, 1989
34. Miller DS, Brady MF, Barrett RJ: A phase II trial of leuprolide acetate in patients with advanced epithelial ovarian cancer. Am J Clin Oncol 15:125, 1992
35. Van den Bossche HV, Moereels H, Koymans LM: Aromatase inhibitors—mechanisms for nonsteroidal inhibitors. Breast Cancer Res Treat 30:43, 1994
36. Cocconi G: First generation aromatase inhibitors—aminoglutethimide and tes-

tosterone. Breast Cancer Res Treat 30:57, 1994

37. Rendina GM, Donadio C, Giovannini M: Steroid receptors and progestinic therapy in ovarian endometrioid carcinoma. Eur J Gynaecol Oncol 3:241, 1982
38. Landoni F, Epis A, Gorga G et al: Hormonal treatment in advanced epithelial ovarian cancer. p. 262 In Panutti F (ed). Anti-oestrogens in Oncology: Past, Present and Prospects. Excerpta Medica, Amsterdam, 1985
39. Schwartz PE, Chambers JT, Kohorn EI et al: Tamoxifen in combination with cytotoxic chemotherapy in advanced epithelial ovarian cancer: a prospective randomized trial. Cancer 36:1074, 1989
40. Kavanagh JJ, Wharton JT, Roberts WS: Androgen therapy in the treatment of refractory epithelial ovarian cancer. Cancer Treat Rep 71:537, 1987
41. Stadel BV: The etiology and prevention of ovarian cancer. Am J Obstet Gynecol 123:772, 1975
42. Helzlsouer KJ, Alberg AJ, Gordon GB et al: Serum gonadotropins and steroid hormones and the development of ovarian cancer. JAMA 274:1926, 1995
43. Jager W, Wildt L, Lang N: Some observations on the effect of a GnRH analog in ovarian cancer. Eur J Obstet Gynecol Reprod Biol 32:137, 1989
44. Kavanagh JJ, Roberts W, Townsend P, Hewitt S: Leuprolide acetate in the treatment of refractory or persistent epithelial ovarian cancer. J Clin Oncol 7:115, 1989
45. Kullander S, Rausing A, Schally AV: LHRH agonist treatment in ovarian cancer. pp. 353. In Klein JGM (ed): Hormonal Manipulation of Cancer: Peptides, Growth Factors and New (Anti)-steroidal Agents. Lippincott-Raven, Philadelphia, 1987
46. Parmar H, Rustin G, Lightman SL et al: Response to d-Trp-6-luteinizing hormone releasing hormone (Decapeptyl) microcapsules in advanced ovarian cancer. Brit Med J 296:1229, 1988
47. Lopez A, Tessadrelli A, Kudelka AP et al: Combination therapy with leuprolide acetate and tamoxifen in refractory ovarian cancer. Int J Gynecol Cancer 6:15, 1996

47a. Long RTL, Evans AM: Diethylstilbestrol as a chemotherapeutic agent for ovarian carcinoma. Mo Med 60:1125, 1963

48. Freedman RS, Saul PB, Edwards CL et al: Ethinyl estradiol and medroxyprogesterone acetate in patients with epithelial ovarian carcinoma: a phase II study. Cancer Treat Rep 70:369, 1986
49. Jakobsen A, Bertlesen K, Sell A: Cyclic hormonal treatment in ovarian cancer: a phase II trial. Eur J Cancer Clin Oncol 23:915, 1987
50. Holt JA, Caputo TA, Kelly KM: Estrogen and progestin binding in cytosols of ovarian adenocarcinomas. Obstet Gynecol 53:50, 1979
51. Schwartz PE, LiVolsi VA, Hildreth N et al: Estrogen receptors in human ovarian epithelial carcinoma. Obstet Gynecol 59:229, 1982
52. Friberg LG, Kullander S, Persian JP et al: On receptors for estrogen (ER) and androgens (DHT) in human endometrial carcinoma and ovarian tumors. Acta Obstet Gynecol Scand 57:261, 1978
53. Galli MC, Giovanni CDE, Nicolletti G et al: The occurrence of multiple steroid hormone receptors in disease-free and neoplastic human ovary. Cancer 47: 1297, 1981
54. Quinn MA, Pearce P, Rome R et al: Cytoplasmic steroid receptors in ovarian tumours. Br J Obstet Gynaecol 89:754, 1982
55. Wurz H, Wassner E, Citoler P et al: Multiple cytoplasmic steroid hormone receptors in benign and malignant ovar-

ian tumors and in disease-free ovaries. Tumor Diagn Ther 4:15, 1983

56. Kuhner R, DeGraff J, Rao BR et al: Androgen receptor predominance in human ovarian carcinoma. J Steroid Biochem Mol Biol 26:393, 1987
57. Kuhner R, Rao R, Poels LG et al: Multiple parameter analyses of human ovarian cancer: morphology, immunohistochemistry, steroid hormone receptors and aromatase. Anticancer Res 8:281, 1988
58. Slotman BJ, Rao BR: The presence of a hitherto undefined high-capacity androgen binding macromolecule in human ovarian cancer tissue. J Steroid Biochem Mol Biol 33:105, 1989
59. Rao BR, Slotman BJ, Geldof AA et al: Correlation between tumor histology, steroid receptor status, and adenosine deaminase complexing protein immunoreactivity in ovarian cancer. Int J Gynecol Pathol 9:47, 1990
60. Rao BR, Slotman BJ: Endocrine factors in common epithelial cancers. Endocrine Rev 12:14, 1991
61. Berqvist A, Kullander S, Thorell J: A study of estrogen and progesterone cytosol receptor concentration in benign and malignant ovarian tumors and a review of malignant ovarian tumors treated with medroxyprogesterone acetate. Acta Obstet Gynecol Scand Suppl 101:75, 1981
62. Timothy I: Progestogen therapy for ovarian carcinoma. Br J Obstet Gynaecol 89:561, 1982
63. Lam HP: Tamoxifen is a calmodulin antagonist in the activation of camp phosphodiesterase. Biochem Biophys Res Commun 118:27, 1984
64. Brandes LJ, Bogdanovic RP: New evidence that the antiestrogen binding site may be a novel growth-promoting histamine receptor (?H^3) which mediates the antiestrogenic and antiproliferative effects of tamoxifen. Biochem Biophys Res Commun 134:601, 1986
65. Slotman BJ: Rationale for the Use of Endocrine Therapy in Ovarian Cancer. Thesis Publishers, Amsterdam, 1990
66. Schwartz PE, Eisenfeld A: Steroid receptor proteins in epithelial ovarian cancer. Proc Felix Rutledge Society, 1978
67. Friedlander ML, Quinn MA, Fortune D et al: The relationship of steroid receptor expression to nuclear DNA distribution and clinicopathological characteristics in epithelial ovarian tumors. Gynecol Oncol 32:184, 1989
68. Kammerman S, Demopoulos RI, Raphael C, Ross J: Gonadotropic hormone binding to human ovarian tumors. Hum Pathol 12:886, 1981
69. Rajaniemi H, Kauppila A, Ronnberg L et al: LH(hCG) receptor in benign and malignant tumors of human ovary. Acta Gynecol Scand Suppl 101:83, 1981
70. Emons G, Pahwa GS, Ortmann O et al: LHRH-receptors and LHRH-agonist treatment in ovarian cancer: an overview. J Steroid Biochem Mol Biol 37:1003, 1990
71. Emons G, Pahwa GS, Grack C et al: Gonadotropin releasing hormone binding sites in human epithelial ovarian carcinomata. Eur J Cancer Clin Oncol 25:215, 1989

71a. Fishman A, Kudelka AP, Tresukosal D et al: Leuprolide acetate for treating refractory or persistent ovarian granulosa cell tumor. J Reprod Med 41:393, 1996

72. Schwartz PE, MacLusky N, Sakamoto H, Eisenfeld A: Steroid receptor proteins in nonepithelial malignancies of the ovary. Gynecol Oncol 15:305, 1983
73. Malik STA, Slevin ML: Medroxyprogesterone acetate (MPA) in advanced granulosa cell tumours of the ovary—a new therapeutic approach? Br J Cancer 63:410, 1991
74. Isaacs R, Foregeson G, Allan S: Progestagens for granulosa cell tumours of the ovary. Br J Cancer 65:140, 1992

75. Schwartz PE, Smith JP: Management of ovarian stromal tumors. Am J Obstet Gynecol 125:402, 1976

76. Flemming P, Wellmann A, Maschek H et al: Monoclonal antibodies against inhibin represent key markers of adult granulosa cell tumors of the ovary even in their metastases: a report of three cases with late metastasis, being previously misinterpreted as hemangiopericytoma. Am J Surg Pathol 19:27, 1995

77. Jobling T, Mamers P, Healy DL et al: A prospective study of inhibin in granulosa cell tumors of the ovary. Gynecol Oncol 55:285, 1994

78. Kauppila A, Bangah M, Burger H, Martikainen H: GnRH agonist analog therapy in advanced/recurrent granulosa cell tumor: further evidence of a role of inhibin in monitoring response to treatment. Gynecol Endocrinol 64:271, 1992

79. Cooper A, Whitehead M: Menopause: refining benefits and risks of hormone replacement therapy. Curr Opin Obstet Gynecol 7:214, 1995

80. Eelles RA, Tan S, Wiltshaw E et al: Hormone replacement therapy and survival after surgery for ovarian cancer. Br Med J 302:259, 1991

81. Colombo N, Chari S, Maggioni A et al: Controversial issues in the management of early epithelial ovarian cancer: conservative surgery and role of adjuvant therapy. Gynecol Oncol 55:S47, 1994

82. Claus E, Schwartz PE: Familial ovarian cancer: update and clinical applications. Cancer 76:1998, 1995

83. Carmichael JA, Shelley WE, Brown LB et al: A predictive index of cure versus no cure in advanced ovarian carcinoma patients—a replacement of second-look laparotomy as a diagnostic test. Gynecol Oncol 27:269, 1987

84. MacLusky N, Voit R, Lazo JS et al: Aromatase activity in human ovarian cancer. Steroids 50:423, 1989

85. Hochberg RB, MacLusky JN, Chambers JT et al: Concentration of 16a-(^{125}I) iodoestradiol in human ovarian tumors in vivo and correlation with estrogen receptor content. Steroids 46:775, 1985

86. Nathan JF, Keefe DL, Weinstein MA et al: Estrogen mustard induces cell cycle arrest of human epithelial ovarian cancer cell lines. J Soc Gynecol Invest 1:97, 1994

CHAPTER 16

INTRAPERITONEAL CHEMOTHERAPY

Maurie Markman
Robert F. Ozols

EDITORS' INTRODUCTION

Regional cytotoxic therapy has been evaluated for approximately 20 years, primarily in ovarian cancer which remains confined to the peritoneal cavity for most of its natural history. Although many drugs have been evaluated in this regional setting, primarily cisplatin, there is still significant controversy regarding the role of this form of therapy as part of primary treatment and to some extent as part of salvage therapy. What has clearly been learned over the past two decades, however, is that intraperitoneal (IP) therapy is of little to no value in patients with bulky disease. Clearly, patients with the best outcome from regional therapy are those with microscopic disease and those with macroscopic disease with no single nodule measuring greater than 0.5 cm.

The pharmacology of this approach is based on a sound scientific rationale with a pharmacologic advantage for IP administration in the 20-fold range for cisplatin to as high as 1000-fold for paclitaxel. Although one might assume that such increments in peak levels to which the tumor is exposed should lead to improvement in outcome, one must also remember that regionally administered chemotherapy does not enter the tumor through the vascular supply but rather by passive diffusion. One obvious potential deficit of this form of therapy is the inability of large organic molecules to penetrate more than a few millimeters into a tumor nodule. In fact, a study utilizing ^{14}C-labeled carboplatin showed penetration of only 0.5 mm.

We asked our experts to comment on the role of regional chemotherapy as part of primary therapy and as salvage therapy in both drug-sensitive and drug-resistant relapse and to discuss the value of adjunctive IP therapy in patients with negative second-look laparotomy.

QUESTIONS

1. What is the role, if any, of intraperitoneal chemotherapy as first-line treatment for advanced-stage epithelial ovarian cancer?
2. What is the role, if any, of intraperitoneal chemotherapy as salvage treatment for refractory epithelial ovarian cancer?
3. What is the value, if any, of intraperitoneal chemotherapy for patients with (1) microscopically positive findings at second-look laparotomy and (2) negative findings at second-look laparotomy?
4. What is the future of intraperitoneal chemotherapy?

QUESTION 1

What is the role, if any, of intraperitoneal chemotherapy as first-line treatment for advanced-stage epithelial ovarian cancer?

MAURIE MARKMAN

The basic goal of IP therapy is to expose cancer present within the peritoneal cavity to higher concentrations of drug for longer durations than are possible with systemic delivery of the same or similar agents.[1] In theory, for chemotherapeutic agents whose cytotoxic activity is influenced by either concentration or duration of exposure, IP drug delivery can optimize the therapeutic potential of the agent against tumors, such as ovarian cancer, that remain principally confined to the peritoneal cavity for most of their natural history.[2,3] As previously stated, pharmacokinetic modeling studies have provided strong support for the concept of IP drug delivery in this clinical setting.[1,2]

Practical and theoretical concerns related to IP chemotherapy

Despite the theoretical appeal of IP therapy, there are a number of important practical and theoretical concerns involving the application of this strategy in the management of ovarian cancer.[2,4–6] These important issues are outlined in Tables 16-1 and 16-2.

Major criticisms of IP chemotherapy as expressed in the medical literature

A number of criticisms have been voiced in the medical oncology literature regarding IP chemotherapy. These include the following.

1. Lack of evidence that responses observed in the salvage (second-line) setting have an impact on survival
2. Lack of evidence that IP drug delivery can overcome demonstrated inherent drug resistance to concentrations of a particular agent when the drug is delivered systemically
3. Small size of patient populations in which this therapeutic strategy can be considered a rational therapeutic option (e.g., only very small-volume residual disease present in a patient demonstrating a major response to initial systemic chemotherapy)

TABLE 16-1
IP Therapy of Ovarian Cancer: Practical Concerns

Requirement for developing drug delivery systems that are convenient, easy to learn, safe, and cost-effective
Difficulty in distributing drug-containing fluid throughout the peritoneal cavity
Development of catheter-associated subcutaneous and peritoneal cavity infections, bowel obstruction, and/or perforation
Risk of chemotherapy-associated chemical peritonitis

TABLE 16-2
IP Therapy of Ovarian Cancer: Theoretical Concerns

Delivery of cytotoxic agent(s) to tumor by capillary flow may be reduced if treatment is delivered via the IP rather than the IV route
Preclinical experience revealing the penetration of cytotoxic drugs directly into tumor tissue is very limited. This strongly suggests that only very small-volume tumors can be successfully treated by the IP route
Even adequate fluid distribution associated with IP delivery cannot expose all tumor-bearing surfaces to the drug-containing fluid

4. Considerable technical requirements associated with catheter placement
5. Justification for accepting the unique complications of this treatment program (e.g., bowel obstruction or perforation, catheter-related infections)
6. Added expense of catheter and requirement for surgical catheter placement

Most of these criticisms are reasonable concerns and can be addressed only by solid data demonstrating the clinical effectiveness of a particular IP treatment strategy.

Initial treatment of small-volume advanced ovarian cancer employing IP cisplatin

Considerable interest in a role for IP chemotherapy in general, and IP cisplatin in particular, has been renewed with the publication of a preliminary report on a large intergroup randomized trial examining IP cisplatin as initial treatment for ovarian cancer.[7] In this important landmark study, more than 600 patients with small-volume residual stage III ovarian cancer (largest disease diameter ≤ 2 cm following tumor debulking were randomized to be treated with either IV or IP cisplatin (100 mg/m^2 in both arms of the study). Intravenous cyclophosphamide 600 mg/m^2 was also administered to all individuals participating in the trial.

At a median follow-up approximately 4 years after entry into the study, patients who received cisplatin by the IP route experienced statistically significant improvement in survival (median 49 months) compared to patients who received systemic treatment with this cytotoxic agent (median 41 months) ($P <$ 0.03). In addition, individuals given IP cisplatin were found to have significantly less neutropenia and clinically relevant hearing loss. This reduction in cisplatin-induced toxicity was presumably due to lower peak levels of the cytotoxic agent present within the systemic compartment after regional administration, compared to intravenous delivery.

Of considerable importance, this large, well-designed, well-conducted randomized trial, which involved numerous institutions (both university- and community-based), has provided strong support for the argument that high peritoneal cavity concentrations of an active cytotoxic agent can improve the clinical effectiveness of treatment of small-volume residual advanced ovarian cancer. Further, it demonstrates that IP therapy can be utilized outside a tertiary research center with an acceptable degree of complications (e.g., catheter-related infections).

At this point it must be noted that the local toxicity of IP treatment is dependent on the specific drug(s) utilized. Thus, the favorable toxicity profile observed in the IP cisplatin trial may not be observed when other cytotoxic drugs or combination IP regimens are employed.

IP cisplatin combined with IV paclitaxel in the treatment of small-volume residual ovarian cancer

The previously noted landmark IP study was started a decade ago, long before paclitaxel was demonstrated to be a major component of the initial chemotherapeutic strategy in treating women with ovarian cancer.[8] Thus, while this trial has established the superiority of IP cisplatin (compared to IV cisplatin) when employed with IV cyclophosphamide in treating small-volume residual advanced ovarian cancer, the clinical utility of IP cisplatin combined with systemically administered paclitaxel is uncertain.

The Gynecologic Oncology Group (GOG) has completed a randomized trial comparing IP cisplatin and IV paclitaxel (preceded by two courses of moderately high-dose single-agent carboplatin) to a standard regimen of IV cisplatin and paclitaxel in the treatment of small-volume residual ovarian cancer. Thus, the clinically relevant question concerning the role of IP cisplatin combined with IV paclitaxel will be at least partially addressed, although the results of this important trial will not be available for several years.

However, based on the available clinical data, it is a reasonable therapeutic strategy to employ IP cisplatin (75 to 100 mg/m² in combination with IV paclitaxel 135 mg/m² over 24 hours as initial chemotherapy for small-volume residual advanced ovarian cancer (largest residual tumor masses ≤0.5 to 1 cm maximum diameter) following tumor debulking surgery.

While available data do not prove the superiority of IP therapy in ovarian cancer, IP delivery of cisplatin as part of an initial chemotherapy strategy (along with systemic paclitaxel) is a reasonable option in women with small-volume (largest tumor mass ≤0.5 to 1 cm maximum diameter at initiation of chemotherapy) residual ovarian cancer. If this approach were employed, a dose of cisplatin of 75 to 100 mg/m² would be reasonable, based on available data.

ROBERT F. OZOLS

The first reported trial of front-line chemotherapy with IP cisplatin was reported in 1989. Investigators at the Istituto Nazionale Tumori in Milan, Italy, started a trial in 1982 exploring the feasibility and activity of five cycles of IP cisplatin combined with IV cyclophosphamide in 24 previously untreated patients with small-volume or no residual disease after initial cytoreductive surgery.[9] In this trial, 25% of patients developed local complications requiring catheter removal before completion of the planned therapy. There were 21 patients evaluable for response, and 71% achieved a pathologic complete remission with median disease-free survival of 29+ months. Two patients who achieved pathologic complete remission relapsed at 20 and 36 months. It was of note that the overall failure rate was 38% and that all failures occurred in the peritoneal cavity. The authors pointed out that since the most favorable cases were selected for IP treatment, the high recurrence rate in the peritoneal cavity raised serious questions regarding the actual contribution of IP cisplatin in the treatment of patients with small-volume residual disease.

In another phase II trial of IP chemotherapy in patients with advanced disease, French investigators did not utilize IP delivery systems such as Tenckhoff catheters or Port-a-Cath systems but instead used a simple needle for lumbar puncture to administer IP chemotherapy in previously untreated patients with stage III ovarian cancer.[10] In their study the IP route was also combined with IV chemotherapy. They also reported a high response rate (76%) with a 4-year actuarial survival of 81% and a disease-free survival of 66%.

These two phase II trials, however, were very limited because of the number of patients treated and because of the potential bias in patients selection. There have been, however, several randomized trials exploring the role of IP chemotherapy versus IV chemotherapy in patients with advanced ovarian cancer. Investigators from the University of California at San Diego performed a phase III study on 62 women with advanced-stage ovarian cancer.[11] In this study, patients were eligible if they had either optimal or suboptimal disease after initial surgery, and patients with stage IV disease were also included. A total of 62 patients were randomized with 29 patients receiving six cycles of IP cisplatin 200 mg/m² plus IP etoposide 350 mg/m² with IV thiosulfate protection given every 4 weeks. Thirty-three patients received six cycles of IV cisplatin 100 mg/m² plus IV cyclophosphamide

600 mg/m^2 administered every 3 weeks. The complete response rate in evaluable patients was 48% in the IP group and 52% in the IV group. Despite the fact that not all women in clinical complete remission had a second-look laparotomy, the overall surgical complete remission rate for all patients in the study was 31% in the IP group and 33% in the IV group. There were no differences in response rates between treatment arms as a function of residual disease, and with a median follow-up of 46 months (range 21 to 70 months) there was no difference in response duration or survival. Both the IP and IV routes were well tolerated, with comparable hematologic and nonhematologic toxicities. The number of patients in this trial clearly was not sufficient to detect clinically important differences in survival.

A somewhat larger randomized trial was reported in abstract form by Conte et al[12] from the clinical trial groups in Italy. Eighty-eight patients with stage II to IV epithelial ovarian cancer with residual disease less than 2 cm after initial surgery were randomized to receive IP cisplatin 50 mg/m^2 in 2 L of normal saline together with epidoxorubicin 45 mg/m^2 IV and cyclophosphamide 600 mg/m^2 IV. Chemotherapy was administered every 28 days. The control arm consisted of all three drugs administered IV at the same doses. There was no severe toxicity related to IP administration, although mild to moderate abdominal pain during infusion was reported in 10% of patients. A surgically confirmed complete remission was observed in 36% of patients receiving IP chemotherapy and in 32% of patients receiving IV chemotherapy. With a median follow-up of over 1 year, 25 patients experienced disease progression (10 patients with IP chemotherapy and 15 with IV chemotherapy). There are no statistically significant differences in median survival or progression-free survival between patients receiving the IP versus IV treatment.

The Italian study likewise is limited by the small number of patients randomized, which precludes identification of a potentially clinically significant improvement in survival. A large phase III trial has been reported in abstract form in which adequate numbers of patients were entered.[7] An intergroup trial (INT 0051) was performed by the Southwestern Oncology Group-Gynecologic Oncology Group-Eastern Cooperative Gynecologic Group (SWOG-GOG-ECOG) in the United States starting in June 1986. Patients eligible for this study had stage III ovarian cancer. After bilateral oophorectomy, total abdominal hysterectomy, omentectomy, and resection of disease, there were no tumor masses greater than 2 cm in the peritoneal cavity. Patients were randomized to receive IP cisplatin 100 mg/m^2 together with IV cyclophosphamide 600 mg/m^2 or IV cisplatin 100 mg/m^2 together with the same dose of IV cyclophosphamide. All chemotherapy was administered in 3-week intervals. From 1986 to 1992, 654 patients were randomized, and 115 patients were ultimately deemed ineligible following surgery or pathology review. Of the 539 eligible patients, 385 had less than 0.5-cm disease (276 in the IV arm and 263 in the IP arm). Patient characteristics were evenly distributed, and median follow-up for living patients was 47 months in the IP arm and 44 months in the IV arm. The surgically confirmed complete remission rate was 40% in the IP arm versus 31% in the IV arm ($P = 0.10$). The median survival for patients in the IP arm was estimated to be 49 months with a 95% confidence interval of 43 to 55 months compared to 41 months with a 95% confidence interval of 34 to 47 months for patients receiving IV chemotherapy. The IP versus IV death hazard ratio was estimated to be 0.76 (95% confidence interval 0.59 to 0.97). Both clinical hearing loss and neutropenia were significantly more frequent and more severe in patients who received both drugs via the IV route. It was concluded that the IP route was associated with superior patient survival and less toxicity in patients with optimal stage III ovarian cancer.

Based on this study, the question as been raised whether IP chemotherapy should now be standard therapy for patients with previously untreated optimal stage III disease. The major limitation of this study relates to the control arm. When this trial was started in 1986, IV cisplatin/cyclophosphamide as used by the investigators was considered standard therapy. However, since that time it has been established in prospective randomized trials that standard therapy for patients with ovarian cancer should be an IV combination of cisplatin and paclitaxel.[8] In a large prospective randomized trial with patients with suboptimal stage III and IV disease, IV cisplatin/paclitaxel led to a median survival of 38 months, compared to 24 months for patients who received IV cisplatin/cyclophosphamide. A major question unanswered at this point is whether the survival advantage produced by IV paclitaxel can be further enhanced if platinum is administered IP. The GOG has already completed a confirmatory trial for this intergroup study. Patients with optimal stage III disease were randomized on GOG protocol 114 to receive IV paclitaxel 135 mg/m^2 in a 24-hour infusion together with IV cisplatin 75 mg/m^2 or to receive a combination consisting of two cycles of carboplatin (dosed to an AUC of 9) followed by six cycles of IV paclitaxel 135 mg/m^2 over 24 hours together with IP cisplatin 100 mg/m^2. If this latter arm produces superior results, it likely will be because of the IP route of administration since it is unlikely that the two cycles of carboplatin have a significant impact, based upon recent studies that have failed to demonstrate that high-dose therapy with platinum compounds in this range is superior.[13] *Until the results of the GOG study mature, standard therapy for patients with optimal stage III disease should consist of IV paclitaxel together with IV administration of a platinum compound, either cisplatin or carboplatin.*

QUESTION 2

What is the role, if any, of intraperitoneal chemotherapy as salvage treatment for refractory epithelial ovarian cancer?

MAURIE MARKMAN

IP cisplatin in the treatment of ovarian cancer

Because of its central role in the management of ovarian cancer, it was natural that most IP chemotherapy in patients with ovarian cancer focused on cisplatin.[2,14,15] Considerable phase II, and now phase III, clinical data are available that directly address the concerns raised about IP therapy with cisplatin in the treatment of ovarian cancer.

In a series reported from Memorial Sloan-Kettering Cancer Center (MSKCC) using combination cisplatin-based therapy as salvage treatment for advanced ovarian cancer, 32% (17 of 50) of individuals whose largest residual tumor mass measured 1 cm or less in maximum diameter at the initiation of IP therapy achieved a surgically documented complete response, compared to only 5% (2 of 39) of patients with at least one tumor mass greater than 1 cm in maximum diameter (Table 16-3).[15] This experience documented the importance of volume of disease in determining an individual patient's opportunity to achieve an objective response to this therapeutic strategy.

However, a second important feature in the MSKCC series was found to strongly predict response to IP cisplatin as salvage therapy. Independent of the size of the largest residual tumor mass at initiation of IP treatment, women who had previously responded to IV cisplatin achieved a 33% (17 of 52) surgically documented complete response rate, compared to only a 3% (1 of 37) complete response rate in individuals whose initial cisplatin-based IV regimen had not resulted in at least partial response.

Of considerable importance regarding the ability of IP cisplatin to overcome inherent drug resistance was the observation that even patients with very small-volume disease (largest tumor mass $\leq$1 cm maximum diameter) at the beginning of second-line IP cisplatin therapy were unable to achieve a significant response rate if they had failed to respond to systemic treatment (surgical complete response rate 7% [1 of 14]). However, in sharp contrast, for those individuals whose largest tumor mass was 1 cm or less and who had also previously responded to systemically delivered cisplatin, the surgically documented complete response rate was 42% (15 of 36) ($P < 0.025$).

Thus, the MSKCC experience,[15] confirmed by several trials conducted by the GOG,[16,17]

TABLE 16-3
MSKCC Experience with IP Cisplatin-Based Salvage Chemotherapy[a]

LARGEST RESIDUAL TUMOR MASS	PRIOR RESPONSE TO SYSTEMIC CISPLATIN	
	YES	NO
Less than 0.5 cm[b]	43% (13/30)	9% (1/11)
Less than 1 cm[c]	42% (15/36)	7% (1/14)

[a] *Surgically defined complete response rate in small-volume residual advanced ovarian cancer.*
[b] *<0.05.*
[c] *<0.025.*

demonstrated that the 10- to 20-fold higher concentrations of cisplatin present in the peritoneal cavity after IP delivery cannot overcome the degree of drug resistance present in tumors shown to be completely resistant (i.e., when treatment fails to achieve at least a partial response) to systemically administered drug. However, in patients with small-volume, partially responsive cancers, a high surgically documented objective response rate can be achieved.

These responses may be associated with prolonged survival times,[18,19] but it remains unknown at present whether such survivals are the direct result of treatment or just represent the natural history of disease in a select group of patients with small-volume residual ovarian cancer. A *definitive answer to the question of a role for IP cisplatin in second-line (salvage) treatment of ovarian cancer must await a randomized clinical trial comparing this strategy to alternative approaches (e.g., continued systemic carboplatin or paclitaxel).*

IP paclitaxel as therapy for ovarian cancer

A number of antineoplastic agents in addition to cisplatin (including carboplatin, doxorubicin, mitoxantrone, etoposide, 5-fluorouracil, a-interferon, g-interferon, and interleukin-2) have been examined for a possible role in the treatment of ovarian cancer via the IP route.[2,14] However, paclitaxel is perhaps the most interesting of all known drugs to be considered for this method of drug delivery. Several characteristics points can be made in support of this statement, including (1) its demonstrated activity in ovarian cancer[8,20], (2) its large size and hepatic metabolism (increasing cavity exposure compared to that of the systemic compartment),[21,22] and (3) its general lack of vesicant properties.[20,23]

Phase I trials conducted under the auspices of the GOG have demonstrated a profound pharmacokinetic advantage (>1000-fold) for peritoneal cavity exposure to paclitaxel (compared to the systemic compartment) after IP delivery.[24,25] Of equal importance, concentrations of paclitaxel known to produce major biological effects have been found to remain in the peritoneal cavity for at least 5 to 7 days after regional drug delivery, suggesting that a weekly IP paclitaxel dosing schedule may permit continuous exposure of thin layers of tumor on the surface of the peritoneal cavity to the drug for the duration of a protracted treatment program.

This strategy is of considerable interest (at least in theory) and might truly be the best method for utilizing paclitaxel, a cycle-specific agent, against cancer cells with their slow doubling times.[20] The GOG has examined the clinical utility of a weekly IP paclitaxel regimen employed as salvage treatment for women with small-volume persistent or recurrent ovarian cancer following initial systemic therapy. It is anticipated that the results of this interesting phase II trial will be available within the next year.

If a favorable surgically documented objective response rate is demonstrated in this trial, it will be appropriate to consider the use of IP paclitaxel as a component of an initial chemotherapy regimen in the management of small-volume residual ovarian cancer. Ultimately, a randomized trial employing IP paclitaxel will be required to define a possible role for this strategy in the standard clinical management of ovarian cancer.

In the salvage (second-line) setting, responses to IP administered cisplatin are observed almost exclusively in individuals with small-volume residual disease (largest tumor mass ≤0.5 to 1 cm maximum diameter) who have previously responded to initial systemic treatment. It is reasonable to consider this second-line treatment strategy for carefully selected patients outside a clinical trial, provided they are informed that the ultimate impact of this approach on long-term disease-free survival has not been established.

If IP cisplatin were employed in this clinical setting, a dose of 75 to 100 mg/m^2 would be reasonable. There are no convincing data available demonstrating that higher doses of either cisplatin or a cisplatin-based combination IP regimen would be superior to a more standard dose single-agent cisplatin program.

It is important to note that patients with cancers resistant to initial systemic chemotherapy or with larger tumor bulk should *not* be treated by the IP route unless they are participating in a clinical trial specifically examining the activity of an antineoplastic agent in chemoresistant disease. The chances of major therapeutic benefit in this clinical setting are (at best) very limited.

ROBERT F. OZOLS

Until recently, phase II trials in ovarian cancer involved a very heterogeneous patient population, however, it has become increasingly apparent that there are distinct prognostic groups of patients who have markedly different outcomes when treated in phase II trials. The most unfavorable group of patients consists of those who did not respond to initial therapy with platinum-based regimens and were left with bulky disease.[26] On the other hand, the most favorable group of patients are those who had a complete remission with IV chemotherapy followed by a long disease-free interval and had a recurrence with small-volume disease. Furthermore, it has also become apparent that even patients considered to have optimal IP disease based on the absence of any tumor nodule greater than 1 cm can be further divided into distinct prognostic groups.[27] Those with diffuse carcinomatosis had a worse prognosis even though no tumor nodule was large, compared to patients in whom there were only a few small tumor nodules scattered throughout the peritoneal cavity. Markman[15] demonstrated that responses to second-line cisplatin-based IP therapy were dependent upon prior response to IV cisplatin and upon volume of disease present at the time IP chemotherapy was administered. In patients who had previously responded to IV cisplatin, the overall response and complete response rates for second-line IP therapy were 56% and 33%, respectively. Patients who never responded to IV cisplatin had only an 11% overall response rate and a 3% complete response rate with IP cisplatin. In the subset of patients who responded to systemic cisplatin and whose largest tumor mass measured less than 1 cm at the time IP therapy with platinum was started, a complete remission rate of 42% was noted, compared to the 7% complete remission rate in patients with the same volume of disease but who had previously failed to respond to systemic cisplatin. These differences in response rates also appeared to translate into differences in survival for patients with microscopic versus macroscopic residual disease at the time IP chemotherapy was administered. Markman et al[19] reported that the median duration of a surgically confirmed complete remission for 10 patients with microscopic residual disease was 32 months, compared with 15 months for 9 patients with macroscopic residual disease. The median overall survival for patients with microscopic disease who responded to IP therapy has not been reached and will exceed 4 years, compared to a 25-month median survival for patients who did not respond to IP therapy. Median survival for patients with small-volume macroscopic disease (largest tumor mass less than 0.5 cm) who responded to IP therapy was 40 months, compared with 19 months for nonresponders.

The importance of volume of disease at time of IP treatment was confirmed in a cooperative group trial. A phase II trial of IP cisplatin plus recombinant human α-interferon was conducted by the GOG with patients with small-volume persistent or recurrent ovarian cancer.[27] In 18 evaluable patients, only one partial response was observed. However, patients could be divided retrospectively into two groups, those with favorable disease (documented response to prior IV cisplatin without diffuse carcinomatosis prior to initiation of IP therapy) and those with unfavorable disease (no prior response to IV cisplatin and/or laparotomy findings of diffuse carcinomatosis prior to IP treatment). In the 15 unfavorable group, only one partial response was observed (7% response rate).

The conclusion from these studies is that IP cisplatin-based chemotherapy is associated with prolonged survival only in patients who had both a prior response to IV cisplatin and small-volume disease at the time IP chemotherapy was administered. The longest survival was reported for those who had microscopic disease at the time IP therapy was administered. It should be pointed out, however, that this is the same group of patients who had extremely favorable responses to retreatment with IV platinum. Relapsed patients who have had a disease-free interval of less than 6 months and have bulky disease are very unlikely to respond to retreatment with platinum.[26] In contrast, patients who have had a long disease-free interval and have small-volume disease are good candidates for retreatment with IV platinum. Consequently there is no debate as to the importance of a patient's prior response to IV platinum with regard to their subsequent ability to respond to second-line treatment. *Without a prospective randomized trial, however, it is impossible to determine whether the route of administration (IP vs IV) is important in this group of patients with favorable response criteria for salvage treatment.*

QUESTION 3

What is the value, if any, of intraperitoneal chemotherapy for patients with (1) microscopically positive findings at second-look laparotomy and (2) negative findings at second-look laparotomy?

MAURIE MARKMAN

Microscopically positive patients can be considered to be in the same category as individuals with very small-volume macroscopic disease (as discussed in Question 2 above) and can be treated in a similar manner.

Patients with negative findings at second-look surgery have a 50% or greater chance of being cured of their malignancy. In concept, IP therapy is certainly a reasonable therapeutic strategy in this specific clinical setting. However, in the absence of data from randomized trials demonstrating the impact of such an approach on survival, IP treatment should not (at this point in time) be considered a standard therapeutic option.

ROBERT F. OZOLS

As previously noted, the longest survival for patients treated with IP therapy has been reported for a group of patients who had only microscopic disease at the time of IP chemotherapy and had had a prior response to IV cisplatin. It must be emphasized, however, that the natural history of patients who have had a prior response to systemic chemotherapy and have only small-volume disease at the time of recurrence is extremely favorable. Consequently, the role of IP chemotherapy in this group of patients remains to be firmly established.

IP cisplatin has also been evaluated in patients who achieve a complete remission. A trial was reported from Israel in which three courses of IP cisplatin were administered together with systemic thiosulfate in 31 stage II to IV ovarian cancer patients who were in clinical complete remission after receiving IV cisplatin-based chemotherapy.[28] The 5-year survival rate was 60% with a median progression-free interval of 35 months. Survival and duration of progression-free interval were significantly superior in patients who achieved a surgically confirmed complete response. A large prospective randomized trial is currently being conducted by the European Organization for Research on Treatment of

Cancer (EORTC) in which patients who achieve a surgically confirmed complete remission are randomized to receive six cycles of IP cisplatin 100 mg/m^2 or observation. No data are currently available from this trial, however, if it demonstrates that patients who have received IP cisplatin have longer survivals, it will not establish unequivocally whether IP therapy was responsible for their improvement. A more scientifically rigorous approach would have been to randomize patients who achieve a surgically confirmed complete remission to either six cycles of IP platinum or six cycles of IV platinum. In this trial continuation of IV platinum in patients who had received prior IV cisplatin-based combination chemotherapy was not considered, based upon toxicity considerations and on the results of previous randomized studies which have failed to demonstrate that more than six cycles of platinum-based chemotherapy is beneficial.[29,30] However, in the randomized trials of 5 versus 10 cycles or 6 versus 12 cycles of IV chemotherapy, the number of patients entered in the trials was not sufficient to detect potentially significant improvements in survival for those who received extended therapy. Despite these limitations, the EORTC study will be important in determining whether IP chemotherapy is useful in preventing or delaying relapses in patients who achieve a surgically confirmed complete remission following IV platinum-based chemotherapy. Until completion of this study, there is no established role for IP therapy as a consolidation treatment for patients who achieve a surgically confirmed complete remission. It should be pointed out that numerous strategies in addition to IP chemotherapy are being studied in clinical trials to determine if they have an impact on disease-free or overall survival in patients who achieve a complete response to initial treatment. Among strategies being studied are IP immunotherapy, IP ^{32}P and prolonged administration of systemic chemotherapy, and whole-abdomen radiation. Furthermore, the same group of patients is being considered for clinical trials of high-dose chemotherapy with peripheral stem cell transplantation. *However, at this time, there is no published information based on a randomized trial supporting a role for any form of consolidation and/or maintenance therapy in patients in a clinical complete remission.*

QUESTION 4

What is the future of intraperitoneal chemotherapy?

MAURIE MARKMAN

On the basis of our current knowledge regarding both the limitations and potential benefits associated with IP delivery of antineoplastic agents in the treatment of ovarian cancer, a number of clinical settings can be proposed in which I believe it is reasonable to consider further exploration of a potential role for this unique therapeutic strategy. These are outlined in Table 16-4, along with possible drug regimens to be considered for examination in these clinical settings.

TABLE 16-4

IP Therapy of Ovarian Cancer: Future Directions for Clinical Research Efforts

1. Initial treatment of small-volume residual disease
   a. IP cisplatin plus IV paclitaxel
   b. IP cisplatin plus IP paclitaxel
   c. IP cisplatin plus IP paclitaxel plus IV paclitaxel
2. Treatment of high-risk, early-stage ovarian cancer (e.g., stage II)
3. Consolidation after achieving a negative second-look laparotomy or laparoscopy when there is a high-risk of recurrence (e.g., stage IIIC, grade 3, tumor)
4. Second-line therapy for individuals with microscopic (or very small-volume macroscopic) disease at second-look laparotomy or laparoscopy with documented major response to initial systemic chemotherapy

ROBERT F. OZOLS

It was nearly two decades ago that the modern era of IP chemotherapy was initiated with large-volume dialysis in patients with ovarian cancer. Since that time, a series of clinical studies have been performed and even large phase III randomized trials have been completed, yet there remains controversy regarding the role of IP therapy in the overall management of ovarian cancer. The large intergroup study shows that the IP route produces an improvement of approximately 20% in median survival for patients with optimal stage III disease compared to IV administration.[7] However, questions remain regarding whether IP platinum adds to the benefit achieved with IV paclitaxel. Even if it is confirmed that IP administration of platinum leads to a 20% improvement in median survival for patients with optimal stage III disease, this will be considered only a relatively modest advance in the overall management of this disease. Whether this improvement in median survival translates into any long-term improvement in overall survival remains to be determined. What is clear, however, is that IP chemotherapy does not provide a curative option for most patients with advanced ovarian cancer. However, the IP route will remain an important avenue in the investigation of new agents, such as paclitaxel, as well as biologic treatments with new targets such as angiogenesis and determinants of metastases. Most importantly, however, ovarian cancer must be considered a systemic disease, and new systemic treatments are needed. Paclitaxel appears to have had a significant impact, but its overall impact upon cure remains to be established. New agents and new strategies will be required in order to make a major impact upon this insidious disease. *IP therapy was a good idea, but after 20 years it can only be considered, at best, to have led to a modest therapeutic benefits for a small number of patients with this disease.* The nature of future studies on IP chemotherapy will be dictated by the results of ongoing clinical trials, but one cannot escape the conclusion that a major improvement in survival will require more than a different route of administration of currently available agents.

EDITORS' COMMENTARY

It is interesting that our two experts, one a staunch critic of IP therapy and the other a strong supporter of good clinical trials utilizing this form of therapy, differ very little in their conclusions regarding regional therapy. Dr. Ozols feels that the value of IP chemotherapy for patients with low-volume disease following primary cytoreductive surgery remains unproven and thinks these patients should still be treated with IV administration of a platinum compound and paclitaxel. Dr. Markman believes that IP therapy in the same group of patients is a "reasonable option" but does not yet consider it standard therapy. We feel that primary IP therapy has potential benefit, however, the technique of IP drug administration depends on experience and should not be routinely employed in such patients. Should the mature data from the large phase III intergroup study continue to show a survival advantage for patients treated with regional platinum over those treated with IV platinum, regional therapy may then become standard for such patients. A recently completed GOG study (GOG protocol 114) will hopefully further address the value of IP therapy. We anxiously await the maturity of the intergroup study and the initial results from this GOG study.

Both authors agree that in the salvage setting IP therapy should not be employed in patients with drug-resistant tumors or in those with persistent or recurrent tumor nodules in excess of 0.5 to 1.0 cm. Dr. Ozols feels that because of the difficulty of IP drug administration, a prospective randomized trial utilizing IP versus IV salvage chemotherapy is necessary before this practice can be recommended. Dr. Markman believes that IP salvage therapy is of value in highly selected patients, with drug-sensitive, low-volume tumors, and feels this is a reasonable approach as long as patients are fully informed that there are no data supporting a survival advantage. We feel that a very small subset of patients with ovarian cancer are candidates for such salvage therapy since most patients are found to have recurrent disease based on symptoms or imaging studies and have a tumor volume that does not lend itself to regional therapy. This, of course, brings up another issue discussed in Ch. 14, as to whether or not serial elevation of CA 125 levels should be a criterion for institution of salvage therapy. Certainly, we feel that if IP therapy were utilized in this patient population, either a laparoscopy or a laparotomy would be needed to verify that the patient has a low-volume recurrence.

Both authors agree that there is no established role for IP chemotherapy as an adjuvant following negative second-look laparotomy. We concur with that approach. A large EORTC trial is addressing this question, but it will be several years before data are available.

Both authors feel that future research in the area of IP therapy is appropriate. Dr. Ozols is less enthusiastic about the potential of IP therapy than is Dr. Markman. Although we agree with the potential clinical trials outlined by Dr. Markman in Table 16-4, there are many competing clinical trials because of the large number of new agents with defined activity in this disease. These agents need to be further evaluated in both primary and salvage therapy. Thus, it is our feeling that unless the results of ongoing or completed and maturing studies show a clear survival benefit, this form of chemotherapy, although a good idea, may not become a standard approach.

References

1. Dedrick RL, Myers CE, Bungay PM, DeVita VT Jr: Pharmacokinetic rationale for peritoneal drug administration in the treatment of ovarian cancer. Cancer Treat Rep 62:1, 1978
2. Markman M: Regional Antineoplastic Drug Delivery in the Management of Malignant Disease. Johns Hopkins University Press, Baltimore, 1991
3. Bergman F: Carcinoma of the ovary: a clinicopathological study of 86 autopsied cases with special reference to mode of spread. Acta Obstet Gynecol Scand 45:211, 1966
4. Pfeifle CE, Howell SB, Markman M, Lucas WE: Totally implantable system for peritoneal access. J Clin Oncol 2:1277, 1984
5. Kaplan RA, Markman M, Lucas WE et al: Infectious peritonitis in patients receiving intraperitoneal chemotherapy. Am J Med 78:49, 1985
6. Davidson SA, Rubin SC, Markman M et al: Intraperitoneal chemotherapy: analysis of complications with an implantable subcutaneous port and catheter system. Gynecol Oncol 41:101, 1991
7. Alberts DS, Liu PY, Hannigan EV et al: Intraperitoneal cisplatin plus intravenous cyclophosphamide versus intravenous cisplatin plus intravenous cyclophosphamide for stage III ovarian cancer. N Engl J Med 335:1950, 1996
8. McGuire WP, Hoskins WJ, Brady MF et al: A phase III randomized study of cyclophosphamide and cisplatin versus paclitaxel and cisplatin in patients with suboptimal stage III and stage IV epithelial ovarian cancer: a Gynecologic Oncology Group study. N Engl J Med 334:1, 1996
9. Zambetti M, Gianni L, Escobedo A et al: First-line chemotherapy with intraperitoneal cisplatin and intravenous cyclophosphamide in ovarian carcinoma. Am J Clin Oncol (CCT) 12(2):118, 1989
10. Zylberberg B, Ravina JH, Baroux-Salat J et al: Chemotherapy by the intravenous and intraperitoneal routes combined in ovarian cancer. Gynecol Oncol 36:271, 1990

11. Kirmani S, Braly PS, McClay EF et al: A comparison of intravenous versus intraperitoneal chemotherapy for the initial treatment of ovarian cancer. Gynecol Oncol 54:338, 1994
12. Conte PF, Bruzzone M, Gadducci A et al: Intraperitoneal vs systemic chemotherapy for advanced ovarian cancer (AOC) patients with minimal residual disease (RD) after initial surgery: preliminary results of a randomized study, abstract 32 Proc Int Gynecol Cancer Soc, 1995
13. Jokobsen A, Bertelsen K, Andersen JE et al: Dose-effect study of carboplatin in ovarian cancer: a Danish ovarian cancer group study. Proc Int Gynecol Cancer Soc, 1995
14. Markman M: Intraperitoneal therapy for treatment of malignant disease principally confined to the peritoneal cavity. Crit Rev Oncol Hematol 14:15, 1993
15. Markman M, Reichman B, Hakes T et al: Responses to second-line cisplatin-based intraperitoneal therapy in ovarian cancer: influence of a prior response to intravenous cisplatin. J Clin Oncol 9:1801, 1991
16. Markman M, Berek JS, Blessing JA et al: Characteristics of patients with small-volume residual ovarian cancer unresponsive to cisplatin-based IP chemotherapy: lessons learned from a Gynecologic Oncology Group phase II trial of IP cisplatin and recombinant alpha-interferon. Gynecol Oncol 45:3, 1992
17. Markman M, Blessing JA, Major F, Manetta A: Salvage intraperitoneal therapy of ovarian cancer employing cisplatin and etoposide: a Gynecologic Oncology Group study. Gynecol Oncol 50:191, 1993
18. Howell SB, Zimm S, Markman M et al: Long term survival of advanced refractory ovarian carcinoma patients with small-volume disease treated with intraperitoneal chemotherapy. J Clin Oncol 5:1607, 1987
19. Markman M, Reichman B, Hakes T et al: Impact on survival of surgically defined favorable responses to salvage intraperitoneal chemotherapy in small volume residual ovarian cancer. J Clin Oncol 10:1479, 1992
20. Rowinsky EK, Donehower RC: Paclitaxel. N Engl J Med 332:1004, 1995
21. Monsarrat B, Mariel E, Crois S et al: Taxol metabolism: isolation and identification of three major metabolites in rat bile. Drug Med Disp 18:895, 1990
22. Monsarrat B, Wright M, Dubois J et al: Taxol metabolism in rat and human bile. p. 123. In Seventh NCI-EORTC Symposium on New Drug Development, Amsterdam, 1992
23. Rowinsky EK, Cazenave LA, Donehower RC: Taxol: a novel investigational antimicrotubule agent. J Natl Cancer Inst 82:1247, 1990
24. Markman M, Rowinsky E, Hakes T et al: Phase 1 trial of intraperitoneal Taxol: a Gynecologic Oncology Group study. J Clin Oncol 10:1485, 1992
25. Francis P, Rowinsky E, Schneider J et al: Phase 1 feasibility and pharmacologic study of weekly intraperitoneal paclitaxel: a Gynecologic Oncology Group pilot study. J Clin Oncol 13:2961, 1995
26. Markman M, Rothman R, Hakes T et al: Second-line platinum therapy in patients with ovarian cancer previously treated with cisplatin. J Clin Oncol 9(3):389, 1991
27. Markman M, Berek JS, Blessing JA et al: Characteristics of patients with small-volume residual ovarian cancer unresponsive to cisplatin-based ip chemotherapy: lessons learned from a Gynecologic Oncology Group phase II trial of IP cisplatin and recombinant a-interferon. Gynecol Oncol 45:3, 1992
28. Menczer J, Ben-Baruch G, Rizel S, Brenner H: Intraperitoneal cisplatin chemotherapy in ovarian carcinoma

patients who are clinically in complete remission. Gynecol Oncol 46:222, 1992

29. Hakes TB, Chalas E, Hoskins WJ et al: Randomized prospective trial of 5 versus 10 cycles of cyclophosphamide, doxorubicin, and cisplatin in advanced ovarian carcinoma. Gynecol Oncol 45:284, 1992
30. Bertelsen K, Jakobsen I, Stroyer K et al: A prospective randomized comparison of 6 and 12 cycles of cyclophosphamide, Adriamycin, and cisplatin in advanced epithelial ovarian cancer: a Danish Ovarian Study Group trial (DACOVA). Gynecol Oncol 49:30, 1993

CHAPTER 17

CLINICAL APPLICATIONS OF BASIC SCIENCE INVESTIGATIONS

Holly H. Gallion
Elise C. Kohn
Gordon B. Mills
Robert C. Bast, Jr.

EDITORS' INTRODUCTION

It has become obvious over the past two decades of treating ovarian cancer that currently used interventions in established disease are likely to cure only a small minority of patients. Clearly a better understanding of the biology of this tumor is needed, with the anticipation that some of these biologic discoveries may lead to better prevention and control, earlier diagnosis, and improved therapy. Major treatises have been published on aspects of the basic biology of ovarian cancer beyond the scope of this book. We have asked four investigators, who study the biology of the disease in the laboratory and see patients with ovarian cancer to address several issues at the interface between the bench and the bedside. To focus this discussion we have asked our contributors to limit their comments to specific areas.

Tumor-associated antigens have been known for over three decades, and the CA 125 marker has been well studied in ovarian cancer over many years. Nevertheless the utility of this marker in screening asymptomatic individuals remains controversial. Even the proper use of this marker in following the course of established disease is unclear, and how one should counsel patients with a rising marker level after apparently successful treatment for their disease is problematic and stress-provoking for both patient and practitioner. We have asked our contributors to discuss these issues and offer their insights into the future of this or other markers as they relate to screening, prognosis, and patient treatment.

As new markers of biologic activity are discovered, it becomes important to assess whether any of them are of sufficient prognostic importance to require stratification in future randomized clinical trials. In breast cancer, for example, steroid receptor status is so important that most clinical studies require its consideration in trial design. Thus, we have asked our experts to consider whether any of the emerging measures of benignancy versus malignancy warrant consideration in the design of future studies.

Only recently have genes been defined that significantly increase a woman's chance of developing either breast or ovarian cancer. Many clinical issues surround this discovery, including screening, alteration of the genome (gene therapy), family planning, prophylactic surgery, and the effect of these genetic mutations on tumor biology. Our contributors will discuss this topic and its many implications, including psychological issues, for the carrier and the real possibility of employment and insurance discrimination.

Frequently patients have samples of tumor submitted for chemoresistance assays. We have asked our contributors to comment on the advisability of submitting such samples and, further, how such information should be used to guide either primary or second-line therapy. Since many patients have this assay performed at their own request, it is prudent that we understand the real meaning of such assays and how they should be used. Further, new compounds are being developed that in vitro appear to alter intrinsic or acquired resistance to cytotoxic drugs frequently used to treat ovarian cancer, including alkylating agents, anthracyclines, and taxanes. We have asked the authors to comment on the potential of these agents for reversing drug resistance and improving therapy.

Gene therapy is often mentioned now in the lay press, although the introduction of genes into tumor cells to alter cellular function is in its infancy. The technology for gene transfer is now available, but whether it will have valid clinical application is mostly a matter of speculation at this point. We have asked the authors to speculate too.

With the explosion of techniques in molecular biology, the nearly daily elucidation of new mechanisms of drug resistance, the anticipated completion of the Human Genome Project, and the rapid development of new drug classes, it is certain that this chapter will become obsolete in a short period of time. Nevertheless, an understanding of where we are now is important to an appreciation of the major strides that will soon be upon us.

QUESTIONS

1. Are there currently any laboratory or molecular markers that should be used routinely in the clinical management of epithelial ovarian cancer? In addition, are there any markers that seem promising for use in the near future?
2. Are there any laboratory or molecular markers that should currently be used as prognostic or stratification factors in the design of randomized clinical trials?
3. On which women should BRCAl testing be performed?
4. Is there any evidence to support the use of resistance modulators in the treatment of ovarian cancer? What about the use of chemoresistance assays?
5. What are the most attractive agents for use in gene therapy?
6. Please discuss future directions in this area.

QUESTION 1

Are there currently any laboratory or molecular markers that should be used routinely in the clinical management of epithelial ovarian cancer? In addition, are there any markers that seem promising for use in the near future?

HOLLY H. GALLION

An ideal tumor marker for ovarian cancer would allow us to accurately follow disease status in patients with cancer and would also provide a screening mechanism for detecting small, potentially curable, early-stage tumors. Such a marker would be secreted by all histologic types of epithelial ovarian cancers, would not be detected in the presence of benign disease or other malignancies, and would accurately reflect the status of disease at all times, even in the presence of minimal disease. Although a number of laboratory markers have been investigated in epithelial ovarian cancer, none of them are ideal. CA 125 is the only currently available tumor marker with proven clinical utility in the treatment of patients with ovarian cancer. Serum levels of this tumor-associated antigen, which is elevated in approximately 80% of patients with ovarian carcinoma, clearly correlate with disease status and are invaluable in monitoring response to chemotherapy, in predicting the presence of residual disease at completion of chemotherapy, and in the early detection of recurrent disease.[1,2] Unfortunately, as serum antigen levels are directly related to tumor volume, CA 125 cannot detect small-volume residual disease in patients with ovarian cancer. In women with advanced-stage disease, as many as 50% of those without clinical or radiologically detectable residual disease following chemotherapy are found to have disease at second-look laparotomy despite a negative CA 125 level (<35 units/ml).[3] Moreover, CA 125 values may not be elevated in patients with mucinous or clear-cell tumors. Although carcinoembryonic antigen (CEA) can be elevated in patients with mucinous tumors, this oncofetal tumor marker has not been shown to correlate well with disease status. Finally, CA 125 has low sensitivity in the detection of early-stage ovarian cancers. Only approximately 50% of clinically detectable stage 1 ovarian tumors are associated with an elevated CA 125 level.[4] This sensitivity is significantly lower than that of transvaginal sonography and seriously limits the usefulness of serum CA 125 as a single screening modality.[5]

Recent developments in monoclonal antibody technology have lead to the identification of several novel tumor-associated antigens, including shed cell surface antigens (GAT, CA 15-3, TAG 72.3, OVX1), hormonal markers [urinary gonadotropin fragment (UGF)], and serum proteins produced by ovarian tumors [macrophage colony stimulation factor (MCSF), NBK 70, and soluble tumor necrosis factor (TNF) receptor], which may ultimately prove to be more useful tumor markers than CA 125. NBK 70, for example, a tumor-associated antigen distinct from CA 125, has the advantage of being elevated in all histologic types of ovarian cancer and may be more sensitive for small-volume disease than CA 125.[6] Similarly, UGF, a cleavage product of the β subunit of human chorionic gonadotropin (HCG), has a greater sensitivity for ovarian cancer than CA 125, and serial UGF levels appear to accurately reflect disease status in patients undergoing therapy for this disease.[7] In screening trials, measurements of serum levels of CA 125, MCSF, and OVX1 in combination yielded a 98% sensitivity for early-stage tumors, suggesting that simultaneous assessment of complementary tumor markers may improve the sensitivity of screening.[8] Similarly, the detection of subclinical recurrent disease has been improved by using CA 125 in combination with other complementary tumor markers.[9] Unfortunately, there are few data on the cost of these tumor markers, particularly when used in the screening setting. Confirmation of the utility of these markers awaits the results of large randomized clinical trials.

A novel direction in tumor marker development is the identification of genetic markers of disease in ovarian cancer. Recent evidence suggests that ovarian cancer is the end result of a complex pathway involving mutations in multiple cancer-associated genes including oncogenes and tumor suppressor genes.[10] The ability to detect specific genetic changes occurring early in ovarian tumorigenesis, for example, by measuring levels of an oncogene product in the serum of patients, could prove invaluable when applied clinically as a detection tool. Similarly, the ability to detect mutations in genes critical for invasion and/or metastasis could be useful in predicting the biologic aggressiveness of the tumor and in monitoring response to chemotherapy in patients. The HER-2/*neu* gene product, which is shed into the sera of some patients with ovarian cancer, is currently being investigated as a potential tumor marker for ovarian cancer.[11] Although currently in its infancy, the measurement of oncogene products as molecular markers of disease is a promising area of research.

GORDON B. MILLS
ROBERT C. BAST, JR.

Serum tumor markers for monitoring the course of epithelial ovarian cancer

Given the distinctive pattern of spread of ovarian cancer over peritoneal surfaces, it is often difficult to monitor the response of residual disease to chemotherapy following cytoreductive surgery. Physical examination, computed tomography (CT), and magnetic resonance (MR) imaging may fail to detect small tumor nodules, and in this setting serum tumor markers can provide clinical information that cannot be obtained by other methods. Several serum markers have been evaluated for their ability to track the tumor burden of ovarian cancer during active treatment and in subsequent follow-up. Among the markers studied to date, CA 125 has proved most useful.[1,12] At diagnosis, CA 125 values have been elevated (>35 units/mL) in serum from more than 80% of patients with epithelial ovarian cancer. When elevated at diagnosis, changes in CA 125 levels have correlated with changes in tumor burden in approximately 90% of instances studied. This correlation has been sufficiently precise that Rustin[13] has suggested that CA 125 be used as a surrogate marker for measurable disease in phase II studies of new cytotoxic drugs.

Approval of CA 125 by the U.S. Food and Drug Administration was based upon the claim that elevation of CA 125 values prior to second-look laparotomy predicts persistence of disease with greater than 95% accuracy. CA 125 levels can, however, return to within normal limits and small amounts of residual disease can still be found in as many as half of patients. Consequently, an elevated CA 125 is a specific marker for persistence of ovarian cancer but is not optimally sensitive. The ability to predict disease persistence has been improved by examining the rate of decrease in CA 125 levels during postoperative chemotherapy. The serum half-life of CA 125 is approximately 4.5 days, and in patients where the apparent half-life of CA 125 exceeded 20 days, persistent ovarian cancer was more likely to be present at second-look laparotomy and survival was shortened.[14]

Repeated measurement of CA 125 following cytoreductive surgery and completion of adjuvant chemotherapy has permitted early detection of disease recurrence with a lead time of approximately 3 months. In theory, early detection of disease recurrence should permit treatment of smaller tumor nodules containing cells that are proliferating more actively and are potentially more susceptible to cytotoxic drugs. In fact, the lack of curative salvage chemotherapy for ovarian cancer has limited the value of CA 125 in detecting disease recurrence or persistence. As more efficacious drugs are developed and more effective strategies identified, information provided by serum markers like CA 125 will attain greater value.

Following detection of recurrent disease, a number of cytotoxic drugs can exert antitumor activity in a fraction of patients. Several of these agents achieve response rates of approximately 20%. A progressively rising CA 125 level despite therapy should prompt a change in treatment, minimizing the morbidity and cost of an inactive agent. Conversely, the side effects and expense of palliative chemotherapy may be justified when CA 125 values continue to decline. Critical studies are needed to determine whether use of CA 125 alone can replace imaging methods in monitoring patients during palliative treatment.

One of the most promising applications of CA 125 is in guiding the appropriate triage of patients prior to surgical exploration. Careful staging and cytoreduction can best be carried out by experienced surgeons with specialized training in gynecologic oncology. Less than 25% of patients with ovarian cancer undergo exploration by a board certified gynecologic oncologist for their initial surgery. Elevation of CA 125 levels (>95 units/ml) in a postmenopausal patient with an adnexal mass strongly suggests that some form of malignancy is present that would benefit from specialized surgical expertise. Indexes have been developed that include clinical and sonographic data in addition to CA 125 values,[15] but elevation of CA 125 levels in a postmenopausal patient should prompt appropriate referral for optimal management in an initial procedure. In our cost-conscious times, more accurate triage of patients should help to maintain the quality of care.

Use of serum tumor markers and transvaginal sonography for early detection of ovarian cancer

Analysis of genetic alterations in primary ovarian cancers and metastases suggests that more than 90% of epithelial ovarian cancers start from a single cell within the ovary.[16,17] Ovarian cancer is not a multifocal disease of the peritoneal cavity but spreads from a primary site, most patients must pass through a stage when cancer cells are in fact localized to the ovary. With conventional methods of diagnosis, metastatic disease is found outside the pelvis in about two-thirds of ovarian cancer patients. In these advanced stages, less than 30% of patients can be cured. When the spread of ovarian cancer is still limited to the ovaries, cure rates can exceed 80% using currently available surgery and chemotherapy or radiotherapy. Consequently, there is reason to believe that early detection might improve prognosis. While this seems reasonable, there is as yet no conclusive trial demonstrating that any of the currently available strategies for early detection actually impact upon the survival of patients with epithelial ovarian cancer.

Detection of asymptomatic ovarian cancer has depended in the past on pelvic examination, but even in the hands of experienced practitioners, pelvic examination is notoriously insensitive. Two approaches have been pursued to detect ovarian cancer in asymptomatic patients at an earlier interval. One uses serum tumor markers such as CA 125, and the other uses transabdominal or transvaginal sonography.

In retrospective studies, elevated CA 125 values have been observed 10 to 60 months prior to conventional diagnosis in women destined to develop ovarian cancer. Despite this lead time, a single determination of CA 125 level does not provide optimal sensitivity or specificity for cost-effective screening. CA 125 values are elevated (>35 units/ml) in only 50% of patients with stage I disease. Specificity is limited in that 2% of apparently healthy postmenopausal women in Stockholm had CA 125 levels of >30 units/ml.[18] Even with a higher threshold of 65 units/ml, 0.4% of apparently healthy nuns from the Archdiocese of Philadelphia had elevated CA 125 values.[19] While this is reasonable specificity for a monitoring test, it is inadequate for screening. Given the prevalence of ovarian cancer in the United States or in Sweden, about 40 laparotomies would be performed for each case of ovarian cancer detected using a cutoff as high as 65 units/ml. Over the last decade several studies have been undertaken to enhance the specificity and sensitivity of CA 125 for screening.

Two approaches have been utilized to improve the specificity of CA 125 in early detection of ovarian cancer. The first combines CA 125 values with sonography, and the second tracks the trend of CA 125 values over time. In a study of 4,000 women in the United Kingdom, Jacobs[20] found that a combination of CA 125 assay and transabdominal sonography provided specificity in excess of 99.7%, which should ensure a positive predictive value of 10%, that is, 10 laparotomies for every case of ovarian cancer detected. In a subsequent trial involving 22,000 postmenopausal women, CA 125 levels were elevated in 340, and abnormal transabdominal ultrasounds prompted laparotomy in 40 patients.[21] Eleven cases of ovarian cancer were detected with several in the early stage. Over the next

2 years eight additional cases of ovarian cancer were detected among women who had had normal CA 125 values at the time of initial screening. Consequently, a combination of CA 125 assay and ultrasound appeared to achieve adequate specificity but was not optimally sensitive. Einhorn and Sjovall[18] conducted a screening trial in Stockholm measuring CA 125 values every 3 months in 5,500 asymptomatic women. Persistently elevated values prompted the use of transabdominal ultrasound and pelvic examination. Only 2% of women over age 50 had abnormal values of CA 125 requiring further workup. Six cases of ovarian cancer were detected, with four in the early stage. With use of the Swedish Tumor Registry, it was possible to identify three additional cases of ovarian cancer occurring in women who had had CA 125 levels of less than 30 to 35 units/ml at the time of initial screening. Consequently, observation of CA125 values over time improved specificity for early detection, but again sensitivity was not optimal.

In following CA 125 values over time, the day-to-day variation in the assay is a critical parameter. The CA 125 antigen is a large molecule with multiple copies of at least two determinants. The original CA 125 radioimmunoassay was a double-determinant sandwich assay that utilized the OC 125 antibody to bind antigen to a bead and radiolabeled OC 125 antibody to detect antigen that had been captured. A second-generation assay has been developed designated CA 125-II that uses the new M11 antibody to bind the CA 125 antigen to a bead and radiolabeled OC 125 as a probe. Serum specimens from the Stockholm trial have been reanalyzed using the CA 125-II assay, and less variation has been observed from day to day than with the standard CA 125 assay. Skates[22] has developed a computer algorithm which utilizes both the slope and intercept of the logarithm of CA 125 values plotted as a function of time. Patients with benign disease tend to have values that fluctuate around a horizontal line, whereas those with ovarian cancer have progressively rising values. With this computer algorithm it is possible to exclude more than 99.7% of individuals who are normal or who have benign disease. Based on data from the Stockholm series the algorithm correctly identified five of six patients with cancer. Although this is much too small a sample to assess the sensitivity of the assay, this specificity should be adequate to permit a trial of sufficient size to test the utility of serial monitoring of CA 125-II levels for early detection of ovarian cancer. The algorithm is currently being tested in such a trial that will involve more than 100,000 women in the United Kingdom.

As only 80% of ovarian cancers express CA 125 as judged by immunohistochemistry, any strategy based only on CA 125 values misses a fraction of cancers even at the advanced stage. Multiple markers have been evaluated for the ability to complement CA 125. Two of the most promising are a mucin determinant, OVX1,[23] and a cytokine, MCSF or CSF-1.[24] A combination of CA 125, OVX1, and MCSF identified 45 of 46 patients with stage I ovarian cancer in one retrospective study.[8] OVX1 and MCSF levels were elevated 11 months prior to detection of a stage IC ovarian cancer in one fortuitous case.[25] Thus, the markers promise to provide lead time as well as a sensitivity in excess of 90% for stage I disease at the time of conventional diagnosis. The combination of three markers exhibited a specificity of 89%.[8] Although this specificity is not adequate to permit screening using blood tests alone, a multistage strategy could be devised employing one or more positive blood tests to trigger ultrasonography.

While studies utilizing CA 125 alone were being conducted, transvaginal sonography was also evaluated in early detection of ovarian cancer. In contrast to transabdominal sonography, the transvaginal approach brings the ultrasound transducer into close proximity with the ovary, permitting a precise estimate of ovarian size and shape. With the use of this technique, more than 95% of stage I disease can be detected. Specificity has, however, posed a major problem. Among 11,283 women screened with transvaginal sonography, 486 laparotomies were performed to diagnose five invasive and eight borderline cancers.[26] Thus 97 laparotomies were required to diagnose each invasive cancer.

For ovarian cancer screening, two technologies have been identified with complementary strengths and weaknesses. CA 125 levels studied over time or in combination with ultrasound are adequately specific but not optimally sensitive. Conversely, ultrasound is quite sensitive but lacks specificity for cost-effective screening. Combining the two techniques might provide a more effective screen. Urban[27] has modeled different alternatives for transvaginal sonography alone, serum markers alone, and a combination of the two modalities. The combination has been shown in this model to be the most cost-effective, falling into a range comparable to that of mammography.[27]

Ultimately, one could imagine an initial screen that uses a panel of two or more serum markers followed by transvaginal sonography. Until definitive studies can be completed, however, neither CA 125 assay nor transvaginal sonography should be utilized for screening in the general population. Both may have a role in the surveillance of individuals with genetic abnormalities strongly predispoing them to the development of ovarian cancer. Such screening is best conducted in the context of a controlled clinical trial with adequate counseling.

QUESTION 2

Are there any laboratory or molecular markers that should currently be used as prognostic or stratification factors in the design of randomized clinical trials?

HOLLY H. GALLION

In the clinical trial arena, tumor stage, grade, histologic cell type, and amount of residual disease are currently used as prognostic or stratification factors in the design of clinical trials. They are used mainly to (1) identify patients with stage I and II tumors at high risk for recurrence who may benefit from adjuvant chemotherapy, (2) identify a subset of patients with stage III and IV tumors who are likely to fail standard chemotherapy, and (3) stratify patients within clinical trials in order to ensure even distribution of prognostic factors. Ideally, prognostic or stratification factors should be reproducible, cost-effective, and independently associated with valid end points. The current standard clinical and pathologic prognostic factors can be subjective in nature. For example, there is significant interobserver and intraobserver variability in assignment of histologic cell type and grade.[28] In more advanced-stage disease, current clinical trials typically stratify or randomize patients based on the amount of residual disease following primary surgery. Certainly, although the volume of residual disease is a powerful prognostic indicator, this measurement is subjective by its very nature and does not take into account the total volume of residual cancer. Moreover, it is possible that the amount of residual disease simply reflects the biologic aggressiveness of the tumor which, if it could be measured, may be a more important predictor of prognosis.

Several studies have clearly shown that flow cytometric analysis of tumor DNA content is an important prognostic indicator in ovarian cancer. Aneuploid tumors have a much poorer prognosis than diploid tumors, and this appears particularly true in borderline tumors and early-stage invasive tumors. In patients with advanced-stage disease, approximately three-fourths of tumors are aneuploid. These women have a median survival of only 4.5 months, compared to 22 months for those with diploid tumors.[29] Similarly, in stage I and II tumors, DNA ploidy as well as degree of proliferative activity in the tumor (S-phase fraction) are significantly related to survival.[30] Moreover, in a series of 370 patients with borderline ovarian tumors, DNA content was the most important independent risk factor. Patients with aneuploid tumors having a 19-fold higher risk of dying from their disease than patients with diploid tumors.[31] *For these reasons, flow cytometric assessment of ploidy and cell proliferation indexes should be incorporated into clinical trials.* The combination of classic prognostic parameters and DNA flow cytometry studies may well improve our ability to predict prognosis in patients with early-stage borderline and invasive ovarian tumors.

As mentioned previously, elucidation of the underlying molecular genetic basis of ovarian cancer may well provide additional useful prognostic factors. Mutation or deletion of the p53 tumor suppressor gene is the most common genetic abnormality identified in ovarian tumors and is clearly related to tumor stage. p53 mutations are detectable in approximately 50% of stage III and IV tumors and are extremely uncommon in early-stage disease. Unfortunately, the rarity of p53 mutations in early-stage tumors and the lack of correlation with prognosis in advanced tumors limits the usefulness of this genetic marker in clinical trial design.[32] Overexpression of the HER-2/*neu* oncogene, which encodes a growth factor receptor structurally similar to epidermal growth factor (EGF) receptor, is found in approximately 10% of stage III and IV epithelial ovarian cancers. In contrast to p53, the HER-2/*neu* oncogene is associated with poor prognosis and poor response to chemotherapy in patients with advanced-stage disease, suggesting that assessment of this oncogene product may be useful in identifying a subset of patients with a particularly high risk of failing standard chemotherapy.[33]

More recently, a preliminary report on the clinicopathologic characteristics of ovarian cancer in women with documented germline mutations in BRCA1 suggests that these hereditary ovarian cancers may have a more indolent clinical course than sporadic tumors.[34] If this is confirmed in a larger series, analysis of the BRCA1 gene or its product may add another prognostic factor to our armamentarium.

Although in its infancy, molecular oncology is expected to provide insight into the molecular genetic mechanisms of ovarian tumorigenesis, which may provide us with new mechanisms for the detection and management of ovarian cancer.

GORDON B. MILLS
ROBERT C. BAST, JR.

The prognostic load of several different genetic and epigenetic changes in ovarian cancer has been identified through retrospective analysis of ovarian cancer cells from patients treated primarily with cisplatin- and, more recently, cisplatin/paclitaxel-based therapy. These predictive markers include increased expression of erbB2, persistent expression of the EGF receptor, novel expression of the MCSF receptor, increased expression of loss of heterozygosity at particular sites, instability assessed by comparative genomic hybridization, abnormalities in comparative genomic hybridization, germline abnormalities in BRCA1, and a number of other changes.[33,35–40] The presence or absence of these predictive markers identifies patients with a relatively better or worse prognosis, however, none of them have proved to be consistently more predictive of outcome than are histology, stage, grade, and residual tumor. Thus these markers are not sufficient to alter current patient treatment strategies. None of the current markers identify early tumors that are likely to recur or not recur and thus do or do not require treatment. Furthermore, these markers do not have sufficient predictive value to identify patients with advanced disease who are likely to be unresponsive to standard therapy and require treatment with alternative approaches. Nevertheless, to determine whether assessing multiple different potential markers in a single tumor through current immunohistochemical approaches or through rapidly emerging genome scanning technologies such as unigene arrays or CHIP technology (see below) can provide results sufficiently robust to modify our current clinical trial design should remain a high priority for laboratory research.

One of the major problems in determining whether markers will be predictive of outcome, particularly in early disease, is the difficulty in obtaining sufficient numbers of samples from patients with stage I or II tumors. As most of these patients are treated in the periphery and early tumors are frequently found by serendipity during surgery for other reasons, it has been difficult to generate tumor banks or libraries that include significant numbers of early tumors. Further, these patients are frequently lost to follow-up. Thus, insufficient studies have been done to determine whether specific markers or, more likely, patterns of markers can identify individuals who do or do not require further therapy.

The lack of an absolute or sufficiently significant correlation between predictive markers and outcome to justify altered patient treatment may be based on the vast majority of epithelial ovarian cancer patients analyzed having received cisplatin-based therapy as first-line therapy. Furthermore, in most cases, only small numbers of patient samples were assessed.[33, 35–40] Thus it is indeed possible that predictive markers or a battery of predictive markers could show sufficient value to justify patient stratification for clinical trials. Most significantly, predictive markers would be identified only if they indicated differential outcomes in response to first-line cisplatin-based therapy. Whether the available markers or combination of available markers is sufficiently powerful to predict the outcome of second-line therapies will require further investigation. It is important to note that in other types of tumors, predictive markers such as steroid receptor levels in breast cancer and kinase-linked receptor levels in breast cancer have proven to be useful in determining whether particular therapies are appropriate for specific patients.[41]

With the rapid emergence of technologies capable of assessing the complete genome for genetic changes[42–44] (see below), it may soon be possible to obtain thousands or even millions of bits of genetic information related to a specific tumor. Tandem mass spectrometry[45] may allow the identification of additional protein markers or even specific postranslational modification of protein markers as predictive factors. The most likely difficulty will be in developing bioinformatics capabilities that can integrate the massive amount of genetic and biochemical data that will be available for patient treatment. Indeed, neural networks, pattern recognition, and other forms of artificial intelligence will be necessary to deal with the amount of information that will be available about a patient's specific tumor.

Given that a number of different potential predictive markers have currently been identified and that multiple new markers are being proposed continuously, it will be essential to design studies that assess the validity of these markers in predicting patient outcome and response to specific therapeutic protocols. Initially, these studies could be retrospective using appropriately annotated and stored tissue, however, any strong predictive patterns will eventually need to be assessed in prospective studies in which patients are stratified for particular markers or patterns of markers. These will need to be compared to the more standard indicators of outcome such as stage, grade, histologic type, and residual tumor to determine the predictive value of markers or sets of markers. Given the investigational nature as well as the labor- and cost-intensive nature of current cell culture, immunohistochemical, loss of heterozygosity, comparative genomic hybridization, and other approaches for identifying and assessing the predictive value of genetic and epigenetic markers, it will likely be necessary to establish collaborative studies in which several different laboratories assess specific markers in a large, well-characterized set of patient samples.[33,35–45] As a first step, it will be essential to establish appropriate quality control for each assay, as well as for prompt cryopreservation of tissue. For example, the ability to detect increased levels of erbB2, and likely other markers, is fraught with considerable potential technical difficulty.[46] Furthermore, the library of samples will need to include sufficient numbers of patients with each histologic type, grade, stage, and residual disease. The patient sample library or tumor bank should also include patients treated with multiple different first- and second-line therapies, which will probably require accumulating tissue in properly annotated prospective tumor banks which can be readily and freely accessed by many laboratories. This tissue will need to be collected in such a manner as to allow histochemistry, DNA, RNA, and protein analysis. Given that ovarian cancer frequently presents with a massive amount of disease and that many assays can be performed on minute amounts of tissue, it should be possible to perform multiple analyses on a single patient sample. Given that tumors recur rapidly and that secondary debulking or at least drainage of ascites is a common component of standard practice, it may be possible to obtain tumor samples before and after specific therapies. It is likely that such a collaborative approach will be required to determine whether predictive markers should be moved into use as stratification for prospective clinical trials.

QUESTION 3

On which women should BRCA1 testing be performed?

HOLLY H. GALLION

Recently, clinical testing for mutations in the BRCA1 gene, which is thought to be responsible for about one-half of inherited breast cancers and almost all inherited ovarian cancers, has become available. For women who have inherited a mutation in the BRCA1 gene, it has been estimated that at age 70 the cumulative risk for developing breast and ovarian cancer are approximately 80% and 60%, respectively.[47] Because of this extremely high risk developing cancer, many women, including those without a family history of the disease, are now requesting BRCA1 mutation screening. Although this cancer susceptibility test is definitely not appropriate for screening asymptomatic individuals in the general population, testing should be considered in women with breast or ovarian cancer whose family history strongly suggests an inherited form of disease. Certainly, this includes women with breast or ovarian cancer who have two or more first or second-degree blood relatives with breast or ovarian cancer and those who have one blood relative with early age of onset (<45 years) breast or ovarian cancer. In addition, women with a personal history of early age of onset breast or ovarian cancer, bilateral breast cancer, or both breast and ovarian cancer may also benefit from testing. Finally, first- or second-degree relatives of persons with documented mutations in the BRCA1 gene should be counseled regarding possible BRCA1 testing. As BRCA1 is not the only gene responsible for inherited breast or ovarian cancer, it is imperative that testing be first done on an affected family member to determine whether it is indeed the responsible gene. If a BRCA1 mutation is identified, testing for the same mutation can then be offered to unaffected close relatives.

The potential benefits of BRCA1 testing are apparent. For women with a positive test, prevention and/or surveillance strategies can be instituted. The options for dealing with breast cancer include prophylactic mastectomy, breast-self examination, regular mammography, and chemoprevention such as the Breast Cancer Prevention Trial. For the prevention of ovarian cancer prophylactic oophorectomy can be considered for women over 35 years of age and for those who no longer desire to bear children. Although the value of screening for ovarian cancer remains unproven, transvaginal sonography and serum CA 125 assay may be useful in detecting ovarian cancer in an early, potentially curable stage. Conversely, women with a negative test can be reassured and can be spared unnecessary prophylactic surgery and excessive screening examinations.

Despite these apparent benefits, genetic testing poses a number of risks. In families where a mutation has been identified, a positive test may lead to undue anxiety, a changed self-image, feelings of guilt for possibly passing the gene on to one's children, and noncompliance with suggested screening strategies. A false positive test, resulting from a benign polymorphism or a laboratory error, could lead to unnecessary anxiety and even to unnecessary prophylactic surgery. Moreover, it is possible that a positive test could compromise patients' insurability, affecting their ability to obtain health, life, or disability coverage. Although the Americans with Disabilities Act offers protection to individuals who carry genes that may predispose them to disease, the full extent of this protection from job discrimination has not yet been tested. Because of this potential, but real, risk of discrimination, confidentiality is a major issue which must be considered by any individual considering BRCA1 testing.

Conversely, there are several inherent risks in interpreting a negative test. In a person with breast or ovarian cancer, it is possible that the cancer may have been the result of a different cancer-related gene such as BRCA2. Alternatively, the cancer may have been sporadic in origin while that of her affected family members was due to BRCA1 mutations. In this case, a negative test may lead to undue complacency in a patient and her family members who may have a marked increased risk of breast and ovarian cancer despite a negative test.

GORDON B. MILLS
ROBERT C. BAST, JR.

Genetic predisposition to ovarian cancer

As cancer is a genetic disease, the identification of genes that are necessary for normal cellular homeostasis and are aberrant in tumor cells may lead to new approaches to preventing cancer development, establishing prognosis, tailoring therapy to the genetic makeup of an individual's cancer, and designing new therapeutic procedures for normalizing the function of aberrant genes or abnormal regulatory cascades. More than 90% of ovarian cancers are clonal[16,17] and thus must arise because of the accumulation of somatic mutations in a single cell resulting in cancer initiation and eventual progression to clinically evident disease. However, for the 5 to 10% of tumors that are familial in nature, one of these mutations is present in the patient's germline, resulting in a high incidence and frequently an early onset of cancer.[47,48] It is important that we develop appropriate management approaches for the identification and care of these high-risk individuals. Furthermore, since the incidence of cancer in individuals with germline mutations in cancer predisposition genes is much higher than in the general population,[47,48] screening or cancer prevention studies on these women may provide a proof of concept for approaches that can then be extended to trials in the general population. Given the difficulty of completing screening and prevention trials in the general population because of the very low rate of "events," we may need to apply results derived from studies on high-risk individuals to the general population without formal scientific evaluation in low-risk individuals. However, it is important to emphasize that the natural history of cancer may be sufficiently different in high- and low-risk populations to preclude the direct extension of studies in high-risk individuals to the normal population without confirmatory evaluation.[40,49]

As similar mutations or mutations in the same regulatory pathways frequently occur in familial and sporadic tumors,[50,51] studies on either sporadic or inherited tumours can provide important information relevant to both types of tumors. At its current stage of development, human cancer genetics has two main goals. The first goal is to determine the identity of the genes involved in the process that renders a cancer cell autonomous from its normal regulatory mechanisms. This requires that we identify the genetic changes that result in tumor initiation and progression and determine the normal mechanism of action of the genes involved. The second goal is to utilize the information that can be generated through molecular genetic technology to determine a patient's prognosis, to devise appropriate treatment strategies, to develop new molecular therapeutic approaches aimed at normalizing cellular functions, and finally to design methods for treating patients with increased susceptibility to the development of cancer.

Cancer is the result of an accumulation of genetic abnormalities that allow the cell to bypass mechanisms aimed at maintaining cellular homeostasis. Thus, mutations contributing to the appearance of a clinically relevant cancer can affect (1) genes that participate in tumor initiation, for example, proto-oncogenes that increase the rate of proliferation of cells and tumor suppressor genes that regulate cell cycle check points; (2) genes that regulate genomic stability, rendering the cell susceptible to additional gene mutations; (3) genes that initiate programmed cell death, increasing cell survival; or (4) genes that regulate cellular senescence, allowing a cell to undergo an increased number of cellular divisions. In addition, a separate set of genetic changes are required for a tumor to progress to a clinically relevant state, including the ability to initiate neovascularization, to invade, and to metastasize. Tumorigenic mutations can either activate or inactivate enzymatic activity in the protein product, render enzymatic activity insensitive to normal regulatory processes, alter the location of the protein, affect the activity of any one protein in a regulatory cascade, alter levels of the protein, or change the temporal expression of the protein.

Discovery of the BRCA1 cancer predisposition gene in 1994 and the BRCA2 cancer predisposition gene in 1995 has allowed the identification of a group of women who are at a greatly increased risk for the development of breast and ovarian cancer.[41,48,52,53] However, whether the identification of individuals at risk for the development of breast and ovarian cancer will facilitate the detection of tumors at an early stage, offer opportunities for prevention or prophylaxis, or increase the quality or duration of life remains to be evaluated. Thus, although we have the technical ability to perform genetic testing for BRCA1 and BRCA2 in individuals with a family or personal history of breast or ovarian cancer, whether such screening is ethically appropriate outside clinical trials at a time when we do not have a scientifically proven treatment option for these women is not clear. Further, the questions of who will pay for genetic testing, screening of high-risk individuals with unproved tests or prophylactic surgery, and whether genetic testing will lead to insurance or employment discrimination render the whole concept of genetic testing an extremely contentious issue. However, it is essential within the ethical limitations of the current situation that we design research protocols to determine the best methods for managing the concerns of women who are at a greatly increased risk of developing cancer either as a result of family history or because of proven mutation in the BRCA1 or BRCA2 cancer predisposition genes. Several consensus conferences and expert reviews have suggested that genetic testing should be performed only as part of a institutional review board approved protocol with hypothesis-driven research and access to appropriate genetic counseling, screening, and prevention strategies.[54,55] However, the availability of commercial testing has begun to render this a moot point. Individuals who have a perception, correctly or incorrectly, that they are risk of developing breast or ovarian cancer are obtaining genetic testing from commercial sources and only then asking for assistance in interpreting the results and in managing the consequences of the results. Given that we know little about the appropriate management for these individuals and the extent to which information obtained from these high-risk individuals can be applied to the general population, all efforts should be made to enroll these women in clinical trials with appropriate counseling and informed consent prior to their obtaining genetic testing. Failing this proactive approach, including these individuals in studies on the efficacy of screening, in prevention or prophylaxis, or at a minimum in registries designed to follow outcomes must remain an important goal.

Overall, women with abnormalities in the BRCA1 gene have up to an 85% chance of developing breast cancer and up to a 60% chance of developing ovarian cancer by the age of 70.[47,48] Individuals with abnormalities in the BRCA2 gene have up to an 80% chance of developing breast cancer and a lower risk, probably in the range of 20%, of developing ovarian cancer by the age of 70.[56] Individuals with abnormalities in these genes may have a smaller but significant increase in the frequency of bowel, pancreatic, or prostate cancer or of ocular melanoma. It is important to note, however, that these predictions are based on studies involving a small number of families with a high frequency of breast and ovarian cancer and probably represent an overestimation of the influence of these abnormalities on tumor development because of an ascertainment bias.[47,48,56] Individuals in these families may have specific high-penetrance mutations in BRCA1 or BRCA2, abnormalities in other cooperating genes, or lifestyles leading to high penetrance. The role that the specific site or type of mutation in these genes plays, in the likelihood that individuals will develop breast or ovarian cancer is only beginning to be elucidated. This is particularly significant in the case of missense mutations which may or may not be polymorphisms and in the case of sequence variations in introns or potential upstream regulatory regions. However, most abnormalities detected in these genes in cancer-prone families are nonsense mutations leading to lack of production of a protein or to production of a truncated protein.[52,53] Until recently these truncation mutations were thought to universally increase an individual's predisposition to developing breast and ovarian cancer. However, recent identification of families with a termination mutation in the carboxy terminus of BRCA2 that does not appear to predispose to the development of cancer, questions even this tenant.[57] Preliminary studies suggest that individuals with mutations in the carboxy terminal third of BRCA1 may have a lesser predisposition to developing ovarian cancer than individuals with abnormalities in the more proximal portions of the gene.[58] Currently, outside these very basic outlines, little is known about the effects of specific abnormalities on the relative risk of developing breast or ovarian cancer, whether particular mutations will lead to tumor development at different ages, or whether particular mutations will predispose to the development of other types of tumors. It is also particularly important to note that genetic testing is not universally predictive. Currently, it does not identify the 20% of patients who, although they carry abnormalities in the BRCA1 or BRCA2 gene, will not develop cancer; it cannot determine at what age an individual will develop cancer; and, finally, negative tests do not eliminate the possibility that an individual will develop cancer either as a consequence of mutation in a different cancer predisposition gene or because of the somatic mutations leading to the approximately 1 in 9 incidence of breast cancer and the 1 in 70 incidence of ovarian cancer in the general population.[47,48,56]

As 20% of individuals with a proven abnormality in BRCA1 or BRCA2 do not develop breast or ovarian cancer, there must be either significant modifying genes that determine the penetrance of mutations in BRCA1 or BRCA2 or environmental effects that modify the action of these genes. These options offer the opportunity to identify other cancer predisposition genes likely to contribute to the multifactorial development of cancer. These genetic changes may represent relatively common, low-penetrance events. One such change may be reflected in the k-*ras* restriction fragment length polymorphism which appears to lead to an increased penetrance of BRCA1 abnormalities.[59] Alternatively, they may reflect environmental effects which if modified could lead to a lower incidence of cancer in these individuals.[60]

Little is known about the function of BRCA1 and BRCA2. BRCA1 levels appear to be influenced by steroids and perhaps as a consequence are elevated during pregnancy and lactation.[61,62] In normal cells, BRCA1 is primarily localized in the nucleus where it likely functions as part of a transcription factor complex or as part of a DNA repair complex.[50,63] Homozygous deletion of BRCA1 by homologous recombination is an embryonal lethal defect in mice.[64,65] However, at least one physiologically normal human patient (other than for developing breast cancer at age 32) has inherited mutations in both copies of BRCA1 from both parents,[66] indicating that it is not required for embryogenesis or development in the human. Thus BRCA1 is either functionally redundant in human development or fulfills a different function in mice and humans. Strikingly, introduction of normal BRCA1 cDNA into breast and ovarian cancer cells both in vitro and in vivo results in a marked decrease in proliferation and tumorigenicity of breast and ovarian cancer cell lines without a similar effect on other tumor lineages, suggesting that BRCA1 has breast- and ovary-specific effects.[58] This has lead to a preliminary phase I trial of gene therapy with BRCA1. Surprisingly, although loss of heterozygosity at or near the BRCA1 and BRCA2 loci is frequently noted in sporadic breast and ovarian tumors, point mutations in BRCA1 and BRCA2 are rare in these tumors.[67–69] BRCA1, however, appears to be localized in the cytosol rather than in the nucleus of sporadic tumors, suggesting that a putative nuclear transport molecule for BRCA1 is aberrant or nonfunctional in sporadic tumors. Thus, although BRCA1 is not mutated in sporadic tumors, its function may be aberrant in such tumors.[50] However, if this is the case, the abnormalities in function may not be concordant in tumors due to germline or sporadic mutations, as preliminary data on a small number of patients suggest that with patients ovarian cancer having germline mutations in BRCA1 have a markedly improved prognosis.[41] This is reminiscent of the situation for individuals with Lynch type II syndrome or hereditary nonpolyposis colon cancer (HNPCC) where germline mutations in the mismatch repair genes result in a high frequency of tumors but these tumors have a better prognosis than in individuals who develop bowel cancers due exclusively to somatic mutations.[49]

Genetic Counseling and Testing

Genetic testing is the most contentious of all the issues related to genetic predisposition to cancer.[54,55,67,70,71] Given our current lack of information on how to treat individuals with abnormalities in BRCA1 and BRCA2, efforts should be made to enroll all women undergoing genetic counseling and testing in clinical trials. Perhaps most importantly, given the current state of our knowledge, genetic testing should be offered only to individuals who have been counseled as to the validity and interpretation of results of genetic testing.[54,55] Further, it is important to emphasize to the patient that no definitive information defining appropriate management of a positive or even a negative genetic test is currently available. Until retrospective and prospective studies have been completed, management is based on expert opinion related to information available on the treatment of low-risk individuals.[54] Effective screening approaches, the outcomes of prophylactic surgery, and potential prevention approaches have not been evaluated in clinical studies on these high-risk individuals. Finally the patient must be apprised of the potential risks of genetic testing related to changes in family relationships, self-perception, insurance eligibility or rates, and employability.[70–72] Further, during counseling patients may learn about issues such as adoption and nonpaternity, which may be as high as 2%, that may alter their family status. Women who decide to undergo genetic testing note that "a need to know," a "feeling of control," and "information about risks for children" are the most important determinants leading individuals to obtain genetic testing.[73]

Given that no definitive management protocols are available, counseling relating to whether an individual wishes to undergo genetic testing needs to be as nondirective as possible. It should thus concentrate on providing the most valid, up-to-date information appropriate to the specific patient in a manner that is understandable and related to the patient's particular family history and ethnic and educational background. It is important to remember that many individuals who request genetic counseling and genetic testing have seen close relatives die, frequently at a young age, of breast or ovarian cancer. Thus their perception of the likelihood of their developing cancer is influenced by a personal experience that has not affected the average person. Indeed, individuals requesting genetic testing frequently greatly overestimate their risk of developing breast and ovarian cancer and are resistant to information provided during intensive genetic counseling.[73] Further, the risk levels that these individuals find comfortable may be very different from those that are acceptable to the general population. Whereas the Breast and Ovarian Cancer Risk Assessment Program at M. D. Anderson Cancer Center classifies a 10% chance of developing breast or ovarian cancer as a high risk, patients not infrequently state they would be comfortable with a 50% chance of developing breast or ovarian cancer and consider a high risk to be over a 80% chance of developing this disease. Many individuals from high-risk families feel that their risk approaches 100% despite the fact that their chance of inheriting an abnormality is 50% and penetrance is approximately 80%. Thus, in the absence of a definite positive genetic test, for an individual the highest risk of developing breast or ovarian cancer by the age of 70 is 40%. Despite this, on repeat visits, a patient may state, "I know, doctor, that you told me my risk is only 20%, but I am one of the 'affected' and my risk is really 80%." Further, although risk estimates are relevant to populations, they are not significant to the patient because they are affected by binary statistics that are either 100% or 0%; that is, they either do or do not have a genetic change or will or will not develop cancer. Nevertheless, counseling related to genetic testing should be aimed at providing information that will empower the patient to make a decision appropriate for her comfort level at the current stage of her life.[73] No matter what the counselor feels is the appropriate approach, in the absence of definitive management options, the decision to undergo genetic testing and which, if any, screening protocol to follow must remain the option of the patient. As there is frequently little urgency to undergo genetic testing, awaiting the results of ongoing trials, changes in the laws regulating insurance, and maturation of our understanding of the best method for treating women with abnormalities in BRCA1 or BRCA2 should always be considered a reasonable alternative.

As many patients are concerned about the likelihood that they may have passed a deleterious mutation on to their children, the question of when to test children arises frequently.[73] Most experts suggest that genetic testing of a minor for a disease that is exceedingly rare before the age of 30 even in high-risk families is inappropriate.[54] Thus for children and most young adults, it is likely that awaiting the outcome of further clinical studies is the best option. Increased awareness, genetic counseling, and potentially genetic testing at 5 years earlier than the age of the youngest cancer patient in the family or at age 30, whichever is the younger, is a reasonable approach given the lack of any other specific information.

More than 100 different genetic changes have been identified in BRCA1, and additional mutations in BRCA1 and BRCA2 are being reported almost daily.[67] Many of these are linked to genetic predisposition to breast and ovarian cancer through cosegregation with cancer in families and soon will likely be linked to specific rates of development of specific cancers and potentially age of onset. As noted above, all termination mutations had been assumed to predispose to genetic predisposition to breast and ovarian cancer, however, recent studies indicate that this may not be correct for all mutations or for all families.[57] Polymorphisms in the coding regions, introns, and potential regulatory regions of BRCA1 and BRCA2 have also been identified.[67] Whether these factors alter the rate of development of cancer is as yet unclear. Nevertheless, the false positive rate is relatively low and is becoming lower as family studies are extended. Unfortunately, the false negative rates of current tests, including DNA sequencing, have not yet been determined but may be fairly high. Current tests assess the sequence either through direct sequencing or sequence-based analysis such as single-strand conformational polymorphism analysis and protein truncation tests of the open reading frame and of part of the introns as well as part of the putative regulatory regions of BRCA1 and BRCA2. As many at 5 to 15% of all mutations in BRCA1 or BRCA2 that predispose to the development of cancer may not be detected by DNA sequencing of these regions. Furthermore, although BRCA1 and BRCA2 account for approximately 80% of the high-penetrance, rare, genetic mutations predisposing to breast and ovarian cancer, additional genetic predisposition genes may exist.[67] Some of these genes may be relatively common but have only a low penetrance and thus may not be identified by current positional cloning techniques. Ovarian cancer is a component of the HNPCC syndrome, and patients with normal BRCA1 or BRCA2 may have mutations in the mismatch repair genes.[73] Usually this can be eliminated by an analysis of the family history. Finally, even if the sequence of all genetic predisposition genes is normal, mutations in somatic cells could still lead to tumor development at the rate observed in the normal population. Thus, unfortunately for most individuals, genetic testing provides only bad news or no news. That is, if genetic testing is positive and detects a specific genetic change known to predispose to the development of cancer, the individual has a lifetime incidence of breast cancer and of ovarian cancer appropriate for that mutation. In the high-risk families so far analyzed, this could be as high as 85% for breast cancer and 60% for ovarian cancer. The data may demonstrate that the mutation contributes to a lower risk of ovarian cancer, such as mutations in BRCA2 or in the carboxy terminal portion of BRCA1.[56,58] Positive test results, although predicting a high lifetime risk of developing cancer, cannot determine if an individual will be among the 20% of mutation carriers who do not develop cancer, or if they do develop cancer at what age it will occur. If genetic testing is negative and fails to detect sequence abnormalities, the individual may still have an abnormality in BRCA1 or BRCA2 that is not detected by testing (i.e., in an intron or a regulatory region), an abnormality in another cancer predisposition gene, or at a minimum the same rate of cancer development as the normal population.[67] However, given that most mutations are detected, a negative test suggests that the chance of the individual carrying a deleterious mutation is much lower than predicted by family history. The only case in which definitive negative results can be delivered to a patient is when a mutation has been identified in another member of the family. The absence of the family-specific mutation makes it highly unlikely that the patient carries an abnormality in BRCA1 or BRCA2. However, it is important to note that at least one individual has inherited independent mutations in BRCA1 from both of her parents.[66] This may be relatively common in Ashkenazi Jewish women in whom the frequency of mutations is much higher than in the normal population.[74–76]

Currently it is not clear which individuals should be tested for abnormalities in BRCA1 or BRCA2 outside research protocols aimed at resolving questions related to penetrance or to the treatment of patients with BRCA1 or BRCA2 mutations. National Institutes of Health (NIH) consensus conferences have suggested that screening for cancer development is appropriate for individuals with a greater than 7% risk of developing this disease.[77] As the incidence of abnormalities in BRCA1 and BRCA2 in the normal population is about 1 in 800, screening of random populations is likely to be expensive, fraught with interpretative difficulties, and complicated by ethical concerns. Thus, screening is generally restricted to individuals with a family history indicative of a potential BRCA1 or BRCA2 mutation or to individuals with early onset of breast or ovarian cancer which increases the chance of finding a mutation in BRCA1 or BRCA2. Given the uncertainty as to how patients with abnormalities in BRCA1 or BRCA2 should be treated, the financial expense of testing, and the potential costs of genetic discrimination, we offer genetic testing to individuals whose family history demonstrates an approximately 10% likelihood of detecting abnormalities in BRCA1 or BRCA2. We also offer testing to individuals considering prophylactic surgery to provide them with additional information in making decisions related to major and possibly mutilating surgery.

As the incidence of specific genetic abnormalities is much higher in some populations such as 185delAG (1%) and5382insC in BRCA1 (0.2%) and 6174delT in BRCA2 (2%) in the Ashkenazi Jewish population and 999del5 in BRCA2 (0.4%) in a population of individuals in Iceland, it would be appropriate to offer analysis for abnormalities at these sites to patients without a strong family history, particularly to women who have had an early onset of breast or ovarian cancer.[74–76,78–80]

Offering testing to relatives of individuals with positive genetic tests also seems to be appropriate. First-degree relatives have a 50% chance of carrying genetic abnormalities, and the risk varies in other individuals depending on the distance of the relationship with the positive proband.

A special case for genetic testing may relate to treatment of an individual with a biopsy-proven breast cancer prior to definitive therapy. While studies have indicated that lumpectomy followed by radiotherapy is an option for women with early breast cancer, the potential for developing second primaries and contralateral tumors suggests that this treatment needs to be reassessed in individuals with mutations in BRCA1 or BRCA2.[67] Until more data are available, the appropriate therapy for these women is not clear.

Although these guidelines can assist in identifying women who would be appropriate for genetic testing, it must be remembered that the designation of 7% for screening and 10% for testing is arbitrary. Decisions related to genetic testing must be the purview of the patient and appropriate for that particular individual.

Screening Protocols for High-risk Individuals

As the National Cancer Institute (NCI) has recommended that screening is appropriate for women with a greater than 7% chance of developing ovarian cancer,[77] identification of individuals with a 10% chance of carrying a mutation in BRCA1 or BRCA2 and enrolling them in screening trials is clearly appropriate. Further, based on family history alone, it is possible to identify individuals with a greater than 7% risk of developing ovarian cancer.[47,48] Thus, women who have a family history predictive of a genetic abnormality, as well as individuals with test-proven abnormalities in BRCA1 or BRCA2, should undergo intensive screening. As noted above, the high number of "events" expected in these at-risk women may not only provide important information related to screening of these individuals or to the penetrance or age of onset of cancers due to specific genetic changes in BRCA1 or BRCA2 but may also provide important information as to the most appropriate screening approaches for the normal population. The difficulty is in identifying and recruiting women who are likely to have abnormalities in BRCA1 and BRCA2 and in delivering accurate, cost-effective molecular diagnostics to those women most likely to benefit from knowledge related to their genetic predisposition to developing breast and ovarian cancer. Although breast self-examination, clinical examination, and mammography lead to early detection of breast cancer in women over the age of 50 and probably improve their quality of life, whether these approaches are effective in premenopausal women remains controversial.[54] As BRCA1 and BRCA2 contribute to an early age of onset of breast and ovarian cancer, with a peak incidence of breast cancer in the forties and an approximately 2% risk per year after the age of 35, it is essential to determine the most appropriate approach in screening for breast and ovarian cancer in these young women.[47,48,67] Although studies comparing the efficacy of mammography with that of other approaches such as ultrasound, position emission tomography (PET) scanning, and MRI imaging in these young, high-risk individuals are under way, definitive results and guidelines will not likely be available in the near future.

The best approach in screening for ovarian cancer outside clinical trials in these at-risk women is even less clear. Given the high risk these individuals have of developing cancer, serial CA 125 measurements and transvaginal ultrasound appear to be reasonable alternatives[1,8,12–15,18–14,25] (see above). Although, guidelines have not been established based on the results of clinical trials, the best current expert advice appears to be to perform an initial CA 125 measurement and a transvaginal ultrasound.[54] If the tests are normal and are followed by normal tests 6 months later, yearly screening is suggested. This may allow patients an opportunity to await the results of studies evaluating the efficacy of prophylactic surgery, cancer prevention, and genetic testing as well as to determine at which point the risk of ovarian cancer development exceeds their own personal comfort level.

It is important to note that these suggestions have not been validated in this high-risk population or indeed in any population.

Prevention

No effective approaches for use in the prevention of breast cancer have yet been defined. However, most individuals who undergo genetic counseling or genetic testing are eligible, based on family history, for enrollment in the Breast Cancer Prevention Trial (using, tamoxifen) or in any other well-designed prevention trials.[81] The birth control pill has been demonstrated to decrease the development of ovarian cancer in the general population.[82,83] A potential increased risk of developing breast cancer may, however, override the benefit related to the prevention of ovarian cancer in this group of individuals.[84] However, in patients with BRCA1 or BRCA2 mutations, the risk of dying of ovarian cancer is greatly increased and may approach or exceed the chance of dying of breast cancer.[47,48,67] If the birth control pill is as effective in preventing cancer in high-risk individuals as it is in the normal population, then it may be a useful alternative for women who wish to retain reproductive potential. Further, it may allow women to delay prophylactic surgery until further data are available.

Prophylactic Surgery

The efficacy of prophylactic surgery in the prevention of breast and ovarian cancer has not been determined. Prophylactic surgery for breast cancer in high-risk individuals defined solely on the basis of family history has a failure rate that may be as high as 5%.[85–87] Given that the population evaluated likely had a 20 to 30% chance of developing breast cancer, the real failure rate for individuals with a BRCA1 or BRCA2 abnormality may be higher. However, this probably represents a significant decrease in the chance of developing breast cancer prophylactic surgery.

Fewer data are currently available on the efficacy of prophylactic oophorectomy in these individuals. Registries have been established, and it is expected that new data will be available soon. Although some individuals who have undergone prophylactic oophorectomy do develop clinically evident peritoneal carcinomatosis indistinguishable from ovarian cancer, the frequency is unclear but is less than 5%, providing significant rates of protection.[88–92] Further, whether this represents a pre-existing ovarian cancer that has metastasized to the peritoneal cavity, a tumor arising in an ovarian remnant, or transformation of the peritoneal mesothelium due to a lack of BRCA1 or BRCA2 function in this related tissue is unknown. In the absence of definitive data, it is likely that prophylactic oophorectomy decreases the chance of developing ovarian cancer, but the magnitude of the protection is unknown.

Genetic Discrimination

Obtaining health, disability, and life insurance involves a commercial transaction between an individual and a company driven by a desire to return a profit to its investors.[71] The insurance company generally distributes the risk of an individual over a broad group and assigns a rate or availability of insurance that is appropriate both for the client and for the owners or investors. It is difficult to argue that automobile insurance should not be based on driving record or "risk" or that smoking should not be considered a risk factor in determining health or life insurance rates. Insurance companies have argued, similarly, that family history has been available and has been used to establish risk in the past and that it is their right and perhaps even their obligation to use this information in determining rates and availability of insurance. The question of whether genetic counseling or identification of a genetic abnormality in a cancer predisposition gene should be used to assess risk remains unresolved. To require that insurance companies not use such information is passing a social obligation on to a commercial entity. Indeed, it could be argued that the insurance rates for individuals with no family history of cancer or for those that test negative for changes in cancer predisposition genes are artificially elevated to account for the development of cancer in high-risk individuals. Nevertheless, it seems that genetic discrimination should be accorded the same significance as discrimination based on racial or ethnic background.

Although a number of states have enacted legislation that decreases the chance that genetic counseling or genetic testing will be used either to increase medical insurance rates or to deny such insurance, current laws are insufficient to provide absolute protection. Further, none of these laws have been tested in the courts. The federal insurance portability law does not provide protection to individuals who lose their employment or to those who do not have employer insurance plans. Further, many proposed or enacted laws do not provide protection against discrimination related to disability or insurability.[70,71] Indeed, several enacted laws specifically permit insurance companies to employ genetic testing or genetic information to determine rates or eligibility for life insurance. Although genetic testing is currently too expensive for most insurance companies to use routinely, CHIP technology (see below) may allow rapid, inexpensive testing insurance companies will consider a reasonable investment. The frequency with which insurance companies utilize family history, which is a fairly accurate method for establishing risk, or the patient having obtained genetic counseling or genetic testing in establishing rates or availability is not clear.[70,71] Thus, until the questions related to genetic predisposition to cancer and insurability have been resolved, it is important to maintain information on patients in as confidential a manner as is possible. At each step, we consult with an ethicist and with legal counsel as to the appropriate approach. Further, all patients are required to sign a series of consent forms stating that they are aware of the potential risks and of the lack of knowledge of how to manage specific genetic changes. Many research protocols approved by the institutional Review Board allow this information to be retained in a separate file not linked to a patient's main chart.

Unlike the situation for most other diseases, in this case genetic counseling and genetic testing can potentially be used by insurance companies to alter rates or availability of insurance to relatives or family members. Thus, testing places not only the patient at risk but can also potentially affect relatives. This opens up a completely new area of ethical and legal concerns which has not been thoroughly explored or resolved.

Confidentiality

In addition to the insurance and genetic discrimination issues described above, confidentiality also potentially affects clinicians. As information obtained through genetic counseling and testing may not only affect the proband but also may be important to the patient's relatives, are clinicians responsible for contacting relatives or encouraging patients to inform relatives? An effort must be made to respect the autonomy of the patient, however, one must also consider our legal requirements for beneficence, our obligation to benefit others, or nonmaleficence, our obligation to not harm others. At the M.D. Anderson Cancer Center, we take the position that our "contract" is with the patients and that our obligation to be fair to them and respect their autonomy takes precedence. Thus, we do not contact relatives directly. Rather patients are empowered to decide whether they wish to make the initial contact and relatives are contacted only after a signed request has been made by both parties. Whether we should encourage patients to contact relatives and suggest that they obtain counseling or testing is under discussion with our ethicist at present. As with all other aspects of genetic counseling at this time, we feel that a nondirective approach is required.

One of the more specific problems that has not been resolved is whether written or even verbal communication with a referring clinician is appropriate. Thus far, we have made this the purview of the patient and do not send a letter to the referring clinician. The patient's primary-care clinician may thus be denied important information that could be integral to the treatment of the patient. This also potentially interferes with the ability to obtain referrals and to achieve the best treatment for other patients. It also hinders the education of primary-care physicians in this rapidly emerging field. These issues have not been resolved and will be resolved only through the passage of time, the passage of appropriate laws, and the decisions of the courts.

Anonymous Testing

In view of the potential risk of genetic discrimination, a possible alternative is to encourage or allow anonymous testing.[93] As noted above, given that extensive genetic counseling is required, that further research studies are needed, and that lifelong surveillance is essential for individuals who test positive, it would be very difficult to provide this information in a truly anonymous manner.

QUESTION 4

Is there any evidence to support the use of resistance modulators in the treatment of ovarian cancer? What about the use of chemoresistance assays?

ELISE C. KOHN

An exciting and equally controversial area in the development of ovarian cancer therapeutics is the question of chemoresistance modulation and chemoresistance or sensitivity testing. The two major chemotherapeutic agents for ovarian cancer, platinum and paclitaxel, appear to be non-cross-resistant and have different mechanisms of resistance. The lack of significantly active second-line chemotherapy for ovarian cancer has spurred interest in the development of chemoresistance-reversing agents and assays for chemoresistance and chemosensitivity. The key questions are (1) Will resistance modulators work in vivo? (2) What are the best clinical trial designs for determining efficacy? (3) Will chemoresistance or chemosensitivity assays accurately predict the in vivo phenotype? (4) Is there a cost benefit of using this approach?

The two predominant proposed mechanisms of chemoresistance to ovarian cancer therapeutics are (1) drug efflux, as in the case of MDR-1, the multidrug resistance P-glycoprotein efflux pump (paclitaxel and doxorubicin), and (2) altered DNA repair (platinum and alkylating agents). Chemoresistance reversal is of increasing therapeutic interest in view of widespread use of the natural product paclitaxel which is a good MDR-1 substrate in vitro.[94] As such, paclitaxel has become the agent of choice in chemoresistance modulator clinical trials. This approach in the treatment of ovarian cancer assumes that MDR-1 overexpression is a primary component of drug resistance, although this assumption has not yet been addressed fully. Although studies performed prior to the broad use of paclitaxel did not indicate high MDR-1 expression de novo in ovarian cancer, there are anecdotal comments on the increased frequency of MDR-1 expression in ovarian cancer patients with a history of paclitaxel treatment.[94–96] This issue is critical in the design, execution, and interpretation of resistance modulator trials.

Of interest during the development of strategies for testing chemomodulators was the observation that just altering the administration schedule of many natural product agents was associated with improved response outcome.[97,98] Trials to date have not demonstrated marked improvement with the chemomodulators. Second-generation agents are now entering trials, and PSC833, a cyclosporin analog, is the most promising.[99] The clinical role of the newer multidrug resistance protein, MRP-1, a transporter of glutathione-conjugated agents, is just now being elucidated.[97] Approaches to overcoming alkylator and cisplatin resistance with the use of glutathione conjugation employing agents such as buthionine sulfoximine (BSO) are now under investigation.[101,101]

Enhanced DNA repair via the nucleotide excision repair pathway is a primary mechanism of resistance to platinum compounds, as is DNA repair via the mismatch repair pathway for alkylating agents.[102] New areas for investigation of resistance to ovarian cancer drugs include genes involved in DNA repair resistance pathways. DNA repair is a critical determinant of platinum chemosensitivity and sensitivity to alkylating agents through the ERCC/XPA nucleotide excision repair system and the mismatch repair genes, respectively.[102,103] Retrospective analysis has demonstrated an increase in ERCC-1 expression in patients who received platinum compounds for treatment of newly diagnosed ovarian cancer and did not attain complete or partial response.[104,105] A synergy in preventing repair of cisplatin-DNA adducts has been shown for paclitaxel, suggesting that chemotherapeutics themselves may be useful in abrogating drug resistance.[103] Further characterization of the role of these enzymes in chemotherapy responsiveness may lead to novel resistance or sensitivity strategies and gene therapy approaches. Studies on glutathione balance and its role in chemosensitivity in ovarian cancer have led to the development of buthionine sulfoximine.[100] This agent has now been investigated in phase I clinical trials, and further development is ongoing.

The next controversy involves the utility and cost-benefit advantages of chemoresistance and chemosensitivity assays. In vitro analysis of the sensitivity or lack thereof of an individual patient's tumor has been studied for several decades. That it is still an investigational and experimental approach, despite the fact that patients can purchase tumor drug testing commercially, in part answers the question. A myriad of tests are under investigation and available for purchase, however, no one technique has been supported by the investigators themselves, let alone by the oncology field. Despite numerous correlative retrospective and some prospective trials, this technology has not been proved or adopted. Do chemosensitivity tests predict accurately? The answer to this question is difficult given that in some experimental designs over half of samples may not reach the final stage of testing because of inadequate numbers of available cells. While most studies confirm the predictive value of the test, its clinical utility has not been confirmed or tested in a randomized prospective fashion. Some interesting observations have been made, however. In lung cancer, for instance, patients whose tumors grew in culture for subsequent chemosensitivity testing had a worse prognosis than those whose tumors did not. Chemosensitivity testing was not found to be better than standard chemotherapy administered to patients whose tumors did not grow or for whom an inadequate amount of tissue was obtained.[106] If a test could be agreed upon and executed reliably, a phase III randomized trial would be necessary to determine if chemosensitivity testing is the proper mechanism for determinating treatment planning. Until adequate support is generated for this procedure, it should be considered experimental. A secondary but important question concerns the cost-benefit advantages of this technique.[107] While ovarian cancer tissue is readily available at debulking laparotomy, the financial cost of this testing and the risk of delay in treatment while awaiting results should be considered.

GORDON B. MILLS
ROBERT C. BAST, JR.

Despite being potentially exciting approaches, resistance modulators and chemoresistance assays have not yet been validated in prospective clinical trials in ovarian cancer. This is not to suggest that further trials are not appropriate but rather that at the present time the use of resistance modulators and chemoresistance assays outside hypothesis-driven clinical trials has not been scientifically justified.

Although drug sensitivity testing is commercially available and frequently obtained, its usefulness in the treatment of ovarian cancer remains controversial.[107] Studies employing a number of model systems have suggested that patterns of drug resistance observed in vitro are frequently recapitulated when cells are assessed in in vivo model systems.[107] However, the converse does necessarily appear to be true. Although cells demonstrate sensitivity to chemotherapeutic drugs when cultured under anchorage-dependent conditions on plastic, they may not necessarily demonstrate the same pattern of sensitivity to chemotherapeutic drugs when studied in vivo.[108] The different pattern of sensitivity to chemotherapeutic drugs in vitro and in vivo may result from (1) lack of appropriate paracrine and autocrine interactions in vitro, (2) lack of cell:cell contact in vitro, (3) failure to form tight junctions in vitro, (4) effects of a chemotherapeutic drug on processes that occur only in vivo such as neovascularization, metastases, and paracrine growth factor production, and (5) failure to obtain similar drug bioavailability in vitro and in vivo. At least in some circumstances, the pattern of sensitivity to cytotoxic drugs in vivo can be recapitulated in vitro by studies of "cellules" which allow analysis of cells in a three-dimensional structure. Similar patterns for both paclitaxel and cisplatin sensitivity and resistance can be observed in sensitive and resistant cell lines in vitro and in vivo utilizing this assay. Whether additional cell lines or freshly isolated patient cells demonstrate a similar concordance between drug sensitivity in cellules and in vivo remains to be established. Furthermore, many fresh patient tumor samples and even cancer cell lines do not form cellules in vitro, potentially limiting the applicability of this approach.

Whether the resistance to drugs in a three-dimensional cellule construct in vitro represents an ability to transport drugs or protective molecules through tight junctions or inherent alterations in sensitivity to programmed cell death induced in a three-dimensional matrix also has not been resolved. As activation of several different growth factor receptors can alter the ability of chemotherapeutic drugs to induce programmed cell death, it is possible that growth factor signaling, expression of growth factor receptors, or production of growth factors can be regulated by three-dimensional structure.[109–111] Indeed, a number of different peptide growth factors, particularly those in the EGF family, are synthesized as active cell surface molecules. Thus cell-cell contact may play a role in their activity. Indeed, antibodies to the epidermal growth factor receptor and to the erbB2 receptor can alter the sensitivity of tumor cells to the effects of various cytotoxic drugs.[109,110] In addition, downregulating the expression of erbB2 by gene therapy-mediated introduction of E1A or intracellular antibodies to erbB2 results in increased sensitivity to chemotherapeutic drugs.[112,113]

Despite the potential advantages of tailoring therapy to drug sensitivity and resistance profiles specific to the patient's own tumor rather than treating ovarian cancer as a homogeneous disease, there are no data suggesting that chemosensitivity testing as currently performed is sufficiently predictive to alter the outcome in ovarian cancer.[107] Further, the requirement that cells be obtained through surgery, laparoscopy, or needle biopsy makes sensitivity testing expensive. It is potentially fraught with difficulties in obtaining cells and delays in therapy while awaiting results of testing. Finally, since cells cannot be cultured from all patients, particularly as cellules or in semisolid media, the outcome of any clinical trial attempting to determine the efficacy of chemosensitivity testing may be biased by being able to assess only patients whose tumors grow under specific culture conditions. It is intriguing, however, that preliminary studies on needle biopsies of patients with ovarian cancer suggest that it may be possible to grow tumor cells from most of these patients. Nevertheless, one study on lung cancer patients demonstrated that although drug sensitivity testing did not successfully predict response to therapy, the ability to grow cells in culture was associated with a worsened outcome.[114]

Research and clinical studies designed to determine whether altering patient treatment based on chemosensitivity testing affects the outcome of therapy in ovarian cancer are clearly warranted. As ovarian cancers are generally highly responsive to initial chemotherapy, it is frequently possible to decrease the tumor burden to very low levels. However, current therapeutic approaches are disappointing in terms of the ability to convert these responses to cures. Nevertheless, a number of different chemotherapeutic drugs have been demonstrated to have activity as second-line approaches in ovarian cancer. Whether the 10 to 20% response rates seen with many second-line therapies represent an effect on the same subset of patients or whether different drugs are active in different subsets of patients is not known. The use of consolidation therapy in patients who have responded to primary therapy is an attractive approach in improving the cure rate in this disease. Thus, studies to determine whether chemosensitivity testing can identify individuals who are likely to respond to particular consolidation therapy or those who are not and should not be subjected to the potential toxicities of chemotherapeutics must have a high priority.

There are two classes of resistance modulators, those that increase the efficacy of a therapeutic drug in tumor cells and those that increase the resistance of targets of toxicity such as bone marrow cells and nerve cells. Given that cisplatin and paclitaxel are the two most widely used drugs in ovarian cancer, drugs that potentially alter the efflux or action of cisplatin (such as modulators of glutathione levels) or potentially alter the efflux of paclitaxel (such as inhibitors of the multidrug resistance [MDR] gene product) are attractive agents for increasing the efficacy of current chemotherapeutic regimens.[98–100,115,116] In addition to altering intracellular concentrations of cisplatin or paclitaxel, therapeutic approaches that alter the sensitivity of cells to the mechanistic action of these drugs (e.g., decreasing the ability of cells to repair cisplatin-induced DNA damage and paclitaxel-induced tubule bundling) are attractive for further investigation of resistance modulation.[102–105] As an alternative approach, both cisplatin and paclitaxel induce programmed cell death; thus agents that alter the ability of cells to enter the programmed cell death pathway are also worth evaluation. These drugs could target signal transduction pathways such as antibodies to EGF receptors which decrease receptor signaling and increase sensitivity to chemotherapeutics or rapamycin which specifically inhibits the activity of FRAP and P70S6 kinase and increases the activity of cisplatin in ovarian cancer cell lines.[109,110,119] Indeed, current patient trials aimed at modulating erbB2 expression or signaling probably function by altering the rate at which cells undergo programmed cell death. These approaches can be used synergistically or at least additively with current cytotoxic drugs. Alternatively, agents that increase the activity of proapoptotic proteins such as members of the BCL2 and ICE protease families may prove to be synergistic with current therapeutics. Whether chemotherapeutic drugs will have altered activities in cells in which intact or aberrant cell cycle progression machinery is a target for further investigation. p53 and induction of the p21 cyclin-dependent kinase inhibitors (CDKI) have been demonstrated to be integrally related to the ability of a number of different cytotoxic drugs and radiation to induce programmed cell death. Although the expression of p53 in ovarian cancer has proven not to be a strong indicator of prognosis or response to therapy,[118] the expression and action of cyclin-dependent kinase (CDK), CDKIs retinoblastoma, and E2F-1 may not only regulate cell cycle progression but may also play an important role in regulating programmed cell death. Thus reintroduction of p53 or CDKIs into cells through gene therapy may not only decrease cell cycle progression but may also alter the sensitivity of tumor cells to the effects of cytotoxic drugs.

Cisplatin does not appear to be transported by the MDR pathway and thus is not an appropriate target for modulation of MDR activity. Furthermore, MDR-1 apparently is not overexpressed in ovarian cancer cells either before or after chemotherapy.[95,96,119] However, paclitaxel is transported by MDR-1. Thus studies on MDR-1 transport inhibitors such as analogs of cyclosporin A seem warranted in the context of paclitaxel. However, despite initial enthusiasm, clinical trials of MDR-1 inhibitors have not yet demonstrated significant activity in studies with other substrates for MDR-1.[98,99]

Analogous to MDR-1, which acts as a drug transporter, MRP-1 may play a role in transport of glutathione-conjugated molecules such as glutathione cisplatin complexes. Glutathione levels correlate with resistance to cisplatin, perhaps through increased transport of cisplatin from cells.[97] BSO, an agent that decreases intracellular glutathione levels by inhibiting γ-glutamylcysteine synthetase, increases toxicity associated with platinum analogs in vitro at least in part by altering transport of glutathione platinum complexes.[100,115,116] Whether or not BSO alters cisplatin activity in vivo remains controversial and probably awaits the results of phase II and III trials. Whether achievable decreases in glutathione levels alter the effect of platinum analogs on ovarian cancer cells without concurrently increasing toxic side effects remains to be evaluated in ongoing trials.[101]

As the mechanisms by which resistance to platinum analogs and paclitaxel are elucidated, it should become possible to alter them through drug discovery or through gene therapy. As noted above, antibodies to the EGF receptor or to erbB2 are undergoing clinical trials for ovarian cancer.[109,110] The initial results suggest that these antibodies can induce responses either directly or in combination with cytotoxic drugs. Gene therapeutic delivery of E1A through viral vectors or through liposome-mediated transfer downregulates the expression of erbB2 through a transcriptional mechanism,[112] and this downregulation renders cells sensitive to programmed cell death mediated by cytotoxic drugs. Virus-mediated introduction of the MDR-1 gene into bone marrow stem cells has resulted in stable overexpression of the MDR-1 gene in bone marrow, and in preclinical models, to increased resistance of bone marrow cells to the action of paclitaxel.[120,121] Phase I studies in humans have demonstrated that MDR-1 can be delivered to bone marrow stem cells ex vivo and that expression can be maintained in cancer patients. No untoward toxicity was identified. Thus gene therapy as a modulator of drug resistance may provide a proof of concept which can either move toward general acceptance of gene therapy approaches or potentially provide an incentive for drug discovery leading to the identification of small-molecule inhibitors which mediate similar actions.

QUESTION 5

What are the most attractive agents for use in gene therapy?

ELISE C. KOHN

The ability to introduce novel genes into hematopoietic cells or tumor cells has opened a new avenue for clinical investigation in gene therapy. Gene introduction targets include using drug resistance genes such as MDR-1 and MRP-1 in hematopoietic cells to allow for increased dose intensity, introduction of immunomodulatory genes into T cells or tumor cells to stimulate local tumor immune response, and introduction of suicide gene constructs which induce cells to undergo apoptosis when exposed to the proper associated drug.[120,122,124] Tumor cells modified with herpes simplex virus thymidine kinase (HSV-TK) are acutely sensitive to the antiviral antibiotic ganciclovir.[122,125] Upon exposure to this drug, these cells die because of their inability to use the phosphorylated form of ganciclovir formed by the activation of HSV-TK. Since a small proportion of cells are successfully infected with the HSV-TK construct, for the large cell kill observed in experimental models to occur, a bystander effect must take place. This approach is now under investigation with protocols approved for studies on ovarian cancer patients.[122,126] Whether or not this technique offers a viable, broadly usable therapeutic intervention is yet to be determined.

An alternative type of gene therapy for which more clinical data have been garnered is the use of MDR genes, allowing chemotherapy dose intensification without the bone marrow toxicity observed with most cytotoxic agents.[120] Transduction of hematopoietic stem cells with MDR-1 has been accomplished with demonstrations in vitro and in vivo of successful gene transcription and translation. Further studies have indicated that this transduced population of cells can be selectively amplified in patient marrow after treatment with marrow-ablative drugs.[127–129] New protocol strategies are under development that use this technique to improve chemotherapy delivery in doses necessary to overcome endogenous or induced expression of MDR-1.

Success with this strategy will lead to similar trials with other multidrug resistance genes such as MRP-1 and nucleotide excision repair genes. The risks imposed upon patients include fewer or even nonreversible secondary toxicities of many cytotoxic agents in use today, including neuropathy, ototoxicity, and cardiopulmonary toxicity. The use of gene therapy in overcoming bone marrow toxicity may lead only to a more serious toxicity profile. Secondarily, if patients were rendered disease-free for long periods of time, we do not know what the random insertion of MDR-1 or other genes into hematopoietic stem cells would do to these cells, underscored by the fact that we do not know what the normal function is for many so-called chemotherapy resistance genes.

GORDON B. MILLS
ROBERT C. BAST, JR.

Several gene therapy approaches for ovarian cancer are being evaluated in preclinical and clinical trials. They are based on (1) changing the resistance of bone marrow stem cells to chemotherapeutic agents through the introduction of MDR or MRP genes, thus allowing dose-intensive treatments; (2) tumor vaccines designed to alter antitumor immune responses through the introduction of putative tumor antigens, cytokines, and costimulatory molecules; (3) suicide constructs such as HSV-TK, bacterial nitroreductase, or other prodrug-converting enzymes; (4) altering expression of cell cycle and programmed cell death regulators; and (5) targeting specific genetic changes occurring tumor cells through (a) reintroduction of tumor suppressor genes such as BRCA1 and p53 or (b) introduction of molecules that alter expression or function of oncogenes such as E1A or intracellular anti-erbB2 antibodies that decrease cell surface expression of erbB2.

The success of gene therapy will depend on the development of appropriate vectors as much as on the identification of targets. It will probably be necessary to target the vector to the appropriate bone marrow stem cell, immune effector cell, or tumor cell, and this targeting can be either at the level of delivery or at the level of expression. It may be necessary to design vectors that preferentially deliver the gene therapeutic to the appropriate target cells without delivery to normal cells in order to generate a therapeutic index. Alternatively and probably in concert, it will be important to design vectors that preferentially express the gene therapeutic in the appropriate target cell. In addition to resolving questions related to specificity, it will likely be necessary to increase the efficiency of transduction of the gene therapeutic prior to gene therapy becoming a practical approach. Most current in vivo techniques, including adenovirus, retrovirus, liposomal, and related technologies, efficiently transduce only a small portion of the target population.

Several studies suggest that bystander effects may occur in which targeting of only a portion of tumor cells can lead to tumor regression.[130–135] In in vitro models, only the tumor is available for assessment. In vivo, the complex interactions involved in tumor growth may be highly sensitive to perturbation of only a small portion of tumor cells. Indeed, the target of gene therapy in vivo need not be restricted to the tumor cell, as paracrine interactions or neovasculature may be required for effective tumor growth and survival. Several studies have suggested that bystander effects occur because the primary target of the gene therapeutic is the tumor microvasculature rather than the malignant cell per se.[135] Alternatively, active drugs converted from prodrugs by suicide genes such HSV-TK or bacterial nitroreductase may be transferred from one cell to another through tight junctions or by release from dying cells and uptake by pinocytosis.[133] The latter mechanism could potentially transfer larger products of gene therapeutics. Furthermore, death and lysis of target cells may lead to the production of cytolytic T cells or of cytokines which can alter immune responsiveness.

Progress is beginning to be made in the identification of cell lineage-specific promoters that drive gene expression in several lineages. For example, the probasin promoter, which appears to be highly expressed in prostate cells but not in other lineages, is an attractive promoter for delivery of gene therapeutics to prostate cancer cells. Unfortunately, ovarian epithelium-specific promoters that can drive a target gene specifically in ovarian epithelium have not yet been identified. Indeed, very little is known about the molecular genetics of ovarian epithelium that could facilitate the development of ovarian epithelium-specific promoters. Most of the genes known to be expressed in ovarian epithelium are widely expressed in a number of other epithelial lineages and in particular in mammary epithelium. Further, promoters or indeed markers capable of distinguishing between ovarian epithelial cancer cells and peritoneal mesothelial cells have not yet been identified. Thus, the identification of ovarian epithelium-specific promoters should remain a high priority for ongoing research.

Methods for specifically targeting only malignant ovarian epithelial cells are not yet available. Retroviruses, which replicate only in proliferating cells, may provide an approach in the regional therapy of ovarian cancer, where most of the proliferating cells in the peritoneal cavity are likely to be of malignant origin. One exciting approach is to utilize cell surface proteins as targets to increase the delivery of gene therapeutics to ovarian cancer cells. This can be accomplished by incorporating targeting mechanisms into the delivery system. Antibodies or even the ligand for cell surface receptors can be incorporated as part of the surface of viral constructs or as integral parts of a liposome.[136–138] The viral construct or liposome preferentially binds to tumor cells and is internalized through receptor-mediated endocytosis. Alternatively, ligand or antibody could be included as part of a DNA-protein complex.[136–138] In this approach, the gene therapeutic is bound to a ligand or to an antibody through a flexible linker. The DNA complex is then delivered to the cell through internalization of the receptor complex via receptor-mediated endocytosis. This technique can be used to deliver gene therapy to cells through any cell surface receptor that is internalized following ligation. Overexpression of the folate and erbB2 receptors by ovarian cancer cells makes them attractive targets as mediators providing cell-specific delivery for gene therapy.[138]

Ovarian cancer cells appear to express unusual splice variants of both CD44 and the EGF receptor.[139,140] If these variants are confirmed to be relatively specific to tumor cells, an alternative approach in generating ovarian cancer-specific expression of gene therapy would be to place the gene therapeutic in an open reading frame downstream of the unique splice acceptor sites present in the tumor-specific CD44 or EGF receptor splice variants. The tumor, but not normal cells, would be expected to process the RNA in such a manner as to produce functional expression of the gene therapeutic in the tumor cell but not in other cell lineages. This would hopefully provide a high therapeutic ratio.

In addition to its use in delivering gene therapy to ovarian cancer cells, erbB2 is an attractive target for gene therapy.[112] Decreasing erbB2 levels either with the E1A adenovirus protein or through intracellular antibodies increases programmed cell death directly and probably renders cells more sensitive to the effects of cytotoxic drugs.[112,113] As elevated erbB2 levels appear to be required to sensitize cells to this activity, normal cells may be spared the effects of these potential gene therapy approaches. This strategy may, however, be restricted to the one-third of tumors that overexpress erbB2.[33]

As p53 is mutated in over 50% of ovarian tumors, it is an attractive target for gene therapy.[118] Ovarian cancer cells can be growth-inhibited both in vitro and vivo by introduction of p53 via adenoviral vectors.[141,142] Further, as p53 is required for the efficient killing of tumor cells by some chemotherapeutic agents, its introduction may induce growth inhibition and sensitize cells to the action of chemotherapy as well. Other cell cycle regulators are attractive mediators for gene therapy. Introduction of the p21, p27, p57, p15, and p16 CDKIs should inhibit cell cycle progression of ovarian cancer, regardless of whether these mediators are aberrant in ovarian cancer cells or not. Indeed, we have demonstrated that retroviral delivery of p16 to ovarian cancer cells inhibits cell cycle progression.[143] The retinblastoma (RB) protein located downstream of CDK-cyclin complexes is regulated by phosphorylation, with nonphosphorylated retinoblastoma protein binding and inactivating the E2F transcription factor complex. An intriguing second-start codon RB protein has been identified[144] which continues to bind and inactivate E2F following phosphorylation, thus inhibiting cell cycle progression. E2F-1 has been demonstrated to program cells for apoptosis so it, along with ICE family proteases and proapoptotic members of the BCL2, provides an attractive approach for gene therapy. In addition to the E2F family of transcription mediators other transcription factors such as Jun, which is inhibited by the Tam67 construct, and PEA3, which may be a major mediator of erbB2 transcription, are intriguing targets for therapy.[145]

Recent studies on the BRCA1 gene suggest that it may prove to be a target for gene therapy. Introduction of this gene in vitro and in vivo inhibits the growth of ovarian cancer cells and of breast cancer cells but not those of other lineages.[58] Further, it appears to be sufficient to initiate programmed cell death.[146] The initial preclinical and animal data have been sufficiently exciting to lead to a phase I human trial.

A number of potential ovarian cancer suppressor genes including SPARC, NOEY2, DOC2, LOT1, OVCA1, and others have been identified by methods aimed at characterizing differential expression of genes in normal ovarian epithelial cells and ovarian cancer cells.[147–149] These genes may not only provide insight into the mechanisms contributing to ovarian tumorigenesis but may also provide attractive targets for gene therapy.

Thus there are several attractive targets for gene therapy for ovarian cancer. Following the development of high-efficiency vectors for selective delivery or expression of these targets in ovarian cancer, it is hoped that preclinical and clinical studies will provide proof of concept for one target or another in the therapy of ovarian cancer. Prior to the development of such vectors preliminary studies aimed at determining potential toxicity and assessing whether the bystander response can be exploited are well justified. In view of the difficulty in delivering large molecules to appropriate targets, whether gene therapy will be the eventual approach or whether gene therapy will provide a proof of concept leading to the development of specific small-molecule molecular mimics awaits the test of time.

QUESTION 6

Please discuss future directions in this area.

ELISE C. KOHN

New directions in the development of treatment approaches for ovarian cancer are clearly needed. The improved responses to first-line therapy observed in the (GOG) trial of paclitaxel and cisplatin are tempered by the continued high-relapse rate in patients with pathologic complete responses at second-look surgery.[151] This is further complicated by the decreasing frequency of secondary surgical assessments and the discontinuation of therapy because of a normal CA 125 value when small-volume disease frequently remains behind. Thus, one area for consideration is identification of more sensitive tumor markers and maintenance or adjuvant therapy after completion of tumor reduction chemotherapy. Options for adjuvant therapy include tumor vaccines, cytostatic agents for response maintenance, and dose-intensive consolidative therapy with marrow reconstitution.

An alternative investigational approach is to utilize the body's internal surveillance system to reduce the remaining tumor burden through stimulation of the immune system. Two systems are under study utilizing tumor vaccines or adoptive immunotherapy through induction of the patient's own tumor cells. These are based on the hypotheses that despite having received chemotherapy, the patient remains immunocompetent and is able to further activate and expand T-cell-mediated immunological memory which recognizes tumor cells as nonself.[123,152–154] Tumor vaccines are created by taking a patient's tumor cells and transducing them with the gene of interest, followed by inactivation and reintroduction into the patient to achieve a specific immunization effect. Alternatively, the patient's T cells are isolated, transduced with immunomodulators, and then reintroduced into the patient. Clinical trials of immunomodulation are ongoing for several tumor types, including ovarian cancer.

Investigation of the invasive biology and potential of ovarian tumors is another important direction for future studies. In colon cancer and breast cancer there is a well established progression from hyperplasia to in situ carcinoma to locally invasive and then metastatic disease, and angiogenesis and invasion are surprisingly early events in this process.[155–157] Angiogenesis is critical for the proliferation of benign and malignant tumor masses larger than 0.125 mm^2 and also provides conduits for the metastasis of cells. Lymphatic conduits are also critical, as they provide a prominent pathway for ovarian cancer dissemination. Hollingsworth and colleagues[158] studied the neovasculature of advanced ovarian cancer specimens and correlated vessel counts with clinical outcome after dose-intensive platinum-based chemotherapy and found a striking correlation between vessel development and overall survival. This supports the hypothesis that antiangiogenic therapies may be useful adjuncts in the treatment of ovarian cancer. Interestingly, all the antiangiogenic therapies under clinical investigation to date are cytostatic agents.[159,160]

Angiogenesis is a provocative target for several other reasons. The observation that vascular endothelial cell-derived growth factor (VEGF) is a mitogen for ovarian cancer in vitro and in animal models and that VEGF antibody treatment in animal models can reduce the ovarian cancer tumor burden opens a new area for potential diagnostics and therapeutics.[161–164] The process of neovascularization is an active one that utilizes the same cellular machinery physiologically as a tumor cell does during invasion.[165] Endothelial cells and tumor cells must interact with their extracellular basement membrane and matrix during activation and capillary sprout formation or the active process of malignant invasion.[156,157,159,163] A key process, necessary but not sufficient for successful angiogenesis or metastasis, is the production and activation of key proteinases for local degradation of the basement membrane.[157] Matrix metalloproteinase-2 (MMP-2), a 72-kDa neutral proteinase, is induced during angiogenesis and malignant invasion. Numerous cancers have increased MMP-2 expression compared with that of the local surrounding tissue. Several novel approaches using translational potential to modulate MMP-2 activity or production have been developed and clinical testing started.[157,166,167] These agents, too, have been found to be cytostatic. First, inhibition of MMP-2 production in ovarian cancer cells and endothelial cells by carboxyamidotriazole (CAI), an inhibitor of calcium influx, has been demonstrated.[167] CAI is a cytostatic antiangiogenesis agent with antiinvasive and antiproliferative properties.[156,160,167–169] Second, drugs targeted at the activation of MMP-2 have been developed and clinical testing started. BB-94 (Batimistat) has been shown to inhibit MMP-2 activity and reduce ascitic burden in ovarian cancer-bearing mice[166,170] and is under clinical investigation as an intraperitoneally administered agent. The development of these two agents suggests that this otherwise controversial area of drug targeting is a viable approach for which further testing is indicated.

Last, better understanding of the genetic progression of ovarian cancer development and dissemination will lead to insight into diagnostic and therapeutic approaches. Further understanding of the risk of BRCA1 mutations as discussed above may lead to improved surveillance of at-risk individuals, which will lead to identification of a population for whom prevention trials may be developed. The development of techniques for gene evaluation requiring microscopic amounts of tissue will expand our ability to discern the molecular basis of ovarian tumorigenesis. As more is known about the molecular genetic makeup of gynecologic cancers, their biochemical and molecular pathways of progression, and their drug responsiveness, newer diagnostic, prognostic, and therapeutic approaches can be developed.

GORDON B. MILLS
ROBERT C. BAST, JR.

Emerging areas of research in ovarian cancer

As described above, research designed to identify new tumor markers and approaches and to assess their role in the early diagnosis of ovarian cancer is an important objective for ongoing research. Patients with an inherited predisposition to ovarian cancer may provide an important resource in determining the best use of early markers in the diagnosis of this disease. Identification of markers that can predict outcome so that patient trials can be stratified on the basis of prognosis remains a high priority. Furthermore, development of therapeutics using either gene therapy or small molecules based on an understanding of the mechanisms by which these markers contribute to prognosis and other genetic abnormalities in tumors should be explored. The rapidly emerging area of genetic predisposition to cancer leads to an incredible number of questions, most importantly, how best to treat individuals with a family history of breast and ovarian cancer as well as those who have positive tests following genetic analysis. Understanding why we can achieve multiple log kills of ovarian cancer cells and a significant frequency of remissions yet rarely induce curative changes in tumour growth is an ongoing problem. Further, treating patients as individuals and tailoring therapy to the molecular genetic changes in their tumors would potentially provide a mechanism for increased efficacy combined with decreased toxicity. Additional targets for therapy, both gene therapy and molecular therapeutics specific to ovarian cancer, remain to be identified. Further studies on differential gene expression, isolation of genes driving amplification and loss of heterozygosity in ovarian cancer, identification and characterization of additional tumor suppressors and proto-oncogenes in ovarian cancer, and understanding of the mechanisms leading to activation of signal transduction pathways regulating cell growth, programmed cell death, senescence, neovascularization, invasion, protease production, metastases, and drug resistance should identify new markers and targets that can be applied to ovarian cancer. However, as detailed below, the greatest challenge for the next 10 years will be the application of our rapidly emerging concepts of the molecular drivers of tumorigenesis to patient treatment, hopefully leading to effective early diagnostics and novel therapeutics for this devastating disease.

Current therapy for ovarian cancer is based on a small set of well-established prognostic criteria such as histologic type, stage, grade, and amount of residual tumor. This treatment has not resulted in a substantial increase in the cure rate for epithelial ovarian cancer, with similar survival rates in the 1990s as were achieved in the 1950s. The vast majority of women with advanced epithelial ovarian cancer currently receive a single initial therapy based on cisplatin and paclitaxel. This treatment ignores the genetic changes and specific characteristics of each patient's tumor and treats epithelial ovarian cancer as a single entity. If we can understand the genetic aberrations that occur during the development of ovarian cancer, we may be able to design strategies that will prevent cancer development, establish prognosis, identify individuals likely to respond to particular therapies, predict response to therapy, and attack the specific genetic abnormalities in the patient's tumor. Less than a generation ago, the idea that we would know the identity of the 80,000 to 100,000 genes in the human genome and that we would soon be able to interrogate ovarian cancer to determine the integrity of each of these genes would have been considered science fiction. Unigene sets, CHIP technology, mass sequencing, and tandem mass spectrometry (see below) will soon provide the ability to determine the status of most if not all of the relevant genes in the human genome at the DNA, RNA, and protein levels in a given tumor. These emerging technologies will provide over a million bits of information related to the genetic changes in a patient's specific tumor. Thus, the challenge will be to determine how to integrate this information into effective, individualized therapy, early cancer detection, and cancer prevention.

Research over the last decade has identified a number of genetic abnormalities that may play a role in the development of ovarian cancer. Most of them were detected using the candidate gene approach based on studying the function, structure, or expression in ovarian cancer of genes identified as potential oncogenes or tumor suppressor genes in other tumor systems. As described above, positional cloning of the BRCA1 and BRCA2 genes has identified two genes that may have a relatively ovarian epithelium-specific function. Further approaches such as representational differential analysis and differential display have identified a number of other candidate genes in our laboratory and in others. These methods are time-consuming and are frequently based on a "best guess" approach. Identification of most of the genes in the genome as a consequence of the Human Genome Project and a rapid increase in our understanding of the function of these genes are likely to lead to a plethora of additional candidate genes for study in ovarian cancer. Furthermore, the development of high-sensitivity, practical genome scanning processes applicable to ovarian tumors is likely to identify an ever-increasing number of genes that play a role in ovarian tumorigenesis. Indeed, over the next several years, it is likely that technologies will arise that will allow us to interrogate a specific patient's tumor to determine the integrity of a significant portion of the genome and to identify several hundred candidate genes of importance. It will be the role of the clinician, through well-designed hypothesis-driven clinical trials, to learn to deal with the wealth of information that will be come available.

Sequencing

High-throughput sequencing now has the ability to sequence hundreds of thousands of base pairs. This already allows us to assess in short periods of time the complete coding sequence and much of the regulatory sequence of cancer predisposition genes in the germline. This technology, although expensive, labor-intensive, and relatively slow, allows us to determine whether any abnormalities exist in candidate genes in the germline or in tumor samples.

Expressed Sequence Tag Arrays

Most of the genes in the human genome have been identified through small sequences present in cDNAs. These expressed sequence tags (ESTs) are being oriented through analysis of independent sequences and overlap into a unigene set which contains at least one representative of most or all of the genes in the human genome.[44] A smaller set of ESTs could be developed that includes all the genes expressed in normal ovarian epithelium and ovarian cancer cells. It will soon be possible to assemble a library of ESTs for candidate genes that may play a role in ovarian cancer or even a random EST library on glass slides. These slides can then be assessed for the expression or integrity of genes at both the DNA and RNA levels.[44] The sole limitation is in the number of ESTs that can be arrayed on several slides. Up to 2,000 genes can be placed on a slide which would allow representation of the complete genome on 100 slides. Only 15% of the genome is expressed in any cell lineage; thus an array of seven or eight slides could provide representation of all the genes expressed in ovarian cancer. By using fluorescent probes from a patient's tumor and comparing the intensity of fluorescence with a different-colored fluorescent probe from normal ovarian epithelium, it is possible to detect changes in level of expression over 3 to 4 logs of dynamic range. These assays may be sufficiently sensitive to detect changes of only two- or threefold.

CHIP Technology

With the use of robotics, it is now possible to create CHIPs containing oriented arrays of hundreds of thousands and possibly millions of specific oligonucleotides.[42–44,150] As in the glass slide technology described above, it is possible to screen these CHIPs with fluorescent probes. Thus a single CHIP can be used to assess the integrity, amplification, or expression of all genes in the genome. As a rapid and inexpensive replacement for DNA sequencing, it is theoretically possible to create CHIPs in which all potential DNA sequences in several hundred cDNAs are represented. Under mutation-sensitive hybridization conditions, it is possible to read the complete sequence of the coding and regulatory regions of candidate genes in minutes using a scanning laser.

Tandem Mass Spectrometry

Tandem mass spectrometry measurement of proteins in serum, urine, or saliva is still in the early developmental stage.[45] However, this technology, which determines the size of enzymatically derived fragments of a protein to the 1/10 or 1/100 Da, has the potential to detect picomolar levels of specific proteins.[45] Tandem mass spectrometry can theoretically determine whether a protein in serum is in its native form or has been modified by posttranslational processing such as enzymatic cleavage or phosphorylation. This technique can readily determine the levels of secreted proteins or of proteins released from cells during cell death, providing new markers for early diagnosis and for determining prognosis.

Bioinformatics

The rapid emergence of new genetic technology capable of analyzing thousands and even millions of genes or proteins in a single step has the ability to provide an overwhelming amount of information about a single tumor. This information if properly utilized has the potential to allow therapy to be individualized to the molecular changes in each tumor. The field of bioinformatics, which deals with this information, will require the development of computer programs, neural nets, pattern recognition, and artificial intelligence to aid clinicians and scientists in applying these data to patient treatment, hopefully improving our ability to cure this devastating disease. Although our ability to assess a patient's tumor is progressing at an exponential rate, translation of this information into patient care has not kept pace. The rapid, ethical application of these data to patient treatment represents an ongoing challenge.

EDITORS' COMMENTARY

All authors agree as do we that the CA 125 marker is the best studied and most useful marker to date. They concur that the test is too insensitive, however, to be used for population screening (80% positivity in advanced disease and only 50% positivity in early and surgical curable disease). Combining this technique with transvaginal ultrasound improves the sensitivity and specificity but not to a degree sufficient to offer it to any large populations as a screen. Thus, we and the authors concur with the current recommendation of the NIH Consensus Conference that these screening procedures be offered only to women from high-risk families or with a genetic predisposition. In terms of prognosis and marker, it is clear that a linear relationship exists between marker value decrements and outcome. Nevertheless, it is disheartening to know that 50% of patients with normal marker levels at the conclusion of therapy have persistent disease at second-look laparotomy. Markers are helpful only in the unfortunate patient in whom marker level does not normalize who may be a candidate for an early change in therapy, although the benefit of this approach has not been put to a clinical trial. Other markers and combinations of markers have used in an attempt to increase the sensitivity and specificity of screening, but no combination to date has a clearly favorable cost/benefit ratio. Markers such as HER-2/*neu* have been promulgated as being prognostic of outcome in breast cancer. Unfortunately, only 10% of ovarian cancers overexpress this oncogene. Finally, the use of rising marker levels after apparently successful primary therapy to guide salvage treatment is very vexing. It is well appreciated that a continued rise of marker levels antedates clinical recurrence on average by 4 months and sometimes 2 years. Many patients demand salvage therapy (with possible toxicity in the absence of symptomatic recurrence) when the marker value begins to rise, although there are no data supporting the notion that early intervention alters outcome. We all anxiously await the results of ongoing trials comparing outcomes for patients who receive treatment when marker values increase versus treatment at the time of symptomatic recurrence.

Neither group of contributors felt strongly that there are any molecular markers so clearly related to prognosis as to deserve a stratification point within clinical trials. Flow cytometry was considered important, and this technique may have its greatest utility in the treatment of borderline tumors (aneuploid tumors are more aggressive). Both p53 and HER-2/*neu* were mentioned but either are expressed in small numbers of tumors and/or are not sufficiently discriminative to justify their use in staging or stratification.

As expected, the discussion of which patients should undergo BRCA1 testing was extensive because of the newness of the test, the uncertain implications of a positive test, and concern that a negative test may give a false sense of security. Additionally, it was pointed out that since screening for ovarian cancer is suboptimal with current methodology, knowledge of a positive result may only generate anxiety without the ability to alter outcome. In sum, however, the contributors *do not* recommend routine testing and caution that, until trials currently under way are complete, physicians be as nondirective as possible in terms of recommending the test and have the capability to counsel patients before and after testing. We agree with this approach and welcome ongoing trials to better understand other factors that work in concert with this gene to increase or reduce the risk of cancer. It is out feeling that *all* such testing should be performed under the auspices of a clinical trial. At the current time this test can be recommended only for patients with a very strong family history (two or more generations afflicted with early breast or ovarian cancer).

No author was in favor of the routine use of chemoresistance assays in guiding either primary or secondary therapy. We fully agree with this approach. It is our opinion that until a randomized clinical trial shows an outcome benefit or an improved cost/benefit ratio this approach should be reserved for the salvage setting. The major value of such testing will very likely be to discard drugs with little chance of efficacy (extreme drug resistance) rather than to assist in selecting active compounds. With regard to resistance modulators there is tempered enthusiasm. The concept is good, however, MDR-1 is not overexpressed in many ovarian cancer, and modifiers of DNA repair mechanisms are untested in terms of clinical efficacy. Additionally, one must be cognizant of multiple clinical trials showing little clinical effect from doubling the intensity of commonly used agents, and it remains to be shown whether such modulators can alter sufficiently the amount of drug targeting macromolecular functions to overcome clinical resistance.

As stated in the introduction, gene therapy is in its infancy. All contributors discuss some of the potential targets of the tumor cell, the bone marrow stem cell to abrogate toxicity, and paracrine and immune functions but conclude that much needs to be learned before this will become a rational strategy for cancer therapeutics. Techniques for transfecting are now clearly available and probably safe, however, the ability to transfect cells has not yet been tested in terms of efficacy and remains in an early experimental stage.

A potpourri of possible new approaches were discussed—none yet ready for the "major leagues" at this point. Inhibitors of angiogenesis are currently being evaluated. These cytostatic agents will require adjunctive use of more classic cytotoxics and low tumor burdens for likely success. There is hope that completion of the Human Genome Project will offer new insights into therapeutics, although the amount of data and the heterogeneity of human tumors make this an awesome task. All contributors discuss the possibilities of some emerging robotics technology that may be capable of making some sense of the huge data base that this project will generate.

In summary, a better understanding of the biology of ovarian cancer is of paramount importance, and the hope is that as more knowledge is gained, the therapeutic envelope will be expanded.

References

1. Bast RC Jr, Klug TL, St. John E et al: A radioimmunoassay using a monoclonal antibody to monitor the course of epithelial ovarian cancer. N Engl J Med 309:883, 1983
2. Berek JS, Knapp RC, Malkasian GD et al: CA 125 serum levels correlated with second-look operations among ovarian cancer patients. Obstet Gynecol 67:685, 1986
3. Gallion HH, Hunter JE, van Nagell JR et al: The prognostic implications of

low serum CA 125 levels prior to the second-look operation for stage III and IV epithelial ovarian cancer. Gynecol Oncol 46:29, 1992

4. Jacobs IJ, Oram DH, Bast RC Jr: Strategies for improving the specificity of screening for ovarian cancer with tumor-associated antigens CA 125, CA 15-3, and TAG 72.3. Obstet Gynecol 80:396, 1992
5. van Nagell JR Jr, Gallion HH, Pavlik EJ, DePriest PD: Ovarian cancer screening. Cancer Suppl 15 76:2086, 1995
6. Petru F, Sevin BU, Averett HF et al: Comparison of three tumor markers—CA 125, lipid associated sialic acid (LSA), and NB/70K—in monitoring ovarian cancer. Gynecol Oncol 38: 181, 1990
7. Cole LA, Schwartz PE, Wang Y: Urinary gonadotropin fragments (UGF) in cancers of the female reproductive system. Gynecol Oncol 31:82, 1988
8. Woolas RP, Xu FJ, Jacobs IJ et al: Elevation of multiple serum markers in patients with stage I ovarian cancer. J Natl Cancer Inst 85:1748, 1993
9. Ward BG, McGuckin MA, Ramm LE et al: The management of ovarian carcinoma is improved by the use of cancer-associated serum antigen and CA 125 assays. Cancer 71:430, 1993
10. Gallion HH, Pieretti M, DePriest PD, van Nagell, JR Jr: The molecular basis of ovarian cancer. Cancer 76:1992, 1995
11. Cane P, Azen C, Lopez E et al: Tumor marker trends in asymptomatic women at risk for ovarian cancer: relevance for ovarian cancer screening. Gynecol Oncol 57:240, 1995
12. Jacobs I, Bast RC Jr: The CA 125 tumour-associated antigen: a review of the literature. Hum Reprod 4:1, 1989
13. Rustin GJ, Nelstrop AE, McClean P et al: Defining response of ovarian carcinoma to initial chemotherapy according to serum CA 125. J Clin Oncol 14:1545, 1996
14. Hunter VJ, Daly L, Helms M et al: The prognostic significance of CA 125 half-life in patients with ovarian cancer who have received primary chemotherapy after surgical cytoreduction. Am J Obstet Gynecol 163:1164, 1990
15. Jacobs IJ, Rivera H, Oram DH et al: Differential diagnosis of ovarian cancer with tumour markers CA 125, CA 15–3 and TAG-72;nd;3. Br J Obstet Gynaecol 100:1120, 1993
16. Jacobs IJ, Kohler MF, Wiseman R et al: Clonal origin of epithelial ovarian cancer: analysis by loss of heterozygosity, p53 mutation and X chromosome inactivation. J Natl Cancer Inst 84: 1793, 1992
17. Mok CH, Tsao SW, Knapp RC et al: Unifocal origin of advanced human epithelial ovarian cancer. Can Res 52:5119, 1992
18. Einhorn N, Sjovall K, Knapp RC et al: Prospective evaluation of serum CA 125 levels for early detection of ovarian cancer. Obstet Gynecol 80:14, 1992
19. Zurawski VR Jr, Broderick SF, Pickens P et al: Serum CA 125 levels in a group of nonhospitalized women: relevance for the early detection of ovarian cancer. Obstet Gynecol 69:606, 1987
20. Jacobs I, Stabile I, Bridges J et al: Multimodal approach to screening for ovarian cancer. Lancet 1:268, 1988
21. Jacobs I, Davies AP, Bridges J et al: Prevalence screening for ovarian cancer in postmenopausal women by CA 125 measurement and ultrasonography. Br Med J 306:1030, 1993
22. Skates SJ, Xu FJ, Yu YH et al: Toward an optimal algorithm for ovarian cancer screening with longitudinal tumor markers. Cancer 76:2004, 1995
23. Xu FJ, Yu YA, Daly L et al: OVX1 radioimmunoassay complements CA

125 for predicting the presence of residual ovarian carcinoma at second-look surgical surveillance procedures. J Clin Oncol 11:1506, 1993

24. Xu FJ, Ramakrishnan S, Daly L et al: increased serum levels of macrophage colony stimulating factor in ovarian cancer. Am J Obstet Gynecol 165: 1356, 1991
25. Woolas R, Xu FJ, Jacobs I et al: Case report: elevated serum levels of macrophage colony stimulating factor and OVX1, 11 months prior to the diagnosis of stage IC ovarian cancer. Int J Gynecol Cancer 6:156, 1996
26. Karlan BY, Platt LD: The current status of ultrasound and color Doppler imaging in screening for ovarian cancer. Gynecol Oncol 55:S28, 1994
27. Urban N, Drescher C, Etzioni R et al: Use of a stochastic simulation model to identify an efficient protocol for ovarian cancer screening. Control Clin Trials, in press
28. Baak JP, Langley FA, Talerman A et al: Interpathologist and intrapathologist disagreement in ovarian tumor grading and typing. Anal Quant Cytol Histol 8:354, 1986
29. Friedlander ML, Headley DH, Taylor I et al: Influence of cellular DNA content on survival in advanced ovarian cancer. Cancer Res 44:397, 1984
30. Wagner TMU, Adler A, Sevelda P et al: Prognostic significance of cell DNA content in early-stage ovarian cancer (FIGO stages I and II/A) by means of automatic image cytometry. Int J Cancer 56:167, 1994
31. Kaern J, Trope CG, Abeler V, Petterson EO: Cellular DNA content: the most important prognostic factor in patients with borderline tumors of the ovary. Can it prevent overtreatment? p. 181. In Sharp F, Mason P, Blackett T, Berek J (eds): Ovarian Cancer 3. Chapman & Hall, London, 1995
32. Marks Jr, Davidoff AM, Kerns BJ et al: Overexpression and mutation of p53 in epithelial ovarian cancer. Cancer Res 51:2979, 1991
33. Berchuck A, Kamel A, Whitaker R et al: Overexpression of HER-2/*neu* is associated with poor survival in advanced epithelial ovarian cancer. Cancer Res 50:4087, 1990
34. Rubin S, Benjamin I, Behbakht K et al: Clinicopathologic characteristics of ovarian cancer in women with documented germline mutations of BRCA1. Gynecol Oncol 60:101, 1996
35. Berchuck A, Rodriguez GC, Kamel A et al: Epidermal growth factor receptor expression in normal ovarian epithelium and ovarian cancer. I. correlation of receptor expression with prognostic factors in patients with ovarian cancer. Am J Obstet Gynecol 164:669, 1991
36. Kacinski BM: CSF-1 and its receptor in ovarian, endometrial and breast cancer. Ann Med 27(1):79, 1995
37. Bellacosa A, de Feo D, Godwin AK et al: Molecular alterations of the AKT2 oncogene in ovarian and breast carcinomas. Int J Cancer 64(4):280, 1995
38. Kim TM, Benedict WF, Xu HJ et al: Loss of heterozygosity on chromosome 13 is common only in the biologically more aggressive subtypes of ovarian epithelial tumors and is associated with normal retinoblastoma gene expression. Cancer Res 54:605, 1994
39. Iwabuchi H, Sakamoto M, Sakunaga H et al: Genetic analysis of benign, low-grade, and high-grade ovarian tumors Cancer Res 55(24):6172, 1995
40. Rubin SC, Benjamin I, Behbakht K et al: Clinical and pathological features of ovarian cancer in women with germline mutations of BRCAI. N Engl J Med 335(19):1413, 1996
41. Jordan VC: Studies on the estrogen receptor in breast cancer—20 years as a target for the treatment and prevention

of cancer. Breast Cancer Res Treat 36(3):267, 1995

42. Hacia JG, Brody LC, Chee MS et al: Detection of heterozygous mutations in BRCA1 using high density oligonucleotide arrays and two-colour fluorescence analysis. Nat Genet 14(4): 441, 1996
43. Chee M, Yang R, Hubbell E et al: Accessing genetic information with high-density DNA arrays. Science 274(5287):610, 1996
44. Sapolsky RJ, Lipshutz RJ: Mapping genomic library clones using oligonucleotide arrays. Genomics 33(3):445, 1996
45. Valaskovic GA, Kelleher NL, McLafferty FW: Attomole protein characterization by capillary electrophoresis mass spectrometry. Science 273(5279): 1199, 1996
46. Press MF, Hung G, Godolphin W et al: Sensitivity of HER-2/*neu* antibodies in archival tissue samples: potential source of error in immunohistochemical studies of oncogene expression. Cancer Res 54:2771, 1994
47. Easton D, Ford D, Bishop DT: Breast Cancer Linkage Consortium. Breast and ovarian cancer incidence in BRCA1 mutation carriers. Am J Hum Genet 56:265, 1995
48. Claus EB, Risch N, Thompson WB: Autosomal dominant inheritance of early onset breast cancer: implications for risk prediction. Cancer 73:643, 1994
49. Sankila R, Aaltonen LA, Jarvinen HJ, Mecklin JP: Better survival rate in patients with MLH1-associated hereditary colorectal cancer. Gastroenterology 110:682, 1996
50. Chen Y, Chen CF, Riley DJ et al: Aberrant subcellular localization of BRCA1 in breast cancer. Science 270:789, 1995
51. Kamb A, Gruis NA, Weaver-Feldhaus J et al: A cell cycle regulator potentially involved in genesis of many tumor types. Science 264(5157):436, 1994
52. Miki Y, Swensen J, Shattuck-Eidens D et al: A strong candidate for the breast and ovarian cancer susceptibility gene BRCA1. Science 266:66, 1994
53. Wooster R, Neuhausen SL, Mangion J et al: Identification of the breast cancer susceptibility gene BRCA2. Nature 378:789, 1995
54. Burke W, Daly M, Garber J: Recommendations for follow-up care of individuals with an inherited predisposition to cancer: 2. BRCA1 and BRCA2 mutations. JAMA (in press)
55. Anonymous: Statement of the American Society of Clinical Oncology: genetic testing for cancer susceptibility. J Clin Oncol 14(5):1730, 1996
56. Wooster R, Neuhausen SL, Mangion J et al: Localization of a breast cancer susceptibility gene, BRCA2, to chromosome 13q12-13. Science 265:2088, 1994
57. Mazoyer S, Dunning AM, Serova O et al: A polymorphic stop codon in BRCA2. Nat Genet 14(3):253, 1996
58. Holt JT, Thompson ME, Szabo C et al: Growth retardation and tumour inhibition by BRCA1. Nat Genet 12:298, 1996
59. Phelan CM, Rebbeck TR et al: Ovarian cancer risk in BRCA1 carries is modified by HRAS1 variable number of Farden repeat (VNTR) locus. Nat Genet 12:7, 1996
60. Narod SA, Goldgar D, Cannon-Albright L et al: Risk modifiers in carriers of BRCA1 mutations. Int J Cancer 64:394, 1995
61. Gudas JM, Nguyen H, Li T et al: Hormone-dependent regulation of BRCA1 in human breast cancer cells. Cancer Res 55:4561, 1995
62. Marquis ST, Rajan JV, Wynshaw-Boris A et al: The developmental pattern of BRCA1 expression implies a role in dif-

ferentiation of the breast and other tissues. Nat Genet 11:17, 1995

63. Chen Y, Farmer AA, Chen CF et al: BRCA1 is a 220-kDa nuclear phosphoprotein that is expressed and phosphorylated in a cell cycle-dependent manner: Cancer Res 56:3168, 1996
64. Hakem R, delaPompa JL, Sirard C et al: The tumor suppressor gene BRCA1 is required for embryonic cellular proliferation in the mouse. Cell 85:1009, 1996
65. Liu CY, Fleskennikitin A, Li S et al: Inactivation of the mouse BRCA1 gene leads to failure in the morphogenesis of the EGG cylinder in early postimplantation development. Gene Dev 10(14):1835, 1996
66. Boyd M, Harris F, McFarlane R et al: A human BRCA1 gene knockout. Nature 375:541, 1995
67. Szabo CI, King MC: Inherited breast and ovarian cancer. Hum Mol Genet 4:1811, 1995
68. Merajver SD, Pham TM, Caduff RF et al: Somatic mutations in the BRCA1 gene in sporadic ovarian tumours. Nat Genet 9:439, 1995
69. Futreal PA, Liu Q, Shattuck-Eldens D et al: BRCA1 mutations in primary breast and ovarian carcinomas. Science 266:120, 1994
70. Weber B: Breast cancer susceptibility genes: current challenges and future promises. Ann Intern Med 124:1088, 1996
71. Cohen MM et al: Background statement: genetic testing and insurance. Am J Hum Genet 56:327, 1995
72. Lerman C, Narod S, Schulman K et al: BRCA1 testing in families with hereditary breast-ovarian cancer. JAMA 275:1885, 1996
73. Lynch HT, Watson P, Lynch JF et al: Hereditary ovarian cancer: heterogeneity in age at onset. Cancer, suppl. 71:573, 1993
74. Friedman LS, Szabo CI, Ostermeyer EA et al: Novel inherited mutations and variable expressivity of BRCA1 alleles, including the founder mutation 185delAG in Ashkenazi Jewish families. Am J Hum Genet 57:1284, 1995
75. Berman DB, Costalas J, Schultz DC et al: A common mutation in BRCA2 that predisposes to a variety of cancers is found in both Jewish Ashkenazi and non-Jewish individuals. Cancer Res 56:3409, 1996
76. Struewing JP, Abeliovich D, Peretz T et al: The carrier frequency of the BRCA1 185delAG mutation is approximately 1 percent in Ashkenazi Jewish individuals. Nat Genet 11:198, 1995
77. Anonymous: NIH Consensus Development Panel on Ovarian Cancer: ovarian cancer—screening, treatment and follow-up. JAMA 273(6):491, 1995
78. Tonin P, Weber B, Offit K et al: Frequency of recurrent BRCA1 and BRCA2 mutations in Ashkenazi Jewish breast cancer families Nat Med 2(11):1179, 1996
79. Thorlacius S, Olafsdottir G, Tryggvadottir L et al: A single BRCA2 mutation in male and female breast cancer families from Iceland with varied cancer phenotypes. Nat Genet 13:117, 1996
80. Johannesdottir G, Gudmundsson J, Bergthorsson JT et al: High prevalance of the 999del5 mutation in Icelandic breast and ovarian cancer patients. Cancer Res 56:3663, 1996
81. O'Shaughnessy JA: Chemoprevention of breast cancer. JAMA 275:1349, 1996
82. Hankinson SE, Colditz GA, Hunter DJ et al: A quantitative assessment of oral contraceptive use and risk of ovarian cancer. Obstet Gynecol 80(4):708, 1992
83. Gross TP, Schlesselman JJ: The estimated effect of oral contraceptive use on the cumulative risk of epithelial

ovarian cancer. Obstet Gynecol 83(3): 419, 1994

84. Anonymous: Collaborative Group on Hormonal Factors in Breast Cancer: breast cancer and hormonal contraceptives—collaborative re-analysis of individual data on 53, 297 women with breast cancer and 100,239 without breast cancer from 54 epidemiological studies. Lancet 347:1713, 1996

85. Goodnight JE, Quagliana JM, Morton DL: Failure of subcutaneous mastectomy to prevent the development of breast cancer. J Surg Oncol 26:198, 1984

86. Eldar S, Meguid MM, Beatty JD: Cancer of the breast after prophylactic subscutaneous mastectomy. Am J Surg 148:692, 1984

87. Wapnir IL, Rabinowitz B, Greco RS: A reappraisal of prophylactic mastectomy. Surg Gynecol Obstet 171:171, 1990

88. Piver MS, Jishi MF, Tsukada Y et al: Primary peritoneal carcinoma after prophylactic oophorectomy in women with a family history of ovarian cancer: a report of the Gilda Radner Familial Ovarian Cancer Registry. Cancer 71:2651, 1993

89. Struewing JP et al: Prophylactic oophorectomy in inherited breast/ovarian cancer families. J Natl Cancer Inst Monogr 17:33, 1995

90. Tobacman JKL, Tucker MA, Kase R: Intraabdominal carcinomatosis after prophylactic oophorrectomy in ovarian cancer-prone families. Lancet 2:795, 1982

91. Nguyen HN, Averette HE, Janicek M: Ovarian carcinoma: a review of the significance of familial risk factors and the role of prophylactic oophorectomy in cancer prevention. Cancer 74:545, 1994

92. Kerlikowske K, Brown JS, Grady DG: should women with familial ovarian cancer undergo prophylactic oophorectomy? Obstet Gynecol 80:700, 1992

93. Mehlman MJ, Kodish ED, Whitehouse P et al: The need for anonymous genetic counseling and testing. Am J Hum Genet 58:393, 1996

94. Bates SE, Regis JI, Robey RW et al: Chemoresistance in the clinic: overview 1994. Bull Cancer, (Paris) 81 81:55S, 1994

95. Bourhis J, Goldstein LJ, Riou G et al: Expression of a human multidrug resistance gene in ovarian carcinomas. Cancer Res 79:5062, 1989

96. Goldstein LJ, Galski H, Fojo A et al: Expression of a multidrug resistance gene in human cancers. J Natl Cancer Inst 81:116, 1989

97. Murren JR, DeVita VT: Another look at multidrug resistance. PPO Updates 9:1, 1995

98. Wilson WH, Bates SE, Fojo A et al: Controlled trial of dexverapamil, a modulator of multidrug resistance in lymphomas refractory to EPOCH chemotherapy. J Clin Oncol 13:1995, 1995

99. Watanabe T, Tsuge H, Oh-Hara T et al: Comparative study on reversal efficacy of SDZ PSC 833, cyclosporin A and verapamil on multidrug resistance in vitro and in vivo. Acta Oncol 34:235, 1995

100. O'Dwyer PJ, Hamilton TC, Young RC et al: Depletion of glutathione in normal and malignant human cells in vivo by buthionine sulfoximine: clinical and biochemical results. J Natl Cancer Inst 84:264, 1992

101. Ozols RF, O'Dwyer PJ, Hamilton TC: Clinical reversal of drug resistance in ovarian cancer. Gynecol Oncol 51:90, 1993

102. Cleaver JE: It was a very good year for DNA repair. Cell 76:1, 1994

103. Reed E, Kohn EC, Sarosy G et al: Paclitaxel (Taxol), cisplatin and cyclophosphamide in human ovarian cancer:

molecular rationale and early clinical results. Semin Oncol 22:90, 1995

104. Dabholkar M, Parker R, Reed E: Determinants of cisplatin sensitivity in non-malignant, non-drug-selected human T cell lines. Mutat Res 274:45, 1992

105. Dabholkar M, Vionnet J, Bostick-Bruton F et al: Messenger RNA levels of XPAC and ERCC1 in ovarian cancer tissue correlate with response to platinum-based chemotherapy. J Clin Invest 94:703, 1994

106. Stevenson H, Gazdar AF, Phelps R et al: Tumor cell lines established in vitro: an independent prognostic factor for survival in non-small-cell lung cancer. Ann Intern Med 113:764, 1990

107. Markman M: Chemosensitivity and chemoresistance assays: are they clinically relevant? J Cancer Res Clin Oncol 121:441, 1995

108. Kobayashi H, Man S, Graham CH et al: Acquired multicellular-mediated resistance to alkylating agents in cancer. Proc Natl Acad Sci USA 90(8):3294, 1993

109. Pietras RJ, Fendly BM, Chazin VR et al: Antibody to HER-2/*neu* receptor blocks DNA repair after cisplatin in human breast and ovarian cancer cells. Oncogene 9(7):1829, 1994

110. Fan Z, Baselga J, Masui H et al: Antitumor effect of anti-epidermal growth factor receptor monoclonal antibodies plus *cis*-diaminedichloroplatinum on well established A-431 cell xenografts. Cancer Res 53(19):4637, 1993

111. Frankel A, Mills GB: Peptide and lipid growth factors decrease cisplatin-induced cell death in human ovarian cancer cells. Clin Cancer Res 2:1307, 1996

112. Yu D, Matin A, Xia W et al: Liposome-mediated in vivo E1A gene transfer suppressed dissemination of ovarian cancer cells that overexpress HER-2/*neu*. Oncogene 11(7):1383, 1995

113. Graus-Porta D, Beerli RR, Hynes NE: Signal-chain antibody-mediated intracellular retention of erbB-2 impairs Neu differentiation factor and epidermal growth factor signaling. Mol Cell Biol 15(3):1182, 1995

114. Stevenson H, Gazdar AF, Phelps R et al: Tumor cell lines established in vitro: an independent prognostic factor for survival in non-small-cell lung cancer. Ann Intern Med 113:764, 1990

115. Raynaud FI, Odell DE, Kelland LR: Intracellular metabolism of the orally active platinum drug JM216: influence of glutathione levels. Br J Cancer 74(3):380, 1996

116. O'Dwyer PJ, Hamilton TC, LaCreta FP et al: Phase I trial of buthionine sulfoximine in combination with melphalan in patients with cancer. J Clin Oncol 14(1):249, 1996

117. Shi Y, Frankel F, Radvanyi L et al: Rapamycin enhances apoptosis and increases sensitivity to cisplatin in vitro. Cancer Res 55:1982, 1995

118. Lukes AS, Kohler MF, Pieper CF et al: Multivariable analysis of DNA ploidy, p53 and HER-2/*neu* as prognostic factors in endometrial cancer. Cancer 79:2380, 1994

119. Goldstein LJ, Gottesman MM, Pastan I: Expression of the MDR1 gene in human cancers. Cancer Treat Res 57: 101, 1991

120. Koc ON, Allay JA, Lee K et al: Transfer of drug resistance genes into hematopoietic progenitors to improve chemotherapy tolerance. Semin Oncol 23: 46, 1996

121. Deisseroth A, Kavanagh J, Champlin R et al: Use of safety-modified retroviruses to introduce chemotherapy resistance sequences into normal hematopoietic cells for chemoprotection during the therapy of ovarian cancer: a

pilot trial. Hum Gene Ther 5:1507, 1994

122. Freemen SM, Whartenby KA, Freeman JL et al: In situ use of suicide genes for cancer therapy. Semin Oncol 23:31, 1996

123. Schirrmacher V: Biotherapy of cancer: perspectives of immunotherapy and gene therapy. J Cancer Res Clin Oncol 121:443, 1995

124. Gilboa E: Immunotherapy of cancer with genetically modified tumor vaccines. Semin Oncol 23:101, 1996

125. Freeman SM, McCune C, Angel C et al: Treatment of ovarian cancer using HSV-TK gene-modified vaccine—regulatory issues. Hum Gene Ther 3:342, 1992

126. Freeman SM, McCune C, Robinson W et al: Treatment of ovarian cancer using a gene-modified vaccine. Hum Gene Ther 6:927, 1995

127. Sorrentino BP, McDonagh KT, Woods D et al: Expression of retroviral vectors containing the human multidrug resistance 1 cDNA in hematopoietic cells of transplanted mice. Blood 86:491, 1995

128. Ward M, Richardson C, Pioli P et al: Transfer and expression of the human multiple drug resistance gene in human CD34 + cells. Blood 84:1408, 1994

129. O'Shaughessy J, Cowan K, Neinhuis A: Retroviral mediated transfer of the human multidrug resistance gene (MDR-1) into hematopoietic stem cells during autologous transplantation after intensive chemotherapy for metastatic breast cancer. Hum Gene Ther 5: 891, 1994

130. Mullen CA: Metabolic suicide genes in gene therapy. Pharmacol Ther 63:199, 1994

131. Culver KW, Ram Z, Wallbridge S et al: In vivo gene transfer with retroviral vector-producer cells for treatment of experimental brain tumors. Science 256:1550, 1992

132. Freeman SM, Abboud CN, Whartenby KA et al: The "bystander effect": tumor regression when a fraction of the tumour mass is genetically modified. Cancer Res 53:5274, 1993

133. Fick J, Barker FG, Dazin P et al: The extent of heterocellular communication mediated by gap junctions is predictive of bystander tumor cytotoxicity in vitro. Proc Natl Acad Sci USA 92:1107, 1995

134. Barba D, Hardin J, Sadelain M et al: Development of anti-tumor immunity following thymidine kinase-mediated killing of experimental brain tumors. Proc Natl Acad Sci USA 91:4348, 1994

135. Ram Z, Walbridge S, Shawker T et al: The effect of thymidine kinase transduction and ganciclovir therapy on tumor vasculature and growth of 9L gliomas in rats. J Neurosurg 81:256, 1994

136. Cristiano RJ, Curiel DT: Strategies to accomplish gene delivery via the receptor-mediated endocytosis pathway, (review). Cancer Gene Ther 3(1):49, 1996

137. Cristiano RJ, Roth JA: Epidermal growth factor mediated DNA delivery into lung cancer cells via the epidermal growth factor receptor. Cancer Gene Ther 3(1):448, 1996

138. Gottschalk S, Cristiano RJ, Smith LC et al: Folate receptor mediated DNA delivery into tumor cells: apoptosomal disruption results in enhanced gene expression. Gene Ther 1(3):185, 1994

139. Cannistra SA, Abu-Jawdeh G, Niloff J et al: CD44 variant expression is a common feature of epithelial ovarian cancer: lack of association with standard prognostic factors. J Clin Oncol 13(8):1912, 1995

140. Moscatello DK, Montgomery RB, Sundareshan P et al: Transformational and altered signal transduction by a

naturally occurring mutant EGF receptor. Oncogene 13(1):85, 1996

141. Mujoo K, Maneval DC, Anderson SC et al: Adenoviral-mediated p53 tumor suppressor gene therapy of human ovarian carcinoma. Oncogene 12(8): 1617, 1996
142. Santoso JT, Tang DC, Lane SB et al: Adenovirus-based p53 gene therapy in ovarian cancer. Gynecol Oncol 59: 171, 1995
143. Fang XJ, Jin X, Xu HJ et al: Expression of P16 induces transcriptional downregulation of the RB gene, submitted.
144. Xu HJ, Zhou Y, Seigne J et al: Enhanced tumor suppressor gene therapy via replication-deficient deficient adenovirus vectors expressing an N-terminal truncated retinoblastoma protein. Cancer Res 56(10):2245, 1996
145. Kim S, Brown PH, Birrer MJ: The inhibitory activity of a transdominant c-Jun mutant fused to the ligand binding domain of the estrogen receptor. Oncogene 12(5):1043, 1996
146. Shao N, Chai YL, Shyam E et al: Induction of apoptosis by the tumor suppressor protein BRCA1. Oncogene 13(1):1, 1996
147. Mok SC, Chan WY, Wong KK et al: SPARC, an extracellular matrix protein with tumor-suppressing activity in human ovarian epithelial cells. Oncogene 12(9):1895, 1996
148. Mok SC, Wong KK, Chan RK et al: Molecular cloning of differentially expressed genes in human epithelial ovarian cancer. Gynecol Oncol 52(2):247, 1994
149. Yu YH, Xu FJ, Fang XJ et al: Differential display of genes expressed in normal ovarian surface epithelium, but not in ovarian cancer, abstract Proc Am Assoc Cancer Res 37:592, 1996
150. Gibbs WW: New chip off the old block—can DNA microprobes do for genetics what microprocessors did for computing. Sci Am 275(3):42, 1996
151. McGuire WP, Hoskins WJ, Brady MF et al: Cyclophosphamide and cisplatin compared with paclitaxel and cisplatin in patients with stage III and stage IV ovarian cancer. N Engl J Med 334:1, 1996
152. Fearon ER, Pardoll DM, Itaya T et al: Interleukin-2 production by tumor cells bypasses T-helper function in the generation of an antitumor response, Cell 60:397, 1990
153. Golumbek PT, Lazenby AJ, Levitsky JL et al: Treatment of established renal cancer by tumor cells engineered to secrete interleukin-4. Science 254:713, 1991
154. Khazaie K, Prifti S, Beckhove P et al: Persistence of dormant tumor cells in the bone marrow of tumor cell vaccinated mice correlates with long term immunological protection. Proc Natl Acad Sci 91:7430, 1994
155. Liotta LA, Kleinerman J, Saidel G: Quantitative relationships of intravascular tumor cells: tumor vessels and pulmonary metastases following tumor implantation. Cancer Res 34:997, 1974
156. Kohn EC, Alessandro R, Spoonster J et al: Angiogenesis: role of calcium-mediated signal transduction. Proc Natl Acad Sci 92:1307, 1995
157. Liotta LA, Steeg PS, Stetler-Stevenson WG: Cancer metastasis and angiogenesis: an imbalance of positive and negative regulation. Cell 64:327, 1991
158. Hollingsworth HC, Kohn EC, Steinberg SM et al: Tumor angiogenesis in advanced stage ovarian carcinoma. Am J Pathol 147:33, 1995
159. Folkman J: Clinical applications of research on angiogenesis. N Engl J Med 333:1757, 1995
160. Kohn EC, Reed E, Sarosy E et al: Clinical investigation of a cytostatic calcium

influx inhibitor in patients with refractory cancers. Cancer Res 56:569, 1996

161. Asano M, Yukita A, Matsumoto T et al: Inhibition of tumor growth and metastasis by an immunoneutralizing monoclonal antibody to human vascular endothelial growth factor/vascular permeability factor 121. Cancer Res 55:5296, 1995

162. Boocock CA, Charnock-Jones DS, Sharkey AM: Expression of vascular endothelial growth factor and its receptors flt and KDR in ovarian carcinoma. J Natl Cancer Inst 87:506, 1995

163. Dvorak HF, Detmar M, Claffey KP: Vascular permeability factor/vascular endothelial growth factor: an important mediator of angiogenesis in malignancy and inflammation. Int Arch Allergy Immunol 107:233, 1995

164. Hatva E, Kaipainen A, Mentula P: Expression of endothelial cell-specific receptor tyrosine kinases and growth factors in human brain tumors. Am J Pathol 146:368, 1995

165. Kohn EC, Liotta LA: Molecular insights into cancer invasion: strategies for prevention and intervention. Cancer Res. 55:1856, 1995

166. Davies B, Brown PD, East N et al: A synthetic matrix metalloproteinase inhibitor decreases tumor burden and prolongs survival of mice bearing human ovarian carcinoma xenografts. Cancer Res 53:2087, 1993

167. Kohn EC, Jacobs W, Kim Y et al: Calcium influx modulates expression of matrix metalloproteinases-2 (72-kDa type IV collagenase, gelatinase A). J Biol Chem 269:21505, 1994

168. Kohn EC, Sandeen MA, Liotta LA: In vivo efficacy of a novel inhibitor of selected signal transduction pathways including calcium, arachidonate, and inositol phosphates. Cancer Res 52:3208, 1992

169. Kohn EC, Felder CC, Jacobs W: Structure function analysis of signal and growth inhibition by carboxyamidotriazole, CAI. Cancer Res 54:935, 1994

170. Davies B, Naylor MS, Balkwill FR: Matrix metalloproteinases and their role in ovarian cancer. P. 243. In Sharp F, Mason P, Blackett T et al (eds): Ovarian Cancer 3. Chapman & Hall, London, 1994

CHAPTER 18

MANAGEMENT OF OVARIAN GERM CELL TUMORS

Stephen Williams
Ling C. Wong
Hextan Y.S. Ngan

EDITORS' INTRODUCTION

Malignant ovarian germ cell tumors account for less than 5% of all ovarian malignancies. The evolution of treatment for these tumors has been one of the true success stories in the annals of oncology. Many, but by no means all, of the recent advances have arisen from the findings of studies on testicular cancer, which is 10-fold more common than ovarian germ cell tumors.

In 1973 the World Health Organization (WHO) introduced the currently accepted classification of ovarian germ cell tumors (Table 18–1). In contradistinction to epithelial tumors, approximately 50 to 75% are stage I, and bilateral ovarian involvement is extremely rare, except in the case of dysgerminoma, for which the incidence of bilaterality is 10 to 15%. Therefore, primary surgery, consisting of resection of the primary tumor and comprehensive surgical staging, usually allows preservation of reproductive potential.

Until the advent of combination chemotherapy in the mid-1960s, the prognosis for most patients with nondysgerminomatous tumors was dismal: virtually all women with advanced disease died. Even in stage I disease, only 5 to 20% of patients survived after treatment with surgery alone. In the early 1970s, the combination of vincristine, dactinomycin, and cyclophosphamide (VAC) was first used for postoperative treatment of these patients. By the early 1980s, it was apparent that this regimen was curative for a high percentage of patients with stage I disease but was successful in less than 50% of patients with advanced-stage tumors. Once Einhorn and Donohue reported their excellent results with the combination of vinblastine, bleomycin, and cisplatin in the treatment of testicular cancer, platinum-containing regimens gradually supplanted the VAC regimen as the preferred treatment. Based on data over the past decade, most experts in the United States consider the combination of bleomycin, etoposide, and cisplatin (BEP) the standard regimen for patients who require postoperative chemotherapy.

Several issues regarding the management of ovarian germ cell tumors, however, remain unresolved. British and European investigators have been pushing the envelope regarding the types of patients who can be safely treated with surgery alone. Other controversies exist, including the optimal number of chemotherapy cycles, the role of second-look surgery, the optimal salvage chemotherapy regimen for those few patients whose primary regimen fails, and the role of secondary cytoreductive surgery.

QUESTIONS

1. Once a malignant ovarian germ cell tumor is diagnosed intraoperatively, how extensive should surgical staging be, particularly with regard to lymph node dissection or sampling?
2. Which patients can be safely treated with surgery alone?
3. How would you treat a patient referred to you with ovarian dysgerminoma seemingly confined to one ovary but with no surgical staging?
4. What should be considered standard postoperative chemotherapy for patients with nondysgerminomatous tumors? Is there any role for high-dose chemotherapy as primary postoperative therapy?
5. What is optimal salvage therapy for a patient with an endodermal sinus tumor who progresses or rapidly relapses after completion of primary therapy? What is optimal salvage therapy for the same patient who relapses 4 months after completion of primary therapy?
6. For which patients do you recommend second-look surgery? For which patients, if any, do you recommend secondary cytoreductive surgery?

TABLE 18-1
WHO Classification of Germ Cell Tumors

Dysgerminoma
Yolk sac tumor (Endodermal sinus tumor)
Embryonal carcinoma
Polyembryoma
Choriocarcinoma
Teratoma
Immature
Mature (dermoid cyst)
Monodermal (struma ovarii, carcinoid)
Mixed forms
Gonadoblastoma

(From Gershenson,[1] with permission.)

QUESTION 1

Once a malignant ovarian germ cell tumor is diagnosed intraoperatively, how extensive should surgical staging be, particularly with regard to lymph node dissection or sampling?

STEPHEN WILLIAMS

This question is in reality two questions. The first, concerning the extent of optimum staging, is relevant for a patient for whom the diagnosis is known or strongly suspected at the time of the initial surgical procedure. The second, concerning the lowest level of acceptable surgical staging, is relevant for patients referred to an oncologist after incomplete staging.

A clear difference between epithelial ovarian cancer and ovarian germ cell tumors is their responsiveness to chemotherapy. In patients with a germ cell tumor, chemotherapy has considerable curative potential. This is usually not true for patients with epithelial ovarian cancer. Further, one can define a group of patients with early epithelial ovarian cancer who have a low risk of recurrence. With some exceptions, however, this is not the case for patients with ovarian germ cell tumors, as most receive chemotherapy regardless of surgical stage. A further issue that must be considered is that not infrequently a germ cell tumor diagnosis is not definitively established at the time of surgery because of the difficulties of pathologic assessment.

In the case of patients with known or suspected germ cell tumor at the time of surgery, surgical staging should be thorough and consistent with that used in published clinical trials. As much as is reasonably possible, patients should have all clinically detectable disease removed. In the experience of the Gynecologic Oncology Group (GOG),[2] women having complete surgical excision and adjuvant chemotherapy nearly always remain free of further clinical progression (91 of 93 patients) regardless of stage. Patients with incompletely resected tumor who subsequently receive chemotherapy have a lower cure rate (60 to 80%).[3] It must be emphasized that this difference may not be due to the surgery but rather to biologic differences between patients who can have their tumor resected versus those that cannot. Nonetheless, it seems prudent that patients who can have their tumor removed with "reasonable" surgical effort should have this done.

In regard to lymph node dissection and sampling, the largest published study on modern adjuvant therapy is the GOG study.[2] In this study, lymph node removal was not required unless there was palpable abnormality present at the time of surgery. The study defined a patient population in which the relapse rate was very low after adjuvant chemotherapy. Further, risk of lymph node involvement is low in such patients. Thus, routine lymph node dissection or sampling does not appear to be necessary. Along these lines, a patient that has not been completely staged but appears to have localized disease receives chemotherapy regardless, and a further operation specifically for tumor staging does not seem warranted.

LING C. WONG
HEXTAN Y.S. NGAN

Surgical staging

Meticulous surgical staging is necessary to define the extent of disease, provide prognostic information, and choose the appropriate form of chemotherapy. This is especially important in an apparent early state of disease. The presence of occult or microscopic disease may alter the choice of postoperative chemotherapy.

A vertical abdominal incision is mandatory for adequate exposure, appropriate staging biopsies, resection of large pelvic tumors, and resection of metastatic disease in the upper abdomen. Ascitic fluid should be aspirated and submitted for cytologic examination. If ascites is absent, peritoneal washing with normal saline should be done before any intraperitoneal manipulation takes place.

Systematic examination of the entire peritoneal cavity and its contents then follows. This procedure usually starts with examination of the subphrenic spaces and continues caudally toward the pelvis. The subdiaphragmatic surface, omentum, colon, small intestine, mesentery, and all peritoneal surfaces should be checked. The retroperitoneal space should be palpated for lymph nodes enlargement. All suspicious areas should be recorded, biopsied, or resected and submitted for pathologic evaluation.

The primary ovarian tumor and pelvic organs should then be inspected. The dimension of the primary tumor, capsular rupture or infiltration, external excrescences, adhesions, and the appearance of the contralateral ovary should be recorded. In localized disease ample staging biopsies from the omentum (partial omentectomy), cul-de-sac, paracolic gutters, lateral pelvic side walls, vesicouterine reflection, and subdiaphragmatic surfaces should be done. All adhesions should be resected for histologic examination.

Any enlarged paraortic or pelvic lymph nodes should be resected for histologic confirmation. In the absence of any lymphadenopathy random sampling of the paraortic and pelvic nodes is recommended.

Extent of primary surgery

Laparotomy is indicated in all patients suspected of having ovarian germ cell tumors. It is diagnostic and therapeutic. The extent of disease and the histology types are essential in deciding whether adjuvant chemotherapy is required and in determining the choice of chemotherapy.

The extent of primary surgery depends on the operative findings. Frozen-section facility is necessary to decide whether bisection and biopsy of the contralateral ovary are required in patients with stage I disease. If the disease is clinically localized to one ovary, unilateral salpingo-oophorectomy with conservation of the contralateral ovary and the uterus is the treatment of choice. The fertility potential can then be preserved. Data from a study by the Armed Forces Institute of Pathology (AFIP)[4–7] in the 1970s and others series[8–11] showed similar cure rates in patients treated with conservative unilateral salpingo-oophorectomy as compared with patients who had bilateral salpingo-oophorectomy with or without abdominal hysterectomy (Table 18–2).

If a frozen section of the ovarian tumor confirms the presence of dysgerminoma, careful examination and biopsy of the contralateral ovary is necessary to exclude bilateral tumor involvement. If there is clinical suspicion of a dysgenetic gonad (e.g., in the case of congenital absence of the uterus) an ovarian biopsy should be performed. The contralateral gonad should be excised if a frozen section confirms the clinical suspicion.

If bilateral ovarian masses are present at surgery, unilateral salpingo-oophorectomy should be performed on the more suspicious side. When the opposite ovary contains malignant germ cell tumor, the other ovary is usually resected. In view of the fact that most malignant germ cell tumors are very chemosensitive, there may be a role for local excision of the smaller tumor of the contralateral ovary and postoperative chemotherapy. There are, however, no data on such conservative treatment.

Advanced disease is found in 30 to 40% of patients. Cytoreductive surgery is the usual surgical treatment, aiming at maximal resection and minimal residual disease. The GOG reported that patients with complete resection did better than patients with incomplete resection. The survival benefit was evident with VAC combination therapy[12] and with vinblastine/bleomycin/cisplatin (PVB).[3] Even in stage III disease, removal of the grossly normal second ovary and the uterus does not change the prognosis.[3]

The advance in in vitro fertilization technology has changed the philosophy of surgical treatment in malignant germ cell disease. Ex-

TABLE 18-2
Actuarial Survival by Type and Stage of Tumor in 263 Patients with Malignant Ovarian Germ Tumors

TUMOR TYPE	NO. OF PATIENTS FOLLOWED	SURVIVAL FOR ALL STAGES (%)	SURVIVAL FOR STAGE I
Dysgerminoma	98	86[a]	90[a]
Immature teratoma	56	63[a]	75[a]
Embryonal carcinoma	14	39[b]	50[b]
Mixed germ cell tumors	28	46[b]	50[b]
Endodermal sinus tumor	67	13[c]	16[c]

[a] *At 10 years.*

[b] *At 5 years.*

[c] *At 3 years.*

(From Kurman and Norris,[6] with permission.)

tensive bilateral ovarian disease can be treated with bilateral salpingo-oophorectomy, maximum cytoreductive surgery, and preservation of the uterus. Intrauterine pregnancy is possible with donor oocyteorembryo transfer and hormonal manipulation. One should no longer deny the patient childbearing. Even if hysterectomy is done, attempts should be made to preserve the second ovary. Aspiration of the oocytes, in vitro fertilization with sperm from her partner, and implantation of the embryo into a surrogate uterus is an alternative way of reproduction.

All malignant germ cell tumors have a propensity for lymphatic spread. Enlarged paraaortic and pelvic lymph nodes should be resected for sectioning. An extensive initial laparotomy, including lymph node dissection, seems unlikely to influence long-term survival in patients with dysgerminoma, but it may identify patients for earlier postoperative therapy.[13] The cure rate of 70 to 96% reported from various series,[3,11,12,14] makes one question the wisdom of routine lymphadenectomy, especially in the management of completely resected disease.

QUESTION 2

Which patients can be safely treated with surgery alone?

STEPHEN WILLIAMS

For many years, appropriate treatment for patients with resected ovarian germ cell tumors has been adjuvant chemotherapy, which has been and continues to be the standard management in such cases. However, recent data have called this recommendation into question for selected patients in certain situations. I do not believe surveillance currently is the standard treatment for any patient (other than those with stage I, grade 1, immature teratoma), but there are emerging data that may change this recommendation.

Patients with embryonal carcinoma, endodermal sinus tumors, and mixed tumors containing these elements are thought to have a very high risk of recurrence without postoperative therapy. In a GOG study, 50 of 51 patients with resected stage I to III tumors of these cell types remained disease-free when three courses of postoperative BEP were given.[2]

The situation for patients with immature teratoma is more complex. Immature teratomas are graded 1, 2, or 3 based upon the amount of immature neuroepithelium present. Prognosis of patients is related to tumor grade. Patients whose tumor is thought to be completely resected have a risk of recurrence related to grade. An early study that attempted to define risk of recurrence according to grade was that of Norris et al.[5] In this study, only 1 of 14 patients with stage I, grade 1, immature teratoma had a recurrence. However, 9 of 20 patients with grade 2 tumors had recurrences, as did 4 of 6 patients with grade 3 tumors. Because of these data, most investigators have not recommended adjuvant therapy for patients with stage I, grade 1, tumors but have done so for those with localized tumors of grade 2 or 3. There were 42 patients with resected high-grade immature teratoma entered in the GOG study and treated with three courses of BEP. Of these, 39 have been continuously disease-free.

Unfortunately, the data from which the recommendation for adjuvant therapy is derived were developed in an era before surgical staging was routinely done. It is conceivable that the relatively high risk of recurrence was not due to biologic aggressiveness of high-grade immature teratoma but rather to underestimation of the extent of disease at the time of initial tumor resection.

Thus, in the modern era of surgical staging of ovarian neoplasms, it might be appropriate to re-evaluate the role of routine adjuvant therapy in such individuals and perhaps define a patient population that may not have a risk of recurrence sufficiently high to warrant such treatment. Obviously, such an approach must be taken with great caution, as surgery followed by adjuvant therapy cures virtually all patients with localized high-grade teratoma. However, it is possible that the risk of relapse will be low in a defined population of well-staged patients and, with careful follow-up, nearly all relapsing patients can be diagnosed with relatively small-volume tumor and cured with subsequent chemotherapy for metastatic disease.

At least three groups of investigators have reported results of surveillance in patients with resected immature teratoma. An intergroup study of the Pediatric Oncology Group and the Children's Cancer Group investigated surveillance after surgical resection in 41 girls with ovarian immature teratoma.[15] Median age was 10 years. Central pathology review confirmed that 31 patients had immature teratoma alone (18 grade 1, 9 grade 2, 4 grade 3) and 10 patients had immature teratoma plus identifiable yolk sac tumor. With a median follow-up of 33 months for the immature teratoma group and 24 months for the combined group, 40 of 41 patients remain continuously disease-free. One patient developed liver metastases, was successfully treated with BEP, and is now disease-free 30 months after chemotherapy.

Investigators at Mt. Vernon and Charing Cross Hospitals in England have observed 15 patients after initial surgical treatment.[16] All had stage IA tumors, but surgical staging was incomplete in some. Nine patients had grade 2 or 3 immature teratoma only, and six also had elements of endodermal sinus tumor. A total of three patients had recurrances, 1 of 9 in the pure immature teratoma group and 2 of 6 in the group that also included endodermal sinus tumor. One patient died of a pulmonary embolus during chemotherapy; all others are currently alive and without evident tumor.

Investigators at the University of Milan followed a group of ovarian immature teratoma patients according to a comprehensive prospective protocol.[17] Patients with stage IA, grade 1 or 2, tumors were observed with examination and ultrasound every 3 months for the first year, every 6 months during the second year, and annually thereafter. Patients with gliomatosis peritonei or with stage IB, IC, II, grade 1 or 2, tumors also underwent laparoscopy every 6 months for the first year. Chemotherapy was to be given to patients with grade 3 or stage III tumors. There was a total of 32 patients, of whom nine had stage IA, grade 2 or 3, tumors and did not receive adjuvant chemotherapy. Of these, 1 patient developed a pelvic relapse which was removed surgically and found to be mature teratoma. Another developed gliosis in follow-up. None of these patients ever received chemotherapy, and all are currently disease-free. There were four other patients with IC tumors who did not receive adjuvant chemotherapy. One had an abdominopelvic relapse which was treated surgically; another developed gliosis in follow-up. None received chemotherapy, and all currently have no evidence of disease (NED) also. Of these 13 patients, follow-up ranges from 11 to 138 months, and only 2 have been followed for less than 2 years.

Thus, it is possible that selected patients with stage I high-grade teratoma can be meticulously followed and not given immediate adjuvant therapy. This approach will be further studied in a GOG protocol in development. At this time, however, the standard of care in my opinion continues to be adjuvant chemotherapy with BEP.

LING C. WONG HEXTAN Y.S. NGAN

Currently only patients with well-documented stage IA, grade 1, pure immature teratoma or stage I pure dysgerminoma should be considered for treatment with surgery alone. Evidence for this conservative approach is based on the AFIP experience.[5,18]

QUESTION 3

How would you treat a patient referred to you with ovarian dysgerminoma seemingly confined to one ovary but with no surgical staging?

STEPHEN WILLIAMS

This situation is one that is troublesome for oncologists and occurs not infrequently. Such a patient should have a determination of human chorionic gonadotropin (HCG) and α-fetoprotein (AFP) and an abdominal computerized tomography (CT) scan. An elevated HCG, level implies persistent ovarian germ cell tumor that requires further therapy. An elevated AFP level connotes the presence of elements other than dysgerminoma and mandates chemotherapy. The CT scan may detect unsuspected residual tumor, particularly in retroperitoneal lymph nodes.

Assuming all these studies are normal, for many patients it is appropriate to observe them and not administer adjuvant chemotherapy. The literature of dysgerminoma is limited in quality because of the rarity of the disease and the paucity of studies that have routinely employed thorough surgical staging. Most patients with dysgerminoma have tumor confined to one ovary at diagnosis, and it is generally stated that the risk of relapse in patients with stage IA dysgerminoma treated with surgery alone is in the range of 15 to 25%.[19] Admittedly these patients have not had complete surgical staging. However, that is also the case for many (or even most) of the patients reported in the literature from which this recommendation is derived. Further, the fact that markers and a CT scan are normal gives one greater confidence that the tumor is truly localized.

It is also clear that patients with recurrent or metastatic dysgerminoma have a very high cure rate with systemic chemotherapy. (BEP). Several series have shown that nearly all patients including those with bulky tumor are cured with such chemotherapy.[14,20]

Considering this information, I believe the most appropriate management for this patient (assuming markers and a CT scan are normal) is careful observation with treatment reserved for relapse, should it occur. Observation should include regular (every 2 months) examination and marker determinations, and an abdominal ultrasound or CT scan every 3 or 4 months for the first year. Follow-up at gradually diminishing frequency should continue for 2 to 5 years. Most relapses occur in the first 2 years and nearly all by 4 years. Should this patient suffer a recurrence, chemotherapy given when tumor is not far advanced will produce a high cure rate.

An alternative course of action is immediate adjuvant chemotherapy with three courses of BEP. As discussed, nearly all such patients remain free of disease. However, use of chemotherapy in patients such as these would expose most of them to unnecessary chemotherapy. Chemotherapy should now be considered only for patients deemed unreliable or for whom relapse would be unacceptable, and for those whose strong preference is to avoid any possibility of relapse. These problems occur infrequently, however, and most such patients should be observed after surgery.

LING C. WONG
HEXTAN Y.S. NGAN

Most gynecologic oncologists working in institutions have been confronted with referrals of patients with disease seemingly localized to one ovary but without adequate surgical staging. Based on the AFIP experience, 15% have contralateral involvement and 20% will have a recurrence.[41] These patients can either be followed up with serial CT scanning for evidence of recurrent or metastatic disease or PVB or BEP therapy can be initiated. The GOG study reported sustained complete remission in 19 of 20 patients with incompletely resected dysgerminoma treated with PVB or BEP therapy.[21] Experience from treatment of dysgerminoma with BEP shows that three or four cycles of therapy are adequate. Thus, to eliminate recurrences, some advocate short-term BEP therapy for dysgerminoma confined to one ovary but with inadequate surgical staging.[22] Routine postoperative BEP therapy in this group may mean unnecessary chemotherapy in 80% of patients who do not develop recurrent disease. Patients should be informed about the available options and be allowed to make their own choice.

QUESTION 4

What should be considered standard postoperative chemotherapy for patients with nondysgerminomatous tumors?

Is there any role for high-dose chemotherapy as primary postoperative therapy?

STEPHEN WILLIAMS

Patients with nondysgerminomatous ovarian tumors can be separated into two prognostic groups: (1) those whose disease is completely resected at the time of the initial surgical procedure, and (2) those that have incompletely resected tumor. In the former group, as discussed previously, nearly all patients should receive postoperative adjuvant chemotherapy. The choice of an appropriate chemotherapy regimen is now quite clear. Patients should receive three courses at 3-week intervals of BEP as follows: cisplatin 20 mg/for days 1 through 5, etoposide (VP-16) 100 mg/m^2 for days 1 through 5, and bleomycin 30 units IV weekly. Several series have shown that patients with completely resected tumor nearly all remain free of cancer after treatment with such chemotherapy. The largest of these studies is the GOG study.[2] In this trial, 91 of 93 patients with completely resected stage I to III ovarian germ cell tumors remain clinically free of progression. While no randomized studies have been done comparing BEP to the earlier VAC regimen, there is no question that BEP is superior. In the largest study using VAC, an earlier GOG trial, 25% of similar patients had recurrences.[23]

Other questions that frequently arise concern the necessity for bleomycin and the relative merits of cisplatin versus carboplatin. There are no randomized trials for ovarian tumors. However, randomized trials in metastatic testis cancer with a good prognosis have shown that bleomycin is an important component of the treatment regimen if only three courses of therapy are given.[24] Also, if only three courses are given, as was the case in the GOG study, serious pulmonary toxicity was not seen. Two other trials [Memorial Sloan-Kettering/Southwest Oncology Group[25] and Medical Research Council/European Organization for Research on Treatment of Cancer (MRC/EORTC)[26]] have shown that carboplatin is inferior to cisplatin in testis cancer and cannot be substituted for cisplatin without worsening the therapeutic outcome.

The issues are somewhat different for patients with incompletely resected tumor. These patients have a finite risk of treatment failure that is probably in the 20 to 40% range. Prognosis is related to amount of residual tumor and the presence or absence of stage IV disease, but not to cell type. Standard therapy consists of four courses of BEP, based upon data from randomized trials in testis cancer. The current GOG trial uses three courses of BEP followed by three courses of VAC, based upon the observation that some patients with persistent tumor after cisplatin-based chemotherapy have meaningful responses to VAC. However, at this time this approach should not be considered standard.

There are almost no data about the role of high-dose therapy with hematopoietic support in ovarian germ cell tumors. The use of such therapy in poor-risk testis cancer patients is now being investigated in an intergroup randomized trial. These patients have a predicted outcome less favorable than that for patients with ovarian germ cell tumor. Considering the absence of data, there is currently no role for high-dose therapy as a component of primary postoperative chemotherapy.

LING C. WONG
HEXTAN Y.S. NGAN

VAC therapy

In 1974 Malkasian et al[27] first reported two objective responses in endodermal sinus tumors treated with VAC combination chemotherapy. Smith and Rutledge[28] also reported responses with a VAC regimen in patients with advanced endodermal sinus tumor and advocated its use prophylactically in early disease. Today the VAC regimen consists of vincristine 1.5 mg/m^2 intravenously on day 1 of the treatment cycle, dactinomycin 0.5 mg daily intravenously for five consecutive days, and cyclosphosphamide 5 to 7 mg/kg daily

TABLE 18-3
VAC Regimen[a]

AGENT	DOSAGE	SCHEDULE
Vincristine	1.5 mg/m² IV	Day 1
Dactinomycin	0.5 mg IV	Days 1–5
Cyclosphosphamide	5–7 mg/kg IV	Days 1–5

[a] *Cycle is repeated once every four weeks.*

for five consecutive days. The treatment cycle is repeated every 4 weeks (Table 18–3). The administration of vincristine has been modified to day 1 of the treatment cycle instead of weekly administration for 12 weeks as proposed in the original report. This change minimizes the incidence of vincristine neurotoxicity.[11,29]

The VAC regimen was widely used in the 1970s and early 1980s, and various reports have confirmed its effectiveness in stage I disease with a high cure rate of over 80%.[11,12,29,31] The final GOG report on VAC treatment of malignant germ cell tumor stated that 15 of 22 patients (68%) with incompletely resected germ cell tumors failed VAC therapy.[12]

PVB therapy

Einhorn and Donohue[31] first report a high remission rate of 70 to 80% in patients, with disseminated testicular cancer treated with PVB regimen (Table 18–4). This regimen soon replaced VAC therapy as the most commonly used combination chemotherapy for germ cell tumor. Willemse et al[32] reported from a review of cumulative series of published data on VAC that the sustained remission rate in stage I and II tumors was 81% and 49% in stage III and IV disease, respectively. A cumulative series from the literature using PVB in previously untreated patients showed 96% long-term remission in stages I and II and 79% in stages III and IV. The GOG reported a 51% disease-free rate at 2 years in 89 patients with advanced or recurrent ovarian germ cell tumors treated by PVB regimen.[3] The Italian group[33] reported a 42% PVB failure rate in patients with measurable disease.

TABLE 18-4
PVB Regimen[a]

AGENT	DOSAGE	SCHEDULE
Cisplatin	100 mg/m² or 20 mg/m² IV	Day 1 Days 1–5
Vinblastine	0.15 mg/kg IV	Days 1 and 2
Bleomycin	10–15 mg daily infusion	Days 1–5

[a] *Cycle is repeated once every three to four weeks.*

BEP regimen

Newland was the first to report the activity of etoposide as a single agent in refractory testicular cancer.[34] A significant remission rate was reported in malignant ovarian teratoma treated with etoposide and cisplatin.[35] In a randomized clinical trial in 261 men with disseminated germ cell tumor, etoposide with cisplatin and bleomycin (Table 18–5) was found to be superior to vinblastine with cisplatin and bleomycin in the treatment of disseminated germ cell tumors because of diminished neuromuscular toxicity and, among patients with advanced disease, better efficacy.[36] The BEP regimen was found to have excellent activity in malignant ovarian germ cell tumor[9,37] with a 96% sustained remission rate in the M.D. Anderson Cancer Center series.

The choice of optimal chemotherapy regimen depends on the initial stage of the disease and the amount of residual tumor after de-

TABLE 18-5
BEP Regimen

AGENT	DOSAGE	SCHEDULE
VP 16-213	100 mg/m² IV infusion	Days 1–5
Cisplatin[a]	100 mg/m² IV infusion or 20 mg/m² IV infusion	Day 1 Days 1–5
Bleomycin	10 mg 24-hr infusion	Day 2

[a] *Precisplatin hydration, 1 L of 0.9% saline over 4 hours; postcisplatin hydration, 1 L of 0.9% saline over 4 hours.*

bulking. For stage I nondysgerminatous malignant ovarian germ cell tumor with no residual disease, the choice is between the VAC and PVB regimens. Though the PVB regimen is more popular, there is no randomized study proving its supremacy over VAC therapy. VAC therapy still has a place in the management of stage I disease since a complete remission rate of about 80% has been reported by various studies.[11,12,29] The toxicity of VAC therapy is much less than that of the PVB regimen. In the 1980s PVB became the standard chemotherapy for advanced malignant germ cell tumor, but whether it should remain the standard treatment is questionable. The Indiana series has demonstrated that the BEP regimen was more effective than the PVB regimen in disseminated testicular germ cell tumor. Excellent results have been reported by the M.D. Anderson Cancer Center group studying malignant ovarian germ cell tumors treated with the BEP regimen.[38] Neurotoxicity was reported to be less when compared with the PVB regimen. In the coming years the treatment of choice for disseminated ovarian germ cell tumor, especially when bulky residual tumors, are involved, may have to shift from a vinblastine-containing (PVB) regimen to etoposide combination (BEP) therapy.

Duration of chemotherapy

In the early 1980s when VAC therapy was used for the treatment of malignant germ cell tumors, the duration of therapy for the responders ranged from 1 year to 2 years.[9,11,12] As experience accumulated and more effective chemotherapy regimens were introduced, the duration of chemotherapy became shorter. The recommended duration of chemotherapy for responders is now between three and six cycles.[1,3,14,32,33,36] Some advocate two more cycles of chemotherapy once the serum tumor marker level has returned to normal.[1]

Primary postoperative high-dose chemotherapy

All patients receiving high-dose chemotherapy with autologous bone marrow rescue experience severe hematologic toxicity with absolute neutropenia, anemia, and thrombocytopenia that require transfusions. Overwhelming infections may develop during the neutropenic phase. Extramyeloid toxicities include mucositis, diarrhea, renal failure, and veno-occlusive disease of the liver.[39] More than 10% of patients treated with high-dose chemotherapy died from treatment-related complications.[39,40] Various reports have shown excellent results, a 80 to 90% cure rate, with primary cisplatin combination therapy in malignant germ cell tumors.[3,14,36,37] There is no justification for primary high-dose chemotherapy which has a treatment-related mortality rate of more than 10%.

QUESTION 5

What is optimal salvage therapy for a patient with an endodermal sinus tumor who progresses or rapidly relapses after completion of primary therapy? What is optimal salvage therapy for the same patient who relapses 4 months after completion of primary therapy?

STEPHEN WILLIAMS

There are almost no data on the treatment of patients who have recurrent, persistent, or progressive disease during or after chemotherapy. Rightly or wrongly, treatment decisions are based on experience gained in patients with the more common testicular germ cell tumor.

In the first situation, the patient is overtly cisplatin refractory. Conventional dose therapy, such as vinblastine, ifosfamide, and cisplatin (VeIP) is illogical and inappropriate. One might consider two courses of high-dose therapy (carboplatin, etoposide with or without cyclophosphamide or ifosfamide) with stem cell support. However, recent detailed analyses of results of high-dose therapy and prognostic factors suggest that the likelihood of long survival is low (< 5%) in cisplatin-refractory patients treated with two courses of high-dose therapy. Given the expense and potential toxicity of such therapy, it is debatable whether or not such therapy should be used. Reasonable therapeutic options are investigational chemotherapy with a phase I or II agent or supportive care.

The second situation is quite different. This patient has active tumor but is not overly cisplatin refractory, that is, has not progressed within 4 weeks of the last dose of cisplatin. Again, there are virtually no data on ovarian germ cell tumor patients, but a testicular cancer patient has a realistic chance for cure with salvage chemotherapy.[41] One option is four courses of VeIP, which includes the drug most active against germ cell tumors (cisplatin) and two new agents that the patient has not previously received. About 30% of testicular cancer patients in this situation have durable complete responses. An approach under investigation in testicular cancer is one or two courses of VeIP followed by two courses of high-dose carboplatin and etoposide with stem cell support. Whether or not this regimen is superior is currently not clear, but early results suggest that it might be. This would be a reasonable treatment option for this patient.

LING C. WONG
HEXTAN Y.S. NGAN

Conventional dose chemotherapy

Cisplatin combination chemotherapy has been demonstrated to be effective in the treatment of patients with persistent or recurrent disease after initial VAC therapy.[3,42,43] BEP therapy has been reported to be effective after VAC failure.[37] Currently the therapy of choice should be BEP therapy; it is a more effective and less toxic regimen than PVB therapy.[35] Since the 1980s most cancer centers have used PVB as the standard primary treatment. In cisplatin combination therapy failures there is a difference between cisplatin-sensitive disease and cisplatin-resistant disease. Patients who respond to cisplatin combination therapy but have a recurrence within months after completion of chemotherapy probably have cisplatin-sensitive disease and can be rechallenged with cisplatin combination therapy. It is logical to choose BEP therapy after PVB failures since it has been demonstrated to be more effective than PVB in the treatment of malignant germ cell tumors. Patients who fail to respond to initial cisplatin combination therapy should be treated with noncisplatin-containing regimens. In the GOG study 5 of 12 PVB failures were salvaged with VAC therapy.[3] Salvage success was reported with a combination of etoposide, methotrexate, dactinomycin, cyclosphosphamide, and vincristine (EMA-CO).[22] Other effective salvage regimens used after PVB failure include a combination of etoposide, doxorubicin, and cyclosphosphamide[44] and combinations of vincristine, dactinomycin, and ifosfamide.[45]

Reports of cisplatin failures in malignant ovarian germ cell tumors are scarce. Most data from the reports on testicular cancer. For platinum-sensitive tumors the most common therapy includes ifosfamide, cisplatin with vinblastine, or etoposide. The complete response rate ranges from 25% to 36% to chemotherapy alone or to chemotherapy followed by surgical resection.[39,46] For patients with platinum-resistant disease a choice should be made from high-dose chemotherapy, phase II drugs, or surgical salvage.

High-dose chemotherapy

The use of high-dose chemotherapy and autologous bone marrow rescue has been useful in the treatment of patients with germ cell tumors that have recurred after conventional dose salvage chemotherapy.[40,47–49] Forty consecutive patients with recurrent or refractory germ cell tumors were treated at Indiana University between 1986 and 1989. All patients received high-dose carboplatin 900 to 2,000 mg/m^2 body surface area and etoposide 1200 mg/m^2. Three patients also received ifosphamide. All patients had autologous bone marrow rescue. Twenty six of the 40 patients in the study received two full courses of therapy. There were 26 (65%) responders, 12 (30%)

achieved a complete response, and 14 (35%) achieved a partial response. Of the 12 complete responders, 5 relapsed and 1 died of treatment-related acute leukemia 27.5 months after treatment without evidence of disease. Six (15%) of the original 40 patients, of whom 3 were refractory to cisplatin, remained in complete remission after at least 24 months of follow-up.[39] Some degree of disease resistance to cisplatin can be overcome with dose escalation of platinum compounds. The Eastern Cooperative Oncology Group reported 5 (30%) of 17 assessable patients achieved sustained complete remission with a minimal follow-up of 1 year.[48] Some advocated earlier intervention with high-dose chemotherapy in poor-risk patients who showed an inappropriately slow decline of serum tumor markers after two cycles of induction cisplatin-based therapy.[50]

QUESTION 6

For which patients do you recommend second-look surgery? For which patients, if any, do you recommend secondary cytoreductive surgery?

STEPHEN WILLIAMS

Second-look laparotomy has been considered by many to be a component of routine treatment of patients with epithelial ovarian cancer to assess disease status after chemotherapy. It is understandable that such an approach has been extrapolated to the treatment of patients with ovarian germ cell tumors. In a series from M. D. Anderson Cancer Center,[51] findings were negative in 52 of 53 patients who underwent this procedure. One patient with negative findings subsequently relapsed and died. Thirteen patients had biopsy-proven evidence of mature teratoma at second-look laparotomy; treatment was discontinued in all patients, and none developed a recurrence.

The GOG experience with second-look laparotomy in ovarian germ cell tumors has been reviewed in a recent publication.[52] All patients in this study were enrolled prospectively in one of three protocols employing relatively brief cisplatin-based chemotherapy after initial surgical staging and cytoreduction when appropriate. Forty-five surgical procedures were performed in patients who received three courses of BEP after initial complete tumor resection. No tumor or mature teratoma was found in 43, and immature teratoma was found in 2 patients. One of the latter patients received further chemotherapy, and one did not. Both these patients and 44 of the total are disease-free. Seventy-two patients were treated with similar chemotherapy for advanced incompletely resected tumor. Forty-eight of these patients did not have teratoma elements in their primary tumor. At surgery, 45 patients had no tumor, and 3 had persistent endodermal sinus tumor or embryonal carcinoma. All three of the latter patients died despite further treatment. Twenty-four patients had teratoma elements in their primary tumor. Of these, 16 had mature teratoma at second-look, surgery, which in 7 was bulky or progressive. Fourteen of the total 16 and six of the seven with bulky residual tumor remain disease-free after surgical resection.

These data prove rather convincingly that second-look laparotomy is not necessary in patients with tumor completely resected initially or in patients with initially incompletely resected tumor that does not contain teratoma. However, enough patients who initially have incompletely resected tumor containing elements of teratoma benefit from the procedure to warrant its general use. Some patients with bulky residual mature teratoma after chemotherapy have progressive teratoma over time that is potentially life-threatening as a result of invasion and compression of adjacent essential structures.[53] A few patients also may develop non-germ cell malignancies that arise in teratoma. Experience in testicular cancer and in smaller numbers of patients with ovarian germ cell tumors suggests that most of these patients do well after complete excision of teratoma.

Secondary cytoreduction of cancer has no place in the treatment of patients with ovarian germ cell tumor. Persistent or recurrent carcinoma (as opposed to teratoma) is typically disseminated and rapidly progressive. It is illogical to incompletely remove tumor, and success or failure of salvage treatment is totally dependent on a subsequent favorable response to chemotherapy and complete tumor resection is rarely possible. There may be a *rare* patient with localized, relatively indolent drug-resistant cancer who can be cured with surgical resection. This is possible with testicular cancer, but only in rare highly selected patients, and there is little or no experience in ovarian germ cell tumors. The recommended surgical procedure in this scenario is not cytoreduction but total meticulous tumor resection.

LING C. WONG
HEXTAN Y.S. NGAN

Second-look laparotomy

Wangensteen et al[38] first described second-look laparotomy in patients with gastrointestinal malignancies. In the 1960s second-look laparotomy was incorporated into the management of ovarian cancer with the goal of documenting the disease-free state or tumor debulking should disease persist. It is not surprising that the same philosophy applies to the management of ovarian germ cell tumor. A review of the literature, however, shows that positive findings in second-look laparotomy are extremely rare. Roberts et al[54] discussed nine second-look laparotomies in patients with germ cell tumor following treatment with VAC; only one patient had residual disease. Slayton reported 27 patients receiving VAC therapy, 16 of whom underwent second-look laparotomy; 10 showed no disease, three had mature teratoma, and three had residual disease.[55] Gershenson et al[22] recently reported negative findings in 52 of 53 patients. Similar findings was reported in Hong Kong, where 15 of 16 patients who underwent second-look laparotomy had negative findings.[11] It seems that in patients with initial raised serum tumor marker levels the profile of the serum tumor marker level accurately reflects the activity of the disease. A second-look procedure is not necessary to document a disease-free status. Second-look laparotomy should be limited to patients with advanced disease and initial negative tumor marker determinations. With more effective chemotherapy and better imaging techniques, the need for second-look laparotomy would be further reduced.

Surgical salvage

A retrospective review on chemorefractory and resectable disseminated germ cell tumors was done on patients treated at Indiana University from 1977 to 1990. A total of 48 patients underwent salvage surgery; 38 (79%) were rendered grossly disease-free, and 29 (60%) achieved serological remission. Ten patients (21%) remained continuously disease-free with no postoperative treatment and a median follow-up of 46 months. Six additional patients who relapsed after salvage surgery were disease-free after further treatment, four with repeat surgery and two with high-dose chemotherapy and autologous bone marrow transplant.[56]

Secondary cytoreductive surgery is indicated only in recurrent or refractory disease where gross tumor has been demonstrated. It is hoped that cytoreduction will make subsequent therapy more effective.

EDITORS' COMMENTARY

With the prognosis of patients with malignant ovarian germ cell tumors already so favorable, controversial or unresolved issues surrounding clinical management principally focus on refinement of existing therapies. As noted, Drs. Williams, Ngan, and Wong generally agree on most issues regarding the questions posed, but there are some differences of opinion.

All authors agree on the advisability of comprehensive surgical staging. Unfortunately, incomplete surgical staging remains a problem in the 1990s. The majority of patients referred to tertiary centers have not undergone comprehensive surgical staging. Several factors account for this phenomenon, not the least of which is the fact that most of these patients are quite young and are operated on by physicians who do not expect to find a malignancy and/or do not understand its biologic behavior. As the answers indicate, there is no standard for lymph node sampling or dissection in this group of tumors. Drs. Wong and Ngan essentially takes the standard position and recommends resection of enlarged nodes or random sampling in the absence of enlarged nodes. Dr. Williams, on the other hand, does not believe that routine lymph node sampling or dissection are essential since, in his opinion, the risk of lymph node involvement is low, and the results are excellent in the absence of lymph node sampling. Until more information is available, some type of lymph node sampling seems recommendable, although complete para-aortic and pelvic lymphadenectomy does not appear to be necessary, especially in the absence of enlarged nodes.

With regard to candidates for treatment with surgery alone, Drs. Wong and Ngan echoes the standard practice in the United States, which consists of postoperative chemotherapy for all patients with ovarian germ cell tumors except those with stage I pure dysgerminoma or stage IA, grade 1, pure immature teratoma. Dr. Williams cites emerging data from the United Kingdom, Italy, and an American intergroup pediatric study indicating that some groups are extending their indications for surgery alone to those with stage I high-grade immature teratomas, and even to those with stage I yolk sac tumors. We agree with Dr. Williams' statement that "such an approach must be taken with great caution." This treatment strategy must be considered investigational. Furthermore, we also must consider what the threshold of acceptance is based on number of recurrences and deaths.

For a patient with incompletely staged dysgerminoma, neither author recommends restaging, with which we agree. Provided serum tumor marker levels and CT scans of the abdomen and pelvis are normal, most experts recommend observation. Both authors make a compelling argument against adjuvant chemotherapy.

In almost all corners of the world, platinum-based chemotherapy is the standard for patients with ovarian germ cell tumors. Drs. Wong and Ngan leaves the door open for treatment of patients with stage I disease with the VAC regimen, but most experts disagree with this opinion. No author sees a current role for high-dose chemotherapy as primary treatment. Unfortunately, the rarity of patients with a poor prognosis precludes a meaningful clinical trial in this area.

As noted by all authors, there is no standard for patients who progress or rapidly relapse after completion of primary chemotherapy, but a platinum-containing regimen—such as a combination of vinblastine/etoposide, ifosfamide, and cisplatin—is recommended for those with relatively late relapse. In general, however, the prognosis for all patients who relapse is rather poor. The role of high-dose chemotherapy with autologous bone marrow transplant or peripheral blood stem cells remains unclear, although preliminary results are not particularly encouraging.

And finally, all authors recommend the restriction of second-look surgery to selected patients. There is, however, no consensus about this issue. As is obvious from their comments, there is also no agreement about the role of secondary cytoreductive surgery for this disease although we believe that selected patients with very limited tumor may benefit.

References

1. Gershenson DM: Management of early ovarian cancer: germ cell and sex cord-stromal tumours. Gynecol Oncol 55: S62–S72, 1994
2. Williams S, Blessing JA, Liao S et al: Adjuvant therapy of ovarian germ cell tumors with cisplatin, etoposide, and bleomycin: a trial of the Gynecologic Oncology Group. J Clin Oncol 12:701–706, 1994

3. Williams SD, Blessing JA, Moore DH et al: Cisplatin, vinblastine, and bleomycin in advanced and recurrent ovarian germ-cell tumors. Ann Int Med 111:22–27, 1989
4. Kurman RJ, Norris HJ: Malignant germ cell tumors of the ovary. Hum Pathol 8:551–564, 1977
5. Norris HJ, Zirkin HJ, Benson WL: Immature (malignant) teratoma of the ovary. Cancer 37:2359–2372, 1976
6. Kurman RJ, Norris HJ: Malignant mixed germ cell tumors of the ovary. Obstet Gynecol 48:579–589, 1976
7. Kurman RJ, Norris HJ: Endodermal sinus tumour of the ovary. Cancer 38:2404–2419, 1976
8. Gershensen DM, Del Junco G, Copeland LJ, Rutledge FN: Mixed germ cell tumours of the ovary. Obstet Gynecol 64:200, 1984
9. Gershenson DM, Del Junco G, Herson J, Rutledge FN: Endodermal sinus tumour of the ovary. The M. D. Anderson experience. Obstet Gynecol 61:194–202, 1983
10. Gershenson DM, Del Junco G, Silva EG et al: Immature teratoma of the ovary. Obstet Gynecol 68:624–629, 1986
11. Wong LC, Ngan HYS, Ma HK: Primary treatment with vincristine, dactinomycin, and cyclosphosphamide in nondysgerminomatous germ cell tumour of the ovary. Gynecol Oncol 34:155–158, 1989
12. Slayton RE, Park RC, Silverberg SG et al: Vincristine, dactinomycin and cyclosphosphamide in the treatment of malignant germ cell tumours of the ovary: a Gynaecologic Oncology Group study (a final report). Cancer 56:243–248, 1985
13. Pfleider A: Therapy of ovarian malignant germ cell tumour and granulosa tumours. Int J Gynaecol Pathol 12:162–165, 1993
14. Gershenson DM, Morris M, Cangir A et al: Treatment of malignant germ cell tumors of the ovary with bleomycin, etoposide, and cisplatin. J Clin Oncol 8:715–720, 1990
15. Cushing B, Giller R, Cohen L et al: Surgery alone is effective treatment of resected ovarian immature teratoma in children: a pediatric intergroup report. Proc ASCO 15:461, 1996
16. Newlands ES, Bower M, Holden L et al: Management of stage I and metastatic ovarian germ cell tumors. Proc ASCO 15:285, 1996
17. Bonazzi C, Peccatori F, Colombo N et al: Pure ovarian immature teratoma, a unique and curable disease: 10 years' experience of 32 prospectively treated patients. Obstet Gynecol 84:598–604, 1994
18. Novak ER, Woodruff JD: p. 367. In Novak ER (ed): Gynecologic and Obstetric Pathology. 6th Ed. Philadelphia, WB Saunders, 1967.
19. Thomas GM, Dembo AJ, Hacker NF, DePetrillo AD: Current therapy for dysgerminoma of the ovary. Obstet Gynecol 70:268–275, 1987
20. Williams SD, Blessing JA, Hatch KD, Homesley HD: Chemotherapy of advanced dysgerminoma: trials of the Gynecolgic Oncology Group. J Clin Oncol 9:1950–1955, 1991
21. Williams SD, Blessing JA, Hatch KD, Homesley HD: Chemotherapy of advanced dysgerminoma: trials of the Gynaecologic oncology Group. J Clin Oncol 9:1950–1955, 1991
22. Gershenson DM: Update on malignant ovarian germ cell tumours. Cancer 71(4):1581–1590, 1993
23. Williams SD, Blessing J, Slayton R, Homesley H et al: Ovarian germ cell tumors: adjuvant trials of the Gynecologic Oncology Group. Proc ASCO 8:150, 1989
24. Loehrer PJ, Johnson D, Elson P et al: Importance of bleomycin in favorable-prognosis disseminated germ cell tu-

mors: an Eastern Cooperative Oncology Group trial. J Clin Oncol 13:470–476, 1995

25. Bajorin DF, Sarosdy MF, Pfister DG et al: Randomized trial of etoposide and cisplatin versus etoposide and carboplatin in patients with good-risk germ cell tumors: a multiinstitutional study. J Clin Oncol 11:598–606, 1993
26. Horwich A, Sleijfer D: Carboplatin-based chemotherapy in good prognosis metastatic non-seminoma of the testis: an interim report of an MRC/EORTC randomised trial. Proc Leeds Germ Cell Tumour Conf, 1994.
27. Malkasian GD, Webbs MJ, Jorgensen EO: Observations on chemotherapy of granulosa cell carcinoma and malignant ovarian teratomas. Obstet Gynecol 44:885–888, 1974
28. Smith J, Rutledge F: Advances in chemotherapy for gnaecologic cancer. Cancer 36:669–674, 1975
29. Gershenson DM, Copeland LJ, Kavangh JJ et al: Treatment of malignant non-dysgerminomatous germ cell tumours of the ovary with vincristine, actinomycin D and cyclosphosphamide. Cancer 56:2756–2761, 1985
30. Schwartz PE: Combination chemotherapy in the management of ovarian germ cell malignancies. Obstet Gynecol 64: 564–572, 1984
31. Einhorn LH, Donohue J: *cis*-Diamminedichloroplatinum, vinblastine and bleomycin combination therapy in disseminated testicular cancer. Ann Intern Med 87:293–298, 1977
32. Willemse PHB, Aalders JG, Bouma J et al: Long-term survival after vinblastine, bleomycin, and cisplatin treatment in patients with germ cell tumours of the ovary: an update. Gynecol Oncol 28:268–277, 1987
33. DePalo G, Zambetti M, Pilotti S et al: Nondysgerminomatous tumours of the ovary treated with cisplatin, vinblastine, and bleomycin: long term results, Gynecol Oncol 47:239–246, 1992
34. Newlands ES, Bagshawe KD: Epipodophyllin derrivatives (VP-16-213) in malignant teratomas and chorocarcinomas. Lancet 2:87, 1977
35. Newlands ES, Begent RHJ, Rustin GJS et al: Teratoma of the ovary. Brit Med J 1213, 1979
36. Williams SD, Bich R, Einhorn LH et al: Treatment of disseminated germ-cell tumours with cisplatin, bleomycin and either vinblastine or etoposide, N Engl J Med 316:1435–1440, 1987
37. Wong LC, Collins RJ, Ngan HYS, Ma HK: Etoposide combination chemotherapy in refractory ovarian malignant germ cell tumour. Gynecol Oncol 39:123–136, 1990
38. Wangesteen OH, Lewis FJ, Tongen LA: The second-look in cancer surgery. Lancet 71:303–307, 1951
39. Broun ER, Nichols CR, Kneebone P et al: Long-term outcome of patients with relapsed and refractory germ cell tumours treated with high-dose chemotherapy and autologous bone marrow rescue. Ann Intern Med 117:124–138, 1992
40. Nichols CR, Anderson J, Wolff SN et al: High dose carboplatin and etoposide with autologous bone marrow transplantation in refractory germ cell cancer: An Eastern Cooperative Group protocol. J Clin Oncol 10:558–563, 1992
41. Loehrer P, Lauer R, Roth B et al: Salvage therapy in recurrent germ cell cancer: ifosfamide and cisplatin plus either vinblastine or etoposide. Ann Int Med 7:540–546, 1988
42. Carlson RW, Sikic BI, Turbow MM, Ballon SC: Combination cisplatin, vinblastine, and bleomycin (PVB) for malignant germ cell tumours of the ovary. J Clin Oncol 1:645–651, 1983
43. Gershenson DM, Kavanagh JJ, Copeland LJ et al: Treatment of malignant

nondysgerminomatous germ cell tumours of the ovary with vinblastine, bleomycin and cisplatin. Cancer 57: 1731–1737, 1986

44. Taylor MH, DePetrillo AD, Turner AR: Vinblastine, bleomycin, and cisplatin in malignant germ cell tumours of the ovary. Cancer 56:1341–1349, 1984
45. Sessa C, Bonazzi C, Landoni F et al: Cisplatin, vinblastine, and blecomycin combination chemotherapy in endodermal sinus tumour of the ovary. Obstet Gynecol 70:220–224, 1987
46. Motzer RJ, Geller NL, Tan C et al: Salvage chemotherapy for patients with germ cell tumours. Cancer 67:12305–12310, 1991
47. Linkesh W, Kuhrer I, Wagner A: rhu-GM-CSF after ultra-high dose carboplatin, VP-16, cyclophosphamide with ABMT in refractory germ cell cancer, abstract. Proc ASCO 9:141, 1990
48. Baume D, Pico JL, Droz JP et al: Value of high dose chemotherapy followed by bone marrow autograft in nonseminomatous germinal tumor with poor prognosis: results of the combination of cisplatin, etoposide and cyclophosphamide (PEC protocol). Bull Cancer 77:160–180, 1990
49. Mulder PO, DeVries EG, Koops HS et al: Chemotherapy with maximally tolerable doses of VP-16-213 and cyclophosphamide followed by autologous bone marrow transplatation for the treatment of relapsed or refractory germ cell tumours. Eur J Cancer Clin Oncol 24:675–679, 1988
50. Motzer RJ, Gulati SC, Crown JP et al: High-dose chemotherapy and autologous bone marrow rescue for patients with refractory germ cell tumours: early intervention is better tolerated. Cancer 69:550–556, 1992
51. Gershenson DM, Copeland LJ, Del Junco G: Second-look laparotomy in the management of malignant germ cell tumors of the ovary. Obstet Gynecol 67:789–794, 1986
52. Williams SD, Blessing JA, DiSaia PJ et al: Second-look laparotomy in ovarian germ cell tumors: the Gynecologic Oncology Group experience. Gynecol Oncol 52:287–291, 1994
53. Geisler JP, Goulet R, Foster RS, Sutton GP: Growing teratoma syndrome after chemotherapy for germ cell tumors of the ovary. Obstet Gynecol 84:719–721, 1994
54. Roberts WS, Hodel K, Rich WM, DiSaia, PJ: Second look laparotomy in the management of gynaecologic malignancies. Gynecol Oncol 13:345–355, 1982
55. Slayton RE, Hershchyshyn MM, Silverberg SG et al: Treatment of malignant ovarian germ cell tumous. Cancer 42:390–398, 1978
56. Murphy BR, Breeden ES, Donohue JP et al: Surgical salvage of chemorefractory germ cell tumours. J Clin Oncol 11:324–329 1993

CHAPTER 19

MANAGEMENT OF SEX CORD-STROMAL TUMORS

Nicoletta Colombo

EDITORS' INTRODUCTION

Ovarian sex cord-stromal tumors account for less than 5% of all ovarian cancers. Table 19-1 shows the World Health Organization (WHO) classification system for these tumors. They may occur at any age, although the age of peak incidence for granulosa cell tumors, the most common cell type, is in the postmenopausal years. Because of their extreme rarity, their multiplicity of histologic patterns and associated confusing terminology, and their variable biologic behavior, the optimal treatment of these tumors remains somewhat of an enigma. No standard therapy exists. Contemporary treatment principles have generally developed based on observations of small groups of patients and on information extrapolated from the clinical management of epithelial tumors.

Surgery remains the cornerstone of treatment for patients with ovarian sex cord-stromal tumors. Reports of large series of patients with granulosa cell tumors and Sertoli-Leydig cell tumors indicate that at least 95% of these neoplasms are unilateral and that at least 95% are confined to the ovary. Thus, conservative surgery with unilateral salpingo-oophorectomy seems to be appropriate treatment for young patients with stage IA disease. For older patients or those with advanced-stage disease or bilateral ovarian involvement, abdominal hysterectomy and bilateral salpingo-oophorectomy are usually indicated. If results of frozen-section analysis suggest the possibility of a stromal tumor, a careful exploration should be conducted for any evidence of metastatic tumor. When any areas suspicious for tumor are detected, the standard practice includes cytoreductive surgery, although there is no definitive evidence supporting this approach. When no suspicious areas are noted, comprehensive surgical staging is appropriate.

In order to select those patients with ovarian sex cord-stromal tumors who should receive postoperative therapy, an understanding of prognostic factors is essential. Unfortunately, available information about these factors is controversial and incomplete. The most commonly used postoperative treatment is platinum-based chemotherapy. However, there are reports of activity with both radiotherapy and hormonal therapy.

QUESTIONS

1. What are the major prognostic factors associated with sex cord-stromal tumors?
2. What are the options for a patient referred to you after surgery for a granulosa cell tumor seemingly confined to the ovary but without surgical staging? Which option do you recommend?
3. Are there stage I patients for whom you recommend postoperative therapy? If so, please describe them.
4. What is currently the treatment of choice for postoperative patients with metastatic (primary advanced-stage or recurrent) sex cord-stromal tumors?
5. What is the role, if any, of radiotherapy in the treatment of patients with sex cord-stromal tumors?
6. What is the role, if any, of hormonal therapy in the treatment of patients with sex cord-stromal tumors?

QUESTION 1

What are the major prognostic factors associated with sex cord-stromal tumors?

NICOLETTA COLOMBO

The term *stromal tumor of the ovary* identifies a variety of neoplasms which are formed of cells derived from the sex cord or mesenchyme of the embryonic gonad and may contain granulosa cells, Sertoli cells, Leydig cells, thecal cells, or fibroblasts of gonadal stromal origin. These neoplasms represent a minority of ovarian malignancies (7%), and their scarcity represents a limitation in our understanding of their natural history, management, and prognosis.

Granulosa cell tumors account for 70% of ovarian stromal tumors. Since these tumors have a propensity for indolent growth and late recurrence (up to 25 years after initial treatment), a true estimate of their malignancy can be obtained only by prolonged surveillance. The overall survival of patients with granulosa cell ovarian tumors is quite good,[1–4] probably because most of these tumors are diagnosed at an early stage. In fact, the only absolute indication of a poor prognosis is the presence of extraovarian spread at the time of initial diagnosis. Other prognostic factors are more debatable: tumor size[5–6] is associated with a poor outcome, but its prognostic value in early-stage disease has not been clearly established; histologic pattern, mitotic count, and atypia have not been proved to be of strict relevance for tumors without extraovarian spread.[4–9] DNA ploidy has recently been correlated with survival. While few studies demonstrated that it was an independent prognostic factor for survival,[10–12] others showed that aneuploidy was significantly associated with other adverse histolopathologic parameters

TABLE 19-1
World Health Organization Classification of Sex Cord-Stromal Tumors

A. Granulosa stromal cell
   1. Granulosa cell
   2. Thecoma-fibroma
B. Androblastomas: Sertoli-Leydig cell tumors
   1. Well differentiated (Pick's adenoma, Sertoli cell tumor)
   2. Intermediate differentiation
   3. Poorly differentiated
   4. With heterologous elements
C. Lipid cell tumors
D. Gynandroblastoma
E. Unclassified

that may be of prognostic value (high stage, vascular invasion, nuclear atypia, high mitotic activity); but aneuploidy by itself is not a useful method to predict the biologic aggressive behavior of granulosa cell tumors.[13–17]

Sertoli and Sertoli-Leydig cell tumors are characterized by onset at an early age (average 27 years). Pure Sertoli cell tumors and pure Leydig cell tumors are benign, while the grade of differentiation is the most important prognostic factor in Sertoli-Leydig tumors: well-differentiated neoplasms always behave in a benign fashion, while poorly differentiatiated neoplasms were associated with a 44% survival rate in a large study.[18] The retiform histologic pattern and the presence of heterologous muscle and cartilage elements confer a poor prognosis.

QUESTION 2

What are the options for a patient referred to you after surgery for a granulosa cell tumor seemingly confined to the ovary but without surgical staging? Which option do you recommend?

NICOLETTA COLOMBO

Although proper staging is warranted in any patient with granulosa cell ovarian tumors, the following considerations should influence the decision for or against laparotomic restaging in a patient with apparent stage I disease.

1. Most patients with granulosa cell ovarian tumors have no evidence of extraovarian spread at surgery. Unlike the situation in epithelial ovarian cancer, 80 to 90% of these neoplasms are at stage I at time of diagnosis.
2. Bilateral ovarian involvement is rare (2%).[1–5,8]
3. Although accurate and complete staging was not performed in most of the published series, overall 10-year survival occurs consistently (70 to 90%), reflecting a low frequency of understaging.
4. No prospective study has been conducted to evaluate the frequency of occult metastases in patients with presumably stage I disease undergoing complete restaging.
5. Granulosa cell tumors have a prolonged natural history and a tendency toward late relapse. Because of their low-grade biology, the average time to recurrence is between 5 and 10 years, but relapses can occur after as long as 25 years.

These considerations make the need for surgical restaging less imperative than it is for epithelial ovarian cancer. In women of reproductive age a unilateral salpingo-oophorectomy is appropriate therapy for stage IA tumors,[7] but dilatation and curettage of the uterus should be performed to exclude coexistent adenocarcinoma of the endometrium. Together with a computerized tomography scan of the pelvis and abdomen, laparoscopy can be a sufficient procedure to rule out spread of tumor. In postmenopausal women a hysterectomy and salpingo-oophorectomy should be performed. If this was not done at the time of first surgery, the benefit of a second laparotomy to remove the internal reproductive apparatus is debatable. Imaging and laparoscopic restaging can be considered adequate to exclude the need for adjuvant chemotherapy.

QUESTION 3

Are there stage I patients for whom you recommend postoperative therapy? If so, please describe them.

NICOLETTA COLOMBO

Granulosa cell tumors should be considered low-grade malignancies, similar to so-called borderline epithelial ovarian cancers. Our understanding of the role of adjuvant therapy in these patients is hampered by a lack of basic information regarding the true incidence of recurrence in stage I disease and the efficacy of different treatment options. Evans[1] reported a 9% risk of recurrence in stage IA. Granulosa cell tumors, which can recur or metastasize, do so in an indolent manner, with one-third of recurrences appearing more than 5 years after diagnosis, one-fifth after 10 years, and possible recurrence at 25 years. Therefore, a true estimate of the risk of recurrence can be obtained only by surveillance for at least 20 years. Moreover, over such a long period of time, a number of patients die of other intercurrent diseases, making a true estimation of the risk of recurrence even more difficult. From the available data, even in the absence of a thorough surgical staging in all patients, survival of patients with stage I granulosa cell tumors is above 90%, making the risk of recurrence very low.

There have been no reports suggesting a benefit from adjuvant chemotherapy in patients with early granulosa cell tumors. In a retrospective series, Bjorkholm[7] reported no benefit from adjuvant irradiation in women with stage I disease.

Currently, there is no basis for recommending adjuvant treatment of any sort following surgery for stage I granulosa cell ovarian tumor.

QUESTION 4

What is currently the treatment of choice for postoperative patients with metastatic (primary advanced-stage or recurrent) sex cord-stromal tumors?

NICOLETTA COLOMBO

Metastatic lesions and recurrences from granulosa cell tumors have been treated with a variety of different antineoplastic agents.

Although responses to a number of combination regimens have been reported, the small number of patients in each series makes it difficult to draw definitive conclusions. Single alkylating agents have been used in the past, producing a 25% partial response rate.[19–20] The few available reports suggest that multidrug regimens may be more effective than single alkylating agents. The combination of actinomycin D, 5-fluorouracil, and cyclophosphamide has shown activity in 2 of 2 patients.[20] More recently, complete responses have been achieved in patients treated with doxorubicin/cisplatin regimens[21] and with doxorubicin/ciplatin/cyclophosphamide.[22–24] The Gynecologic Oncology Group used a combination of vincristine, actinomycin D, and cyclophosphamide in the treatment of advanced or recurrent granulosa cell ovarian tumors and achieved only a 20% partial response rate.[25] The highest activity has been demonstrated with the cisplatin/vinblastine/bleomycin (PVB) regimen. We reported six complete and three partial responses in 11 previously untreated patients with recurrent and/or metastatic granulosa cell tumors using this regimen,[26] and these results have been confirmed by other reports.[27–28] This regimen has been associated with significant myelotoxicity and a few septic deaths, however. In the treatment of germ cell tumors, the substitution of etoposide for vinblastine might produce lower myelotoxicity while retaining similar efficacy. We suggest therefore the following regimen for the treatment of metastatic and/or recurrent granulosa cell ovarian tumors (Table 19-2).

TABLE 19-2
Recommended Regimen for the Treatment of Metastatic and/or Recurrent Granulosa Cell Ovarian Tumors[a]

AGENT	DOSAGE
Bleomycin	15 units/m²/day 1,15 every 3 weeks
Etoposide	100 mg/m²/day for 5 days every 3 weeks
Cisplatin	20 mg/m²/day for 5 days every 3 weeks

[a] *Five cycles are generally recommended, with the suggestion that bleomycin be withdrawn after cycle 3.*

Because of the rarity of Sertoli-Leydig cell tumors and the infrequent finding of advanced or recurrent disease, there is even less experience with chemotherapy for these tumors. Active regimens reported in the literature include vincristine/actinomycin D/cyclophosphamide (VAC) and cisplatin/Adriamycin/cyclophosphamide (PAC) regimens.[18,29] Other active drugs include methotrexate, vinblastine, and bleomycin.[30] Although it is not possible to draw definitive conclusions from the above isolated cases, it is apparent that Sertoli-Leydig tumors may respond to chemotherapy regimens that utilize cisplatin, cyclophosphamide, doxorubicin, actinomycin, vinblastine, or bleomycin in various combinations. It seems reasonable, therefore, to adopt for advanced Sertoli-Leydig tumors the same treatment regimen previously described for granulosa cell ovarian tumors.

QUESTION 5

What is the role, if any, of radiotherapy in the treatment of patients with sex cord-stromal tumors?

NICOLETTA COLOMBO

There are few data on the role of radiotherapy in the management of sex cord-stromal tumors. In a retrospective series Bjorkholm[7] reported no benefit from adjuvant irradiation in patients with stage I granulosa cell tumors. There is little information concerning the use of radiotherapy in advanced or recurrent tumors. Although most reported series include patients treated with radiotherapy, the lack of uniformity in the staging and treatment program precludes any definitive conclusion. It seems reasonable to conclude that this modality may represent an alternative to chemotherapy only in patients with small-volume residual disease and that pelvic radiation can be utilized for palliative treatment of isolated pelvic recurrences.

QUESTION 6

What is the role, if any, of hormonal therapy in the treatment of patients with sex cord-stromal tumors?

NICOLETTA COLOMBO

The rationale for using hormonal treatment relies on the observation that receptors for follicle stimulating hormone (FSH) have been demonstrated in granulosa cell tumors, and FSH has been shown to support the growth of this tumor in nude mice. In lung metastases one transient response to gonadotropin releasing hormone (GnRH) agonist analog therapy after failure of surgery and cytotoxic chemotherapy has been reported.[31] Another report showed a partial response in five patients with advanced granulosa cell tumors resistant to chemotherapy.[32] Besides these few observations there is essentially no experience in the systematic use of hormonal manipulation in the treatment of advanced or recurrent granulosa cell ovarian tumors.

EDITORS' COMMENTARY

We agree with Dr. Colombo regarding her perspective on prognostic factors in this group of tumors. Unfortunately, for granulosa cell tumors, the only known reliable predictor of survival is stage. The literature on all other factors is quite confusing. Therefore, in a patient with stage I granulosa cell tumor, the prognostic significance of such factors as tumor size, tumor rupture, mitotic count, and presence of atypia remains unclear. Furthermore, the literature is also in conflict regarding the prognostic value of DNA ploidy. For Sertoli-Leydig cell tumors, in addition to stage, histologic differentiation, presence of heterologous elements, and presence of the retiform pattern all appear to be prognostic. For example, the incidence of recurrence is essentially negligible in patients with well-differentiated Sertoli-Leydig tumors and approximately 60% in those with poorly differentiated tumors.

We also agree with Dr. Colombo that a restaging operation in a patient with a sex cord-stromal tumor with disease seemingly confined to the ovary but with incomplete surgical staging can be avoided in most instances. Bilateral ovarian involvement is rare—less than 5%—and most patients have stage I disease. For such patients, our usual management consists of obtaining a computerized tomography scan of the abdomen and pelvis, and serum tumor marker assays appropriate to the tumor (CA 125 and inhibin for granulosa cell tumor, and CA 125 and α-fetoprotein for Sertoli-Leydig cell tumor). Of course, for all these tumors, even if there are no peripheral stigmata of a feminizing or virilizing process, it is probably prudent to obtain serum levels of estradiol and testosterone as a baseline. Dr. Colombo does mention laparoscopy, and this procedure may be indicated in some situations.

Dr. Colombo nicely outlines the difficulties in decision making regarding patients with stage I granulosa cell tumors, including their long natural history and the lack of meaningful information in the literature. Although she does not discuss Sertoli-Leydig cell tumors, the pathology literature indicates that the recurrence rate in patients with poorly differentiated tumors is approximately 60%. Therefore, this group seems to be a reasonable one to include a prospective study using adjuvant therapy.

Dr. Colombo indicates that the treatment of choice for patients with metastatic sex cord-stromal tumors is a platinum-based combination chemotherapy regimen. Her recommendation of choice is a combination of bleomycin, etoposide, and cisplatin. Clearly, this regimen is the most popular in the United States for treatment of such patients. On average, however a population older than those with malignant germ cell tumors is involved, and deaths from bleomycin lung toxicity have been reported. Recently, we and other investigators have observed promising antitumor activity with paclitaxel in patients with refractory ovarian sex cord-stromal tumors. Therefore, a combination of paclitaxel and a platinum drug may be a reasonable candidate for future study.

It is difficult to evaluate the efficacy of radiotherapy in treating this group of tumors. This problem is related to the fact that several patients reported in the literature were treated in an adjuvant fashion or were treated with a combination of radiotherapy and chemotherapy. On the other hand, definite examples of the activity of this modality have been reported. There are also a handful of reports on antitumor activity with hormonal therapy for management of these tumors. Both treatment deserve further study.

In summary, there is a tremendous gap in our knowledge about ovarian sex cord-stromal tumors related to their extreme rarity and, in the case of granulosa cell tumors, their potential long natural history. As in the case of other types of ovarian cancers, genetic and molecular studies will undoubtedly unlock some of the mysteries associated with these interesting neoplasms.

References

1. Evans AT, Gaffey TA, Malkasian GD, Annegers JF: Clinicopathologic review of 118 granulosa and 82 theca cell tumors. Obstet Gynecol 55:231, 1980
2. Norris HG, Taylor HB: Prognosis of granulosa-theca tumors of the ovary. Cancer 21:255, 1968
3. Pankratz E, Boyes DA, White GW et al: Granulosa cell tumors. Obstet Gynecol 52:718, 1978
4. Stenwig JT, Hazekamp JT, Beecham JB: Granulosa cell tumors of the ovary. Gynecol Oncol 7:136, 1979
5. Fox H, Agrawal K, Langley FA: A clinicopathological study of 92 cases of granulosa cell tumor of the ovary with special reference to the factors influencing prognosis. Cancer 35:231, 1975
6. Sjostedt S, Wahlen T: Prognosis of granulosa cell tumors. Acta Obstet Gynecol Scand, suppl 6. 40:3, 1961

7. Bjorkholm E, Petterson F: Granulosa cell and theca cell tumours: the clinical picture and long term outcome for the Radiumhemmet series. Acta Obstet Gynecol Scand 59:361, 1980
8. Bjorkholm E, Silfverswald C: Prognostic factors in granulosa cell tumors. Gynecol Oncol 11:261, 1981
9. Young RE, Scully RE: Ovarian sex cord-stromal tumors with bizarre nuclei: a clinicopathologic analysis of seventeen cases. Int. J Gynecol Pathol 1:325, 1983
10. Holland DR, LeRiche J, Swenerton KD et al: Flow cytometric assessment of DNA ploidy as a useful prognostic factor for patients with granulosa cell ovarian tumors. Int J Gynecol Cancer 1:227, 1991
11. Haba R, Miki H, Kobayashi S, Ohmori M: Combined analysis of flow cytometry and morphometry of ovarian granulosa cell tumor. Cancer 72(11):3258, 1993
12. Klemi PJ, Joensuu H, Salmi T: Prognostic value of flow cytometric DNA content analysis in granulosa cell tumor of the ovary. Cancer 65(5):1189, 1990
13. Chadha S, Cornelisse CJ, Schaberg A: Flow cytometric DNA ploidy analysis of ovarian granulosa cell tumors. Gynecol Oncol 36(2):240, 1990
14. Suh KS, Silverberg SG, Rhame JG, Wilkinson DS: Granulosa cell tumor of the ovary: histopathologic and flow cytometric analysis with clinical correlation. Arch Pathol Lab Med 114:496, 1990
15. Jacoby AF, Young RH, Colvin RB et al: DNA content in juvenile granulosa cell tumors of the ovary: a study of early and advanced stage disease. Gynecol Oncol 46(1):97, 1992
16. Evans MP, Webb MJ, Gaffey TA et al: DNA ploidy of ovarian granulosa cell tumors lack of correlation between DNA index or proliferative index and outcome in 40 patients. Cancer 75(9):2295, 1995
17. Roush GR, El Naggar AK, Abdul-Karim FW: Granulosa cell tumor of the ovary: a clinicopathologic and flow cytometric DNA analysis. Gynecol Oncol 56(3): 430, 1995
18. Young RH, Scully RE: Ovarian Sertoli-Leydig cell tumors: a clinicopathological analysis of 207 cases. Am J Surg Pathol 9:543, 1985
19. Malkasian GD, Webb MJ, Jorgensen EO: Observation on chemotherapy of granulosa cell carcinomas and malignant ovarian teratomas. Obstet Gynecol 44: 885, 1974
20. Schwartz PE, Smith JP: Treatment of ovarian stromal tumors. Am J Obstet Gynecol 125:402, 1976
21. Jacobs HJ, Deppe G, Cohen CJ: Combination chemotherapy of ovarian granulosa cell tumor with cisplatinum and doxorubicyn. Gynecol Oncol. 14:294, 1982
22. Canlibel F, Caputo TA: Chemotherapy of granulosa cell tumors. Am J Obstet Gynecol 145:763, 1983
23. Neville AJ, Gilchrist KW, Davis TE: The chemotherapy of granulosa cell tumors of the ovary: experience of the Wisconsin Clinical Cancer Center. Med Pediatr Oncol 12:397, 1984
24. Pectasides D, Alevizakos N, Athanassiou AE: Cisplatin-containing regimen in advanced or recurrent granulosa cell tumours of the ovary. Ann Oncol 3(4):316, 1992
25. Slayton RE: Management of germ cell and stromal tumors of the ovary. Semin Oncol. 11:299, 1984
26. Colombo N, Sessa C, Landoni F et al: Cisplatin, vinblastine, and bleomycin combination chemotherapy in metastatic granulosa cell tumor of the ovary. Obstet Gynecol 67:265, 1986
27. Chiara S, Merlini L, Campora E et al: Cisplatin-based chemotherapy in recurrent or high risk ovarian granulosa cell tumor patients. Eur J Gynaecol Oncol 14(4):314, 1993

28. Zambetti M, Escobedo A, Pilotti S, De Palo G: Cisplatin/vinblastine/bleomycin combination chemotherapy in advanced or recurrent granulosa cell tumors of the ovary. Gynecol Oncol 36(3):317, 1990

29. Zaloudek C, Norris HJ: Sertoli-Leydig tumors of the ovary: a clinicopathologic study of 64 intermediate and poorly differentiated neoplasms. Am J Surg Pathol 8:409, 1984

30. Pride GL, Pollock WJ, Norgard MJ: Metastatic Sertoli- Leydig cell tumor of the ovary during pregnancy treated by BV-CAP chemotherapy. Am J Obstet Gynecol 143:231, 1982

31. Martikainem H, Penttinem J, Huhtaniemi I, Kauppila A: Gonadotropin-releasing hormone agonist analog therapy effective in ovarian granulosa cell malignancy. Gynecol Oncol 35(3):406, 1989

32. Kauppila A, Bangah M, Burger H, Martikainem H: GnRH agonist analog therapy in advanced/recurrent granulosa cell tumours: further evidence of a role of inhibin in monitoring response to treatment. Gynecol Endocrinol 6(4):271, 1992

CHAPTER 20

PATHOLOGY OF OVARIAN CANCER

Robert E. Scully
Elvio Silva

EDITORS' INTRODUCTION

Ovarian cancer, often considered by the uneducated to be a single entity, actually consists of many types and subtypes of malignancies, each with its unique histologic appearance and biologic behavior. The most widely used classification scheme is that of the World Health Organization (WHO). Over the past several decades, the histologic description and nomenclature of ovarian neoplasms has continued to evolve and to be refined.

The correct histologic diagnosis of an ovarian malignancy is obviously of paramount importance to a clinician. Along with other prognostic factors, such as stage and residual tumor diameter, histologic type and grade (when applicable) help guide physicians in selecting the appropriate treatment or research protocol. Of course, the correct diagnosis is directly related to proper specimen examination, tissue sectioning, and processing, and to review by a competent pathologist. Unfortunately, a small but significant proportion of patients referred to university medical centers or cancer centers following surgery have had their tumors incorrectly classified. It is therefore very important prior to treatment planning, for pathologists or clinicians to liberally seek second opinions regarding the histologic diagnosis of an ovarian tumor, especially when it might represent a rare type.

To address some of the most important controversies surrounding the pathology of ovarian cancer, we have selected two world-class gynecologic pathologists. As the reader will note, many of the controversies in the literature are at least partially related to lack of reproducibility. This accounts for the fact that much current research in this area focuses on the development of standardized quantitative tests with which to clearly distinguish among different neoplasms.

Among the most critical issues regarding the pathology of ovarian cancer are the current status of histologic typing and grading, the state of our knowledge and technology involving the use of molecular markers and DNA ploidy analysis, and the prognostic implications associated with two rare tumor types—borderline epithelial tumors and granulosa cell tumors.

QUESTIONS

1. With so many different systems of histologic grading of surface epithelial tumors being used throughout the world, is it time to attempt to better standardize grading? Is it possible?
2. Please discuss your views on the current status of the definition, terminology, and significance of borderline tumors.
3. What is the evidence that, within the surface epithelial tumor classification, different cell types are associated with different prognoses? How should this information be used in designing clinical trials?
4. In the current analysis of ovarian tumors, are there any types for which a gynecologic pathologist should routinely use DNA ploidy or molecular markers? Are there any such studies now under way that may be of benefit in the near future?
5. What is the evidence, if any, that histopathologic factors are prognostic for ovarian granulosa cell tumors? Is DNA ploidy useful and should it be routinely studied in these tumors?

QUESTION 1

With so many different systems of histologic grading of surface epithelial tumors being used throughout the world, is it time to attempt to standardize grading? Is it possible?

ROBERT E. SCULLY

Almost all investigators of prognostic factors in cases of epithelial ovarian cancer have concluded that grade is a predictor of relapse-free interval, survival, or both, although there is less agreement on whether it is an independent prognostic parameter.[1] The great majority of grading studies have been performed on series of cases that have included all subtypes of epithelial cancer. Some investigations have been based on cancers of all stages, others on low-stage cancers, and still others on advanced cancers. The criteria for grading have been architectural (pattern); nuclear; architectural combined with nuclear; and combined architectural and nuclear with the evaluation of additional features such as capsular penetration, appearance of the tumor margin, and vascular invasion.[2] It is difficult to compare the relative efficacy of these approaches because of insufficient detail about the method of grading in most studies, the different subsets of cases analyzed, and the lack of uniform therapy among and within most series.[1] In one cooperative study in which there was a strong correlation with prognosis independent of extent of disease, the participating pathologists utilized whatever criteria they were accustomed to using, without any attempt at standardization.[3] Therefore, there is no way to discern from the literature whether one method of grading ovarian carcinomas is better than another.

Several other problems are involved in standardizing criteria for grading epithelial ovarian tumors. One group of investigators have concluded that grade is prognostically meaningful for serous carcinomas but not for endometrioid and mucinous carcinomas[4], and several other groups have found that grading of clear cell carcinomas is of little value.[5–7] Therefore, the uncommon as well as the common forms of epithelial cancer require subtype-specific recommendations for either the optimal method of grading or no grading. Subtyping these tumors and separating them from borderline forms, however, is at present not highly reproducible.[8,9] For example, the authors of a number of grading studies have interpreted borderline tumors as grade 1 carcinomas, spuriously increasing the prognostic value of grading by enhancing the number of survivors in the grade 1 category.[1] Another problem has been the use of different criteria for the diagnosis of epithelial cancers, especially undifferentiated and mixed carcinomas. The WHO defines an undifferentiated carcinoma as one with no differentiation or very rare, minor foci of differentiation,[10] and other authors,[11] as a tumor that lacks differentiation over one-half of its area. The WHO defines a mixed tumor as one in which one or more components in addition to the predominant component account for at least 10% of the epithelial content of the tumor.[10] According to FIGO,[12] however, a mixed tumor is one in which no specific subtype predominates. Obviously, use of these different definitions affects the reported efficacy of grading, particularly of the most common serous subtype. If the above issues could be resolved, formulators of a grading system would face the greatest problem, that of interobserver and intraobserver reproducibility. Several studies on reproducibility of grading systems have shown it to be poor.[13,14] Also, in most reported studies grading has been done retrospectively by one or two pathologists who examined a large number of tumors in a limited period of time, with an opportunity to compare and review problem cases. Reproducibility studies are performed in a somewhat similar manner, with pathologists reviewing cases within a specified period of time. Reproducibility is obviously worse in everyday practice, when a pathologist grades individual tumors prospectively at intervals that may range from days to months. It is highly probable that competent pathologists can identify reproducibly obvious examples of grade 1 and grade 3 tumors, but that tumors that approach grade 2 in their degree of differentiation cannot be graded reproducibly. Therefore, unless a pathologist expresses certainty about the grade being assigned, it must be considered a soft criterion on which to base clinical management.

The magnitude of the task of standardizing criteria for grading epithelial cancers and the low probability of its success should lead pathologists to explore alternative approaches in evaluating the degree of malignancy of these cancers.

European investigators have been the leaders in the use of morphometry in examining the degree of malignancy of epithelial ovarian tumors.[15–20] Baak and coworkers[15,16] reported that evaluation of the mitotic index and the volume percentage of epithelium yielded three prognostic groups in patients with stage I tumors with 89%, 71%, and 52% survival rates. These measurements were found to be more reproducible and more accurate in evaluating prognosis than nonquantitative grading by several expert pathologists.[15] Nevertheless, in separate studies, Carey et al[4] and Vergote et al[20] achieved results comparable to those of Baak et al using the latter approach. The relatively simple morphometric analyses mentioned above deserve further investigation in carefully designed studies because their reproducibility is probably greater than that of grading. Future investigations should concentrate on stage I cases, in which the results are most likely to have the greatest impact on clinical management.[21]

Baak et al.[22] have successfully used more complex morphometry (mitotic index, volume percentage of epithelium, and analysis of nuclear shape) to predict the outcome of borderline ovarian tumors in a small series of cases (which enigmatically included one case of carcinoma); details regarding stage and other prognostic factors were not given in their report. This approach deserves further investigation, particularly in evaluating the peritoneal implants of serous borderline tumors, in the presence of which the results might have therapeutic importance.[23] Routine use of morphometry for stage I borderline tumors would not be cost-effective because of the rarity of their malignant behavior.

ELVIO SILVA

Different types of common epithelial ovarian tumors are morphologically different; they have different associations and different prognoses. It will be very difficult to standardize their grading. We must consider each type individually instead of evaluating them together as a single group.

Different grading systems have been used for serous neoplasms.[2,14,24–30] Some studies were based on the Broder system designed for/cervical carcinomas[25,26], whereas other investigators used a grading system based on percentage of solid tumor area. However, this widely used grading system does not take into consideration some very important characteristics of serous neoplasms, cytologic changes. For serous neoplasms, we use a grading system based on cytologic atypia and mitoses. Tumors with mild or moderate atypia or fewer than 10 mitoses per 10 high-power fields are designated low grade. Tumors with severe atypia or more than 10 mitoses per 10 high-power fields are high grade. Table 20–1 summarizes the cases we studied using this grading system. Most serous carcinomas are high grade and prognosis is extremely poor, with only 9% of patients surviving 5 years. Patients with low-grade serous carcinoma have a 30% 5-year survival rate. With the use of a cytologic grading system based on atypia and mitosis, it is possible to find a serous carcinoma with solid areas, which is still a low-grade lesion, or a serous carcinoma without solid areas, which is a high-grade lesion.

Some investigators have graded mucinous carcinomas using percentage of solid tumor area.[30] We do not grade mucinous carcinomas, as we believe that there are no histologic features that identify different groups of mucinous tumors with different prognoses.

Endometrioid tumors are graded similarly to endometrial carcinomas. Based on the percentage of solid tumor area, they are graded as I (<5% solid area), II (5 to 50% solid area), and III (>50% solid area). In the ovary, as well as in the uterus, marked cytologic atypia can be used to upgrade a grade I carcinoma to grade II.

Undifferentiated, clear-cell, and transitional cell carcinomas are considered high-grade neoplasms. Undifferentiated carcinomas are solid tumors with a high nuclear grade. Clear-cell carcinomas have different patterns and at least focally have a high nuclear grade. Some studies have reported a relationship between the presence of solid areas and prognosis. We believe that most transitional cell carcinomas are high-grade tumors and that rare low-grade carcinomas with a transitional cell carcinoma pattern are related to Brenner tumors.

QUESTION 2

Please discuss your views on the current status of the definition, terminology, and significance of borderline tumors.

ROBERT E. SCULLY

The WHO defines a borderline tumor[10] as "one that has some, but not all, of the morphological features of malignancy; those present include in varying combinations: stratification of the epithelial cells, apparent detachment of cellular clusters from their sites of origin, and mitotic activity and nuclear abnormalities intermediate between those of clearly benign and unquestionably malignant tumours of a similar cell type; on the other hand, obvious invasion of the adjacent stroma is lacking. Tumours with epithelial cell proliferation or atypicality of a minor degree should not be placed in the borderline category." The international committee that recently revised the

TABLE 20-1
Survival of Serous Carcinoma: Stages II to IV

GRADE	NO. OF CASES	1 YEAR (%)	2 YEARS (%)	3 YEARS (%)	4 YEARS (%)	5 YEARS (%)	10 YEARS (%)
Low	39	97	72	54	44	31	18
High	101	70	30	13	9	5	4

WHO classification has retained this definition.

The same year the WHO classification was published, Hart and Norris[31] of the Armed Forces Institute of Pathology coauthored an article introducing a more complex set of criteria for distinguishing borderline tumors from carcinomas, specifically those in the mucinous category. These authors accepted obvious invasion as a valid criterion for the diagnosis of carcinoma but in its absence were satisfied with architectural abnormalities in the epithelium lining the cysts, placing greatest emphasis on stratification of the nuclei to four or greater. Later, Hart[32] added the presence of stroma-free cellular papillae, a cribriform pattern, and a frankly malignant appearance of the lining cells as criteria for the diagnosis of carcinoma in the absence of obvious invasion. Subsequently, many pathologists, particularly in the United States, have utilized the Hart-Norris criteria for subdividing mucinous malignant tumors, and to a lesser extent for subclassifying malignant tumors of other epithelial cell types. In contrast, many pathologists elsewhere have followed the WHO criteria. This discrepancy in diagnostic criteria has confused pathologists attempting to distinguish borderline tumors from carcinomas as well as gynecologists treating patients with these neoplasms.

In a recent study[33] the survival rate of patients with stage I mucinous borderline tumors diagnosed by the WHO criteria was compared with that of similar patients whose tumors were diagnosed as borderline based on the Hart-Norris criteria. No difference in survival was appreciable in a cumulative review of the literature, suggesting that the latter criteria do not distinguish a subgroup of noninvasive mucinous tumors that have a worse prognosis and warrant the designation *carcinoma*. In contrast, a small number of investigators[34–36] (but not all) who have focused on the distinction between the mucinous borderline tumor and the mucinous carcinoma without obvious invasion of Hart and Norris have found that, in comparison to the former, the latter tend to present at a higher stage, have a poorer prognosis, or both. These studies involved small numbers of cases, and one of the problems in some series was inadequate sampling of tumors to exclude the presence of invasion in cases in which only cyst linings had the features of carcinoma.

In order to clarify the biologic behavior of the various gradations of histologic malignancy in mucinous tumors and of other epithelial cell types, more precise subclassification of these tumors after they have been adequately sampled for microscopic examination is necessary. To achieve this goal and promote uniformity of terminology throughout the literature, we shall propose in the upcoming Armed Forces Institute of Pathology fascicle dealing with ovarian tumors that the WHO diagnostic criteria for distinguishing between borderline tumors and carcinomas be retained, with the following amplification: (1) borderline tumor (no obvious invasion)—with intraepithelial carcinoma; (2) carcinomas (obvious invasion).

Another problem in the diagnosis of borderline ovarian neoplasms involves mucinous tumors associated with pseudomyxoma peritonei. In many such cases these tumors are accompanied by mucinous lesions of the appendix, and whether the ovarian tumor is an independent primary tumor or is secondary to the appendiceal lesion is controversial. A survey of 25 recently reported cases in which ovarian tumors interpreted as having microscopic features of borderline tumors were associated with pseudomyxoma peritonei disclosed synchronous mucinous lesions of the appendix in 15 cases (60%) and a microscopically normal appendix in the remaining 10 cases.[37–42] Arguments supporting an independent primary origin as well as those supporting a secondary nature of ovarian tumors in cases in which both organs are involved have been presented in detail in the literature.[43–46] Preliminary molecular genetic studies have provided conflicting evidence regarding the nature of ovarian tumors in such cases.[47,48] Until the question of the primary or secondary nature of ovarian tumors in cases of pseudomyxoma peritonei accompanied by appendiceal lesions is resolved, such tumors should continue to be staged as ovarian neoplasms, with the realization that their clinical behavior may not accurately reflect that of mucinous borderline tumors of unquestionable ovarian origin.

The biologic malignancy of borderline tumors has been overstated in the literature by some investigators, and in several cases the chemotherapy or radiotherapy administered rather than the tumor itself has caused the death of the patient. In an attempt to portray borderline tumors in a more benign light, several authors.[49,50] have recommended alternative designations such as *proliferating*, and *atypically proliferating*. These terms are undesirable, however, for several reasons. First, a minority of borderline tumors are clinically malignant. They often spread to the peritoneum; they can invade vascular spaces in their stroma;[51] they can metastasize to regional lymph nodes,[52,53] to distant lymph nodes (rarely), and via the bloodstream (exceptionally) (RE Scully, personal observations); and they can cause the death of the patient.[54] Omission of the word *malignancy* or *malignant* in the designation of these tumors fails to transmit to the physician their malignant potential and could result in clinical mismanagement. Second, use of the alternative terms would result in a failure to report these tumors to cancer registries, eliminating avenues of future research. Third, like other changes in the terminology of tumors, such alterations would cause a great problem for epidemiologists and other scientists investigating these neoplasms.

Introduction of a category of borderline tumors by the International Federation of Gynecology and Obstetrics in 1961 (and its adoption by WHO 12 years later) initiated a major advance in understanding the pathology and biology of ovarian neoplasms. Knowledge that these tumors are associated with a much better prognosis than carcinomas means that the former can be treated more conservatively than the latter. Conservative treatment is particularly important for young women, many of whom wish to retain their reproductive capacity.[55] The distinction between borderline tumors and carcinomas is also important for all women with advanced stage disease in terms of both prognosis and therapy.[23,56]

ELVIO SILVA

The concept of borderline tumors was proposed in 1929 when semimalignant tumors were described by Taylor.[57] The WHO adopted the term *tumor of low malignant potential* (LMP) or *borderline* in 1959.[58] As with any new term, it has taken 30 years to reach the point where LMP or borderline tumors are well recognized and treated in a fairly uniform way. Some authors have proposed that since recurrences are rare in LMP neoplasms, it would be better to designate these lesions as atypically proliferating tumors.[59–62] Our view is that such a designation would be misleading because many LMP neoplasms have areas of tumor outside the ovary and some recur.[23]

We will discuss serous and mucinous neoplasms. Endometrioid, clear-cell, and transitional cell types are exceptionally rare. Serous neoplasms might be associated with areas of endosalpingiosis and implants in the peritoneum; the recurrence rate of these tumors varies according to the patient's age, tumor stage, and type of implant but ranges between 5% and 30%. Authors who support the term *atypically proliferating* believe that the extraovarian lesions in these cases are independent tumors or multicentric lesions.[59–62] We believe that this issue is important in understanding the natural history of this disease, but treatments for metastatic versus multicentric lesions currently do not differ. Therefore, for practical purposes this distinction is not necessary. As far as we know, there are no reliable histologic features that can be used to determine which cases will recur and to separate them from those that will not recur.

Mucinous tumors are divided into two categories, endocervical and intestinal categories. Endocervical lesions do not occur very frequently, but they can be associated with similar lesions in the peritoneum. Because of this extraovarian component, it is better to continue using the term *LMP* or *borderline*. Intestinal lesions can be associated with pseudomyxoma, and many of them might represent metastases from the appendix. If the appendix has been resected and found to be normal but

TABLE 20-2
Ovarian Serous LMP Neoplasms

INITIAL STAGE	NO. OF CASES	MICROINVASION
I	12	2 (16%)
II	7	1 (14%)
III	18	8 (44%)

there is pseudomyxoma ovarii, it is important to consider the tumors mucinous LMP because they might recur as pseudomyxoma peritonei. If the appendix is normal and there is no evidence of pseudomyxoma ovarii, the ovarian neoplasm is probably benign.

Our view is that before changing the name of these neoplasms it will be necessary to review cases with a long (>5 and >10-year) follow-up. Many studies on these tumors with follow-ups shorter than 5 years have been reported in the literature, and this has been the basis for erroneous conclusions. We now believe that microinvasion and endosalpingiosis have some clinical relevance because in our study of serous LMP neoplasms that recurred, we found a relationship between microinvasion and tumor stage and between endosalpingiosis and recurrence. Table 20–2, from a study on 37 serous LMP neoplasms that recurred, and Table 20–3, from a study on 27 cases of stage I disease,[63] summarize our findings. Had we reviewed only cases with a short follow-up, however, we would not have found these relationships.

QUESTION 3

What is the evidence that, within the surface epithelial tumor classification, different cell types are associated with different prognoses? How should this information be used in designing clinical trials?

TABLE 20-3
Ovarian Serous LMP Neoplasms

STATUS[a]	NO. OF CASES	ENDOSALPINGIOSIS
Recurred	11	8 (73%)
Did not recur	16	2 (13%)

[a] *Follow-up of 15 years or more.*

ROBERT E. SCULLY

The findings in the literature relating to the prognostic significance of cell type in epithelial cancers are controversial. Epithelial cell type was an important prognostic feature in most of the studies reported prior to 1988 and reviewed by Silverberg.[1] Multivariate analysis of prognostic factors, however, generally downgraded and often eliminated the significance of cell type. The usual findings in univariate analyses were a relatively good prognosis for mucinous and endometrioid carcinomas, a poor prognosis for serous carcinomas, and the worst prognosis for undifferentiated carcinomas. Clear cell carcinomas were considered favorable tumors in about half the studies and unfavorable in the other half. The 1991 annual report of FIGO[54] showed a poor prognosis for clear cell carcinoma (Table 20–4), and two recent studies have confirmed this finding for stage I and II clear cell carcinomas.[64,65] Another investigation, which specifically compared clear cell and serous carcinomas, found the former to be associated with poorer survival stage for stage.[66]

Most studies evaluating the prognostic importance of cell type have antedated those from the M. D. Anderson Cancer Center showing a far better response to chemotherapy and a longer survival of patients with a predominance of transitional cell carcinoma in their tumors than of patients with a predominance of carcinomas of other cell types.[67–69]

Problems in evaluating the importance of epithelial cell type include variations in their definitions and suboptimal reproducibility of their differentiation,[8,9] as discussed in the answer to Question 1. Clinical trials should be designed to determine the comparative malignant behavior and response to therapy of the

TABLE 20-4
Five-Year Survival Figures for Ovarian Carcinomas According to Stage and Cell Type

CELL TYPE	STAGE I	STAGE II	STAGE III	STAGE IV
Serous	76	56	25	9
Mucinous	83	55	21	9
Endometrioid	78	63	24	6
Clear cell	69	55	14	4
Undifferentiated	68	40	17	6

(Adapted from Petersson,[54] with permission.)

cellular subtypes of epithelial cancer. Unfortunately, accumulation of adequate numbers of cases of the rarer subtypes poses a problem.

ELVIO SILVA

Unfortunately, most studies on ovarian epithelial tumors have included all histologic types together and have evaluated prognosis as that of only one tumor, ovarian carcinoma. We believe that there are different prognoses for the different histologic types of ovarian epithelial neoplasms. The differences involve not only pathologic features but also clinical manifestations. Endometrioid, clear-cell, and mucinous tumors are usually low-stage lesions, while serous, transitional, and undifferentiated tumors are usually high-stage lesions. Endometrioid tumors are associated with endometriosis, ovarian adenofibromas, and endometrial tumors.[70] Clear-cell tumors are also associated with endometriosis and clear-cell adenofibromas in the ovary.[71] Mucinous neoplasms can be of two different types. The endocervical type is strongly associated with endometriosis, while this association is rare in the intestinal type.[72] There are different types of serous carcinomas. Surface papillary serous carcinomas of the ovary and peritoneum are associated with similar lesions in the endometrium but involve endometrial polyps, while in the usual type of serous ovarian carcinoma, where a large tumor mass is formed, this association is very rare.[73,74] These characteristics are important for prognosis because, for example, it is possible that endometrioid lesions recur because the patient has areas of endometriosis which can be the origin of new lesions. We believe that these differences among the types of ovarian epithelial neoplasms might be important in understanding the natural history of these tumors and should be considered when clinical trials are designed.

We also think that some ovarian epithelial tumors might have a different response to chemotherapy. Tumors with a predominant transitional cell carcinoma pattern might have a better response to traditional chemotherapy for ovarian tumors than would papillary serous carcinomas.[67,69,75]

Clinical trials need to categorize patients according to their histologic tumor types. By doing this, we will be able to determine whether response to chemotherapy is different for each tumor type. Also, the surgical treatment of these patients might be affected; more aggressive debulking might be indicated in patients having tumors that have shown some response to chemotherapy.

Clinical trials designed for ovarian carcinoma considered one tumor type are never informative in assessing the possibility that different histologic types might have a different response to chemotherapy.

QUESTION 4

In the current analysis of ovarian tumors, are there any types for which a gynecologic

pathologist should routinely use DNA ploidy or molecular markers? Are there any such studies now under way that may be of benefit in the near future?

ROBERT E. SCULLY

There have been numerous discrepancies in the conclusions drawn about the prognostic significance of DNA ploidy, DNA index, and increase in the S-phase fraction in carcinomas.[76] and borderline tumors[77,78] of the ovary. Reasons for these discrepancies include variations in study design, in techniques utilized to determine ploidy, and in interpretation of histograms, including the definition of aneuploidy, about which even authorities disagree.[76,79] Although the technique for performing flow cytometry retrospectively on paraffin-embedded material is well standardized, there are problems with its use, particularly the presence of debris in paraffin blocks, which can alter the histogram and obscure some examples of aneuploidy. For this reason, some authorities believe that the use of fresh tissue is more desirable; however, its use is associated with an inability to make an accurate histologic correlation with the tissue being analyzed and is difficult to use in retrospective studies. Finally, flow cytometry may overlook small populations of aneuploid cells that can be detected by image analysis,[80] and ploidy is heterogeneous in 20% or more of tumors,[76] indicating that several samples should be analyzed before excluding aneuploidy.

Aneuploidy has been documented in 50 to 80% of ovarian carcinomas.[81] Compared to diploidy, it has been shown in most studies to be associated with a higher stage, a higher grade, a shorter survival time, a lower survival rate, or a combination of these findings, but the independent prognostic significance of ploidy has been more controversial.[76] At the present time there is no convincing evidence in the literature that tumor ploidy should influence the management of advanced-stage disease. It is possible, however, that it may have a role in the management of stage I tumors. In a recent report[20] it was shown that grade of tumor was the most powerful prognostic determinant but that evaluation of ploidy yielded additional prognostic information. For example, in that study there were no relapses in patients with stage I well-differentiated diploid tumors, in contrast to a 14% rate of relapse in patients with well-differentiated nondiploid tumors (aneuploid, tetraploid, and multiploid). Higher rates of relapse were also demonstrated in patients with higher-grade nondiploid tumors than in those with higher-grade diploid tumors.

The most extensive study of DNA ploidy in borderline tumors has been performed at the Norwegian Radium Hospital, which has identified it as the single most powerful indicator of prognosis associated with these tumors.[77] Unfortunately, borderline tumors of all cell types were grouped together in the analysis even though cellular subtypes of borderline tumors vary considerably in their clinicopathologic features. An examination of the authors' data indicates the strong probability that their conclusions were based mostly on analysis of the nonserous group of borderline tumors, the great majority of which were mucinous. Another problem is that cases of pseudomyxoma peritonei in which appendiceal mucinous lesions as well as ovarian mucinous tumors were present were probably included in the series of cases analyzed.[82] It is currently controversial whether the ovarian tumor is primary or secondary in such cases.[43–46] Other investigators, in contrast, have found no relation between DNA ploidy and survival in cases of borderline neoplasms.[78,83] (It is interesting that borderline tumors analyzed by flow cytometry of fresh tissue have been diploid almost without exception.[79])

One problematic area in which DNA ploidy analysis may have an impact on therapy is in the treatment of stage II and III serous borderline tumors. It has been shown by some investigators[23,56] that the presence or absence of invasion of the peritoneal implants is an important prognostic finding in such cases, suggesting that chemotherapy should be reserved for patients with invasive implants.

Two groups have recently reported that DNA ploidy analysis of the implants may be more helpful in distinguishing between high-stage borderline tumors with good prognosis and those with poor prognosis.[84,85]

Until the discrepancies in the literature are resolved, DNA studies cannot be recommended for routine use in the laboratory workup of ovarian malignant tumors. If an individual institution has shown that its technique yields important prognostic information, it can appropriately continue to rely on it. Carefully designed clinical trials on ovarian carcinomas and borderline tumors should optimally include studies to determine the prognostic value of DNA ploidy and its impact on therapy. It is possible that with improved standardization of histogram interpretation, uniformity of tissue sampling, and well-designed clinical trials, flow cytometry will have a more widespread role in the determination of prognosis and possibly therapy.

Numerous oncogenes and tumor suppressor genes have been investigated for their pathogenetic role and possible prognostic significance when amplified or overexpressed in ovarian cancers, with generally conflicting results. One of the oncogenes that has been studied most extensively in ovarian epithelial cancer is erbB2 (HER-2/*neu*), which has been reported to be overexpressed in 0 to 72% and amplified in 0 to 32% of cases.[86] There is disagreement, however, whether overexpression or amplification confers a poor prognosis on the tumor.[87–92] A variety of other oncogenes have been investigated less extensively for their role in the initiation or progression of ovarian cancer. Attempts to correlate the findings with the prognosis have resulted in similarly conflicting or negative results or have been too few to warrant firm conclusions. The tumor suppressor gene p53 has been the most widely investigated gene in ovarian cancer, with most of the studies devoted to the frequency of its overexpression or amplification and its role in initiation or progression. Overexpression has been reported in 50 to 89% of ovarian carcinomas.[93,94] The few studies that have addressed its prognostic significance have yielded inconclusive results.[95–97]

Improved standardization of techniques and study designs for evaluation of the prognostic significance of genetic alterations with agreement on results are necessary before these techniques can be stated to have prognostic significance or a role in the treatment of patients with ovarian cancer.

ELVIO SILVA

DNA ploidy and molecular markers have been used to investigate different aspects of ovarian neoplasms, including origin and prognosis. In regard to origin, when two neoplasms are resected from one patient, it is important to know whether they are independent primaries or if one has metastasized from the other. Different parameters have been examined in this situation, including loss of heterozygosity, inactivation of an X chromosome, p53 status, and ras mutations.[98–103] These studies in general have confirmed that many endometrioid tumors involving the endometrium and ovary are independent primaries. Mucinous tumors involving the appendix and ovary also appear to be independent primaries. In addition, these studies have confirmed previously proposed suggestions that in patients with a large ovarian mass, small areas of tumor in the peritoneum represent metastases from the ovarian tumor because they have similar clones. However, when small lesions involve not only the peritoneum but also the ovarian surface, or what is known as surface papillary carcinomas, clonality studies demonstrate that tumors from different areas are polyclonal, meaning that they represent independent primaries.[104] This information can be very important because resection of a large ovarian carcinoma and the metastases should result in cure of the patient. However, if the patient has small lesions in the peritoneum and ovary or has several independent primaries, the entire peritoneal surface will be at risk for developing new tumors because there is a field effect involving the peritoneum, and even the removal of all visible lesions will not result in a cure.

The use of DNA ploidy or molecular markers to determine the prognosis in ovarian carcinoma cases is very preliminary because these techniques have only recently been simplified enough to allow their use at many centers; more time will be needed to find a practical use for each technique and to confirm the results. Some studies have shown that aneuploidy and high expression of some oncogenes are associated with tumor recurrences and high-grade neoplasms.[83,85,91,105–114]

One of the main obstacles in DNA and molecular studies is that it is not known whether ovarian carcinomas are entirely monoclonal. Each of these techniques studies only a minimal portion of a large ovarian mass; even if two or three areas are studied entirely, they might not represent more than 1% of the entire tumor. Therefore, it is difficult to rule out the possibility that a different clone might be present in a tumor and that this clone might be the part that metastasizes or the part that is resistant to therapy. We are familiar with tumors that have different components in the ovary (e.g., transitional cell carcinoma mixed with serous carcinoma and endometrioid carcinoma mixed with serous carcinoma), but that often have only one component, serous carcinoma, in the metastasis. This probably means that the most aggressive component is the one found in the metastases. If the tissue obtained for DNA and molecular studies contains only the transitional cell carcinoma or endometrioid carcinoma components, the results can be misleading. An example of the polyclonal population in ovarian tumors is the trisomy found in the granulosa cell tumor, where areas with bizarre nuclei have a trisomy not found in other areas.[116] Another disadvantage of DNA ploidy and molecular studies is that a patient might have a weak point in a chromosome throughout the body that might break or translocate as a result of injury. This lack of chromosome stability can create similar changes in different tumors which might affect different organs, but because of similar results from molecular studies might mislead us. An example is the case of small cell carcinoma found in the endometrium in a patient with carcinoma of the cervix. Both tumors were independent, but both had identical ras mutations.[116]

QUESTION 5

What is the evidence, if any, that histopathologic factors are prognostic for ovarian granulosa cell tumors? Is DNA ploidy useful and should it be studied routinely in these tumors?

ROBERT E. SCULLY

The literature is confusing with regard to the correlation between histologic findings in granulosa cell tumors and survival. These tumors are known to recur late in a high proportion of cases, and therefore the results of series in which a large number of patients have not been followed for prolonged periods are subject to criticism. Second, it is highly probable that undifferentiated carcinomas or adenocarcinomas have been misdiagnosed as granulosa cell tumors in some series and have accounted at least partly for the correlation of mitotic activity and nuclear atypicality with a poor prognosis. Series in which there is a high percentage of stage II to IV cases or in which unusual numbers of patients have died within 1 or 2 years of diagnosis are particularly suspected of including cases of carcinoma since high stage and a short clinical course to recurrence or death are atypical of granulosa cell tumors.

The three histologic features that have been evaluated in studies on large series of apparently valid granulosa cell tumors have been pattern, mitotic activity, and nuclear atypia. Kottmeier reported significantly better survival of patients with well-differentiated patterns such as follicular or "cylindromatous" than of those with a more poorly differentiated (sarcomatoid) pattern.[117] The difference in survival at 5 years was 87% versus 64%, and at 10 years, 82% versus 29%. Several other investigators, however, did not confirm the prognostic importance of pattern in granulosa cell tumors.[119–121] In one of these studies,[121] tumors with two or fewer mitotic figures per 10 high-power fields were associated with a 70% 10-year survival in contrast to only a 37% survival for those with three or more.[121] In another investigation,[119] tumors with numerous mitotic figures were associated with a worse prognosis than those with few, but the differences were not statistically significant for patients with stage I tumors. Another group of investigators were unable to correlate the degree of mitotic activity with the prognosis.[120] In one study,[119] the 5-year survival of patients whose tumors had no nuclear atypicality was 92%, slight atypicality 80%, and moderate atypicality 30%.[121] In another investigation,[118] there was an 80% 25-year survival in patients whose tumors had grade 1 nuclear atypicality, in contrast to only a 60% survival associated with grade 2 atypicality. In both studies nuclear atypicality was the most reliable prognostic finding in stage I cases; in higher-stage cases nuclear atypicality and mitotic rate were of similar significance.

The prospect of pathologists' identification of histologic features in granulosa cell tumors that can be correlated with prognosis is discouraging. The reproducibility of mitotic counting and grading nuclear atypia in these tumors has not been reported but is probably as poor as it is in evaluating similar findings in epithelial cancers. Also, since granulosa cell tumors are relatively rare even in pathology practice at a university hospital with an active gynecologic oncology service, reproducibility in clinical practice is expected to be even less optimal. Finally, the question arises whether the reported differences in survival based on assessment of mitotic activity and nuclear atypia, even if reproducible, would be great enough to alter the clinical management of these generally indolent, late-recurring tumors.

At least eight ploidy studies have been performed on granulosa cell tumors, six on the adult form and two on the juvenile type.[76, 122–124] In most of these series aneuploidy was detected in 5 to 20% of adult granulosa cell tumors, and in two series, in 45 and 46% of juvenile granulosa cell tumors.[76] The prevailing conclusion was that aneuploidy does not predict adverse outcome. In one study in which aneuploidy was claimed to be predictive,[123] almost two-thirds of the neoplasms were higher than stage I, indicating a high probability that carcinomas were erroneously included in the series, and in another study[124] the aneuploid tumors had very high mitotic rates, two of them being high stage and one showing squamous metaplasia, which does not occur in granulosa cell tumors.

ELVIO SILVA

In ovarian granulosa cell tumors, there is no unequivocal evidence that histopathologic factors are important prognostic indicators.[119,123,125–127] However, this may be because of the low incidence of this tumor and the long interval to recurrence. No single institution has enough cases with a follow-up long enough to really determine the prognostic value of histopathologic indicators. Adult granulosa cell tumors occur more frequently than the juvenile type, but the incidence of the former is approximately 3% of ovarian malignancies, and less than 25% of these tumors recur. The only feature related to tumor recurrence is stage.[119, 123, 125–127] The pathologic features reported in most granulosa cell tumors, because they might be related to tumor recurrence, are tumor size, nuclear pleomorphism, and number of mitoses. Several studies have investigated the relationship between tumor ploidy and recurrence.[123,125,126] Promotors and detractors of the prognostic value of these features can be found in different studies. We have also found that granulosa cell tumors with Call Exner bodies recur less frequently than those without Call Exner bodies. This observation could be interpreted as the opposite of the presence of a sarcomatous pattern, which is associated with tumor recurrence. Call Exner bodies can be interpreted as a sign of differentiation, while a sarcomatous pattern represents lack of differentiation.

In regard to ploidy, the results of different studies have been disparate because in addition to the low incidence of tumor and the long interval to recurrence, the technical aspects of this procedure also are important.[123,125,126] Usually only a small portion of the tumor is studied for DNA ploidy; therefore, since we know that these tumors are not always homogeneous, because the atypia can be very focal, it is possible that the results of DNA ploidy analysis also depend on the area examined.

Only the study of large series of cases with long follow-ups can determine the value of histopathologic factors. However, until this is achieved, the histopathologic factors discussed need to be reported in order to investigate their value in the follow-up of patients with stage I disease.

EDITORS' COMMENTARY

Although there is general agreement that histologic grade is an important prognostic factor, a standardized classification system for the histologic typing and grading of ovarian cancers has thus far eluded experts. As both authors indicate, there are several methods of classification based on either nuclear or architectural features or on a combination of these two parameters. Dr. Scully is somewhat pessimistic that standardization of histologic grading will ever occur; instead, he recommends evaluation of alternative approaches. The use of morphometry, popularized by Baak and colleagues, is one such method under study.

Likewise, there continues to be controversy surrounding the importance of histologic type. Information about this parameter is often confounded by other factors, such as histologic grade and stage. In patients with advanced-stage disease, there is mounting evidence that clear-cell carcinoma is a very aggressive cell type with a poor prognosis. There is also information suggesting that advanced-stage transitional cell carcinoma is associated with better chemosensitivity and survival compared with serous carcinoma. Endometrioid tumors are usually of low grade and early stage and are associated with a favorable prognosis. Similarly, mucinous tumors tend to occur in early-stage disease. In our experience, however, advanced-stage mucinous tumors have tended to be chemoresistant and associated with a poor prognosis.

The current controversy regarding ovarian borderline tumors has also been addressed. Both Dr. Scully and Dr. Silva agree that, although these tumors rarely exhibit malignant behavior, they do so frequently enough to resist the trend toward classifying them as atypically proliferating or benign. In our experience, borderline serous ovarian tumors with peritoneal implants have a recurrence rate of approximately 30%. As addressed elsewhere in this text, however, the impact of postoperative treatment in this group of patients remains unclear. One of the major challenges for investigators is to identify molecular or genetic markers that will assist clinicians in selecting patients for appropriate postoperative therapy.

Despite the plethora of publications on the topic of DNA ploidy and the study of molecular markers in ovarian cancer, neither author recommends their routine clinical use. If one surveys the literature, the prognostic significance of DNA ploidy, p53 status, and overexpression of HER-2/*neu*, to name a few of the more widely studied markers, remains unresolved. As pointed out, tumor heterogeneity and methodological variations may account for the lack of consensus regarding some of these markers. In the near future, however, as we become more sophisticated about the molecular biology and genetics of ovarian cancer, it is probable that such tests will become part of our standard diagnostic workup.

And finally, both authors agree that pathologic studies have failed to identify any unequivocal prognostic factors in ovarian granulosa cell tumors. The rarity of these tumors and their long natural history significantly complicate these investigations. In our estimation, however, it is more than likely that molecular biomarkers will eventually allow us to select patients for postoperative therapy based on prognosis.

References

1. Silverberg SG: Prognostic significance of pathologic features of ovarian carcinoma. p. 85. In Nogales F (ed): Current

Topics in Pathology: Ovarian Pathology. Springer-Verlag, Berlin, 1989

2. Bichel P, Jakobsen A: A new histologic grading index in ovarian carcinoma. Int J Gynecol Pathol 8:147, 1989
3. Henson DE: The histological grading of neoplasms. Arch Pathol Lab Med 112:1091, 1988
4. Carey MS, Dembo AJ, Simm JE et al: Testing the validity of a prognostic classification in patients with surgically optimal ovarian carcinoma: a 15-year review. Int J Gynecol Cancer 3:24, 1993
5. Kennedy AW, Biscotti CV, Hart WR, Tuason LJ: Histologic correlates of progression-free interval and survival in ovarian clear cell adenocarcinoma. Gynecol Oncol 50:334, 1993
6. Montag AG, Jenison EL, Griffiths CT et al: Ovarian clear cell carcinoma: clinicopathologic analysis of 44 cases. Int J Gynecol Pathol 8:85, 1989
7. O'Brien MER, Schofield JB, Tan S et al: Clear cell epithelial ovarian cancer (mesonephroid): bad prognosis only in early stages. Gynecol Oncol 49:250, 1993
8. Cramer SF, Roth LM, Ulbright TM et al: Evaluation of the reproducibility of the World Health Organization classification of common ovarian cancers. Arch Pathol Lab Med 111:819, 1987
9. Stalsberg H, Abeler V, Blom GP, et al: Observer variation in histologic classification of malignant and borderline ovarian tumors. Hum Pathol 19:1030, 1988
10. Serov SF, Scully RE, Sobin LH: International Histological Classification of Tumors (No. 9): Histological Typing of Ovarian Tumors. Geneva, World Health Organization, 1973
11. Silva EG, Tornos C, Bailey MA, Morris M: Undifferentiated carcinoma of the ovary. Arch Pathol Lab Med 115:377, 1991
12. Pettersson F: Annual report of results of treatment in gynecological cancer. Vol 20. International Federation of Gynecology and Obstetrics, Stockholm, 1988.
13. Baak JPA, Langley FA, Talerman A, Delemarre JFM: Interpathologist and intrapathologist disagreement in ovarian tumor grading and typing. Anal Quant Cytol Histol 8:354, 1986
14. Bertelsen K, Hølund B, Andersen E: Reproducibility and prognostic value of histologic type and grade in early epithelial ovarian cancer. Int J Gynecol Cancer 3:72, 1993
15. Baak JPA, Wisse-Brekelmans ECM, Langley FA et al: Morphometric data to FIGO stage and histological type and grade for prognosis of ovarian tumours. J Clin Pathol 39:1340, 1986
16. Baak JPA, Chan KK, Stolk JG, Kenemans P: Prognostic factors in borderline and invasive ovarian tumours of the common epithelial type. Pathol Res Pract 182:755, 1987
17. Haapasalo H, Collan Y, Atkin NB et al: Prognosis of ovarian carcinomas: prediction by histoquantitative methods. Histopathology 15:167, 1989
18. Haapasalo H, Collan Y, Seppä A et al: Prognostic value of ovarian carcinoma grading methods—a method comparison study. Histopathology 16:1, 1990
19. Ludescher C, Weger AR, Lindholm J et al: Prognostic significance of tumor cell morphometry, histopathology, and clinical parameters in advanced ovarian carcinoma. Int J Gynecol Pathol 9:343, 1990
20. Vergote IB, Kaern J, Abeler VM et al: Analysis of prognostic factors in stage I epithelial ovarian carcinoma: importance of degree of differentiation and DNA ploidy in predicting relapse. Am J Obstet Gynecol 169:40, 1993
21. Hreshchyshyn MM, Park RC, Blessing JA et al: The role of adjuvant therapy

in stage I ovarian cancer. Am J Obstet Gynecol 138:139, 1980

22. Baak JPA, Fox H, Langley FA, Buckley CH: The prognostic value of morphometry in ovarian epithelial tumors of borderline malignancy. Int J Gynecol Pathol 4:186, 1985
23. Bell DA, Weinstock MA, Scully RE: Peritoneal implants of ovarian serous borderline tumors: histologic features and prognosis. Cancer 62:2212, 1988
24. Baak JPA, Langley FA, Talerman A, Delemarre JFM: The prognostic variability of ovarian tumor grading by different pathologists. Gynecol Oncol 27:166, 1987
25. Decker DG, Malkasian Jr, Taylor WF: Prognostic importance of histologic grading in ovarian carcinoma. Natl Cancer Inst Monogr 42:9, 1975
26. Malkasian GD Jr, Decker DG, Webb MJ: Histology of epithelial tumors of the ovary: clinical usefulness and prognostic significance of the histologic classification and grading. Semin Oncol 2:191, 1975
27. Ozols RF, Garvin AJ, Costa J et al: Histologic grade in advanced ovarian cancer. Cancer Treat Rep 63:255, 1979
28. Swenerton KD, Hislop TF, Spinelli J et al: Ovarian carcinoma: a multivariate analysis of prognostic factors. Obstet Gynecol 65:264, 1985
29. Taylor HC Jr: Studies in the clinical and biological evolution of adenocarcinoma of the ovary. J Obstet Gynaecol 66:827, 1959
30. Mauch PM, Ehrmann RL, Griffiths T et al: Radiation therapy in stage II ovarian carcinoma: the influence of histologic grade. Cancer 45:1344, 1980
31. Hart WR, Norris HJ: Borderline and malignant mucinous tumors of the ovary: histologic criteria and clinical behavior. Cancer 31:1031, 1973
32. Hart WR: Ovarian epithelial tumors of borderline malignancy (carcinomas of low malignant potential). Hum Pathol 8:541, 1977
33. Siriaunkgul S, Robbins KM, McGowan L, Silverberg SG: Ovarian mucinous tumors of low malignant potential: a clinicopathologic study of 54 tumors of intestinal and müllerian type. Int J Gynecol Pathol 14:198, 1995
34. Chaitin BA, Gershenson DM, Evans HL: Mucinous tumors of the ovary: clinicopathologic study of 70 cases. Cancer 55:1958, 1985
35. Sumithran E, Susil BJ, Looi LM: The prognostic significance of grading in borderline mucinous tumors of the ovary. Hum Pathol 19:15, 1988
36. Watkin W, Silva EG, Gershenson DM: Mucinous carcinoma of the ovary: pathologic prognostic factors. Cancer 69:208, 1992
37. Kaern J, Tropé CG, Abeler VM: A retrospective study of 370 borderline tumors of the ovary treated at the Norwegian Radium Hospital from 1970 to 1982: a review of clinicopathologic features and treatment modalities. Cancer 71:1810, 1993
38. Costa MJ: Pseudomyxoma peritonei: histologic predictors of patient survival. Arch Pathol Lab Med 118:1215, 1994
39. Prayson RA, Hart WR, Petras RE: Pseudomyxoma peritonei: a clinicopathologic study of 19 cases with emphasis on site of origin and nature of associated ovarian tumors. Am J Surg Pathol 18:591, 1994
40. Kahn MA, Demopoulos RI: Mucinous ovarian tumors with pseudomyxoma peritonei: a clinicopathologic study. Int J Gynecol Pathol 11:15, 1992
41. Ronnett BM, Kurman RJ, Zahn CM et al: Pseudomyxoma peritonei in women: a clinicopathologic analysis of 30 cases with emphasis on site of origin, prognosis, and relationship to ovarian mucinous tumors of low malignant potential. Hum Pathol 26:509, 1995

42. Michael H, Sutton G, Roth LM: Ovarian carcinoma with extracellular mucin production: reassessment of "pseudomyxoma ovarii et peritonei." Int J Gynecol Pathol 6:298, 1987

43. Seidman JD, Elsayed AM, Sobin LH, Tavassoli FA: Association of mucinous tumors of the ovary and appendix: a clinicopathologic study of 25 cases. Am J Surg Pathol. 17:22, 1992

44. Seidman JD, Elsayed AM, Sobin LH, Tavassoli FA: Authors reply to the editor. Am J Surg Pathol 17:1070, 1993

45. Young RH, Gilks CB, Scully RE: Mucinous tumors of the appendix associated with mucinous tumors of the ovary and pseudomyxoma peritonei: a clinicopathological analysis of 22 cases supporting an origin in the appendix. Am J Surg Pathol 15:415, 1991

46. Young RH, Gilks CB, Scully RE: Pseudomyxoma peritonei, letter. Am J Surg Pathol 17:1068, 1993

47. Chuaqui R, Zhuang Z, Emmert-Buck MR et al: Genetic analysis of synchronous tumors of ovary and appendix to determine site of origin, abstract. Mod Pathol 8:87A, 1995

48. Cuatrecasas M, Matias-Guiu X, Prat J: Synchronous mucinous tumors of the appendix and the ovary associated with pseudomyxoma peritonei: a clinicopathologic study of six cases with comparative analysis of c-Ki-ras mutations. Am J Surg Pathol 22:739, 1996

49. Russell P: Surface epithelial-stromal tumors of the ovary. p. 705. In Kurman RJ (ed): Blaustein's Pathology of the Female Genital Tract. 4th Ed. Springer-Verlag, New York, 1994

50. Barnhill DR, Kurman RJ, Brady MF, et al: The behavior of stage I ovarian serous tumors of low malignant potential: a Gynecology Oncology Group study. Trans Am Gynecol Oncol Soc 13:35, 1994

51. Bell DA, Scully RE: Ovarian serous borderline tumors with stromal microinvasion: a report of 21 cases. Hum Pathol 21:397, 1990

52. Leake JF, Rader JS, Woodruff JD, Rosenshein NB: Retroperitoneal lymphatic involvement with epithelial ovarian tumors of low malignant potential. Gynecol Oncol 42:124, 1991

53. DiRe F, Paladini D, Fontanelli R et al: Surgical staging for epithelial ovarian tumors of low malignant potential. Int J Gynecol Cancer 4:310, 1994

54. Pettersson F: Annual Report of the Results of Treatment in Gynecological Cancer. Vol. 20. International Federation of Gynecology and Obstetrics, Stockholm, 1991

55. Lim-Tan SK, Cajigas HE, Scully RE: Ovarian cystectomy for serous borderline tumors: a follow-up study of 35 cases. 72:755, 1988

56. McCaughey WTE, Kirk ME, Lester W, Dardick I: Peritoneal epithelial lesions associated with proliferative serous tumours of the ovary. Histopathology 8:195, 1984

57. Taylor HC Jr: Malignant and semimalignant tumours of the ovary. Surg Gynaecol Obstet 48:204, 1929

58. Taylor HC Jr: Studies in the clinical and biological evolution of adenocarcinoma of the ovary. J Obstet Gynecol Br Common 66:827, 1959

59. Kurman RJ, Trimble CL: The behavior of serous tumor of low malignant potential: are they ever malignant? Int J Gynecol Pathol 12:120, 1993

60. Russell P: The pathological assessment of ovarian neoplasms, II: the proliferating "epithelial" tumours. Pathology 11:251, 1979

61. Russell P, Merkur H: Proliferating ovarian "epithelial tumours: a clinicopathological analysis of 144 cases." Aust N Z J Obst Gynaecol 19:45, 1979

62. Russell P: Ovarian epithelial tumours with atypical proliferation. p. 299. In Lowe D, Fox H (eds): Advances in

Gynaecologic Pathology. Churchill Livingstone, Edinburgh, 1992

63. Silva E, Tornos C, Zhuang A et al: Tumor recurrence in stage I ovarian serous low malignant potential neoplasms, abstract. United States and Canadian Academy of Pathology, Washington DC, 1996
64. Young RC, Walton LA, Ellenberg SS et al: Adjuvant therapy in stage I and stage II epithelial ovarian cancer. N Engl J Med 322:1021, 1990
65. Rubin SC, Wong GYC, Curtin JP: Platinum-based chemotherapy of high-risk stage I epithelial ovarian cancer following comprehensive surgical staging. Obstet Gynecol 82:143, 1993
66. Jenison EL, Montag AG, Griffiths CT et al: Clear cell adenocarcinoma of the ovary: a clinical analysis and comparison with serous carcinoma. Gynecol Oncol 32:65, 1989
67. Robey SS, Silva EG, Gershenson DM et al: Transitional cell carcinoma in high-grade high-stage ovarian carcinoma: an indicator of favorable response to chemotherapy. Cancer 63:839, 1989
68. Silva EG, Robey-Cafferty SS, Smith TL, Gershenson DM: Ovarian carcinomas with transitional cell carcinoma pattern. Am J Clin Pathol 93:457, 1990
69. Gershenson DM, Silva EG, Mitchell MF et al: Transitional cell carcinoma of the ovary: a matched control study of advanced-stage patients treated with cisplatin-based chemotherapy. Am J Obstet Gynecol 168:1178, 1993
70. Hughesdon PE: Benign endometrioid tumours of the ovary and the müllerian concept of ovarian epithelial tumours. Histopathology 8:970, 1984
71. Crozier MA, Copeland LJ, Silva EG et al: Clear cell carcinoma of the ovary: a study of 59 cases. Gynecol Oncol 35:199, 1989
72. Young RH, Bell DA, Clement PB: Recent advances in the pathology of ovarian tumors. Mod Pathol 8:930, 1995
73. Silva EG, Jenkins R: Serous carcinoma in endometrial polyps. Mod Pathol 3:120, 1990
74. Mulhollan TJ, Silva EG, Tornos C et al: Ovarian involvement by serous surface papillary carcinoma. Int J Gynecol Pathol 13:120, 1994
75. Austin RM, Norris HG: Malignant Brenner tumor and transitional cell carcinoma of the ovary: comparison. Int J Gynecol Pathol 6:29, 1987
76. Bell DA: Flow cytometry of ovarian neoplasms. p. 337. In N. Sasano (ed.) Current Topics in Pathology. Vol. 85. Springer-Verlag, Berlin, 1992
77. Kaern J, Tropé CG, Kristensen GB et al: DNA ploidy: the most important prognostic factor in patients with borderline tumors of the ovary. Int J Gynecol Cancer 3:349, 1993
78. Harlow BL, Fuhr JE, McDonald TW: Flow cytometry as a prognostic indicator in women with borderline epithelial ovarian tumors. Gynecol Oncol 50: 305, 1993
79. Rice LW, Mark SD, Berkowitz RS et al: Clinicopathologic variables, operative characteristics, and DNA ploidy in predicting outcome in ovarian epithelial carcinoma. Obstet Gynecol 86: 379, 1995
80. Kaern J, Wetteland J, Tropé CG et al: Comparison between flow cytometry and image cytometry in ploidy distribution assessments in gynecologic cancer. Cytometry 13:314, 1992
81. Brady PS, Klevecz RR: Flow cytometric evaluation of ovarian cancer. Cancer 71S:1621, 1992
82. Kaern J, Tropé CG, Abeler VM: A retrospective study of 370 borderline tumors of the ovary treated at the Norwegian Radium Hospital from 1970 to 1982: a review of clinicopathologic fea-

tures and treatment modalities. Cancer 71:1810, 1993

83. Seidman JD, Norris HJ, Griffin JL, Hitchcock CL: DNA flow cytometric analysis of serous ovarian tumors of low malignant potential. Cancer 71:3947, 1993

84. deNictolis M, Montironi R, Tommasoni S et al: Serous borderline tumors of the ovary: a clinicopathologic, immunohistochemical, and quantitative study of 44 cases. Cancer 70:152, 1992

85. Padberg BC, Stegner HE, von Sengbusch S et al: DNA-cytophotmetry and immunohistochemistry in ovarian tumours of borderline malignancy and related peritoneal lesions. Virchows Archiv 421:497, 1992

86. Singleton TP, Perrone T, Oakley G et al: Activation of c-erb B2 and prognosis in ovarian carcinoma: comparison with histologic type, grade, and stage. Cancer 73:1460, 1994

87. Kacinski BM, Mayer AG, King BL et al: Neu protein overexpression in benign, borderline, and malignant ovarian neoplasms. Gynecol Oncol 44: 245, 1992

88. Rubin SC, Finstad CL, Wong GY et al: Prognostic significance of HER-2/*neu* expression in advanced epithelial ovarian cancer: a multivariate analysis. Am J Obstet Gyneol 168:162, 1993

89. Scambia G, Benedetti Panici P, Ferrandina G et al: Expression of HER-2/*neu* oncoprotein, DNA-ploidy and S-phase fraction in advanced ovarian cancer. Int J Gynecol Cancer 3:271, 1993

90. Meden H, Marx D, Rath W et al: Overexpression of the oncogene c-erb B2 in primary ovarian cancer: evaluation of the prognostic value in a Cox proportional hazards multiple regression. Int J Gynecol Pathol 13:45, 1994

91. Slamon DJ, Godolphin W, Jones LA et al: Studies of the HER-2/*neu* proto-oncogene in human breast and ovarian cancer. Science 244:707, 1989

92. Berchuck A, Kamel A, Whitaker R et al: Overexpression of HER-2/*neu* is associated with poor survival in advanced epithelial ovarian cancer. Cancer Res 50:4087, 1990

93. Kupryjanczyk J, Thor AD, Beauchamp R et al: p53 gene mutations and protein accumulation in human ovarian cancer. Proc Natl Acad Sci USA 90:4961, 1993

94. Kiyokawa T: Alteration of p53 in ovarian cancer: its occurrence and maintenance in tumor progression. Int J Gynecol Pathol 13:311, 1994

95. Henriksen R, Strang P, Wilander E et al: p53 expression in epithelial ovarian neoplasms: relationship to clinical and pathological parameters, Ki-67 expression and flow cytometry. Gynecol Oncol 53:301, 1994

96. Klemi PJ, Takahashi S, Joensuu H et al: Immunohistochemical detection of p53 protein in borderline and malignant serous ovarian tumors. Int J Gynecol Pathol 13:228, 1994

97. Hartmann LC, Podratz KC, Keeney GL et al: Prognostic significance of p53 immunostaining in epithelial ovarian cancer. J Clin Oncol 12:64, 1994

98. Bast RC Jr: Perspectives on the future of cancer markers. Clin Chem 39(11):2444, 1993

99. Diebold J, Baretton G, Felcher M et al: bcl-2 expression, p53 accumulation, and apoptosis in ovarian carcinomas. Am J Clin Pathol 105:34, 1996

100. Dodson MK et al: Comparison of loss of heterozygosity patterns in invasive low-grade and high-grade epithelial ovarian carcinomas. Cancer Res. 53:4456, 1993

101. Dodson MK et al: Evidence of functional RB protein in epithelial ovarian carcinomas despite loss of heterozygosity at the RB locus. Cancer Res 54:610, 1994

102. Lau CC, Mok SC, Tsao SW et al: Further evidence for the unifocality of advanced stage human epithelial ovarian carcinoma, abstract. Gynecol Oncol 52:126, 1994
103. Mok CH, Tsao SW, Knapp RC et al: Unifocal origin of advanced human epithelial ovarian cancers. Cancer Res 52:5119, 1992
104. Muto MG, Welch WR, Mok SC et al: Evidence for a multifocal origin of papillary serous carcinoma of the peritoneum, abstract. Gynecol Oncol 52:127, 1994
105. Bell DA, Flotte TJ, Pastel-Levy C et al: DNA ploidy of ovarian serous borderline tumors (SBT) and their extraovarian implants, abstract. Mod Pathol 2:8, 1989
106. Enomoto T et al: K-ras activation occurs frequently in mucinous adenocarcinomas and rarely in other common epithelial tumors of the human ovary. Am J Pathol 139:777, 1991
107. Friedlander ML, Russell P, Taylor W et al: Flow cytometric analysis of cellular DNA content as an adjunct to the diagnosis of ovarian tumors of borderline malignancy. Pathology 16:301, 1984
108. Fujita M, Enomoto T, Wada H et al: Applicaton of clonal analyis: differential diagnosis of synchronous primary ovarian and endometrial cancers and metastatic cancer. Am J Clin Pathol 105:350, 1996
109. Kim TM et al: Loss of heterozygosity on chromosome 13 is common only in the biologically more aggressive subtypes of ovarian epithelial tumors and is associated with normal retinoblastoma gene expression. Cancer Res 54:605, 1994
110. Marks JR et al: Overexpression and mutation of p53 in epithelial ovarian cancer. Cancer Res 51:2979, 1991
111. Medl M, Sevelda P, Czerwenka K et al: DNA amplification of HER-2/*neu* and INT-2 oncogenes in epithelial ovarian cancer. Gynecol Oncol 59: 321, 1995
112. Mok SC et al: Mutation of K-ras protooncogene in human ovarian epithelial tumors of borderline malignancy. Cancer Res 53:1489, 1993
113. Okamoto N, Sameshima Y, Yokoyama S et al: Frequent allelic losses and mutations of the p53 gene in human ovarian cancer. Cancer Res 51:5171, 1991
114. Padberg BC, Arps H, Franke U et al: DNA cytophotometry and prognosis in ovarian tumors of borderline malignancy. Cancer 69:2510, 1992
115. Gaffey MJ, Frierson HJ Jr, Mills SE et al: Ovarian granulosa cell tumors with bizarre nuclei (GCT-BN): an immunohistochemical and fluorescence in situ hybridization (FISH) study. Mod Pathol 90A:8, 1995
116. Steinhoff MM, King TC: Synchronous small cell and endometrioid carcinomas of common clonal origin. Mod Pathol 97A, 1995
117. Kottmeier HL: Carcinoma of the female genitalia: the Abraham Flexner lectures. No 11. Williams and Wilkins, Baltimore, 1953
118. Björkholm E, Silfverswärd C: Prognostic factors in granulosa-cell tumors. Gynecol Oncol 11:261, 1981
119. Fox H, Agrawal K, Langley FA: A clinicopathologic study of 92 cases of granulosa cell tumor of the ovary with special reference to the factors influencing prognosis. Cancer 35:231, 1975
120. Norris HJ, Taylor HB. Prognosis of granulosa-theca tumors of the ovary. Cancer 21:255, 1968
121. Stenwig JT, Hazekamp JT, Beecham JB: Granulosa cell tumors of the ovary: a clinicopathological study of 118 cases with long-term follow-up. Gynecol Oncol 7:136, 1979
122. Evans MP, Webb MJ, Gaffey TA et al: DNA ploidy of ovarian granulosa cell

tumors: lack of correlation between DNA index or proliferative index and outcome in 10 patients. Cancer 75:2295, 1995

123. Klemi PK, Joensuu H, Salmi T: Prognostic value of flow cytometric DNA content analysis in granulosa cell tumor of the ovary. Cancer 65:1189, 1990

124. Haba R, Miki H, Kobayashi S, Ohmori M. Combined analysis of flow cytometry and morphometry of ovarian granulosa cell tumor. Cancer 72:3258, 1993

125. Chadha S, Cornelisse CJ, Schaberg A: Flow cytometric DNA ploidy analysis of ovarian granulosa cell tumors. Gynecol Oncol 36:240, 1990

126. Hitchcock CL, Norris HJ, Khalifa MA, Wargotz ES: Flow cytometric analysis of granulosa tumors. Cancer 64:2127, 1989

127. Malmstrom H, Hogberg T, Risberg B, Simonsen E: Granulosa cell tumors of the ovary: prognostic factors and outcome. Gynecol Oncol 52:50, 1994

INDEX

Page numbers followed by *f* indicate figures; those followed by *t* indicate tables.

H

O

P

S

T

Z

GWUMC
P16V4D
DATE DUE
AUG 2 6 1998